THE HARRIET LANE HANDBOOK OF PEDIATRIC ANTIMICROBIAL THERAPY

THE HARRIET LANE HANDBOOK OF PEDIATRIC ANTIMICROBIAL THERAPY

Second Edition

Julia A. McMillan, MD
Professor of Pediatrics
Associate Dean for Graduate Medical Education
Johns Hopkins University School of Medicine
Baltimore, Maryland

Carlton K. K. Lee, PharmD, MPH
Clinical Pharmacy Specialist, Pediatrics
Program Director, Pediatric Pharmacy Residency
Department of Pharmacy
The Johns Hopkins Hospital;
Associate Professor, Pediatrics
Johns Hopkins University School of Medicine
Baltimore, Maryland

George K. Siberry, MD, MPH
Assistant Professor
Department of Pediatrics
Johns Hopkins University School of Medicine
Baltimore, Maryland

Karen C. Carroll, MD
Director, Division of Medical Microbiology
Director, Medical Microbiology Fellowship Program
Professor of Pathology
Johns Hopkins University School of Medicine
Baltimore, Maryland

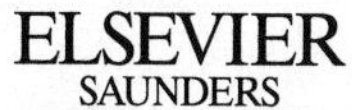

ELSEVIER
SAUNDERS

1600 John F. Kennedy Blvd.
Ste 1800
Philadelphia, PA 19103-2899

THE HARRIET LANE HANDBOOK OF PEDIATRIC ANTIMICROBIAL THERAPY, SECOND EDITION

ISBN: 978-0-323-11247-5

NOTICES

Knowledge and best practice in this field are constantly changing. As new research and experience broaden our understanding, changes in research methods, professional practices, or medical treatment may become necessary.

Practitioners and researchers must always rely on their own experience and knowledge in evaluating and using any information, methods, compounds, or experiments described herein. In using such information or methods they should be mindful of their own safety and the safety of others, including parties for whom they have a professional responsibility.

With respect to any drug or pharmaceutical products identified, readers are advised to check the most current information provided (i) on procedures featured or (ii) by the manufacturer of each product to be administered, to verify the recommended dose or formula, the method and duration of administration, and contraindications. It is the responsibility of practitioners, relying on their own experience and knowledge of their patients, to make diagnoses, to determine dosages and the best treatment for each individual patient, and to take all appropriate safety precautions.

To the fullest extent of the law, neither the Publisher nor the authors, contributors, or editors, assume any liability for any injury and/or damage to persons or property as a matter of products liability, negligence or otherwise, or from any use or operation of any methods, products, instructions, or ideas contained in the material herein.

Previous edition copyrighted 2009

Library of Congress Cataloging-in-Publication Data

The Harriet Lane handbook of pediatric antimicrobial therapy / [edited by] Julia A. McMillan ... [et al.]—2nd ed.
p. ; cm.
Handbook of pediatric antimicrobial therapy
Includes bibliographical references and index.
ISBN 978-0-323-11247-5 (pbk.)
I. McMillan, Julia A. II. Johns Hopkins Hospital. Children's Center. III. Title: Handbook of pediatric antimicrobial therapy.
[DNLM: 1. Anti-Infective Agents—therapeutic use—Handbooks. 2. Adolescent. 3. Child. 4. Infant. QV 39]
RM262
615'.1—dc23

2013003412

Content Strategist: James Merritt
Content Development Specialist: Andrea Vosburgh
Publishing Services Manager: Pat Joiner
Design Manager: Steven Stave

Printed in the United States of America

Last digit is the print number: 9 8 7 6 5 4 3 2 1

DEDICATION

We dedicate this second edition of *The Harriet Lane Handbook of Pediatric Antimicrobial Therapy* to the clinicians and investigators whose work has allowed continued improvement in our ability to treat and to prevent infections in infants and children.

Contributors

Karen C. Carroll, MD
Director, Division of Medical Microbiology
Director, Medical Microbiology Fellowship Program
Professor of Pathology
Johns Hopkins University School of Medicine
Baltimore, Maryland

Lisa A. Degnan, PharmD, BCPS
Clinical Assistant Professor
Ernst Mario School of Pharmacy
Rutgers, The State University of New Jersey;
Clinical Pharmacy Specialist, Pediatrics
Hackensack University Medical Center
Hackensack, New Jersey

Swathi Gowtham, MD
Clinical Fellow
Division of Pediatric Infectious Diseases
Division of Clinical Pharmacology
Johns Hopkins University School of Medicine
Baltimore, Maryland

Angela M. Helder, PharmD, BCPS
Clinical Pharmacy Specialist
Pediatric Emergency Medicine
Department of Pharmacy
The Johns Hopkins Hospital
Baltimore, Maryland

Hiwot Hiruy, MD
Clinical Fellow
Division of Pediatric Infectious Diseases
Johns Hopkins University School of Medicine
Baltimore, Maryland

Carlton K. K. Lee, PharmD, MPH
Clinical Pharmacy Specialist, Pediatrics
Program Director, Pediatric Pharmacy Residency
Department of Pharmacy
The Johns Hopkins Hospital;
Associate Professor, Pediatrics
Johns Hopkins University School of Medicine
Baltimore, Maryland

Melissa D. Makii, PharmD, BCPS
Clinical Pharmacy Specialist
Pediatric Oncology
Department of Pharmacy
Rainbow Babies and Children's Hospital
Cleveland, Ohio

Julia A. McMillan, MD
Professor of Pediatrics
Associate Dean for Graduate Medical Education
Johns Hopkins University School of Medicine
Baltimore, Maryland

Kristine A. Parbuoni, PharmD, BCPS
Clinical Pharmacy Specialist
Pediatric Critical Care
University of Maryland Medical Center
Baltimore, Maryland

George K. Siberry, MD, MPH
Assistant Professor
Department of Pediatrics
Johns Hopkins University School of Medicine
Baltimore, Maryland

Elizabeth A. Sinclair, PharmD, BCPS
Clinical Pharmacist
Pediatric Critical Care
Riley Hospital for Children at Indiana University Health
Indianapolis, Indiana

Paul K. Sue, MD
Clinical Fellow
Division of Pediatric Infectious Diseases
Johns Hopkins University School of Medicine
Baltimore, Maryland

Preface

This second edition of *The Harriet Lane Handbook of Pediatric Antimicrobial Therapy* was, like the first edition, a collaboration that included the disciplines of pediatric infectious diseases, microbiology, and clinical pharmacology. We recognize that decisions regarding effective antimicrobial therapy require the knowledge and experience of all three of these disciplines, particularly when caring for children whose infections are complications of underlying conditions or the compromised immunity that results from chemotherapy or surgery.

For this edition, our microbiology expert was Dr. Karen C. Carroll, who kindly agreed to replace Dr. James Dick, who is now retired. Dr. Carroll reviewed and significantly revised Chapter 4, Mechanisms of Action and Routes of Administration of Antimicrobial Agents, and Chapter 5, Mechanisms of Drug Resistance. The other faculty authors for the first edition have participated in this one, but the pediatric infectious diseases fellows, Drs. Hiwot Hiruy, Swathi Gowtham, and Paul K. Sue, all contributed for the first time. Their dedication to excellence in the care of their patients is reflected in the care with which they have reviewed and revised Chapter 2, Recommended Empiric Antimicrobial Therapy for Selected Clinical Syndromes.

Because decision-making about antimicrobial selection and dosage requires more than matching a "drug" to a "bug," we are particularly proud to that Dr. Carlton K. K. Lee was able to recruit former Pediatric Pharmacy residents Drs. Lisa A. Degnan, Angela M. Helder, Melissa D. Makii, Elizabeth A. Sinclair, and Kristine A. Parbuoni to assist in revising Chapter 3, Drug Dosing in Special Circumstances; Chapter 6, Therapeutic Drug Monitoring; Chapter 7, Adverse Drug Reactions; and Chapter 9, Antimicrobial Desensitization Protocols.

We have reviewed available evidence and current guidelines from expert panels to provide recommendations that are as accurate and as contemporary as is possible. We realize, however, that new evidence and guidelines will emerge during the life of this second edition, so we urge readers to consult additional resources, particularly for unusual infections or for suspected antimicrobial resistance.

Decisions regarding antimicrobial therapy for children require an understanding of biologic development, mechanisms of resistance, and pharmacology. We hope that this handbook will help clinicians in their efforts to provide the most effective therapy for each individual circumstance.

Karen C. Carroll, MD
Carlton K. K. Lee, PharmD, MPH
Julia A. McMillan, MD
George K. Siberry, MD, MPH
Swathi Gowtham, MD
Hiwot Hiruy, MD
Paul K. Sue, MD
Lisa A. Degnan, PharmD, BCPS
Angela M. Helder, PharmD, BCPS
Melissa D. Makii, PharmD, BCPS
Kristine A. Parbuoni, PharmD, BCPS
Elizabeth A. Sinclair, PharmD, BCPS

Contents

Notes and Abbreviations Used in Tables

TABLE 1-1

*Some recommendations are for antibiotics that are not approved by the U.S. Food and Drug Administration (FDA) for use in children, and some may not be approved for treatment of the pathogen listed. Recommendations are based on published evidence of efficacy.

A/C, Amoxicillin/clavulanic acid (Augmentin); *AG*, aminoglycoside; *APCS*, antipseudomonal cephalosporin; *APPN*, antipseudomonal penicillin; *aq*, aqueous; *BL/BLI*, β-lactam plus β-lactamase inhibitor combination; *BT*, bioterrorism; *CDC*, Centers for Disease Control and Prevention; *Ceph*, cephalosporin; *1st Ceph*, first generation cephalosporin; *2nd Ceph*, second generation cephalosporin; *3rd Ceph*, third generation cephalosporin; *CGD*, chronic granulomatous disease; *CHL*, chloramphenicol; *CNS*, central nervous system; *CSF*, cerebrospinal fluid; *EM*, erythema marginatum; *ESBL*, extended-spectrum β-lactamase producer; *FQ*, fluoroquinolone; *GI*, gastrointestinal; *HUS*, hemolytic uremic syndrome; *IM*, intramuscular; *IV*, intravenous; *IVIg*, intravenous immunoglobulin; *LP*, lumbar puncture; *MIC*, minimum inhibitory concentration; *NSAID*, nonsteroidal anti-inflammatory drug; *OCS*, oral cephalosporin; *OCS1*, first generation oral cephalosporin; *OCS2*, second generation oral cephalosporin; *OCS3*, third generation oral cephalosporin; *PCS*, parenteral cephalosporin; *PCS1*, first generation parenteral cephalosporin; *PCS2*, second generation parenteral cephalosporin; *PCS3*, third generation parenteral cephalosporin; *PCS4*, fourth generation parenteral cephalosporin; *PenG*, penicillin G; *Pen VK*, penicillin VK (oral); *PID*, pelvic inflammatory disease; *Pip/tazo*, piperacillin/tazobactam (Zosyn); *PO*, by mouth; *PPI*, proton pump inhibitor; *R/O*, rule out; *RE*, reticuloendothelial; *SS-Pen*, semisynthetic penicillin (nafcillin, oxacillin); *Tic/clav*, ticarcillin/clavulanic acid (Timentin); *TMP/SMX*, trimethoprim/sulfamethoxazole; *UTI*, urinary tract infection; *WBC*, white blood cell.

TABLE 1-2

Some recommendations are for antibiotics that are not approved by the U.S. Food and Drug Administration for use in children, and some may not be approved for treatment of the pathogen listed. Recommendations are based on published evidence of efficacy.

*Public health authorities should be notified if an individual has newly diagnosed latent infection.

†Intramuscular streptomycin is usually recommended; if not available, kanamycin, amikacin, or capreomycin can be used.
‡Recommendations are for presumptive therapy and no recommendation for duration is provided. Controlled trials are limited, and susceptibility testing may not correlate with clinical response. Guidance from a specialist in treating mycobacterial infection is recommended.
§Doxycycline should be prescribed for children <8 years old only if the benefits outweigh the risks.
ART, Antiretroviral therapy; *DOT*, directly observed therapy; *TB*, tuberculosis; *TMP/SMX*, trimethoprim-sulfamethoxazole; *TST*, tuberculin skin test.

TABLE 1-3

Some recommendations are for antibiotics that are not approved by the U.S. Food and Drug Administration for use in children, and some may not be approved for treatment of the pathogen listed. Recommendations are based on published evidence of efficacy.
CMV, Cytomegalovirus; *CNS*, central nervous system; *GI*, gastrointestinal; *HSV*, herpes simplex virus; *IM*, intramuscular; *IV*, intravenous; *PO*, by mouth.

TABLE 1-4

Some recommendations are for antibiotics that are not approved by the U.S. Food and Drug Administration for use in children, and some may not be approved for treatment of the pathogen listed. Recommendations are based on published evidence of efficacy.
*Recommendations for duration of treatment often cannot be provided because optimal duration depends on disease severity and immune status of the patient.
†Unless a specific recommendation is made, decisions regarding the appropriate formulation of amphotericin B should be made based on a need to reduce toxicity associated with amphotericin B deoxycholate. Lipid complex and liposomal formulations are associated with fewer adverse events, but they do not enhance efficacy. Amphotericin B deoxycholate is the preferred formulation for treating neonates and other patients with renal involvement because lipid complex and liposomal forms do not achieve effective concentration in the kidneys.
‡*Candida albicans* is generally susceptible to fluconazole; *C. krusei* is resistant to fluconazole; *C. glabrata* is often resistant to fluconazole but may be susceptible to high doses; *C. lusitaniae* may be resistant to amphotericin B.
§Includes *Absidia* spp., *Mucor* spp., *Rhizomucor* spp., *Rhizopus* spp., *Mortierella* spp., *Cunninghamella* spp., *Penicillium* spp., *Acremonium* spp., and *Fusarium* spp.

TABLE 1-6

Some recommendations are for antibiotics that are not approved by the U.S. Food and Drug Administration for use in children, and some may not be approved for treatment of the pathogen listed. Recommendations are based on published evidence of efficacy.

[a]Available from Leiters Park Avenue Pharmacy, San Jose, CA (800-292-6773).

[b]Approved drug but considered investigational for this indication.

[c]Not recommended during pregnancy and for children younger than 8 yr.

[d]Can be obtained from the CDC Drug Service (404-639-3670 or 404-639-2888 evenings and weekends).

[e]Fumagillin is made by Mid-Continent Agrimarketing, Inc., Olathe, KS (800-547-1392).

[f]Not available commercially. This drug can be compounded as a service by Medical Center Pharmacy, New Haven, CT (203-688-6816), or by Panorama Compounding Pharmacy, 6744 Balboa Blvd., Van Nuys, CA 91406 (800-247-9767).

[g]Triclabendazole is available from Victoria Pharmacy, Zurich, Switzerland (41-1-211-24-32).

[h]Available in limited supply from WHO.

[i]Not marketed in the United States.

[j]Not recommended in pregnant or breastfeeding women.

[k]Miltefosine is manufactured by Paladin (Montreal, Quebec, Canada) and is not available in the United States.

[l]Artemether/lumefantrine is contraindicated during the first trimester of pregnancy; safety during the second and third trimester has not been established. It should not be used in patients with cardiac arrhythmias, bradycardia, severe cardiac disease, or prolonged QT interval, and it should not be given concomitantly with drugs that prolong the QT interval or are metabolized by CYP2D6.

[m]If quinidine is unavailable, call Eli Lilly (800-821-0538) or the CDC Malaria Hotline (770-488-7788).

CDC, Centers for Disease Control and Prevention; *CNS*, central nervous system; *FDA*, U.S. Food and Drug Administration; *GI*, gastrointestinal; *IM*, intramuscular; *IV*, intravenous; *LP*, lumbar puncture; *PO*, by mouth; *WHO*, World Health Organization.

TABLE 2-1

*Pharmacokinetics of Synercid (quinupristin plus dalfopristin) and daptomycin have not been studied, and use in children has been limited.

†Spectinomycin is not available in the United States.

‡Li PK, Szeto CC, Piraino B, et al. Peritoneal dialysis-related infections recommendations: 2010 update. Perit Dial Int 2010;30:393-423.

A/C, Amoxicillin/clavulanic acid; *AG*, aminoglycoside; *AP pen*, antipseudomonal penicillin; *BAL*, bronchoalveolar lavage; *BL/BLI*, β-lactam plus β-lactamase inhibitor; *CGD*, chronic granulomatous disease; *CMV*, cytomegalovirus; *CNS*, central nervous system; *CSF*, cerebrospinal fluid; *CT*, computed tomography; *EBV*, Epstein-Barr virus; *FDA*, U.S. Food and Drug Administration; *FQ*, fluoroquinolone; *GAS*, group A streptococcus; *GBS*, group B streptococcus; *GI*, gastrointestinal; *GU*, genitourinary; *HSV*, herpes simplex virus; *IVIg*, intravenous immunoglobulin; *MRSA*, methicillin-resistant *Staphylococcus aureus*; *MRSE*, methicillin-resistant *Staphylococcus epidermidis*; *MSSA*, methicillin-susceptible *Staphylococcus aureus*; *NSAID*, nonsteroidal anti-inflammatory drug; *OCS2/3*, second generation oral cephalosporin; *OCS3*, third generation oral cephalosporin; *OM*, otitis media; *PCN*, penicillin; *PCR*, polymerase chain reaction; *PCS3*, third generation parenteral cephalosporin; *Pip/tazo*, piperacillin/tazobactam; *RFQ*, respiratory fluoroquinolone (levofloxacin, moxifloxacin); *RSV*, respiratory syncytial virus; *STI*, sexually transmitted infection; *TB*, tuberculosis; *Tic/clav*, ticarcillin/clavulanic acid; *TMP/SMX*, trimethoprim/sulfamethoxazole; *UTI*, urinary tract infection.

TABLE 3-1

*Pharmacogenomic polymorphisms should be taken under consideration for potential altered net effect.

†Works cooperatively with transporters (e.g., MDR-1 or P-glycoprotein).

↑, Increased; ↓, decreased; ?, unknown; *BSA*, body surface area; *CNS*, central nervous system; *GI*, gastrointestinal.

TABLE 3-3

*Route in parentheses indicates secondary route of excretion.

†Subsequent doses are best determined by measurement of serum levels and assessment of renal insufficiency.

‡May add to peritoneal dialysate to obtain adequate serum levels.

§For a glomerular filtration rate (GFR) ≥5 mL/min, give full dose as first dose; for a GFR <5 mL/min, give 33% of full dose as first dose.

¶May inactivate aminoglycosides in patients with renal impairment.

‖Rate of acetylation of isoniazid.

**If using high-flux hemodialysis (polysulfone polyamide and polyacrylonitrile), give supplemental dose after dialysis.

?, Unknown; *CrCl*, creatinine clearance; *D*, dose reduction; *DI*, dose reduction and interval extension; *D,I*, dose reduction or interval extension; *He*, hemodialysis; *I*, interval extension; *N*, no; *N/A*, not applicable; *NRTI*, nucleoside reverse transcriptase inhibitor; *P*, peritoneal dialysis; *Y*, yes.

TABLE 3-4

CAVH, Continuous arteriovenous hemodialysis; *CAVHD,* continuous arteriovenous hemodialysis, *CF,* cystic fibrosis; *CrCl,* creatinine clearance rate; *CNS,* central nervous system; *CVVH,* continuous venovenous hemofiltration; *CVVHD,* continuous venovenous hemodialysis; *IV,* intravenous; *PCP, Pneumocystis* pneumonia; *PO,* by mouth.

TABLE 3-7

+, Use with caution in the presence of hepatic impairment; *IM*, intramuscular; *INR,* international normalized ratio; *IV*, intravenous.

TABLE 3-8

ABW, Adjusted body weight (kg); Cl_{Cr}, creatinine clearance (mL/min/1.73m^2); *CrCl*, creatine clearance; *IBW*, ideal body weight (kg); *MIC*, minimum inhibitory concentration; *TBW*, total or actual body weight (kg); *Vd*, volume of distribution (L/kg).

TABLE 3-9

+/–, Yes in some studies, no in others; *BBB,* blood–brain barrier; *CNS,* central nervous system; *CSF,* cerebrospinal fluid; *IM,* intramuscular; *IV,* intravenous; *MIC,* minimum inhibitory concentration; *NRTI,* nucleoside reverse transcriptase inhibitor; *PI,* protease inhibitor.

TABLE 4-1

*Unique among β-lactams; binds to PBP2a, so it has methicillin-resistant *Staphylococcus aureus* activity.

†Ophthalmic drops or retinal administration.

‡Vaginal cream.

HBV, Hepatitis B virus; *IM*, intramuscular; *INHAL*, inhalation; *IV*, intravenous; *mRNA*, messenger RNA; *PBP*, penicillin-binding protein; *PO*, by mouth; *rRNA*, ribosomal RNA; *T*, topical; *tRNA*, transfer RNA.

TABLE 6-1

*Assuming normal renal function.

†Terminal half-life.

‡These steady-state times are achieved regardless of whether a loading dose is administered.

§Data for specific peak and trough levels and efficacy are not well established. Trough concentration at four to five times the minimum inhibitory concentration (MIC) has been recommended with higher concentrations; may be needed for sequestered infections or situations of poor vancomycin tissue penetration.

‖Postconceptual age: the sum of gestational age at birth and chronologic age.

¶Nonlinear pharmacokinetics exhibited in adults and children because of saturation of voriconazole metabolism and higher than proportional

increase in exposure observed with an increasing dose; however, linear pharmacokinetics has been reported in younger children.
CNS, Central nervous system; *IV*, intravenous; *MRSA*, methicillin-resistant *Staphylococcus aureus; N/A*, not applicable; *SSTI*, skin and soft tissue infection.

TABLE 6-2

*Reflects free-drug concentration measurements.
AUC/MIC, Area under the serum concentration versus time curve to minimum inhibitory concentration ratio; C_{max}*/MIC*, maximum serum concentration to MIC ratio; *T > MIC*, duration of the dosing interval with serum concentrations exceeds the MIC; *PD*, pharmacodynamics; *PK*, pharmacokinetics.

TABLE 6-3

AUC/MIC, Area under the serum concentration versus time curve to minimum inhibitory concentration ratio; *PD*, pharmacodynamics; *PK*, pharmacokinetics.

TABLE 6-4

AUC/MIC, Area under the serum concentration versus time curve to minimum inhibitory concentration ratio; C_{max}*/MIC*, maximum serum concentration to MIC ratio; *PD*, pharmacodynamics; *PK*, pharmacokinetics.

TABLE 6-5

*Postantifungal effects have been identified for certain drugs within the indicated antifungal drug class and specific *Candida* strain.
AUC/MIC, Area under the serum concentration versus time curve to minimum inhibitory concentration ratio; C_{max}*/MIC*, maximum serum concentration to MIC ratio; *T > MIC*, duration of the dosing interval with serum concentrations exceeds the MIC; *PD*, pharmacodynamics; *PK*, pharmacokinetics.

TABLE 8-1

CDC, Centers for Disease Control and Prevention; *CMV,* cytomegalovirus; *CSF,* cerebrospinal fluid; *DTaP,* diphtheria and tetanus toxoids and acellular pertussis vaccine; *Ig,* immunoglobulin; *IM,* intramuscular; *IV,* intravenous; *IVIg,* intravenous immunoglobulin; *max,* maximum; *Td,* adult-type diphtheria and tetanus toxoids vaccine; *Tdap,* tetanus toxoid, reduced diphtheria toxoid, and acellular pertussis vaccine; *TMP/SMX,* trimethoprim/sulfamethoxazole; *TST,* tuberculin skin test.

TABLE 9-1

Observe patient for 30 min, then give full therapeutic dose by the desired route.

*Interval between doses is 15 min.

TABLE 9-2

Observe patient for 30 min, then give full therapeutic dose by the desired route.

*Interval between doses is 15 min.

TABLE 9-3

Observe patient for 30 min, then give full therapeutic dose by the desired route.

*Interval between doses is 15 min.

TABLE 9-4

*Interval between doses is 30 min.

TABLE 9-5

Protocol for intravenous desensitization to all cephalosporins with a goal dose of 1 and 2 g.

TABLE 9-6

Protocol for intravenous desensitization to all cephalosporins with a goal dose of 2 g.

*Interval between doses is 15 min.

TABLE 9-7

*Interval between doses is 30 min. Dose is expressed as sulfamethoxazole portion of trimethoprim/sulfamethoxazole (TMP/SMX). If an allergic reaction occurs, formal desensitization should be performed.

NA, Not applicable.

TABLE 9-10

Drink 180 mL water after each dose of trimethoprim/sulfamethoxazole (TMP/SMX). Subjects tolerating this protocol were prescribed 800/160 mg TMP/SMZ every Monday, Wednesday, and Friday for low-dose *Pneumocystis jiroveci (carinii)* prophylaxis.

NA, Not applicable.

TABLE 9-11

*Administer doses as continuous 15-min infusions, except for the last three doses, which are given as 30-min infusions with no intervals between the doses.

TABLE 9-12

*Interval between doses is 15 min.
NA, Not applicable.

TABLE 9-14

*Beginning on day 7, doses infused consecutively.
IV, Intravenously.

TABLE 9-17

*Interval between doses is 8 hours.

TABLE 9-18

*Goal interval between doses is 20 minutes.
NA, Not applicable.

TABLE 9-19

*Interval between doses is 30 minutes.

THE HARRIET LANE HANDBOOK OF PEDIATRIC ANTIMICROBIAL THERAPY

Chapter 1

Infectious Agents and Drugs of Choice

Julia A. McMillan, MD, and
George K. Siberry, MD, MPH

I. RECOMMENDED TREATMENT FOR BACTERIAL INFECTIONS

TABLE 1-1

RECOMMENDED TREATMENT FOR BACTERIAL INFECTIONS (for notes and abbreviations used in this table, see p. xiii.)

Pathogen	Host Category	Indication/Type of Infection	Recommended Treatment	Duration	Alternative Treatment	Duration	Comments
Acinetobacter spp.	All	Respiratory, bacteremia	Imipenem	≥14 days (depending on site of infection)	Other carbapenem *or* Ampicillin/ sulbactam *or* Colistin *or* Tigecycline	≥14 days (depending on site of infection)	Variably but often highly resistant—susceptibility results guide final choice; colistin used in some highly resistant cases. Tigecycline and doripenem not FDA approved for <18 yr old.
Aggregatibacter actinomycetemcomitans (formerly *Actinobacillus* sp.)	All	Any	3rd ceph	Variable (endocarditis, 4–6 wk)	Penicillin + gentamicin *or* Ampicillin + gentamicin *or* Ciprofloxacin	Variable endocarditis, 4–6 wk	Common coinfection with *Actinomyces.* May add AG or rifampin to 3rd ceph for endocarditis.
Actinomyces israeli and other species	All	Any	IV PenG *or* Ampicillin, then oral amoxicillin	4–6 wk 6–12 mo	PCS3 *or* PCS *then* Oral: Erythromycin, Doxycycline, or Clindamycin	3 wk 4 wk 6–12 mo	Surgical debridement. Prolonged antibiotics essential. Failure of erythromycin, doxycycline, or clindamycin may be caused by presence of *Aggregatibacter.*

Aeromonas hydrophila	All	Gastroenteritis	TMP/SMX	5 days?	FQ *or* Tetracycline	5 days? 5 days?	Unclear benefit of antimicrobial treatment.
		Invasive	3rd ceph + gentamicin	≥10 days (depending on site of infection)	Carbapenem *or* Tetracycline *or* Ciprofloxacin	≥10 days (depending on site of infection)	Debridement
Achromobacter xylosoxidans (formerly *Alcaligenes xylosoxidans*)	All	Any	Ceftazidime *or* Meropenem	≥10 days (depending on site of infection)	Other Carbapenem *or* TMP/SMX	≥10 days (depending on site of infection)	Variable activity of Pip/tazo, Tic/clav, FQ, ceftobiprole. Initial therapy guided by local susceptibility patterns.
Anaplasma phagocytophila (formerly *Ehrlichia phagocytophila*)	All	Disseminated	Doxycycline	≥7 days *and* 3 days afebrile	Tetracycline *or* Rifampin	≥7 days *and* 3 days afebrile	Doxycycline is drug of choice regardless of age. No evidence of teeth staining after ≤2-wk course of doxycycline. Chloramphenicol not recommended. Levofloxacin active in vitro.
	Pregnant	Disseminated	Rifampin *or* Doxycycline	All: ≥7 days *and* 3 days afebrile	—		Limited clinical data about efficacy of rifampin vs. potential negative effect of doxycycline on bones and teeth of fetus.

Continued

TABLE 1-1

RECOMMENDED TREATMENT FOR BACTERIAL INFECTIONS (Continued)

Pathogen	Host Category	Indication/Type of Infection	Recommended Treatment	Duration	Alternative Treatment	Duration	Comments
Arcanobacterium haemolyticum	All	Pharyngitis	Erythromycin	Unknown	Clindamycin *or* Tetracycline *or* Penicillin	Unknown	TMP/SMX resistant Test for penicillin susceptibility and tolerance.
		Invasive disease	PenG +/– AG	10 days?	Clindamycin *or* Ceph *or* Macrolide	Variable	AG may be warranted if endocarditis suspected.
Bacillus anthracis (potential BT agent)	All	Cutaneous	Doxycycline *or* Ciprofloxacin	All: 7–10 days (60 days if BT)	Levofloxacin *or* Amoxicillin (see comments) *or* Penicillin (see comments)	All: 7–10 days (60 days if BT)	Potential BT agent. Penicillin or amoxicillin can be used to complete therapy for children <8 yr old with naturally acquired anthrax or proven penicillin-susceptible after initial treatment with doxycycline or ciprofloxacin.
		Gastrointestinal; pulmonary; invasive	[Doxycycline *or* Ciprofloxacin] + [Rifampin *and/or* Clindamycin]	60 days	[Levofloxacin or ofloxacin] + [Rifampin *and/ or* clindamycin]		Potential BT agent. Cephalosporins and TMP/SMX not reliable.
Bacillus cereus	All	Food poisoning	None				Supportive care only
		Invasive	Vancomycin	Variable	Ciprofloxacin *or* Meropenem *or* Imipenem *or* Clindamycin	Variable	Debridement and hardware removal. Uniformly resistant to β-lactams.

Bacteroides: fragilis group	All	Above diaphragm	Clindamycin	Depends on site and ability to drain/débride	Pip/tazo *or* Tic/clav *or* A/C *or* Ampicillin/ sulbactam *or* Carbapenem		Debridement/drainage important for therapy.
		Below diaphragm	Metronidazole	Depends on site and ability to drain/débride	Pip/tazo *or* Carbapenem *or* Cefoxitin	Depends on site and ability to drain/débride	Debridement/drainage important for therapy. Increasing clindamycin resistance.
		Intracranial	Metronidazole	Unknown	Carbapenem?	Unknown	Duration depends on clinical and radiologic response.
Bartonella henselae (cat scratch disease)	Immunocompetent	Adenitis	None *or* Azithromycin	— 5 days	Rifampin *or* Ciprofloxacin *or* TMP/SMX	2–3/wk 2–3/wk 7–10 days	Needle aspiration of suppurative lymph node for relief. Reserve antibiotic treatment for severe cases.
		Severe systemic cat scratch disease	TMP/SMX *and/or* Rifampin *and/or* IV Gentamicin (see Comments)	All: ≥2 weeks?	Ciprofloxacin *or* Doxycycline	All: ≥2 weeks?	Preferred therapy unclear. Some experts advocate gentamicin until defervescence followed by TMP/SMX + rifampin for 2–4 weeks. (Florin et al. *Pediatrics* 2008).[†]

Continued

TABLE 1-1

RECOMMENDED TREATMENT FOR BACTERIAL INFECTIONS (Continued)

Pathogen	Host Category	Indication/Type of Infection	Recommended Treatment	Duration	Alternative Treatment	Duration	Comments
Bartonella henselae or *quintana*	Any	Endocarditis	Ceftriaxone + gentamicin +/− doxycycline	Prolonged	Doxycycline + gentamicin	Prolonged	Gentamicin for at least 14 days based on adult studies.
	Immunocompromised	Bacillary peliosis (liver, other RE sites) Bacillary angiomatosis	Erythromycin +/− rifampin *or* Doxycycline +/− rifampin	2–3 mo (angiomatosis) 4 mo (peliosis)	Azithromycin +/− rifampin	2–3 mo (angiomatosis) 4 mo (peliosis)	
Bartonella bacilliformis (bartonellosis *or* Carrion's disease)	All	Acute (Oroya fever)	CHL +/− Pen G *or* Ciprofloxacin +/− ceftriaxone	10 days after fever resolves	Doxycycline	Unknown	Seen in the Andes mountains. Chloramphenicol or ciprofloxacin preferred for prevention of secondary salmonellosis. Use second agent for severe or nonresponsive illness.
		Chronic (Verruga peruana)	Rifampin	14–21 days	Azithromycin *or* Erythromycin *or* Ciprofloxacin	7–14 days 7–14 days 7–14 days	Seen in the Andes mountains. Unclear benefit of treatment. Surgery.
Bordetella pertussis, parapertussis	All	Respiratory	Erythromycin *or* Azithromycin *or* Clarithromycin	14 days 5 days 7 days	TMP/SMX	14 days	Increased pyloric stenosis with erythromycin use <2 wk old; not studied for other macrolides. Azithromycin preferred for infants <1 mo old.

Borrelia burgdorferi	Nonpregnancy, ≥8 yr old	Early localized disease/EM	Doxycycline *or* Amoxicillin	14–21 days	Amoxicillin *or* Cefuroxime *or* Erythromycin	14–21 days 14–21 days 14–21 days	Amoxicillin preferred alternative.
		Multiple EM	Doxycycline	21 days	Amoxicillin *or* Cefuroxime *or* Erythromycin	21 days 21 days 21 days	Amoxicillin preferred alternative.
		Isolated facial palsy	Doxycycline	14–21 days	Amoxicillin *or* Cefuroxime *or* Erythromycin	14–21 days 14–21 days 14–21 days	Amoxicillin preferred alternative. Antibiotic treatment prevents late disease but has no impact on facial palsy outcome. Steroids not helpful.
		Arthritis—initial	Doxycycline	28 days	Amoxicillin *or* Cefuroxime *or* Erythromycin	28 days 28 days 28 days	Amoxicillin preferred alternative.
		Arthritis—recurrent or persistent	Repeat initial prescription *or* Ceftriaxone	28 days 14–28 days	Penicillin IV *or* Cefotaxime	14–28 days 14–28 days	No clear option for patients intolerant of penicillin and ceftriaxone.

Continued

TABLE 1-1

RECOMMENDED TREATMENT FOR BACTERIAL INFECTIONS (Continued)

Pathogen	Host Category	Indication/Type of Infection	Recommended Treatment	Duration	Alternative Treatment	Duration	Comments
Borrelia burgdorferi (Continued)	Child <8 yr old, or pregnancy	Early localized disease/EM	Amoxicillin	14–21 days	Cefuroxime *or* Erythromycin	14–21 days 14–21 days	
		Multiple EM	Amoxicillin	21 days	Cefuroxime *or* Erythromycin	21 days	
		Isolated facial palsy	Amoxicillin	14–21 days	Cefuroxime *or* Erythromycin	14–21 days 14–21 days	Antibiotic treatment prevents late disease but has no impact on facial palsy outcome. Steroids not helpful.
		Arthritis—initial	Amoxicillin	28 days	Cefuroxime *or* Erythromycin	28 days 28 days	NSAIDs helpful adjunctive therapy.
		Arthritis—recurrent or persistent	Repeat initial prescription *or* Ceftriaxone	28 days 14–28 days	Penicillin IV *or* Cefotaxime	14–28 days 14–28 days	No clear option for patients intolerant of penicillin and ceftriaxone.
	All	Carditis	Ceftriaxone *or* Penicillin IV	14–21 days 14–28 days			If asymptomatic, alternative would be same oral regimen as for early disease.
		Meningitis or encephalitis	Ceftriaxone *or* Cefotaxime	14–28 days 14–28 days	Penicillin IV *or* Doxycycline	14–28 days 14–28 days	Repeated or prolonged antibiotic course not helpful. Doxycycline alternative only for patients ≥8 yr old, nonpregnant.
		Encephalitis, other late neurologic complications	Ceftriaxone	14–28 days	Penicillin IV *or* Cefotaxime	14–28 days 14–28 days	

Borrelia recurrentis	<8 yr old, or pregnant	Relapsing fever—louse-borne	Penicillin *or* Erythromycin	Single dose Single dose	Chloramphenicol	Single dose	
	Nonpregnant, ≥8 yr old		Doxycycline	Single dose	Penicillin *or* Erythromycin	Single dose Single dose	
Borrelia hermsii and *turicatae*	<8 yr old, or pregnant	Relapsing fever—tickborne	Penicillin *or* Erythromycin	5–10 days 5–10 days	CHL	5–10 days	Monitor for Jarisch–Herxheimer reaction.
	Nonpregnant, ≥8 yr old		Doxycycline	5–10 days	Erythromycin *or* Penicillin	5–10 days 5–10 days	
Brucella abortus and other species	Nonpregnant, ≥8 yr old	Brucellosis	Doxycycline + rifampin	6 wk 6 wk	Doxycycline + gentamicin *or* TMP/SMX + rifampin	6 wk 2 wk 6 wk 6 wk	
	<8 yr old, or pregnant		TMP/SMX + rifampin	6 wk 6 wk	TMP/SMX + gentamicin	4–8 wk 2 wk	
	Nonpregnant, ≥8 yr old	Meningitis or endocarditis	Doxycycline + rifampin + gentamicin	4–6 mo 4–6 mo 2 wk	—		
	<8 yr old, or pregnant		TMP/SMX + rifampin + gentamicin	4–6 mo 4–6 mo 2 wk	Doxycycline + rifampin + gentamicin	4–6 mo 4–6 mo 2 wk	

Continued

TABLE 1-1

RECOMMENDED TREATMENT FOR BACTERIAL INFECTIONS (Continued)

Pathogen	Host Category	Indication/Type of Infection	Recommended Treatment	Duration	Alternative Treatment	Duration	Comments
Burkholderia cepacia	All	Any	Meropenem	14 days?	TMP/SMX *or* Imipenem *or* Minocycline *or* Ceftazidime *or* Quinolones *or* Chloramphenicol	14 days? (all)	Combination therapy with meropenem + 1 or 2 agents from alternative list (e.g., meropenem + TMP/SMX may be needed for multiresistant strains).
Burkholderia mallei (potential BT agent)	All	Glanders	Sulfadiazine	Unknown	Doxycycline *or* FQ *or* Tobramycin *or* Gentamicin *or* Imipenem *or* Ceftazidime *or* TMP/SMX	Unknown	Limited clinical evidence for treatment recommendations.
Burkholderia pseudomallei (potential BT agent)	Southeast Asia, Australia, India, Central America	Melioidosis	Ceftazidime *or* Meropenem Followed by oral: doxycycline *or* TMP/SMX	10–14 days 10–14 days 4–6 mo 4–6 mo	Parenteral phase: imipenem *or* CHL Oral phase: Amox/clav	 10–14 days 10–14 days 4–6 mo	After IV therapy, give prolonged oral therapy.
Campylobacter jejuni	Children	Gastroenteritis	Erythromycin *or* Azithromycin	5–7 days 5 days	Doxycycline (≥8 yr old)	5–7 days	
	Adults		Azithromycin	5 days	Erythromycin *or* Ciprofloxacin *or* Doxycycline	5–7 days 5–7 days 5–7 days	FQ resistance is increasing.

All *Campylobacter* spp.	All	Invasive	Carbapenem *and/or* Gentamicin	Variable	3rd ceph	Variable	
Capnocytophaga canimorsus	All	Any	Penicillin *or* A/C	Variable	Pip/tazo *or* Clindamycin *or* Erythromycin	Variable	Dog oral flora. Consider splenic dysfunction. Susceptible to penicillin but may prefer A/C for coinfection with other dog oral flora.
Capnocytophaga ochracea	All	Any	Clindamycin *or* A/C	Variable	Carbapenem *or* Pip/tazo *or* FQ	Variable	Human oral flora.
Cardiobacterium hominis			3rd ceph	Variable	Penicillin + gentamicin	Variable	Penicillin/gentamicin only if penicillin susceptibility confirmed.
Chlamydophila (*Chlamydia*) *pneumoniae*	<8 yr old	Pneumonia	Azithromycin	5 days	Erythromycin *or* Clarithromycin	10–21 days 10 days	
	≥8 yr old	Pneumonia	Doxycycline *or* Azithromycin	14 days 5 days	Erythromycin *or* FQ *or* Clarithromycin	10–21 days 10 days 10 days	

Continued

TABLE 1-1

RECOMMENDED TREATMENT FOR BACTERIAL INFECTIONS (Continued)

Pathogen	Host Category	Indication/Type of Infection	Recommended Treatment	Duration	Alternative Treatment	Duration	Comments
Chlamydophila (*Chlamydia*) *psittaci*	<8 yr old	Psittacosis	Azithromycin *or* Erythromycin	10–14 days after fever resolved	Clarithromycin	10–14 days after fever resolved	
	≥8 yr old	Psittacosis	Doxycycline		Erythromycin *or* Azithromycin *or* Clarithromycin		
Chlamydia trachomatis	Infant	Conjunctivitis or pneumonia	Erythromycin *or* Azithromycin	14 days 3–5 days	Sulfonamide (oral)	14 days?	Increased risk for pyloric stenosis with erythromycin in infants <6 wk old. Sulfonamide for conjunctivitis, not pneumonia. Avoid sulfonamides in infants <4 wk old.
	All	Urethritis, cervicitis, proctitis	Doxycycline *or* Azithromycin	7 days 1 dose (1 g)	Erythromycin *or* Ofloxacin *or* Levofloxacin	7 days 7 days 7 days	6 mo to 12 yr: erythromycin or azithromycin. Pregnancy: erythromycin, azithromycin, or amoxicillin.
	All	PID					See PID treatment recommendations in Chapter 2 (includes recommendations for *C. trachomatis*).
	All	Epididymitis	Doxycycline	10 days			

Chromobacterium violaceum	All	Any	Initial phase: [TMP/SMX *or* FQ *or* Imipenem] *then* Oral phase: TMP/SMX	 2–3 wk 2–3 wk 2–3 wk 4 wk to several mo	Initial phase: [CHL + Gentamicin] Oral phase: Doxycycline *or* CHL	 2–3 wk 4 wk to several mo 4 wk to several mo	R/O CGD. Erythromycin resistant, even if appears susceptible in vitro. Preferred treatment not well established. Two- to 3-wk initial phase (parenteral) followed by prolonged oral phase. Two drugs from list used by some for first 2–3 wk. Relapse common.
Citrobacter spp.	All	Non-CNS and other less serious infections	Carbapenem *or* [PCS3 +/– gentamicin]	Variable (all)	OCS3 *or* Pip/tazo *or* FQ	Variable	PCS3 (ceftriaxone) alone preferred for *C. koseri*; resistance more common for *C. freundii* (*ampC* β-lactamase producer).
		CNS, other serious infections	Meropenem *or* [PCS3 + aminoglycoside]	See Comments	Imipenem	See Comments	Non-CNS infections: 10–14 days. CNS infections: ≥21 days; ≥4–6 wk if abscesses.
Clostridium botulinum	Infant	Infant botulism	Human-derived botulism immunoglobulin intravenous (BabyBIG) as soon as possible; ordering info at http://www.infantbotulism.org/ or 510-231-7600				Do *not* use antibiotics, especially aminoglycosides! BabyBIG active against botulinum toxin types A and B.

Continued

TABLE 1-1

RECOMMENDED TREATMENT FOR BACTERIAL INFECTIONS (Continued)

Pathogen	Host Category	Indication/Type of Infection	Recommended Treatment	Duration	Alternative Treatment	Duration	Comments
Clostridium botulinum (Coutinued)	All	Wound or foodborne botulism	Equine-derived heptavalent (HBAT) botulinum antitoxin from local health department or CDC. [If local health department unavailable, contact CDC at 800-232-4636 or http://emergency.cdc.gov/agent/botulism/clinicians/index.asp				HBAT active against all botulinum toxin types (A–F).
Clostridium difficile	All	Colitis	Oral metronidazole	10 days	Oral vancomycin *or* IV metronidazole	10 days 10 days	Stop other antibiotics. Limited data for nitazoxanide. Fidaxomicin an option for adults, but no data available for children. Positive toxin in infant may not signify disease.
Clostridium tetani	All	Tetanus	Metronidazole + antitoxin	10–14 days	PenG IV + antitoxin	10–14 days	Human tetanus immunoglobulin (TIG) 3000–6000 units IM. Some experts infiltrate part of TIG into wound.
Clostridium perfringens, other species	All	Food poisoning (*perfringens*)	None (supportive)				
		Septicemia, necrotizing myositis/fasciitis	PenG + clindamycin + surgery	Variable	[Clindamycin *or* Metronidazole *or* Carbapenem] + surgery	Variable	Surgery essential. Hyperbaric oxygen may be helpful.

Corynebacterium diphtheriae	All	Any	Antitoxin + [erythromycin *or* PenG aq *or* PenG procaine]	Antibiotic: 14 days			Before IV antitoxin is given, a scratch test with 1 : 1000 dilution of antitoxin in saline solution should be performed, followed by an intradermal test if the scratch test is negative. Dose of antitoxin depends on severity of clinical presentation. Desensitization required if patient sensitive. Antitoxin and specific instructions available from the CDC (770-488-7100 or http://www.cdc.gov/vaccines/vpd-vac/diphtheria/dat/dat-main.htm#how). Document eradication by 2 consecutive negative cultures at least 24 hr after beginning treatment. Repeat erythromycin if culture is positive.
Corynebacterium jeikeium, other species	All	Any	Vancomycin	Variable	[Pen + AG] *or* Clindamycin *or* Erythromycin	Variable	Use vancomycin until specific susceptibilities are known.

Continued

TABLE 1-1

RECOMMENDED TREATMENT FOR BACTERIAL INFECTIONS (Continued)

Pathogen	Host Category	Indication/Type of Infection	Recommended Treatment	Duration	Alternative Treatment	Duration	Comments
Coxiella burnetii	All	Q fever	Doxycycline	10–14 days	FQ *or* TMP/SMX	10–14 days 10–14 days	May not need treatment in mild illness; TMP/SMX in pregnancy.
		Endocarditis	Doxycycline + hydrochloroquine	≥18 mo	[Doxycycline *or* Ofloxacin] + rifampin	3 yr	
Edwardsiella tarda	All	Gastroenteritis	None				Similar to *Salmonella*. More common in warm climates.
		Invasive	PCS3	≥10–14 days	FQ	≥10–14 days	
Ehrlichia chaffeensis and *Ehrlichia ewingii*	All	Any	Doxycycline	5–10 days *and* afebrile ≥3 days	Rifampin (pregnancy *only*)	5–10 days *and* afebrile ≥3 days	Doxycycline is drug of choice even in children <8 yr old. Consider alternative only for pregnant women.
Eikenella corrodens	All	Any	Ampicillin *or* Penicillin *or* A/C	7–10 days (all)	Ureidopenicillin *or* TMP/SMX *or* 3rd ceph *or* Carbapenem	7–10 days (all)	A/C better than penicillin or ampicillin for occasional strain that produces β-lactamase. All resistant to clindamycin and metronidazole.
Elizabethkingia (formerly *Chryseobacterium*) *meningosepticum*	All	Health care–associated invasive	Vancomycin + rifampin	Unknown	[TMP/SMX *or* Levofloxacin *or* Minocycline] + rifampin	Unknown	Formerly *Flavobacterium*; susceptibility testing may be unreliable.

Enterobacter spp.	All	Any	Ureidopenicillin + aminoglycoside	≥10–14 days	Carbapenem *or* FQ *or* Tic/clav *or* Pip/tazo *or* [PCS3 + AG]	≥10–14 days	Nosocomial strains may be multiresistant. Laboratory should test for ESBL. Consider meropenem for CNS infection.
Enterococcus faecalis and *faecium* (not vancomycin resistant)	All	Urinary tract	Ampicillin *or* Nitrofurantoin	7–14 days 7–14 days	Vancomycin	7–14 days	
		Sepsis, meningitis, endocarditis	Ampicillin + gentamicin *or* Penicillin + gentamicin	≥2 wk (sepsis) 2–3 wk (CNS) 4–6 wk (endocarditis)	Vancomycin + gentamicin	≥2 wk (sepsis) 2–3 wk (CNS) 4–6 wk (endocarditis)	Low-dose gentamicin for synergy. No gentamicin if high-level resistance, in which case, longer course (8–12 wk for endocarditis).
Enterococcus, vancomycin resistant (VRE) (usually *E. faecium*)	All	Urinary tract	Linezolid *or* Quinupristin/dalfopristin	7–14 days 7–14 days	Nitrofurantoin *or* FQ (if susceptible)	7–14 days 7–14 days	Most VRE are *E. faecium.* Quinupristin/dalfopristin *not* active against *E. faecalis.*
		Sepsis, meningitis endocarditis, other invasive infection	Linezolid *or* Daptomycin	≥2 wk (sepsis) 2–3 wk (CNS) 8–12 wk? (endocarditis)	Quinupristin/dalfopristin	≥2 wk (sepsis) 2–3 wk (CNS) 8–12 wk? (endocarditis)	Quinupristin/dalfopristin *not* active against *E. faecalis.* Expect higher relapse rate for endocarditis.
Erysipelothrix rhusiopathiae	All	Sepsis *or* Endocarditis	PenG *or* Ampicillin	4–6 wk 4–6 wk	PCS3 *or* FQ *or* Imipenem	4–6 wk 4–6 wk 4–6 wk	Oral antibiotics and shorter course for erysipeloid. Intrinsic vancomycin resistance.

Continued

TABLE 1-1

RECOMMENDED TREATMENT FOR BACTERIAL INFECTIONS (Continued)

Pathogen	Host Category	Indication/Type of Infection	Recommended Treatment	Duration	Alternative Treatment	Duration	Comments
Escherichia coli	All	Meningitis	PCS3	≥21 days	Meropenem *or* Cefepime	≥21 days ≥21 days	Treat for at least 21 days *and* at least 14 days from first negative CSF culture. Meropenem preferred if ESBL suspected.
		Sepsis	PCS3	≥14 days	FQ *or* Pip/Tazo *or* Carbapenem	≥14 days	Carbapenem if ESBL suspected.
		Cystitis	Amoxicillin *or* TMP/SMX	7–10 days 7–10 days	Sulfisoxazole *or* Nitrofurantoin *or* Oral ceph	7–10 days 7–10 days 7–10 days	Many oral options, based on susceptibility, including amoxicillin. Shorter courses of 3–5 days appropriate for adolescents and adults.
		Pyelonephritis	PCS 3 *or* OCS3	14 days 14 days	Ampicillin + gentamicin *or* FQ *or* TMP/SMX *or* Gentamicin *or* BL/BLI	7–14 days 14 days 14 days 14 days 14 days	Transition to oral antibiotics to complete 14-day course.

		Intra-abdominal	PCS3 *or* BL/BLI	For all: 7 days	Carbapenem *or* FQ *or* Cefoxitin	For all: 7 days	Carbapenem if ESBL suspected. If polymicrobial (gut flora) infection likely, add metronidazole to PCS3 or FQ to improve anaerobic coverage. Seven days adequate provided signs of infection have resolved (i.e., afebrile, normal WBC counts, oral intake resumed.) (Infectious Diseases Society of America Clinical Practice Guidelines: Clin Infect Dis 2010; 50:625–663)
Escherichia coli—enterohemorrhagic (STEC)	All	Diarrhea (risk for HUS)	None				Antibiotic therapy has no proven benefit and may increase risk for HUS.
Escherichia coli—enteroinvasive	All	Dysentery	Azithromycin	5 days	FQ	3 days	TMP/SMX resistance common.
Escherichia coli—enterotoxigenic	All	Traveler's diarrhea	Azithromycin	5 days	FQ	3 days	TMP/SMX resistance common.
Francisella tularensis	All	Tularemia	Gentamicin	10 days (longer if more severe illness)	Streptomycin *or* Ciprofloxacin *or* CHL	All: 10 days (longer if more severe illness)	More relapses with tetracyclines. 3rd ceph poor despite in vitro susceptibility.
		Tularemia with meningitis	CHL + [streptomycin *or* gentamicin]	≥10–14 days	Doxycycline + [streptomycin *or* gentamicin]	≥14 days	Recommendations based on few cases.

Continued

TABLE 1-1

RECOMMENDED TREATMENT FOR BACTERIAL INFECTIONS (Continued)

Pathogen	Host Category	Indication/Type of Infection	Recommended Treatment	Duration	Alternative Treatment	Duration	Comments
Fusobacterium spp.	All	Bacteremia (septic jugular vein thrombosis/ Lemierre syndrome)	Pip/tazo *or* Ticarcillin/clav *or* Meropenem *or* Imipenem	4–6 wk 4–6 wk 4–6 wk 4–6 wk	Clindamycin IV *or* Metronidazole IV	4–6 wk 4–6 wk	Can switch IV to PO if ≥14 days, stable and good response. Role of anticoagulation unclear. Penicillin or other agents often used with metronidazole because co-infection with microaerophilic oral flora common.
Gardnerella vaginalis (see Bacterial Vaginosis in Chapter 2)							
Haemophilus ducreyi		Chancroid	Ceftriaxone *or* Azithromycin	1 dose 1 dose	Ciprofloxacin *or* Erythromycin	3 days 7 days	
Haemophilus influenzae—type b, occasionally other types, rarely nontypeable	All	Meningitis	Ceftriaxone *or* Cefotaxime	10 days 10 days			
		Other invasive, non-CNS	PCS3 *or* Ampicillin/ sulbactam IV	10 days 10 days	PCS2 *or* FQ IV	10 days 10 days	

Haemophilus influenzae — nontypeable		Otitis, otitis-conjunctivitis, sinusitis	A/C	10 days	OCS2 *or* OCS3 *or* Azithromycin *or* Clarithromycin *or* FQ *or* Ceftriaxone	10 days 10 days 5 days 10 days 10 days 1 dose	Some experts treat for only 5 days in children ≥6 yr old.
Haemophilus influenzae—aegyptius, other nontypeable	All	Conjunctivitis	FQ ophthalmic *or* Polymyxin/TMP	5–10 days 5–10 days	Gentamicin *or* Tobramycin	5–10 days 5–10 days	
Haemophilus parainfluenza, haemolyticus, aphrophilus, other species	All	Endocarditis	Ceftriaxone	4 wk	Ampicillin + gentamicin *or* Ampicillin/sulbactam + gentamicin	4 wk	Use ampicillin/sulbactam/gentamicin instead of ampicillin + gentamicin for β-lactamase producers. *H. aphrophilus* renamed *Aggregatibacter aphrophilus*.
Helicobacter pylori	All	Gastritis, gastric, and duodenal ulcers	Amoxicillin + [clarithromycin *or* metronidazole] + PPI *or* Amoxicillin + metronidazole + bismuth	14 days 14 days	Amoxicillin + PPI *followed by* clarithromycin + PPI + [metronidazole *or* tinidazole]	5 days each for initial and follow-on regimen	PPI options include omeprazole, lansoprazole, esomeprazole, pantoprazole, rabeprazole. Increasing clarithromycin resistance.

Continued

TABLE 1-1

RECOMMENDED TREATMENT FOR BACTERIAL INFECTIONS (Continued)

Pathogen	Host Category	Indication/Type of Infection	Recommended Treatment	Duration	Alternative Treatment	Duration	Comments
Kingella kingae, other species	All	Osteomyelitis, arthritis	PCS 1/2/3 *or* PenG *or* BL/BLI	≥14 days ≥14 days ≥14 days	AG *or* FQ *or* TMP/SMX *or* Oxacillin	≥14 days ≥14 days ≥14 days ≥14 days	2–3 weeks for arthritis; 3–6 weeks for osteomyelitis. PenG drug of choice if no β-lactamase. Vancomycin resistance uniform; clindamycin resistance common.
		Endocarditis	*PenG + gentamicin *or* *Ampicillin + gentamicin *or* Ceftriaxone	≥28 days ≥28 days ≥28 days	Ampicillin/sulbactam + gentamicin *or* Other BL/BLI + gentamicin	≥28 days ≥28 days	Course 4–7 weeks. PenG or ampicillin only if no β-lactamase. For regimens with gentamicin, use gentamicin for whole course.
Klebsiella spp.	All	Cystitis, other minor infections	OCS 1/2/3 *or* A/C	3–5 days 3–5 days	TMP/SMX *or* FQ	7–10 days 7–10 days	For ESBL-positive strains, carbapenem drug of choice. Can use FQ if susceptible in vitro. Failure of BL/BLI (e.g., Pip/tazo) for ESBL-positive strains despite in vitro susceptibility. Meningitis: CSF cultures may be positive up to 2 wk despite treatment. Treat CNS infection ≥21 days *and* ≥10–14 days from first negative CSF culture.
		Pyelonephritis, bacteremia, sepsis (NO CNS)	PCS3 *or* FQ	7–14 days 7–14 days	Gentamicin Carbapenem BL/BLI	≥14 days ≥14 days ≥14 days	
		Meningitis	PCS3 +/– AG	≥21 days	FQ Meropenem Pip/Tazo	≥21 days ≥21 days ≥21 days	

		ESBL-positive	Carbapenem	As above for type of infection	FQ	As above for type of infection	
Klebsiella (formerly *Calymmatobacterium*) *granulomatis*	Nonpregnant	Granuloma inguinale; donovanosis	Doxycycline	≥3 wk	TMP/SMX *or* Ciprofloxacin Erythromycin *or* Azithromycin (weekly)	≥3 wk ≥3 wk ≥3 wk ≥3 wk	Should have response within 7 days; if not, add gentamicin.
	Pregnant		Erythromycin *or* Azithromycin	≥3 wk ≥3 wk	—		
Legionella pneumophila	Healthy	Mild to moderate illness	Azithromycin *or* FQ	5–10 days 14–21 days	Doxycycline *or* TMP/SMX *or* Erythromycin	14–21 days 14–21 days 14–21 days	
	Immunocompromised and/or severe illness		FQ	≥14–21 days	Azithromycin	≥10 days	
Leptospira spp. (Leptospirosis)	All	Mild illness	Amoxicillin *or* Doxycycline	7–14 days 7–14 days	Azithromycin	5 days	Jarisch–Herxheimer reaction common after therapy initiation.
		Hospitalized or severe illness	PenG	14 days	Doxycycline *or* Ceftriaxone *or* Cefotaxime	14 days 14 days 14 days	

Continued

TABLE 1-1

RECOMMENDED TREATMENT FOR BACTERIAL INFECTIONS (Continued)

Pathogen	Host Category	Indication/Type of Infection	Recommended Treatment	Duration	Alternative Treatment	Duration	Comments
Leuconostoc spp.	All	Any	PenG +/– AG *or* Ampicillin	Variable Variable	Macrolide *or* Tetracycline *or* Clindamycin	All: variable	Intrinsic vancomycin resistance. High rates of resistance to FQ and quinupristin/dalfopristin.
Listeria monocytogenes	Any	Meningitis	Ampicillin + gentamicin	≥21 days	TMP/SMX	≥21 days	Intrinsic ceph resistance. No good alternative for neonates and late pregnancy. Failures reported with vancomycin and CHL; FQ and linezolid—minimal clinical data.
	Neonatal	Non-CNS	Ampicillin + gentamicin	14–21 days			
	Older	Sepsis, pneumonia	Ampicillin + gentamicin	14 days	TMP/SMX	14 days	
Moraxella catarrhalis	All	Noninvasive	A/C *or* TMP/SMX *or* OCS2,3	All: variable	Azithromycin *or* Clarithromycin *or* FQ *or* Doxycycline	All: variable	Duration depends on site of infection: for example, shorter for otitis media than for sinusitis.
Morganella	All	Cystitis; other less serious infections	OCS3 *or* FQ	Variable Variable	TMP/SMX	7–10 days for UTI; others, variable	Duration depends on site of infection.
		Invasive and/or severe illness	PCS4 + AG *or* FQ *or* Carbapenem	≥10 days ≥10 days ≥10 days	TMP/SMX *or* Pip/tazo	≥10 days ≥10 days	PCS3 can select spontaneous AmpC-derepressed mutants during therapy and lead to treatment failure.

Mycobacterium TB and others—Table 1.2 of this chapter							
Mycoplasma hominis	All	Any	Doxycycline *or* Clindamycin	≥10 days ≥10 days	FQ	≥10 days	Duration depends on site of infection. *M. hominis* is intrinsically resistant to macrolides. IVIG has been suggested for agammaglobulinemic patients.
Mycoplasma pneumoniae	All	Lower respiratory tract infection	Azithromycin	5 days	Doxycycline *or* Erythromycin *or* Clarithromycin *or* FQ	7–10 days 7–10 days 7–10 days 7–10 days	Best response if started within first 3–4 days of illness. Appropriate therapy for extrapulmonary disease not well defined.
Neisseria gonorrhoeae	All	Urethritis, pharyngitis, proctitis, epididymitis	Ceftriaxone + azithromycin *or* Ceftriaxone once + doxycycline	Once 7 days	Cefixime + azithromycin *or* Cefixime + doxycycline High-dose azithromycin (2 g)	Once 7 days Once	Ceftriaxone dose always 250 mg. Ceftriaxone strongly preferred. If alternative regimen used, patient should have test of cure 1 week after treatment. Fluoroquinolones *not* recommended unless susceptibility of infecting strain is documented.

Continued

TABLE 1-1

RECOMMENDED TREATMENT FOR BACTERIAL INFECTIONS (Continued)

Pathogen	Host Category	Indication/Type of Infection	Recommended Treatment	Duration	Alternative Treatment	Duration	Comments
Neisseria gonorrhoeae (Coutinued)		Conjunctivitis	Ceftriaxone	Once	Cefotaxime	Once	Cefotaxime for neonates with hyperbilirubinemia or if neonate receiving IV calcium. Plus local irrigation. Add treatment for *C. trachomatis.*
		PID	See PID treatment recommendations in Chapter 2 (includes treatment for gonorrhea)				Add treatment for *C. trachomatis.*
		Disseminated, arthritis	Ceftriaxone	7 days	Cefotaxime	7 days	Test and/or treat for *C. trachomatis.*
		Meningitis	Ceftriaxone	10–14 days	Cefotaxime	10–14 days	Cefotaxime may be preferred in newborns with increased bilirubin levels.
		Endocarditis	Ceftriaxone	≥4 wk	—		125 mg IM in term infant; 25–50 mg/kg (maximum 125 mg) IM in preterm infant.
		Exposed infant	Ceftriaxone	Once			
Neisseria meningitidis	All	Meningitis, sepsis, pneumonia	PenG *or* PCS 3	5–7 days 5–7 days	Ampicillin *or* Meropenem *or* CHL	5–7 days 5–7 days 5–7 days	Some experts use PCS3 until susceptibilities known because of increasing penicillin resistance in some areas (especially Spain). CHL or meropenem only if very severe β-lactam allergy.

Nocardia brasiliensis, asteroides, other species	Normal	Noninvasive	TMP/SMX	6–12 wk	Minocycline *or* A/C	6–12 wk 6–12 wk	Linezolid also active.
	Immunocompromised	Invasive	TMP/SMX + imipenem	≥6–12 mo	[Amikacin + imipenem] *or* [Amikacin + ceftriaxone] *or* [Amikacin + TMP/SMX]	≥6–12 mo	
	All	CNS or severe	TMP/SMX + Amikacin + Ceftriaxone	≥6–12 mo 1–3 mo 1–3 mo	[TMP/SMX + imipenem + amikacin] *or* [Imipenem + amikacin + ceftriaxone]	≥6–12 mo 1–3 mo 1–3 mo ≥6–12 mo ≥1–3 mo 1–3 mo	
Pasteurella multocida	All	Localized	PenVK *or* Amoxicillin	7–10 days 7–10 days	Azithromycin *or* TMP/SMX *or* OCS2 *or* Doxycycline *or* FQ	5 days 10–14 days 10–14 days 10–14 days 10–14 days	PCS3 susceptible in vitro but clinical data lacking.
		Invasive or severe	PenG *or* Ampicillin	10–14 days 10–14 days	PCS2 *or* FQ *or* Doxycycline	10–14 days 10–14 days 10–14 days	

Continued

TABLE 1-1

RECOMMENDED TREATMENT FOR BACTERIAL INFECTIONS (Continued)

Pathogen	Host Category	Indication/Type of Infection	Recommended Treatment	Duration	Alternative Treatment	Duration	Comments
Pediococcus spp.	All	Any	PenG +/– AG	Variable	Other β-lactam *or* Erythromycin *or* Minocycline *or* Imipenem *or* Clindamycin *or* Daptomycin	Variable	Intrinsic vancomycin resistance. High rates of resistance to quinupristin/dalfopristin. Susceptibility testing important for choosing therapy as susceptibility of individual isolates varies.
Plesiomonas shigelloides	All	Diarrhea	TMP/SMX *or* FQ	3 days 3 days	A/C *or* CS2/3 *or* Carbapenem	3 days 3 days 3 days	Probable diarrheal pathogen.
	All	Invasive	PCS3	Variable	Carbapenem	Variable	Definitive antibiotic therapy should be guided by susceptibility testing.
Prevotella spp.	All	Oral, respiratory	Clindamycin	≥10 days	Pip/tazo *or* Ampicillin/sulbactam *or* Ticar/clav	≥10 days ≥10 days ≥10 days	β-lactamase production common. Longer duration if undrainable abscesses.
		GI, genitourinary	Metronidazole	≥10 days	Clindamycin *or* Cefoxitin *or* Carbapenem *or* BL/BLI	≥10 days ≥10 days ≥10 days ≥10 days	Longer duration if undrainable abscesses.

Propionibacterium acnes	All	Acne vulgaris (inflammatory)	Erythromycin topical *or* Clindamycin topical	Many weeks Many weeks	Doxycycline PO *or* Minocycline PO	Many weeks Many weeks	Plus nonantibiotic topical antiacne. Oral agents used for nonresponse to topicals or severe acne.
		Invasive	PenG (high dose) *or* Vancomycin	Variable Variable	Clindamycin *or* Doxycycline *or* PCS3 *or* Linezolid	Variable Variable Variable Variable	Usually associated with hardware. Consistently resistant to metronidazole. Increasing clindamycin resistance.
Proteus mirabilis	All	Cystitis, other nonserious	Ampicillin	5–7 days	TMP/SMX *or* OCS *or* FQ	5–7 days 5–7 days 5–7 days	Proteus UTI associated with urolithiasis.
		Pyelonephritis, other invasive	Ampicillin *or* FQ	≥10 days ≥10 days	PCS3 *or* AG *or* Carbapenem	≥10 days ≥10 days ≥10 days	Isolates from urine/blood/CSF should be tested for ESBL.
Proteus vulgaris and other indole-positive species	All	Cystitis, other nonserious	PCS3 *or* FQ	5–7 days 5–7 days	A/C	5–7 days	Carbapenem if ESBL suspected.
		Pyelonephritis, other invasive	PCS3 + AG *or* FQ + AG	≥10 days ≥10 days	Carbapenem *or* BL/BLI	≥10 days ≥10 days	
Providencia spp.	All	Cystitis, other nonserious	TMP/SMX *or* A/C	5–7 days 5–7 days	OCS3	5–7 days	
		Pyelonephritis, other invasive	PCS3 + AG *or* FQ	≥10 days ≥10 days	Carbapenem *or* BL/BLI	≥10 days ≥10 days	

Continued

TABLE 1-1

RECOMMENDED TREATMENT FOR BACTERIAL INFECTIONS (Continued)

Pathogen	Host Category	Indication/Type of Infection	Recommended Treatment	Duration	Alternative Treatment	Duration	Comments
Pseudomonas aeruginosa, other species	All	Uncomplicated UTI, other nonserious	FQ (ciprofloxacin) *or* APCS *or* APPN	≥10 days ≥10 days ≥10 days	AG Carbapenem	≥10 days ≥10 days	
		Pneumonia, bacteremia, sepsis	APCS3/4 +/– AG *or* APPN + AG	≥14 days ≥14 days	Carbapenem +/– AG FQ + AG	≥14 days ≥14 days	
		Meningitis	APCS3/4 +/– AG *or* APPN + AG	≥14 days ≥14 days	Carbapenem +/– AG	≥14 days	Cultures negative at least 10 days.
Rickettsia rickettsii	All	Rocky Mountain Spotted Fever	Doxycycline	7–10 days	CHL	7–10 days	Treat until at least 3 days afebrile. Doxycycline drug of choice even <8 yr old. Use doxycycline for pregnant women if severe illness and/or chloroquine not available.
Rickettsia akari	All	Rickettsialpox	Doxycycline	3–5 days	CHL	3–5 days	Treat until at least 3 days afebrile.
Rickettsia prowazekii	All	Epidemic typhus	Doxycycline	7–10 days	CHL *or* FQ	7–10 days 7–10 days	Treat until at least 3 days afebrile. Doxycycline drug of choice even <8 yr old.

Rickettsia typhi	All	Endemic typhus	Doxycycline	5–10 days	CHL	5–10 days	Treat until at least 3 days afebrile. Doxycycline drug of choice even <8 yr old.
Rickettsia—other species	All		Doxycycline	7–10 days	CHL	7–10 days	Treat until at least 3 days afebrile.
Salmonella typhi (type D)	All	Typhoid fever	PCS3 *or* FQ IV	10–14 days 10–14 days	Azithromycin	10–14 days	High rates of FQ resistance in some geographic areas. Dexamethasone may be appropriate adjunctive therapy. May switch to oral therapy to complete course once improvement established. Clinical failure despite in vitro activity of 1st ceph and 2nd ceph, AG, furazolidone.
		Typhoid fever—mild	Azithromycin PO *or* PCS3 *or* FQ PO	7 days 7–14 days 7–14 days	Amoxicillin PO *or* TMP/SMX PO *or* CHL PO	10–14 days 10–14 days 10–14 days	Shorter courses for milder disease in nonimmunocompromised host may be effective.

Continued

TABLE 1-1

RECOMMENDED TREATMENT FOR BACTERIAL INFECTIONS (Continued)

Pathogen	Host Category	Indication/Type of Infection	Recommended Treatment	Duration	Alternative Treatment	Duration	Comments
Salmonella, non-*typhi*	All	Enteric fever, bacteremia	Same as for typhoid fever				
		Localized, nonmeningeal disease (osteomyelitis, abscess)	PCS3	≥4 wk	FQ	≥4 wk	May change to ampicillin IV if isolate proved susceptible.
		Meningitis	PCS3	6 wk			May change to ampicillin IV if isolate proved susceptible.
	Normal	Gastroenteritis	No antibiotics				Supportive treatment only.
	Infant <3 mo old; sickle cell; splenic dysfunction	Gastroenteritis	PCS3 *or* Amoxicillin *or* TMP/SMX	5 days 5 days 5 days	FQ *or* Azithromycin	5 days	FQ may be first choice in adults. Avoid amoxicillin and TMP/SMX in areas of prevalent resistance unless susceptibility proved.

Serratia marcescens	All	Invasive (bacteremia, meningitis, pneumonia)	Imipenem + AG *or* Meropenem + AG	All: variable, ≥21 days for meningitis	PCS3/4 + AG *or* APPN + AG *or* FQ	All: variable, ≥21 days for meningitis	For neonatal meningitis, perform daily CSF cultures until sterile. Treat 10–14 days after first sterile CSF culture. Susceptibility testing should guide therapy. Consider CGD evaluation for non-neonates.
Shigella sonnei, Shigella dysenteriae, Shigella boydii, Shigella flexneri	Child	Gastroenteritis, dysentery	Azithromycin *or* Cefixime *or* FQ	5 days 3 days 5 days	Ampicillin *or* Ceftriaxone	2–5 days 2–5 days	Ampicillin and TMP/SMX resistance high in many areas; indicated if susceptibility confirmed. Mixed results for efficacy of cefixime. Treat for 7–10 days in immunocompromised hosts.
	Adult	Gastroenteritis, dysentery	FQ *or* Azithromycin	5 days 5 days	TMP/SMX *or* Ceftriaxone	5 days 2 days	TMP/SMX if susceptibility confirmed.
	All ages	Bacteremia, invasive	Ceftriaxone	≥10 days	FQ	≥10 days	Invasive disease is uncommon.

Continued

TABLE 1-1

RECOMMENDED TREATMENT FOR BACTERIAL INFECTIONS (Continued)

Pathogen	Host Category	Indication/Type of Infection	Recommended Treatment	Duration	Alternative Treatment	Duration	Comments
Staphylococcus aureus; methicillin-susceptible *S. aureus* (MSSA)	All	Superficial	1st ceph *or* SS-pen *or* BL/BLI *or* Macrolide	10 days 10 days 10 days 10 days	Clindamycin *or* TMP/SMZ *or* Doxycycline	10 days 10 days	
		Osteomyelitis	SS-pen IV *or* 1st ceph IV	4–6 wk 4–6 wk	Clindamycin IV *or* Vancomycin IV	4–6 wk 4–6 wk	Switch from IV to PO when good clinical response.
		Arthritis	SS-pen IV *or* 1st ceph IV	3–4 wk 3–4 wk	Clindamycin IV *or* Vancomycin IV	3–4 wk 3–4 wk	
		Bacteremia/sepsis/ pneumonia/ empyema	SS-pen IV	≥3 wk	Vancomycin IV	≥3 wk	Some experts add rifampin and/or gentamicin in selected cases.
		Endocarditis (native valve)	SS-pen IV + gentamicin	4–6 wk (gentamicin 3–5 days)	Vancomycin + gentamicin	4–6 wk (gentamicin 3–5 days)	
		CNS	SS-pen IV +/– rifampin	10 days from negative culture	Vancomycin IV +/– rifampin	10 days from negative culture	
		Toxic shock syndrome	SS-pen IV + clindamycin	10 days	Vancomycin + clindamycin	10 days	Eliminate either antibiotic once stable and can complete PO. Some experts recommend adding IVIg.

Staphylococcus aureus; methicillin-resistant *S. aureus* (MRSA)	All	Superficial	Clindamycin *or* TMP/SMZ	10 days 10 days	Vancomycin IV *or* Doxycycline (≥8 yr) *or* Linezolid	10 days 10 days 10 days	
		Osteomyelitis, arthritis	Clindamycin IV *or* Vancomycin IV	All: 6 wk (osteomyelitis) 3–4 wk (arthritis)	Linezolid *or* Daptomycin	All: 6 wk (osteomyelitis) 3–4 wk (arthritis)	Switch from IV to PO when good clinical response. Confirm clindamycin susceptibility with D-test.
		Bacteremia/sepsis/ pneumonia/ empyema	Vancomycin IV	≥3 wk	Linezolid IV Daptomycin	≥3 wk ≥3 wk	May add rifampin and/or gentamicin. No daptomycin for pneumonia. Ceftaroline approved for adults, but no data in children.
		Endocarditis (native valve)	Vancomycin IV	4–6 wk	Linezolid *or* Daptomycin	4–6 wk 4–6 wk	Gentamicin +/– rifampin for first 3–5 days for synergy.
		CNS	Vancomycin IV +/– rifampin	10 days from negative culture			Add rifampin for shunt infections.
		Toxic shock syndrome	Vancomycin + clindamycin	10 days			Confirm clindamycin susceptibility with D-test if erythromycin resistant.

Continued

TABLE 1-1

RECOMMENDED TREATMENT FOR BACTERIAL INFECTIONS (Continued)

Pathogen	Host Category	Indication/Type of Infection	Recommended Treatment	Duration	Alternative Treatment	Duration	Comments
Stenotrophomonas maltophilia	All	Pneumonia, bacteremia	TMP/SMX	≥10 days	Tic/clav *or* Ceftazidime	≥10 days ≥10 days	Minocycline or moxifloxacin often used if resistant to preferred and alternative agents. Duration depends on site and severity of infection.
Streptobacillus moniliformis	All	Rat bite fever	PenG procaine IM *or* PenG IV	7–10 days for all regimens	Ampicillin IV *or* Cefuroxime IV *or* PCS3 *or* Erythromycin *or* Doxycycline *or* Clindamycin	7–10 days for all regimens	Course can be completed orally once patient stable and with good response.
Streptococcus pneumoniae	All	Sinopulmonary infections, otitis media, pneumonia (non-CNS, noninvasive, nonsevere)	Amoxicillin, high dose *or* Cefuroxime *or* Cefdinir *or* Cefpodoxime	10 days for all regimens	Azithromycin *or* Clindamycin *or* PCS3	5 days 10 days 10 days (1 day for otitis media)	Parenteral choices for more severe illnesses. Shorter courses (5–7 days) of oral β-lactams for acute, uncomplicated otitis media in healthy children age ≥6 yr without recent otitis.
		Bacteremia, severe pneumonia (invasive, non-CNS)	PCS3	≥10 days (longer if focus of infection, e.g., bone)	Vancomycin IV *or* Clindamycin IV *or* Linezolid IV *or* Carbapenem IV	All ≥10 days (longer if focus of infection, e.g., bone)	Can switch to PO when stable in many cases. Susceptibility testing guides antibiotic options.

	Meningitis, penicillin and PCS3 susceptible	PCS3 *or* AqPenG	14 days 14 days	Carbapenem IV *or* Vancomycin +/– rifampin	14 days 14 days	Susceptibility testing guides antibiotic options. Vancomycin + PCS3 until susceptibilities known. If severe β-lactam allergy requires use of vancomycin, consider addition of rifampin.
	Meningitis: penicillin nonsusceptible and PCS3 susceptible	PCS3	14 days	Carbapenem IV *or* Vancomycin +/– rifampin	All: 14 days	If severe β-lactam allergy requires use of vancomycin, consider addition of rifampin. Vancomycin + PCS3 until susceptibilities known. Susceptibility testing guides antibiotic options.
	Meningitis: penicillin and PCS3 nonsusceptible	Vancomycin + PCS3 +/– rifampin	14 days	CHL *or* Vancomycin + rifampin *or* Linezolid	All: 14 days	Susceptibility testing guides antibiotic options. Repeat LP 48–72 hr, especially if inadequate clinical improvement. Rifampin if clinical worsening, high-level cefotaxime/ceftriaxone resistance (MIC ≥ 4 mcg/mL), and/or persistently positive CSF, **but** only if rifampin susceptible.

Continued

TABLE 1-1

RECOMMENDED TREATMENT FOR BACTERIAL INFECTIONS (Continued)

Pathogen	Host Category	Indication/Type of Infection	Recommended Treatment	Duration	Alternative Treatment	Duration	Comments
Group A *Streptococcus*		Pharyngitis	PenVK PO *or* Amoxicillin PO *or* PenG benzathine IM	10 days 10 days One dose	OCS1 *or* Erythromycin *or* Azithromycin *or* Clarithromycin	5–10 days 10 days 5 days 10 days	PenVK BID and amoxicillin BID or once daily acceptable. Some data for 5 days OCS1.
		Toxic shock syndrome, necrotizing fasciitis, other invasive	PenG IV + clindamycin	≥10 days	Ceftriaxone + clindamycin *or* Vancomycin + clindamycin	≥10 days ≥10 days	Simplify to single antibiotic when patient stable. Adjunctive surgery often needed. Duration depends on site of infection.
Group B *Streptococcus*	All	Invasive (nonmeningitis, not sepsis)	Ampicillin *or* PenG	All: ≥10 days, depending on site of infection	PCS3 *or* Vancomycin	All: ≥10 days, depending on site of infection	
		Meningitis, sepsis	Ampicillin + gentamicin *or* Penicillin + gentamicin	14–21 days (ampicillin or penicillin) 2–3 days (gentamicin)	PCS3 *or* Vancomycin	14–21 days 14–21 days	High-dose ampicillin or penicillin used for meningitis. Gentamicin used until clinical response and CSF/blood sterile.
Group C, G *Streptococcus*	All	Pharyngitis; other noninvasive	PenVK PO	10 days	OCS1, OCS2, *or* TMP/SMX	10 days 10 days	
	All	Invasive, nonendocarditis	PenG IV	>10 days	PCS1, 2, 3 *or* Vancomycin	>10 days >10 days	May add gentamicin if tolerance suspected.

	All	Endocarditis	PenG IV + gentamicin *or* Ceftriaxone + gentamicin	4–6 wk (β-lactam) + 2 wk (gentamicin)	Vancomycin	4–6 wk	Once-daily gentamicin not studied in pediatric endocarditis. If prosthetic valve/material or less susceptible organism, use 6 wk instead of 4. For highly resistant isolate, use 6 wk of [penicillin or ceftriaxone] *plus* 6 wk of gentamicin. Vancomycin *only* if penicillin and ceftriaxone contraindicated.
Viridans streptococci	All	Dental, soft tissue, noninvasive	Penicillin PO *or* Amoxicillin *or* Ampicillin	All: variable	OCS *or* PSC *or* Vancomycin	All: variable	Ceftriaxone preferred PCS. Must consider possible polymicrobial infections; vancomycin preferred by some experts for oncology patients because of growing PCN resistance.
	Usually neonate, altered immunity or intravascular catheter	Bacteremia, other invasive	Penicillin IV *or* Ampicillin IV *or* Ceftriaxone	10–14 days 10–14 days 10–14 days	Vancomycin IV	10–14 days	Increasing penicillin-resistant strains, especially in oncology patients.
		Native valve endocarditis, highly susceptible (Pen MIC ≤0.1)	PenG IV *or* Ceftriaxone IV *or* PenG IV+ gentamicin *or* Ceftriaxone + gentamicin	4 wk 4 wk 2 wk 2 wk	Vancomycin IV	4 wk	Vancomycin only if intolerant of other regimen.

Continued

TABLE 1-1

RECOMMENDED TREATMENT FOR BACTERIAL INFECTIONS (Continued)

Pathogen	Host Category	Indication/Type of Infection	Recommended Treatment	Duration	Alternative Treatment	Duration	Comments
Viridans streptococci *(Coutinued)*		Native valve endocarditis, relatively resistant (Pen MIC >0.12 g/mL to ≤0.5 g/mL)	PenG IV/ gentamicin *or* Ceftriaxone/ gentamicin	4 wk/2 wk 4 wk/2 wk	Vancomycin IV	4 wk	Vancomycin only if intolerant of other regimen.
		Native valve endocarditis, resistant	Ampicillin IV + gentamicin *or* Penicillin IV+ gentamicin *or* Vancomycin IV + gentamicin	4–6 wk 4–6 wk 6 wk	—	—	Same as for enterococcal endocarditis. Vancomycin only if intolerant of other regimen.
		Prosthetic valve endocarditis, susceptible (Pen MIC ≤0.12)	Pen G IV *or* Ceftriaxone	6 wk 6 wk	Vancomycin IV	6 wk	Gentamicin often added to Pen G or ceftriaxone for first 2 wk of treatment. Vancomycin only if intolerant of other regimen.
		Prosthetic valve endocarditis, relatively or fully resistant (Pen MIC >0.12)	Pen G IV + gentamicin *or* Ceftriaxone + gentamicin	6 wk 6 wk	Vancomycin IV	6 wk	Gentamicin used for all 6 wk of PenG or ceftriaxone therapy. Vancomycin only if intolerant of other regimen.

Treponema pallidum (syphilis)	Infants	Proven or probable congenital syphilis	PenG IV 50,000 units/kg/dose Q12 hr (<8 days old) or Q8 hr (>7 days old)	10 days	PenG procaine IM 50,000 units/kg once daily	10 days	Close clinical and serologic follow-ups essential.
		Mother's treatment or response inadequate, but infant evaluation normal	PenG IV *or* PenG procaine IM *or* PenG benzathine IM	10 days 10 days Once			Close clinical and serologic follow-ups essential, especially if single-dose regimen used.
		Mother adequately treated and infant evaluation normal	PenG benzathine IM *or* no antibiotic	Once			Close clinical and serologic follow-ups essential, especially if no treatment given.
	Beyond infancy	Primary; secondary; latent <1 yr	PenG benzathine IM	Once	Doxycycline *or* Tetracycline	14 days 14 days	Doxycycline and tetracycline only used for penicillin-allergic, nonpregnant patients. Penicillin-allergic pregnant women must be desensitized and treated with penicillin.
	Beyond infancy	Latent ≥1 yr; latent unknown duration; tertiary *without* neurosyphilis	PenG benzathine IM	Once weekly for 3 wk	Doxycycline *or* Tetracycline	28 days 28 days	

Continued

TABLE 1-1

RECOMMENDED TREATMENT FOR BACTERIAL INFECTIONS (Continued)

Pathogen	Host Category	Indication/Type of Infection	Recommended Treatment	Duration	Alternative Treatment	Duration	Comments
Treponema pallidum (syphilis) *(Coutinued)*	Beyond infancy	Neurosyphilis; syphilitic eye disease	AqPenG IV	10–14 days	[PenG procaine IM + probenecid] *or* Ceftriaxone	10–14 days 10–14 days	Penicillin-allergic pregnant women must be desensitized and treated with penicillin. Ceftriaxone only in nonpregnant women if penicillin cannot be used.
Ureaplasma urealyticum	All	Urethritis	Doxycycline PO	7 days	Erythromycin PO *or* Azithromycin PO	7 days 1 dose	Erythromycin ×14 days preferred for children <8 yr old.
	Preterm neonates	Symptomatic respiratory	Erythromycin IV/PO	10 days	Azithromycin (?) PO/IV	10 days	Route depends on degree of illness. Pyloric stenosis risk with erythromycin. Scant data for azithromycin treatment.
		Symptomatic CNS	Doxycycline IV	10–14 days	CHL IV	10–14 days	Very limited data.
Vibrio cholerae	All	Moderate to severe illness	TMP/SMX PO *or* Doxycycline PO *or* Ciprofloxacin PO *or* Azithromycin PO	3 days 1 dose 1 dose 1 dose	Tetracycline PO *or* Furazolidone PO *or* Erythromycin PO *or* Ofloxacin PO	3 days 3 days Unknown Unknown	Fluid/electrolyte most important part of prescription. Tetracycline and doxycycline preferred for patients ≥8 yr old. Ciprofloxacin if ≥18 yr old. Variable resistance. Azithromycin preferred during pregnancy.

Vibrio vulnificus, Vibrio parahaemolyticus, other species	All	Bacteremia/sepsis Wound	Doxycycline + ceftazidime	Variable	FQ *or* PCS3	Variable Variable	Prompt debridement for wound infections and necrotizing fasciitis.
Yersinia enterocolitica, Yersinia pseudotuberculosis	Normal	Enterocolitis Pseudoappendicitis Mesenteric adenitis	None				Antibiotics may limit duration of shedding, but no clinical benefit.
	Immunocompromised	Enterocolitis	TMP/SMX *or* PCS3 *or* FQ	Variable	Tetracycline *or* Doxycycline *or* Piperacillin *or* AG	Variable	Tetracycline and doxycycline for ≥8 yr old. FQ for ≥18 yr old. *Y. enterocolitica*: consider iron overload syndromes.
	All	Sepsis or other invasive illness	TMP/SMX *or* PCS3 *or* FQ	Variable	Tetracycline *or* Doxycycline *or* Piperacillin *or* AG	Variable	
Yersinia pestis (plague)		Bubonic/pneumonic plague	Streptomycin IM Gentamicin IM/IV	≥7–10 days ≥7–10 days	Tetracycline IV *or* Doxycycline IV	≥7–10 days ≥7–10 days	Treat until afebrile several days.
		Meningitis, endophthalmitis, or shock	CHL IV	≥7–10 days	—	—	

1

II. RECOMMENDED TREATMENT FOR MYCOBACTERIAL INFECTIONS

TABLE 1-2

RECOMMENDED TREATMENT FOR MYCOBACTERIAL INFECTIONS (for notes and abbreviations used in this table, see p. xiii.)

Pathogen	Host Category	Indication/Type of Infection	Recommended Treatment	Duration	Alternative Treatment	Duration	Comments
*Mycobacterium tuberculosis**	Immunocompetent	Latent infection (positive TST, no disease); isoniazid-susceptible	All ages: Isoniazid *or* (if ≥12 yr) Isoniazid + rifapentine	 9 mo 12 wk 12 wk	2–11 yr old: Isoniazid + rifapentine *or* Rifampin <2 yr old: Rifampin	 12 wk 12 wk 6 mo 6 mo	12-wk combination therapy equally preferred if ≥12 yr; alternative if 2–11 yr old (limited data); not recommended if <2 yr old. Isoniazid alone is given by DOTS daily or twice weekly; isoniazid plus rifapentine combination is given weekly by DOTS.
		Latent infection; isoniazid-resistant	Rifampin	6 mo			
		Latent infection; isoniazid and rifampin-resistant	Treat only after consultation with a TB specialist				
	Pregnancy and breast-feeding	Latent infection	Isoniazid + pyridoxine	9 mo 9 mo			Treatment with isoniazid should be avoided during the first trimester. However, for those at increased risk for progression to active disease, isoniazid treatment should not be delayed based on pregnancy alone, including during the first trimester. Isoniazid is secreted in human milk, but no adverse effects to infants have been detected.

Immunocompromised, HIV-infected	Latent infection	Isoniazid + pyridoxine	9 mo 9 mo		12-wk isoniazid-rifapentine can be considered for HIV-infected children not taking ART and other immunocompromised children. Beware of ART and other drug interactions with rifampin and rifapentine. Consultation with a specialist is recommended. DOT is advised.
All	Pulmonary and extrapulmonary, **drug-susceptible disease** (excluding meningitis or disseminated/ miliary TB)	Isoniazid + rifampin + pyrazinamide + ethambutol	6 mo 6 mo 2 mo 2 mo	Aminoglycoside (streptomycin; alternative: kanamycin, amikacin, capreomycin) may be used in place of ethambutol	May discontinue 4th drug if isolate is fully drug-susceptible *and* disease is not considered high burden (pulmonary TB with extensive parenchymal involvement, cavitary disease). **Corticosteroids** may be considered as adjunctive therapy for 4–6 wk for patients with pleuritis or pericarditis.

Continued

TABLE 1-2

RECOMMENDED TREATMENT FOR MYCOBACTERIAL INFECTIONS (Continued)

Pathogen	Host Category	Indication/Type of Infection	Recommended Treatment	Duration	Alternative Treatment	Duration	Comments
*Mycobacterium tuberculosis** *(Coutinued)*		Pulmonary and extrapulmonary disease—possibly multidrug-resistant or extensively drug resistant isolate	Treat only after consultation with a TB specialist				
		Meningitis or disseminated/ miliary TB	Isoniazid + rifampin + pyrazinamide + [ethionamide *or* ethambutol *or* aminoglycoside]	9–12 mo 9–12 mo 2 mo 2 mo 2 mo 2 mo			If susceptibility to isoniazid, rifampin, and pyrazinamide is confirmed, the fourth drug can be discontinued. Usual aminoglycoside: streptomycin; alternatives: kanamycin, amikacin, capreomycin. Corticosteroid (2 mg/kg/day prednisone, maximum 60 mg/day for 4–6 wk followed by taper) is also indicated for meningitis once anti-TB therapy is begun.
	Pregnancy	Pulmonary and extrapulmonary disease	Isoniazid + rifampin + ethambutol + pyridoxine	9 mo 9 mo 2 mo 9 mo	Isoniazid + rifampin + pyrazinamide + pyridoxine	6 mo 6 mo 2 mo 6 mo	Although teratogenicity data are not available, pyrazinamide can probably be used safely during pregnancy and is recommended by the World Health Organization and the International Union against Tuberculosis and Lung Disease. If pyrazinamide is not included in initial treatment regimen, treatment should be for at least 9 mo.

	Congenital infection	Pulmonary and extrapulmonary disease	Isoniazid + rifampin + pyrazinamide + amikacin	Treat as above for TB disease, depending on antibiotic susceptibility.			Add corticosteroid if meningitis is confirmed. Send placenta for TB culture and pathologic examination.
NONTUBERCULOUS MYCOBACTERIA†							
Mycobacterium bovis	All	Pulmonary and extrapulmonary disease, excluding meningitis	Isoniazid + rifampin	9–12 mo 9–12 mo			Recommended treatment for *M. bovis* is based on treatment trials for *M. tuberculosis.* All strains of *M. bovis* are resistant to pyrazinamide. Usual aminoglycoside: streptomycin; alternatives: kanamycin, amikacin, capreomycin.
		Meningitis	Isoniazid + rifampin + ethionamide *or* ethambutol *or* aminoglycoside†	At least 12 mo At least 12 mo 2 mo 2 mo 2 mo			
Mycobacterium avium complex	Immunocompetent	Lymphadenitis	Excision of affected node(s)		[Clarithromycin *or* Azithromycin] + [ethambutol *and/or* (rifampin *or* rifabutin)]	≥3 mo ≥3 mo ≥3 mo ≥3 mo ≥3 mo	Pharmacologic therapy is recommended if excision is incomplete or if disease recurs.

Continued

TABLE 1-2

RECOMMENDED TREATMENT FOR MYCOBACTERIAL INFECTIONS (Continued)

Pathogen	Host Category	Indication/Type of Infection	Recommended Treatment	Duration	Alternative Treatment	Duration	Comments
Mycobacterium avium complex *(Coutinued)*	Immunocompetent or immunocompromised	Pulmonary infection	[Clarithromycin *or* Azithromycin] + ethambutol + [rifampin *or* rifabutin]	12 mo 12 mo 12 mo 12 mo			Amikacin or streptomycin can be added initially for severe disease.
		Disseminated disease	Treat only in consultation with an expert. Initial recommended therapy with 3–4 drugs, including [clarithromycin or azithromycin] + ethambutol + [rifampin or rifabutin] +/– [amikacin or streptomycin] +/– ciprofloxacin				Treatment for 12 mo followed by suppressive therapy.
Mycobacterium kansasii	All	Pulmonary infection	[Rifampin + ethambutol + isoniazid]	≥3 mo ≥3 mo ≥3 mo			Resistant to pyrazinamide.
		Osteomyelitis	Surgical debridement + Rifampin + ethambutol + isoniazid	All: prolonged, variable			
Mycobacterium marinum	All	Cutaneous infection	Rifampin *or* TMP/SMX *or* Clarithromycin *or* Doxycycline	≥3 mo ≥3 mo ≥3 mo ≥3 mo			Minor infection may heal without therapy. Extensive lesions may require surgical debridement. Isoniazid and pyrazinamide resistant.

Mycobacterium ulcerans	All	Cutaneous and bone infection	Excision of tissue +		Excision of tissue +		
			Rifampin +	8 wk	rifampin +	8 wk	
			streptomycin	8 wk	ciprofloxacin	8 wk	
Mycobacterium fortuitum	All	Cutaneous infection	Excision of tissue				
		Serious infection	Amikacin + meropenem, followed by [clarithromycin *or* doxycycline[§] *or* TMP/SMX *or* ciprofloxacin]	See Comment			Duration of therapy should be determined in consultation with an infectious disease specialist.
		Catheter infection	Catheter removal + Amikacin + meropenem, followed by [clarithromycin *or* doxycycline[‡] *or* TMP/SMX *or* ciprofloxacin]	See Comment			Definitive therapy should be based on susceptibility testing. Duration of therapy should be determined in consultation with an infectious disease specialist.

Continued

1

TABLE 1-2

RECOMMENDED TREATMENT FOR MYCOBACTERIAL INFECTIONS (Continued)

Pathogen	Host Category	Indication/Type of Infection	Recommended Treatment	Duration	Alternative Treatment	Duration	Comments
Mycobacterium abscessus	All	Otitis media	Clarithromycin + amikacin + cefoxitin	Variable	Meropenem may be used in place of cefoxitin.		May require debridement. Susceptibility testing should be performed—amikacin resistance occurs in 50% of isolates.
	Patients with cystic fibrosis	Pulmonary infection	Clarithromycin + amikacin + cefoxitin	Variable	Meropenem may be used in place of cefoxitin.		Surgical resection may be required. Susceptibility testing should be performed. May not always require treatment as it is difficult to establish if mycobacteria are only colonizers or true pathogens.
Mycobacterium chelonae	All	Catheter infection	Catheter removal + tobramycin + clarithromycin	Variable			
		Disseminated cutaneous infection	[Tobramycin + (meropenem *or* linezolid) + clarithromycin]	Variable			

III. RECOMMENDED TREATMENT FOR VIRAL INFECTIONS

TABLE 1-3

RECOMMENDED TREATMENT FOR VIRAL INFECTIONS (for notes and abbreviations used in this table, see p. xiv.)

Pathogen	Host Category	Indication	Recommended Treatment	Alternative Treatment	Comment
Cytomegalovirus	Immunocompromised	GI tract, lungs, viremia	Ganciclovir, IV for 14–21 days	Foscarnet IV *or* Cidofovir IV *or* Valganciclovir PO	For treatment of pulmonary or GI infection, immunoglobulin or CMV immunoglobulin may be used together with ganciclovir. Long-term suppressive therapy is used to prevent relapse in patients with HIV infection. Cidofovir should be administered with probenecid and hydration.
		Ocular infection	Ganciclovir IV	Valganciclovir PO *or* Foscarnet IV *or* Cidofovir IV	
		Long-term suppression of ocular infection	Ganciclovir, IV indefinitely	Foscarnet IV *or* Cidofovir IV *or* Valganciclovir PO	Suppressive therapy for HIV-infected patients should continue until immune reconstitution has been achieved.
	Neonate	Symptomatic congenital infection involving the central nervous system ≤28 days of life	Ganciclovir, IV for 6 wk	Valganciclovir	Data to support optimal use and duration of ganciclovir for this indication are controversial.

Continued

TABLE 1-3

RECOMMENDED TREATMENT FOR VIRAL INFECTIONS (Continued)

Pathogen	Host Category	Indication	Recommended Treatment	Alternative Treatment	Comment
Hepatitis B		Chronic disease with evidence of ongoing viral replication	Interferon alpha-2b *or* pegylated Interferon alpha-2a, subcutaneously	Lamivudine (for children >2 yr old); adefovir (for children >11 yr old); Telbivudine (for those >16 yr old)	Treatment of chronic hepatitis B infection in children is under continued investigation, and some drugs used to treat adults are not approved for children. Specialists in hepatology should be consulted. If lamivudine is used to treat children coinfected with HIV and hepatitis B, the lamivudine dose used should be the approved dose for treating HIV infection.
Hepatitis C		Chronic infection, ≥3 yr old	[Interferon alpha-2b *or* pegylated Interferon alpha, subcutaneously or IM] + ribavirin, PO, for 12–48 wk depending on virologic response and virus genotype		Children with symptomatic hepatitis C disease or histologically advanced pathologic features should be considered for treatment in consultation with a gastroenterologist or infectious disease consultant. All patients with hepatitis C should be immunized against hepatitis A and B.
Herpes simplex (HSV)	Immunocompetent	Genital (first episode)	[Acyclovir PO *or* Famciclovir PO *or* Valacyclovir PO] for 7–10 days *or* Acyclovir IV for 5–7 days		Famciclovir and valacyclovir are licensed only for adolescents and adults. May switch to PO to complete.

	Genital (recurrent)	[Acyclovir PO *or* Famciclovir PO *or* Valacyclovir PO] for 5 days *or* Acyclovir IV for 5–7 days		Famciclovir and valacyclovir are licensed only for adolescents and adults. May switch to PO to complete.
	Suppression of recurrent mucocutaneous outbreaks	Acyclovir PO (400 mg BID) *or* Famciclovir PO (250 mg BID) *or* Valacyclovir PO (1000 mg/day)] for as long as 12 mo continuously		Famciclovir and valacyclovir are licensed only for adolescents and adults.
	CNS (encephalitis) (postneonatal)	Acyclovir IV (30–45 mg/kg/day divided into 3 doses) for at least 21 days		
Neonate	Any	Acyclovir IV (60 mg/kg/day divided into 3 doses) for 14 (skin, eye, mucous membrane involvement) to 21 days (disseminated or CNS involvement)		
Immunocompromised	Any non-CNS site	Acyclovir IV (30 mg/kg/day divided into 3 doses) for 7–14 days	Foscarnet IV	Use foscarnet for HSV infection resistant to acyclovir. Treat until infection resolves.
	Mucocutaneous	Acyclovir PO for 7–14 days *or* Famciclovir PO *or* Valacyclovir PO	Foscarnet IV	Use foscarnet for HSV infection resistant to acyclovir.

Continued

TABLE 1-3

RECOMMENDED TREATMENT FOR VIRAL INFECTIONS (Continued)

Pathogen	Host Category	Indication	Recommended Treatment	Alternative Treatment	Comment
Herpes simplex (HSV) *(Coutinued)*	All	Keratoconjunctivitis	[Trifluridine *or* Iododeoxyuridine *or* Vidarabine] topical		Consult an ophthalmologist.
Influenza A and B	≥2 weeks of age	Treatment	Oseltamivir PO for 5 days		Most effective if treatment is initiated within 48 hr of onset of symptoms. Treatment may be beneficial if initiated after 48 hr in patients with severe, complicated, or progressive illness or those requiring hospitalization. Amantadine and rimantadine have been used to treat influenza A, but most isolates since 2006 have been resistant. For current recommendations see www.cdc.gov/flu/professionals/antivirals/index.htm or www.aapredbook.org/flu.
	≥7 yr of age	Treatment	Oseltamivir PO for 5 days *or* Zanamivir, inhalation, for 5 days		Most effective if treatment is initiated within 48 hr of onset of symptoms. Treatment may be beneficial if initiated after 48 hr in patients with severe, complicated, or progressive illness or those requiring hospitalization. Amantadine and rimantadine have been used to treat influenza A, but most isolates since 2006 have been resistant.

Parvovirus	Immunocompromised with persistent anemia		IVIG		
Respiratory syncytial virus		Bronchiolitis/pneumonia, severe	Ribavirin, aerosol via small-particle generator, 18 hr/day for 3–7 days		Longer treatment may be required for some patients. Effectiveness has been questioned. Not routinely recommended.
Varicella	Immunocompetent	Varicella	Acyclovir PO or IV for 5 days		Begin within 24 hr of symptoms. Treatment is indicated only for individuals at increased risk for moderate to severe varicella.
		Zoster	Acyclovir PO or IV for 5–7 days	Famciclovir PO for 7 days *or* Valacyclovir PO for 7 days	Famciclovir and valacyclovir are licensed only for adolescents and adults.
	Immunocompromised	Varicella	Acyclovir IV for 7–10 days	Foscarnet IV	Use of oral acyclovir instead of or to complete an IV therapy course is used by some experts for patients thought to be at low risk for severe disease. Use foscarnet for varicella infection resistant to acyclovir.
		Zoster	Acyclovir PO or IV for 7–10 days	Famciclovir PO for 7 days *or* Valacyclovir PO for 7 days *or* Foscarnet IV for up to 3 wk	Famciclovir and valacyclovir are licensed only for adolescents and adults. Use foscarnet for varicella infection resistant to acyclovir.

1

IV. RECOMMENDED TREATMENT FOR FUNGAL INFECTIONS

Fungal pathogens are listed according to clinical and laboratory presentation on pp. 77–78.

A. Systemic Treatment

TABLE 1-4

RECOMMENDED TREATMENT FOR FUNGAL INFECTIONS: SYSTEMIC TREATMENT* (for notes and abbreviations used in this table, see p. xiv.)

Fungus	Host Category	Indication	Recommended Treatment	Duration*	Alternative Treatment	Duration*	Comments
Alternaria spp. (phaeohyphomycosis)	Immunocompromised	Locally invasive infection (mycotic keratitis, paranasal sinusitis, osteomyelitis, cutaneous infection)	Voriconazole		Itraconazole for localized cutaneous disease Amphotericin B†		Surgical debridement with or without granulocyte transfusion may be helpful additional modes of therapy.
Aspergillus spp.	Immunocompromised	Invasive infection (pulmonary, sinus, disseminated, CNS)	Voriconazole	≥12 wk	Amphotericin B† (preferred in neonates) *or* caspofungin *or* micafungin *or* anidulafungin	≥12 wk	Surgical debridement for sinusitis. Consult infectious disease specialist regarding possible combination therapy.

	Immunocompetent	Allergic bronchopulmonary aspergillosis	Corticosteroid	Itraconazole may be helpful to reduce need for corticosteroid
		Allergic sinusitis	Surgical drainage, antibiotic for secondary bacterial infection, topical corticosteroid	
		Pulmonary aspergilloma	Surgical removal may be required; endobronchial instillation of amphotericin B or itraconazole has been used	
		Otomycosis	Debridement; topical clotrimazole or econazole nitrate	
Bipolaris spp.	Immunocompromised or after trauma	Disseminated infection; sinusitis	Voriconazole *or* itraconazole *or* amphotericin B[†] Surgical excision or debridement may be required	Itraconazole for cutaneous infection

Continued

TABLE 1-4

RECOMMENDED TREATMENT FOR FUNGAL INFECTIONS: SYSTEMIC TREATMENT (Continued)

Fungus	Host Category	Indication	Recommended Treatment	Duration*	Alternative Treatment	Duration*	Comments
Blastomyces dermatitidis (blastomycosis)	All	Disseminated, life-threatening disease	Amphotericin B[†] (total dose: 15 mg/kg; maximum: 1.5–2.5 g) followed by itraconazole *or* fluconazole	2 wk of amphotericin B,[†] followed by 6 mo of itraconazole or fluconazole	Fluconazole		Consider fluconazole therapy only for patients unable to tolerate amphotericin B. If itraconazole is used, serum concentration should be measured and adherence should be assessed.
		CNS disease	Amphotericin B[†]	Daily for 4–6 wk (total dose 30–40 mg/kg) followed by amphotericin B,[†] 3 times weekly for 1–3 mo			Treatment recommendations for children are extrapolated from adult studies. Consultation with infectious disease specialist is advised.

Immunocompromised	Cutaneous, pulmonary, bone disease	Amphotericin B† (total dose: 15 mg/kg; maximum 1.5–2.5 g), followed by itraconazole *or* fluconazole	2 wk of Amphotericin B,† followed by 6 mo of Itraconazole or Fluconazole Bone infection should be treated for a total of 12 mo	Fluconazole *or* Itraconazole	6 mo Bone infection should be treated for a total of 12 mo	If itraconazole is used, serum concentration should be measured and adherence should be assessed. Treatment recommendations for children are extrapolated from adult studies. Consultation with infectious disease specialist is advised.
Immunocompetent	Mild to moderate skin, pulmonary, or bone infection	Itraconazole	6–12 mo (12 mo recommended for bone infections)	Fluconazole		Observation alone may be appropriate for mild or resolving disease.
	Severe pulmonary disease	Amphotericin B† (total dose 1.5–2.5 g) *or* Amphotericin B† (total dose 15 mg/kg over 2 wk) followed by itraconazole *or* fluconazole	If azole is used, it should be continued for 6–12 mo	Fluconazole		If itraconazole is used, serum concentration should be measured and adherence should be assessed.

Continued

1

TABLE 1-4

RECOMMENDED TREATMENT FOR FUNGAL INFECTIONS: SYSTEMIC TREATMENT (Continued)

Fungus	Host Category	Indication	Recommended Treatment	Duration*	Alternative Treatment	Duration*	Comments
Candida spp.‡	Immunocompromised	Oropharyngeal (thrush)	Fluconazole	7–21 days	Voriconazole *or* Posaconazole *or* Itraconazole *or* Caspofungin *or* Micafungin *or* Anidulafungin *or* Amphotericin B†	7–21 days	
		Esophagitis	Fluconazole *or* Amphotericin B† *or* Caspofungin *or* Micafungin *or* Anidulafungin	21 days (or at least 14 days after resolution of symptoms)	Itraconazole *or* Voriconazole		Alternative drugs should be used for refractory cases; prolonged therapy may be required.

	Catheter-associated infection (intravascular or peritoneal)	Catheter removal + amphotericin B[†]	Until blood/peritoneal cultures are negative for at least 14 days; longer treatment course for granulocytopenic and severely immunocompromised patients; at least 14 days for peritonitis	Fluconazole *or* Caspofungin *or* Micafungin *or* Anidulafungin	Until blood/peritoneal cultures are negative for at least 14 days; longer treatment course for granulocytopenic and severely immunocompromised patients; at least 14 days for peritonitis	Intraperitoneal infusion of amphotericin B is alternative for patients with candidal peritonitis; flucytosine provides synergistic therapy for *C. albicans* but not demonstrated for other *Candida* species; alternative agents should not be used until the infecting species is known to be susceptible.

Continued

1

TABLE 1-4

RECOMMENDED TREATMENT FOR FUNGAL INFECTIONS: SYSTEMIC TREATMENT (Continued)

Fungus	Host Category	Indication	Recommended Treatment	Duration*	Alternative Treatment	Duration*	Comments
Candida spp.‡ *(Coutinued)*		Disseminated infection	[Amphotericin B† +/– flucytosine] *or* Caspofungin *or* Micafungin *or* Anidulafungin	Varies with site of infection, clinical response, and presence or absence of neutropenia	Fluconazole	Varies with site of infection, clinical response, and presence or absence of neutropenia	Flucytosine provides synergistic therapy for *C. albicans* but not demonstrated for other *Candida* species. Alternative agents should not be used until the infecting species is known to be susceptible. Amphotericin B is preferred in neonates.
		Endocarditis	Valve replacement + amphotericin B† *or* Caspofungin *or* Micafungin *or* Anidulafungin	6 wk after valve replacement			Lifelong suppressive therapy with fluconazole may be an alternative if valve replacement is not possible.

	Meningitis	[Amphotericin B† +/– flucytosine] *or* Caspofungin *or* Micafungin *or* Anidulafungin	At least 4 wk after resolution of signs and symptoms			Fluconazole has been used for follow-up therapy and long-term suppression. Data on success are limited.
	Chronic mucocutaneous candidiasis	Fluconazole *or* Itraconazole *or* Voriconazole	Lifelong	Amphotericin B† (0.3 mg/kg/day IV)	Lifelong	
	Congenital/disseminated candidiasis of newborn	Amphotericin B†	Total dose of 10–25 mg/kg over 21 days	Caspofungin *or* Micafungin *or* Anidulafungin *or* Fluconazole	3 wk	Experience with echinocandins and fluconazole in newborns is limited. Some lipid formulations of amphotericin B have questionable renal penetration and should not be used to treat disseminated disease.
Immunocompetent	Oropharyngeal (thrush)	Nystatin *or* clotrimazole	7–10 days	Fluconazole	7–10 days	

Continued

1

TABLE 1-4

RECOMMENDED TREATMENT FOR FUNGAL INFECTIONS: SYSTEMIC TREATMENT (Continued)

Fungus	Host Category	Indication	Recommended Treatment	Duration*	Alternative Treatment	Duration*	Comments
Candida spp.[‡] *(Continued)*		Vulvovaginal	Topical agents, including Clotrimazole *or* Miconazole *or* Butoconazole *or* Terconazole *or* Tioconazole *or* Nystatin *or* Fluconazole (oral), single dose	1–14 days, depending on the agent used	Oral agents: Fluconazole (single dose *or* for refractory cases, Itraconazole *or* Ketoconazole)	7–14 days	
		Diaper dermatitis	Nystatin, topical	7–10 days	Topical Miconazole *or* Clotrimazole *or* Naftifine *or* Ketoconazole *or* Econazole *or* Ciclopirox	7–10 days	
		Intertrigo, paronychia	Topical agents, including Clotrimazole, miconazole, and nystatin	Prolonged therapy may be required			Surgical drainage is important for paronychia.
		IV catheter-associated candidemia	Catheter removal + Fluconazole *or* Caspofungin *or* Micafungin *or* Anidulafungin *or* Amphotericin B[†]	14 days if blood cultures are negative after catheter removal			

Coccidioides immitis (coccidioidomycosis)	Severe infection; immunocompromised patients	Pulmonary disease	Amphotericin B† (total dose, 10–100 mg/kg; maximum 1 g), followed by fluconazole *or* itraconazole	1–12 mo, total, depending on clinical and immunologic response; lifelong for HIV patients	Itraconazole *or* Fluconazole for milder disease	1–12 mo, depending on clinical and immunologic response; lifelong for HIV patients	The majority of immunocompetent patients with coccidioidomycosis do not require treatment. Dose and duration of amphoteracin B depend on host of factors, severity of disease, and rapidity of response to therapy.
		Nonmeningeal, extrapulmonary disease	Amphotericin B† (total dose, 10–100 mg/kg; maximum 1 g), followed by fluconazole *or* itraconazole	At least 12 mo and 3 mo beyond resolution of symptoms	Fluconazole *or* Itraconazole	At least 12 mo and 3 mo beyond resolution of symptoms	Absorption of itraconazole is unpredictable; serum concentrations should be measured. Dose and duration of amphoteracin B depend on host of factors, severity of disease, and rapidity of response to therapy.
		CNS Infection	Fluconazole	Lifelong	Amphotericin B† IV and in the intrathecal, ventricular, or cisternal space	Lifelong	Dose of fluconazole should be in the upper end of the recommended range. Periodic CSF examination should be performed for 2 yr.

Continued

TABLE 1-4

RECOMMENDED TREATMENT FOR FUNGAL INFECTIONS: SYSTEMIC TREATMENT (Continued)

Fungus	Host Category	Indication	Recommended Treatment	Duration*	Alternative Treatment	Duration*	Comments
Curvularia spp.		Eumycotic mycetoma	Surgical excision + voriconazole *or* itraconazole *or* amphotericin B*	≥10 mo (or at least 3 mo after inflammation has resolved)			May be a cause of disseminated infection in neutropenic patients.
		Phaeohyphomycosis	Amphotericin B *or* Voriconazole *or* Itraconazole	Unknown; prolonged therapy required depending on the host and the site of infection	Voriconazole	Unknown; prolonged therapy required depending on the host and the site of infection	Surgical excision may be required.
Cryptococcus neoformans		Disseminated disease without CNS involvement	[Amphotericin B[†] (1 mg/kg/day) + flucytosine (25 mg/kg/dose given 4 times/ day) for 2 weeks] followed by fluconazole (12 mg/kg/d on day 1 for 2 weeks, then 6–12 mg/kg [maximum 800 mg] daily for 8–10 weeks)	Lifelong prophylaxis in individuals with HIV infection Daily Fluconazole *or* Itraconazole *or* weekly Amphotericin B for lifelong suppressive therapy			CSF should be examined to rule out occult meningitis; maintain flucytosine serum concentration at 40–60 mcg/mL. Discontinuation of therapy after 6 mo may be considered in asymptomatic children who have achieved immune reconstitution through antiretroviral therapy.

	Meningitis	[Amphotericin B† (1 mg/kg/day) + flucytosine (25 mg/kg/dose given 4 times/day) for 2 weeks] followed by fluconazole (12 mg/kg/d on day 1, then 6–12 mg/kg [maximum 800 mg] daily for 8–10 weeks or until CSF is sterile).	Lifelong prophylaxis in individuals with HIV infection Fluconazole (6 mg/kg/day) should be administered lifelong	Amphotericin B† alone for 4–6 wk. *or* [Fluconazole + flucytosine] for 6 weeks	Lifelong prophylaxis in individuals with HIV infection Daily Fluconazole *or* Itraconazole *or* weekly Amphotericin B may be used for lifelong suppressive therapy	Manage increased intracranial pressure with repeat lumbar puncture; reassess CSF after 2 wk of therapy; intrathecal amphotericin B may be required. Maintain flucytosine serum concentration at 40–60 mcg/mL. Discontinuation of therapy after 6 mo may be considered in asymptomatic children who have achieved immune reconstitution through antiretroviral therapy.
Exophiala spp.	Eumycotic mycetoma; sinusitis	Catheter removal + Voriconazole *or* Posaconazole *or* Itraconazole *or* Amphotericin B†	≥10 mo (or at least 3 mo after inflammation has resolved)			

Continued

TABLE 1-4

RECOMMENDED TREATMENT FOR FUNGAL INFECTIONS: SYSTEMIC TREATMENT (Continued)

Fungus	Host Category	Indication	Recommended Treatment	Duration*	Alternative Treatment	Duration*	Comments
Exserohilum spp.		Eumycotic mycetoma; sinusitis	Surgical excision *and* [Itraconazole *or* Amphotericin B]	≥10 mo (or at least 3 mo after inflammation has resolved)	Voriconazole	≥10 mo (or at least 3 mo after inflammation has resolved)	
Fusarium spp.	Immunocompromised	Disseminated disease (fungemia, skin lesions, multiple organ involvement)	Voriconazole *or* Posaconazole		High-dose Amphotericin B *or* lipid formulation of Amphotericin B		Granulocyte transfusion and granulocyte colony-stimulating factor may be beneficial.
	Immunocompetent	Locally invasive infection (mycotic keratitis, endophthalmitis, sinusitis, subcutaneous infection)	Voriconazole *or* Posaconazole		High-dose Amphotericin B *or* lipid formulation of Amphotericin B		
Histoplasma capsulatum (Histoplasmosis)	Immunocompromised	Disseminated infection	Liposomal Amphotericin B,[†] 30 mg/kg (total) over 4–6 wk, followed by itraconazole for 12 wk	Lifelong itraconazole in individuals with HIV and congenital immunodeficiencies	Amphotericin B for 1–2 wk followed by itraconazole	Lifelong itraconazole in individuals with HIV and congenital immunodeficiencies	Monitor urine or serum antigen concentration monthly; should decrease with effective therapy.

	Meningitis	Amphotericin B† for 3 mo, then itraconazole for 12 mo				
Immunocompetent	Severe acute pulmonary disease	Amphotericin B† for 1–2 wk followed by itraconazole for 12 wk	Total therapy: 13–15 wk or until urine *Histoplasma* antigen is <4 units	Amphotericin B† followed by fluconazole	Total therapy: 12 wk or until urine *Histoplasma* antigen is <4 units	Primary pulmonary infection does not require treatment in most individuals. If respiratory complications develop during treatment, methylprednisolone can be added.
	Progressive disseminated histoplasmosis	Amphotericin B† for 6–12 wk followed by itraconazole	Total therapy 6–18 mo	Amphotericin B for 2–3 wk followed by itraconazole	Total therapy 6–18 mo	
	Granulomatous mediastinitis	[Corticosteroids + itraconazole]	6–12 wk			Surgical drainage may be required for large, necrotic masses, but excision of fibrotic pulmonary lesions risks uncontrolled hemorrhage.

Continued

1

TABLE 1-4

RECOMMENDED TREATMENT FOR FUNGAL INFECTIONS: SYSTEMIC TREATMENT (Continued)

Fungus	Host Category	Indication	Recommended Treatment	Duration*	Alternative Treatment	Duration*	Comments
Exserohilum spp. *(Coutinued)*		Pericarditis, erythema nodosum, arthritis	NSAID; antifungal therapy not required	2–12 wk			Pericardial drainage may be required.
Madurella spp. (South Asia)		Eumycotic mycetoma	Surgical excision *and* Ketoconazole	≥10 mo (or at least 3 mo after inflammation has resolved)	Surgical excision *and* Griseofulvin		
Malassezia spp.	Immunocompromised (including neonates)	Catheter-associated fungemia	Catheter removal + discontinuation of IV lipid + Amphotericin B	Depends on persistence of fungemia, presence/absence of metastatic foci			
	Immunocompetent	Pityriasis versicolor	Topical selenium sulfide (2.5%)	1–2 wk; then monthly	Topical ketoconazole (2%) *or* Oral fluconazole *or* ketoconazole *or* Itraconazole	Single application Single dose 5 days	

Paracoccidioides brasiliensis	All	GI infection; disseminated disease	Itraconazole *or* Amphotericin B	6–12 mo	Voriconazole	6–12 mo	Trimethoprim-sulfamethoxazole is used in resource-poor countries, but maintenance therapy must be used for ≥2 yr to avoid relapse.
Penicillium marneffei	Immunocompromised (HIV+)	Pneumonitis; disseminated infection	Itraconazole *or* Amphotericin B				Common in AIDS patients in Southeast Asia.
Pneumocystis jiroveci	Immunocompromised	Severe pneumonia (pO_2 <70 mm Hg or alveolar-arterial gradient of >35)	Trimethoprim-sulfamethoxazole + prednisone	21 days (prednisone should be administered for 5–7 days at 1 mg/kg (maximum 80 mg), then tapered over 21 days)	IV Pentamidine		Prednisone should be started within 72 hr after starting specific antibiotic therapy.
		Mild to moderate pneumonia	Trimethoprim-sulfamethoxazole	21 days—oral therapy may be substituted for IV therapy once clinically stable	[Dapsone + trimethoprim] *or* Atovaquone *or* [Trimetrexate + leucovorin] *or* [Primaquine + clindamycin]		

Continued

TABLE 1-4

RECOMMENDED TREATMENT FOR FUNGAL INFECTIONS: SYSTEMIC TREATMENT (Continued)

Fungus	Host Category	Indication	Recommended Treatment	Duration*	Alternative Treatment	Duration*	Comments
Pneumocystis jiroveci (Coutinued)	HIV infection	Prophylaxis	Trimethoprim-sulfamethoxazole	Depends on age and CD4$^+$ T-lymphocyte count	Dapsone *or* [Dapsone + pyrimethamine + folinic acid] *or* Atovaquone *or* aerosolized Pentamidine monthly	Depends on age and CD4$^+$ T-lymphocyte count	HIV+ adults/adolescents can discontinue primary or secondary prophylaxis if CD4 >200 for at least 6 mo. HIV+ children >12 mo old can stop primary prophylaxis if CD4 exceeds age-related minimum required for prophylaxis for 6 mo. All infants born to HIV-infected mothers should receive prophylaxis from 4–6 weeks of age until 12 mo of age unless HIV diagnosis in the infant has been excluded presumptively or definitively.

Pseudoallescheria boydii	Immunocompromised	Pneumonia; disseminated infection	Surgical excision *and* Voriconazole	Indefinitely	Itraconazole	Indefinitely	Usually resistant to amphotericin B. If oral therapy is used, serum concentration should be measured and adherence should be assessed.
	Immunocompetent	Eumycotic mycetoma; other localized infections (pneumonia, septic arthritis, osteomyelitis, sinusitis)	Surgical excision *and* Itraconazole	3–6 mo if local excision is possible; otherwise, years	Surgical excision *and* Posaconazole *or* Voriconazole	3–6 mo if local excision is possible; otherwise, years	Usually resistant to amphotericin B. If oral therapy is used, serum concentration should be measured and adherence should be assessed.
Trichosporon spp. (trichosporonosis)	Immunocompromised	Disseminated infection	Voriconazole	Varies with site of infection, clinical response, and presence or absence of neutropenia	Itraconazole *or* Amphotericin B[†]		

Continued

TABLE 1-4

RECOMMENDED TREATMENT FOR FUNGAL INFECTIONS: SYSTEMIC TREATMENT (Continued)

Fungus	Host Category	Indication	Recommended Treatment	Duration*	Alternative Treatment	Duration*	Comments
Wangiella (Exophiala)	Immunocompromised	Sinusitis; cutaneous lesions; disseminated infection	Voriconazole; surgical excision	Varies with site of infection, clinical response, and presence or absence of neutropenia	Itraconazole *or* Amphotericin B[†]		
Zygomycetes (mucormycosis)[§]	Immunocompromised, diabetes mellitus, metabolic aciduria, renal failure, neutropenia	Rhinocerebral, pulmonary, cutaneous, GI, or disseminated infection	Amphotericin B at maximum tolerated dose (1–1.5 mg/kg/day) + surgical excision of infected necrotic tissue		Posaconazole		Important considerations in association with antifungal therapy include reduction or discontinuation of immunosuppressive medication, correction of acidosis, and discontinuation of iron chelation therapy.

B. Therapy for Superficial Cutaneous Infections

TABLE 1-5

RECOMMENDED TREATMENT FOR FUNGAL INFECTIONS: THERAPY FOR SUPERFICIAL CUTANEOUS INFECTIONS

Site of Infection	Common Fungal Cause	Recommended Treatment	Duration	Alternative Treatment	Duration	Comments
Scalp (tinea capitis)	*Trichophyton tonsurans, Microsporum canis, Microsporum audouinii, Microsporum gypseum, Trichophyton mentagrophytes, Trichophyton violacea, Trichophyton soudanense*	Griseofulvin (ultramicronized) *or* Terbinafine	4–8 wk, or at least 2 wk after clinical resolution 6 wk	Itraconazole *or* once-weekly Fluconazole	2–4 wk	Selenium sulfide or ketoconazole shampoo may reduce infectivity, but they are not sufficient for treatment; corticosteroid treatment may enhance resolution of kerion if used in conjunction with antifungal therapy. Kerion should be treated with terbinafine **only** if Trichophyton is the pathogen.
Tinea pedis	*T. mentagrophytes, Trichophyton rubrum, Epidermophyton floccosum*	Topical Terbinafine (twice daily) *or* Clotrimazole *or* Miconazole *or* Econazole *or* Oxiconazole *or* Sertaconazole *or* Ketoconazole (once or twice daily)	1–4 wk	Itraconazole *or* Terbinafine *or* Griseofulvin	4 wk 4 wk 4 wk	Burrow solution can be used together with antifungal for vesicular lesions. For dry, scaly variant ("moccasin" type), use longer course of oral agents.
Tinea corporis	*T. rubrum, T. tonsurans, T. mentagrophytes, Microsporum canis, E. floccosum, M. gypseum*	[Topical miconazole *or* Clotrimazole *or* Terbinafine *or* Tolnaftate *or* Naftifine *or* ciclopirox] (twice daily) *or* [topical Ketoconazole *or* Econazole *or* Oxiconazole *or* Butenafine *or* Sulconazole] (once daily)	4 wk (all regimens)	Griseofulvin *or* Itraconazole *or* Fluconazole *or* Terbinafine	4 wk (all regimens)	

Continued

TABLE 1-5

RECOMMENDED TREATMENT FOR FUNGAL INFECTIONS: THERAPY FOR SUPERFICIAL CUTANEOUS INFECTIONS (Continued)

Site of Infection	Common Fungal Cause	Recommended Treatment	Duration	Alternative Treatment	Duration	Comments
Tinea cruris (jock itch)	*T. rubrum, T. mentagrophytes, E. floccosum*	[Topical Clotrimazole *or* Miconazole *or* Terbinafine *or* Tolnaftate *or* Ciclopirox] (twice daily) *or* [topical Econazole *or* Ketoconazole *or* Naftifine *or* Oxiconazole *or* Butenafine *or* Sulconazole] (once daily)	4–6 wk (all regimens)	Griseofulvin *or* Itraconazole *or* Fluconazole *or* Terbinafine	2–6 wk (all regimens)	Burrow solution should be used to dry weeping areas of skin; concomitant topical corticosteroid treatment should be avoided.
Tinea favosa (chronic scalp infection)	*Trichophyton schoenleinii, Trichophyton violaceum, M. gypseum*	Griseofulvin (ultramicronized)	4–8 wk, or at least 2 wk after clinical resolution	Itraconazole *or* Terbinafine *or* weekly Fluconazole	2–4 wk (all regimens)	Selenium sulfide or ketoconazole shampoo may reduce infectivity, but they are not sufficient for treatment; corticosteroid treatment does not enhance resolution of kerion, and corticosteroids enhance clinical symptoms in the absence of antifungal treatment.
Tinea unguium	*T. mentagrophytes, T. rubrum, E. floccosum*	Itraconazole *or* Terbinafine	6–12 wk			Pulse therapy used in adults: 500 mg terbinafine daily for 1 wk each month for 2 mo (fingernails) or for 4 mo (toenails); has not been studied in children.

1. Groupings of Fungal Genera by Clinical Presentation
a. Cutaneous: Superficial, Not Inflammatory
   (1) **Tinea versicolor (Pityriasis versicolor):** *Malassezia (M. furfur)*
b. Cutaneous: Inflammatory
   (1) **Dermatophytes:** *Trichophyton, Microsporum, Epidermophyton*
   (2) **Primary cutaneous candidiasis:** *Candida*
c. Mucosal
   (1) *Candida*
d. Subcutaneous
   (1) **Sporotrichosis:** *Sporothrix*
   (2) **Phaeohyphomycosis:** *Alternaria, Bipolaris, Curvularia, Exophiala, Exserohilum, Wangiella*
   (3) **Chromomycosis:** *Fonsecaea, Cladophialophora, Phialophora, Rhinocladiella*
   (4) **Mycetoma:** *Madurella, Pseudallescheria, Acremonium, Exophiala, Leptosphaeria*
e. Pulmonary +/– Dissemination
   (1) **Abnormal cell-mediated immunity:** *Cryptococcus, Histoplasma, Pneumocystis, Coccidioides, Penicillium (P. marneffei)*
   (2) **Neutropenia/Neutrophil dysfunction:** *Aspergillus, Fusarium, Pseudallescheria*
f. Sinusitis
   (1) **Zygomycosis:** *Rhizopus, Mucor, Absidia, Rhizomucor, Cunninghamella*
   (2) **Aspergillosis:** *Aspergillus*
   (3) **Phaeohyphomycoses:** *Alternaria, Bipolaris, Curvularia, Exophiala, Exserohilum, Wangiella*

2. Groupings of Fungal Genera by Laboratory Report
   Direct examination of tissues (pathology or fungal stain in microbiology) reveals the following:
a. **Yeast:** *Candida, Sporothrix, Malassezia, Histoplasma, Cryptococcus, Saccharomyces, Blastomyces, Paracoccidioides, Penicillium (P. marneffei)*
b. **Hyphae**
   (1) **No melanin:** *Aspergillus; Scedosporium; Pseudallescheria;* Hyalohyphomycoses agents *(Fusarium, Acremonium, Paecilomyces)*
   (2) **Melanin (dark):** Phaeohyphomycosis agents *(Alternaria, Bipolaris, Curvularia, Exophiala, Exserohilum, Wangiella)*
c. **Hyphae and yeast:** *Candida*
d. **Grains or granules:** *Mycetoma (Madurella, Pseudallescheria, Acremonium, Exophiala, Leptosphaeria)*
e. **Pigmented (melanin) sclerotic cells/bodies:** Chromomycosis agents *(Fonsecaea, Cladophialophora, Phialophora, Rhinocladiella)*
f. **Spherules seen in tissue:** *Coccidioides*
g. **Cysts and trophozoites:** *Pneumocystis*

Laboratory culture reveals the following:

a. **Yeast growing in culture**
   (1) *Candida*
   (2) *Cryptococcus*
   (3) *Malassezia* (*M. pachydermatis* only)
   (4) *Trichosporon*
   (5) *Saccharomyces*

b. **Dimorphic fungi (recovered as a filamentous fungus but also displays yeast form):**
   (1) *Paracoccidioides*
   (2) *Blastomyces*
   (3) *Histoplasma*
   (4) *Sporothrix*
   (5) *Penicillium* (*P. marneffei* only)

c. **Fungi only as filamentous fungi**
   (1) **Darkly pigmented (melanin) hyphae (Dematiaceous):** Phaeohyphomycoses agents *(Alternaria, Bipolaris, Curvularia, Exophiala, Exserohilum, Wangiella)* and chromomycosis agents *(Fonsecaea, Cladophialophora, Phialophora, Rhinocladiella)*
   (2) **Pale or brightly colored hyphae lacking dark pigment:** *Aspergillus, Scedosporium, Pseudallescheria,* Hyalohyphomycoses agents *(Fusarium, Acremonium, Paecilomyces)*
   (3) **Zygomycosis/Mucormycosis agents:** *Rhizopus, Mucor, Absidia, Rhizomucor, Cunninghamella*
   (4) **Coccidioidomycosis:** *Coccidioides* (also a dimorphic fungus but without a yeast form)

d. **Fungal growth from blood culture**
   (1) **Yeast:** *Candida* (especially *C. albicans, C. parapsilosis*), *Malassezia*; *Cryptococcus,* Histoplasma,* Paracoccidioides,* Blastomyces**
   (2) **Filamentous:** *Fusarium, Pseudallescheria*

*Growth not reliably detected in broth blood culture systems that depend on abundant CO_2 production to detect growth of pathogen.

V. RECOMMENDED TREATMENT FOR PARASITIC AND PROTOZOAL INFECTIONS

Pathogen listing by category is provided on p. 122.

TABLE 1-6

RECOMMENDED TREATMENT FOR PARASITIC AND PROTOZOAL INFECTIONS (for notes and abbreviations used in this table, see p. xv.)

Parasite/Where Infection Acquired	Host Category	Indication	Recommended Treatment	Duration	Alternative Treatment	Duration	Comments
Acanthamoeba/ Worldwide	Immunosuppressed	Granulomatous amebic encephalitis, disseminated infection	Usually susceptible in vitro to Pentamidine, Ketoconazole, Amphotericin B. [Fluconazole *or* Itraconazole], Sulfadiazine, Sulfamethoxazole, and Rifampin have been used in combination	Unknown			Therapy is rarely successful. Susceptibility testing is advisable. Combination IV and intraventricular therapy may be of benefit but should be undertaken only in consultation with an infectious diseases specialist.
	Immunocompetent	Keratitis	[Topical 0.1% Propamidine isethionate (Brolene) + 0.15% Dibromopropamidine]	Weeks to months	[Topical 0.02% Polyhexamethylene biguanide[a] + chlorhexidine gluconate]	Weeks to months	Topical corticosteroids are sometimes recommended once clinical improvement is noted. Successful treatment depends on early diagnosis.
Ancylostoma braziliense (dog hookworm)/Southeast Asia, Caribbean, Puerto Rico	Symptomatic patient	Cutaneous larva migrans	Thiabendazole (topical) *or* Albendazole[b] *or* Ivermectin[b]	Until lesions inactivated 3 days 1–2 days			Disease is usually self-limited, lasting weeks to months without therapy.
Ancylostoma caninum (dog hookworm)/Worldwide		Eosinophilic enterocolitis	Mebendazole *or* Albendazole[b]	100 mg BID × 3 days or 500 mg once 400 mg once	Pyrantel pamoate	3 days	Endoscopic removal of the parasite may be required.

Continued

TABLE 1-6

RECOMMENDED TREATMENT FOR PARASITIC AND PROTOZOAL INFECTIONS (Continued)

Parasite/Where Infection Acquired	Host Category	Indication	Recommended Treatment	Duration	Alternative Treatment	Duration	Comments
Ancylostoma caninum, Ancylostoma ceylanicum, Ancylostoma duodenale (hookworm)/Worldwide (*A. caninum*, predominantly Australia and United States; *A. ceylanicum*, predominantly Southeast Asia and India; *A duodenale*, worldwide)	Symptomatic patient	Dermatitis, anemia, nonspecific GI complaints	Mebendazole *or* Albendazole[c]	100 mg BID × 3 days 400 mg once	Pyrantel pamoate	3 days	WHO recommends half the adult dose of mebendazole or albendazole[b] for children <2 yr old.
Angiostrongylus cantonensis (visceral larva migrans)/ Southeast Asia, Hawaii, Pacific Islands, Philippines, China, Taiwan	Symptomatic patient	Eosinophilic meningitis					No treatment is well established; most infections are self-limited. Corticosteroids and analgesics may be helpful.
Angiostrongylus costaricensis/Central and South America	Symptomatic patient	Fever, eosinophilia, abdominal pain					No treatment is well-established. Mebendazole treatment has resulted in modest success in experimental animals. Corticosteroids may be helpful.
Anisakis/Japan	Symptomatic patient	Viscera larva migrans	Endoscopic removal of the parasite				

Ascaris lumbricoides/ Worldwide	All		Mebendazole *or* Albendazole[b] *or* Pyrantel pamoate	100 mg BID × 3 days *or* 500 mg once 400 mg once 3 days	Ivermectin[b] *or* Nitazoxanide[b]	150–200 mcg once 100 mg twice daily for 3 days (<3 yr old); 200 mg twice daily for 3 days (4–11 yr old); 500 mg twice daily (>12 yr old)	Mineral oil or Gastrografin (orally or by nasogastric tube) may cause relaxation of the worms and allow passage without surgery. Albendazole or mebendazole can then be administered safely.
Babesia microti/ United States and Europe	Asplenic or normal host	Parasitemia	[Quinine + clindamycin] *or* [Atovaquone + azithromycin]	7–10 days 7–10 days	Europe only: Pentamidine + TMP/SMX		Most infections acquired in the United States are self-limited and require no specific therapy. Exchange blood transfusion may be required in cases of rapidly increasing parasitemia and massive hemolysis.
Balamuthia mandrillaris/ Worldwide	Immunosuppressed	Granulomatous amebic meningoencephalitis	[Clarithromycin + fluconazole + sulfadiazine + flucytosine + pentamidine]	Unknown		Unknown	Recommendation is based on limited clinical experience. Surgical resection of CNS lesions may contribute to survival.

Continued

TABLE 1-6

RECOMMENDED TREATMENT FOR PARASITIC AND PROTOZOAL INFECTIONS (Continued)

Parasite/Where Infection Acquired	Host Category	Indication	Recommended Treatment	Duration	Alternative Treatment	Duration	Comments
Balantidium coli/ Worldwide	Symptomatic patient	Intestinal infection	Tetracycline[c]	10 days	Metronidazole *or* Iodoquinol	5 days 20 days	Healthy infected individuals usually are asymptomatic; malnourished or immunosuppressed hosts are more likely to suffer severe disease.
Baylisascaris procyonis (raccoon ascaris)/ United States	Symptomatic patient	Eosinophilic meningitis; ocular infection					No effective treatment has been documented. Albendazole, mebendazole, thiabendazole, levamisole, or ivermectin might theoretically be helpful. Albendazole has been recommended as preventive therapy after known exposure. Steroid therapy has been used to reduce CNS and/or ocular inflammation. Laser photocoagulation has been used to destroy intraretinal larvae.

Blastocystis hominis/ Worldwide	Symptomatic patient	Intestinal infection	Metronidazole	10 days	Iodoquinol *or* Furazolidone *or* TMZ/SMX *or* Nitazoxanide	20 days Not established Not established Not established	*B. hominis* has not been established as a cause of symptoms. Treatment should be initiated only if all other more likely causes of symptoms have been investigated and ruled out. In vitro metronidazole resistance has been observed. [*Note:* This organism has recently been reclassified as a fungus.]
Brachiola vesicularum (microsporidiosis)/ Not defined	All	Disseminated microsporidiosis	Albendazole[b] *or* Metronidazole[b] *or* Atovaquone[b] *or* Nitazoxanide[b] *or* Fumagillin[b]	Duration unknown for all regimens			There is no known effective therapy for microsporidial infection. Albendazole and other listed therapies may reduce symptoms. HIV+ patients may benefit from highly active antiretroviral therapy to improve their own immunity.

Continued

TABLE 1-6

RECOMMENDED TREATMENT FOR PARASITIC AND PROTOZOAL INFECTIONS (Continued)

Parasite/Where Infection Acquired	Host Category	Indication	Recommended Treatment	Duration	Alternative Treatment	Duration	Comments
Brugia malayi (filariasis)/ Southeast Asia	All	Lymphatic infection	Diethylcarbamazine[d] Day 1: 1 mg/kg after a meal (max 50 mg) Day 2: 1 mg/kg (max 50 mg) TID Day 3: 1–2 mg/kg (max 100 mg) TID Days 4–14: 2 mg/kg (max 100 mg) TID	14 days			Antihistamines or corticosteroids may be required to decrease allergic reaction to microfilarial disintegration. Full doses can be given from day 1 for patients with no microfilariae in the blood.
		Tropical pulmonary eosinophilia	Diethylcarbamazine[d] 2 mg/kg (max dose 100 mg) TID	21 days			Antihistamines or corticosteroids may be required to decrease allergic reaction to microfilarial disintegration.

Brugia timori (filariasis)/ Indonesia		Lymphatic infection	Diethylcarbamazine[d] Day 1: 1 mg/kg (max 50 mg) Day 2: 1 mg/kg TID (max 50 mg) TID Day 3: 1–2 mg/kg TID (max 100 mg) TID Days 4–14: 2 mg/kg (max 100 mg) TID	14 days			Antihistamines or corticosteroids may be required to decrease allergic reaction to microfilarial disintegration. Full doses can be given from day 1 for patients with no microfilariae in the blood.
		Tropical pulmonary eosinophilia	Diethylcarbamazine[d]	21 days			Antihistamines or corticosteroids may be required to decrease allergic reaction to microfilarial disintegration. Multiple courses of therapy may be required.
Capillaria philippinensis/Philippines, Thailand	Symptomatic patient	Intestinal capillariasis (diarrhea, protein-losing enteropathy)	Mebendazole[b]	20 days	Albendazole[b]	10 days	
Clonorchis sinensis (Chinese liver fluke)/Far East, Eastern Europe, Russian Federation	All	Biliary tract involvement	Praziquantel *or* Albendazole[b]	2 days 7 days			

Continued

TABLE 1-6

RECOMMENDED TREATMENT FOR PARASITIC AND PROTOZOAL INFECTIONS (Continued)

Parasite/Where Infection Acquired	Host Category	Indication	Recommended Treatment	Duration	Alternative Treatment	Duration	Comments
Cryptosporidium/ Worldwide	Immunocompromised patient	Diarrhea	Nitazoxanide	3 days (based on studies in immunocompetent children)	Paromomycin alone *or combined with* Azithromycin	Unknown Unknown	Most infections in immunocompetent individuals are self-limited and do not require treatment. Longer courses of nitazoxanide (up to 14 days) may be required. Effective antiretroviral therapy is the most important treatment for HIV-infected individuals.
Cyclospora/ Nepal, Peru, Haiti, Guatemala, Indonesia	Immunocompetent patient	Diarrhea	TMP/SMX	7–10 days	Ciprofloxacin	7 days	
	Immunocompromised patient	Diarrhea	TMP/SMX	10 days	Ciprofloxacin	7–10 days	Recurrence can often be prevented using prophylactic TMP/SMX given 3 times per week.
Cystoisospora belli (formerly *Isospora belli*)/Tropical and subtropical climates	Immunocompetent	Diarrhea	TMP/SMX	10 days	Pyrimethamine with leucovorin *or* Ciprofloxacin	10 days 10 days	

	Immunocompromised	Diarrhea	TMP/SMX	Administer QID × 10 days, followed by BID × 3 wk	Pyrimethamine with leucovorin *or* Ciprofloxacin	75 mg/day for 10 days followed by 25 mg/day for 7 days 10 days?	Prolonged therapy may be required to control symptoms.
Dientamoeba fragilis/ Worldwide	Symptomatic patient	Diarrhea	Iodoquinol[b] *or* Paromomycin[b] *or* Metronidazole[b] *or* Tetracycline[c]	20 days 7 days 10 days 10 days			
Diphyllobothrium latum (fish tapeworm)/Worldwide	All	Diarrhea, abdominal pain, intestinal obstruction	Praziquantel[b]	1 dose	Niclosamide	1 dose	Cobalamin injections and oral folic acid are indicated for individuals with evidence of vitamin B_{12} deficiency.
Dipylidium caninum (dog tapeworm)/Worldwide	All	Proglottids in stool	Praziquantel[b]	1 dose	Niclosamide	1 dose	Retreatment is indicated if proglottids are evident in stools ≥1 wk after initial therapy. Cobalamin injections and oral folic acid are indicated for individuals with evidence of vitamin B_{12} deficiency.

Continued

TABLE 1-6

RECOMMENDED TREATMENT FOR PARASITIC AND PROTOZOAL INFECTIONS (Continued)

Parasite/Where Infection Acquired	Host Category	Indication	Recommended Treatment	Duration	Alternative Treatment	Duration	Comments
Dracunculus medinensis (Guinea worm)/Africa	Symptomatic patient	Emerging worm from cutaneous lesion	Metronidazole	10 days			There is no curative therapy other than gradual removal of the worm, but metronidazole reduces local inflammation and facilitates removal.
Echinococcus granulosus/ South America, Eastern Africa, Eastern Europe, Middle East, Mediterranean, China, Central Asia, Australia, New Zealand, Southeastern United States	All	Hydatid cyst of the liver or other site	Albendazole	3–6 mo	Mebendazole	10 days	Surgical excision of cysts may be required. Praziquantel has been used perioperatively. In uncomplicated patients, percutaneous aspiration, infusion of scolicidal agents, and reaspiration (PAIR) should be performed a few days after initiation of albendazole therapy.
Echinococcus multilocularis/ Europe, Russia, Central Asia, Western China, Northwest Canada, Western Alaska	All	Liver disease, alveolar echinococcosis	Albendazole[b]	Prolonged therapy			Surgical excision provides the only reliable cure.

Encephalitozoon hellem (microsporidiosis)/ Not defined	All	Ocular microsporidiosis	Albendazole[b] + fumagillin[a,b,e] (eye drops)	There is no known effective therapy for microsporidial infection. Fumagillin is used to control microsporidial disease in honeybees; fumagillin eye drops have been helpful in some HIV-infected patients. Albendazole may reduce symptoms. HIV+ patients may benefit from highly active antiretroviral therapy to improve their own immunity.
	All	Disseminated microsporidiosis	Albendazole[b]	There is no known effective therapy for microsporidial infection. Albendazole may reduce symptoms. HIV+ patients may benefit from highly active antiretroviral therapy to improve their own immunity.

Continued

TABLE 1-6

RECOMMENDED TREATMENT FOR PARASITIC AND PROTOZOAL INFECTIONS (Continued)

Parasite/Where Infection Acquired	Host Category	Indication	Recommended Treatment	Duration	Alternative Treatment	Duration	Comments
Encephalitozoon cuniculi (Microsporidiosis)/ Not defined	All	Ocular microsporidiosis	Albendazole[b] + fumagillin[a,b,e] (eye drops)				There is no known effective therapy for microsporidial infection. Fumagillin is used to control microsporidial disease in honeybees, and fumagillin eye drops have been helpful in some HIV-infected patients. Albendazole may reduce symptoms. HIV+ patients may benefit from highly active antiretroviral therapy to improve their own immunity.
	All	Disseminated microsporidiosis	Albendazole[b]				There is no known effective therapy for microsporidial infection. Albendazole may reduce symptoms. HIV+ patients may benefit from highly active antiretroviral therapy to improve their own immunity.

Encephalitozoon [Septata] intestinalis (microsporidiosis)/ Not defined	All	Intestinal microsporidiosis	Albendazole[b]				There is no known effective therapy for microsporidial infection. Albendazole may reduce symptoms. HIV+ patients may benefit from highly active antiretroviral therapy to improve their own immunity.
		Disseminated microsporidiosis	Albendazole[b]				There is no known effective therapy for microsporidial infection. Albendazole may reduce symptoms. HIV+ patients may benefit from highly active antiretroviral therapy to improve their own immunity.
Entamoeba dispar/ Worldwide							No treatment is needed. This organism does not cause human disease.
Entamoeba histolytica (amebiasis)/Worldwide	All	Asymptomatic cyst excreters (intraluminal infection)	Iodoquinol *or* Paromomycin	20 days 7 days	Diloxanide furoate[f]	10 days	These agents provide intraluminal therapy only. Corticosteroids and antimotility drugs can worsen symptoms and disease.

Continued

TABLE 1-6

RECOMMENDED TREATMENT FOR PARASITIC AND PROTOZOAL INFECTIONS (Continued)

Parasite/Where Infection Acquired	Host Category	Indication	Recommended Treatment	Duration	Alternative Treatment	Duration	Comments
Entamoeba histolytica (amebiasis)/Worldwide *(Continued)*		Mild to moderate intestinal disease	Metronidazole followed by [iodoquinol *or* paromomycin]	7–10 days 20 days 7 days	Tinidazole (50 mg/kg/day; maximum 2 g/day divided into 3 doses) followed by [iodoquinol *or* paromomycin]	3 days 20 days 7 days	Corticosteroids and antimotility drugs can worsen symptoms and disease.
		Amebic colitis, liver abscess	Metronidazole +/– chloroquine followed by [iodoquinol *or* paromomycin]	7–10 days 20 days 7 days	Tinidazole (50 mg/kg/day; maximum 2 g/day divided into 3 doses) +/– chloroquine followed by [iodoquinol *or* paromomycin]	3 days 20 days 7 days	Corticosteroids and antimotility drugs can worsen symptoms and disease. Dehydroemetine followed by iodoquinol or paromomycin should be considered if other therapies fail. Large liver abscesses may require surgical or percutaneous aspiration if response to medical therapy is poor. Repeat stool examination after treatment is recommended, and stool examination should be performed for household members, and other contacts should be tested.

Entamoeba polecki/Tropics	All		Metronidazole	10 days	
Enterocytozoon bieneusi (microsporidiosis)/ Not defined	All	Intestinal microsporidiosis	Fumagillin[e] (oral)		Octreotide may provide symptomatic relief for patients with large-volume diarrhea. Treatment with oral fumagillin has resulted in thrombocytopenia. There is no known effective therapy for microsporidial infection. HIV+ patients may benefit from highly active antiretroviral therapy to improve their own immunity.
Enterobius vermicularis (pinworm)/ Worldwide	All		Pyrantel pamoate *or* Mebendazole *or* Albendazole[b]	Give 1 dose; repeat in 2 wk	When multiple or repeated symptomatic infections occur, family members should be treated as a group.
Fasciola buski (intestinal fluke)/Far East	All		Praziquantel[b] 75 mg/kg/day divided into 3 doses	3 doses in 1 day	

Continued

TABLE 1-6

RECOMMENDED TREATMENT FOR PARASITIC AND PROTOZOAL INFECTIONS (Continued)

Parasite/Where Infection Acquired	Host Category	Indication	Recommended Treatment	Duration	Alternative Treatment	Duration	Comments
Fasciola hepatica (sheep liver fluke)/ Tropics and temperate areas	All		Triclabendazole[g] 10 mg	Once	Bithionol,[d] 30–50 mg/kg *or* Nitazoxanide[b]	Give on alternate days for 10–15 doses 7 days	Triclabendazole is a veterinary medication that may be safe and effective, but there is limited information about its use in humans.
Giardia lamblia/ Worldwide	Symptomatic patient	Diarrhea, abdominal pain, anorexia	Nitazoxanide *or* Metronidazole[b] *or* Tinidazole	3 days 5 days 1 dose	Furazolidone *or* Paromomycin[b] *or* Quinacrine[f]	7–10 days 7 days 5 days	Treatment of asymptomatic patients is generally not recommended. Because paromomycin is not absorbed from the GI tract, it may be particularly useful to treat giardiasis in pregnant women.

Gnathostoma spinigerum/ Thailand, Asia, Mexico	All	Ocular larva migrans, eosinophilic meningitis, subcutaneous swelling	Albendazole[b] *or* Ivermectin[b]	21 days 2 days			Surgical removal of the worm may be performed in addition to or as an alternative to pharmacotherapy.
Gongylonema spp./ Worldwide	All		Albendazole[b]	10 mg/kg/day for 3 days			Surgical removal of the worm is an alternative to pharmacotherapy.
Heterophyes heterophyes (intestinal fluke)/ Egypt, Far East, Southeast Asia	All		Praziquantel[b]	3 doses in 1 day			
Hymenolepis nana (dwarf tapeworm)/Worldwide	All		Praziquantel[b]	1 dose	Niclosamide	7 days	Repeat treatment may be necessary.
Isospora belli (see *Cystoisospora belli*)							

Continued

TABLE 1-6

RECOMMENDED TREATMENT FOR PARASITIC AND PROTOZOAL INFECTIONS (Continued)

Parasite/Where Infection Acquired	Host Category	Indication	Recommended Treatment	Duration	Alternative Treatment	Duration	Comments
Leishmania spp./Worldwide	All	Visceral leishmaniasis (kala-azar)	Liposomal amphotericin B IV *or*	3 mg/kg/day IV on days 1–5, day 14, and day 21	Amphotericin B IV *or*	1 mg/kg on alternate days for a total of 2 g (adults)	Side effects of pentavalent antimonial drugs are common. Serious adverse effects include hepatotoxicity, pancreatitis, and cardiotoxicity.
			Sodium stibogluconate[d,h] IV or IM *or*	Minimum of 4 wk	paromomycin sulfate[b] IM	21 days	Antimonial resistance is high in India and Nepal, so sodium stibogluconate should not be used for patients infected in South Asia. Relapses should be treated for at least twice the time period of the initial course.
			Meglumine antimonate[i] IV or IM *or*	Minimum of 4 wk			
			Miltefosine[j,k] PO	Minimum of 4 wk			

Cutaneous leishmaniasis	Sodium stibogluconate[d,h] IV or IM *or* Meglumine antimonate[i] IV or IM *or* Miltefosine[j,k] PO	20 days 20 days 28 days	Pentamidine IM or IV *or* Paromomycin (topical)	Daily or every other day for 4–7 doses Twice daily for 10–20 days	Treatment decision should be made after consultation with infectious disease specialist or with CDC (404-639-3670). Use topical paromomycin only in geographic regions where cutaneous leishmaniasis species have low likelihood for mucosal spread. Should not be used for treating *L. braziliensis, L. guyanensis, L. panamensis, L. amazonensis*, or *L. aethiopica*.
Mucosal leishmaniasis	Sodium stibogluconate[d,h] IV or IM *or* Meglumine antimonate[i] IV or IM *or* *miltefosine*[j,k] PO *or* amphotericin B	28 days 28 days 28 days 0.5–1 mg/kg daily or every other day for up to 8 weeks			

Continued

TABLE 1-6

RECOMMENDED TREATMENT FOR PARASITIC AND PROTOZOAL INFECTIONS (Continued)

Parasite/Where Infection Acquired	Host Category	Indication	Recommended Treatment	Duration	Alternative Treatment	Duration	Comments
Loa loa (filariasis)/ West and Central Africa	All		Diethylcarbamazine[d]	9 mg/kg/day in 3 doses for 12 days			Antihistamines or corticosteroids may be required to decrease allergic reaction to microfilarial disintegration. Apheresis may reduce the risk for encephalopathy associated with rapid microfilarial killing if blood microfilarial burden is high. Full doses of therapy can be given beginning on day 1 for patients with no microfilariae in the blood. For patients with high microfilarial burden, initial dose should be 0.5 mg/kg with doubling of the dose every 8 hours until 3 mg/kg dose is reached.
Malaria—see Plasmodium							

Mansonella ozzardi (filariasis)/ South and Central America, Caribbean	All	Ivermectin 200 mcg/kg	1 dose	Antihistamines or corticosteroids may be required to decrease allergic reaction to microfilarial disintegration. Most infected persons are asymptomatic.
Mansonella perstans (filariasis)/ Africa, South and Central America	All	Mebendazole[b] *or* Albendazole[b]	30 days 10 days	Most infected persons are asymptomatic. Antihistamines or corticosteroids may be required to decrease allergic reaction to microfilarial disintegration.
Mansonella streptocerca (filariasis)/West and Central Africa	All	Diethylcarbamazine[d] 6 mg/kg *or* Ivermectin, 150 mcg/ kg	14 days 1 dose	Antihistamines or corticosteroids may be required to decrease allergic reaction to microfilarial disintegration. Diethylcarbamazine kills both microfilariae and adult worms; ivermectin kills only microfilariae.
Metagonimus yokogawai (intestinal fluke)/ Far East, Spain, Greece, Balkans	All	Praziquantel[b] 75 mg/ kg/day in 3 doses	1 day	
Metorchis conjunctus (North American liver fluke)/North America	All	Praziquantel[b] 75 mg/ kg/day in 3 doses	1 day	

Continued

TABLE 1-6

RECOMMENDED TREATMENT FOR PARASITIC AND PROTOZOAL INFECTIONS (Continued)

Parasite/Where Infection Acquired	Host Category	Indication	Recommended Treatment	Duration	Alternative Treatment	Duration	Comments
Microsporidia/ Not defined	Immunocompetent	Keratopathy, diarrhea, myositis, encephalitis	(See specific organisms.) No therapy has demonstrated consistent benefit. Albendazole is beneficial for some. Metronidazole, Atovaquone, Nitazoxanide, Fumagillin have been used with some success.				
Microsporidia spp./ Worldwide	Immunocompromised (HIV-infected)	Keratopathy, diarrhea, myositis, encephalitis, disseminated disease, sinusitis, osteomyelitis, urinary tract infection, peritonitis	(See specific organisms.) No therapy has demonstrated consistent benefit. Albendazole is beneficial for some. Metronidazole, Atovaquone, Nitazoxanide, Fumagillin have been used with some success.				HIV+ patients may benefit from highly active antiretroviral therapy to improve their immune function.

Naegleria fowleri/Worldwide	All	Amebic meningoencephalitis	Amphotericin B[b] + [miconazole *or* fluconazole]	Uncertain	Amphotericin B[b] + azithromycin	Treatment is usually unsuccessful. Combined therapy with IV and intrathecal amphotericin B, intrathecal miconazole, and oral rifampin has been reported successful. Dexamethasone may be used to control cerebral edema.
Nanophyetus salmincola (fluke)/Pacific northwestern United States	All		Praziquantel[b] 60 mg/kg/day in 3 doses	1 day		
Necator americanus (hookworm)/ Western hemisphere, sub-Saharan Africa, Southeast Asia, Pacific Islands	All	Dermatitis, anemia, nonspecific GI complaints	Mebendazole *or* Albendazole[b] *or* Pyrantel pamoate[b]	100 mg BID × 3 days or 500 mg once 400 mg once 11 mg/kg daily for 3 days		WHO recommends half the adult dose of mebendazole or albendazole for children <2 yr old.
Oesophagostomum bifurcum/ Togo, Ghana	All		Albendazole[b] *or* Pyrantel pamoate[b]			Efficacy of these drugs is uncertain.

Continued

TABLE 1-6

RECOMMENDED TREATMENT FOR PARASITIC AND PROTOZOAL INFECTIONS (Continued)

Parasite/Where Infection Acquired	Host Category	Indication	Recommended Treatment	Duration	Alternative Treatment	Duration	Comments
Onchocerca volvulus (river blindness) (filariasis)/ Africa, South and Central America	All	Subcutaneous nodules, dermatitis, lymphadenitis, ocular disease	Ivermectin[j]	150 mcg/kg × 1; repeat every 6–12 mo until asymptomatic			Prevention: annual treatment with ivermectin, 150 mcg/kg. A 6-wk course of doxycycline is sometimes used as adjunctive therapy for individuals ≥8 yr old and nonpregnant adults. Diethylcarbamazine should **not** be used to treat this infection.
Opisthorchis viverrini (Southeast Asian liver fluke)/ Thailand, Kampuchea, Laos	All	Biliary tract involvement	Praziquantel[b] 75 mg/kg/day in 3 doses	2 days			
Paragonimus westermani (lung fluke)/ Worldwide, especially Far East	All	Pulmonary, cardiac, CNS, cutaneous involvement	Praziquantel[b] 75 mg/kg/day in 3 doses	2 days	Bithionol[i]	30–50 mg/kg on alternate days for 10–15 doses	A short course of corticosteroids should be given together with praziquantel when treating CNS disease.

Plasmodium falciparum/ Tropical areas worldwide	Uncomplicated or mild malaria	Oral therapy for infections acquired in areas where chloroquine resistance is reported	Atovaquone/proguanil *or* Artemether/lumefantrine *or* Quinine sulfate + [doxycycline[b,c] *or* tetracycline[b,c] *or* clindamycin[b]]	3 days 3 days 3 or 7 days 7 days 7 days 7 days	Mefloquine *or* Artesunate[i] + [atovaquone/proguanil *or* doxycycline[b,c] *or* clindamycin *or* mefloquine]	1 day 3 days	The longer course of quinine (7 days) should be used for patients who acquired infection in Southeast Asia. Clindamycin is the preferred adjunct to quinine sulfate for pregnant individuals. Atovaquone should be taken at least 45 min after eating. Mefloquine should not be used in pregnancy; it should not be given together with quinine or quinidine. Artemether/lumefantrine is contraindicated during the first trimester; safety during the second and third trimester has not been established. It should not be used in patients with cardiac arrhythmias, bradycardia, severe cardiac disease, or prolonged QT interval, and it should not be given concomitantly with drugs that prolong the QT interval or are metabolized by CYP2D6.

Continued

TABLE 1-6

RECOMMENDED TREATMENT FOR PARASITIC AND PROTOZOAL INFECTIONS (Continued)

Parasite/Where Infection Acquired	Host Category	Indication	Recommended Treatment	Duration	Alternative Treatment	Duration	Comments
Plasmodium falciparum/ Tropical areas worldwide *(Continued)*							Artesunate is not available in the United States except from the CDC through an investigational protocol in IV form. Caution is required in treating patients with quinine or quinidine if they have received mefloquine as prophylaxis. **If in doubt, consult CDC malaria hotline at 770-488-7788** Monday–Friday, 9:00 AM to 5:00 PM. Off-hours, weekends, and federal holidays, call 770-488-7100 and ask to have the malaria clinician on-call paged.

Plasmodium vivax/ Tropical areas worldwide	Uncomplicated or mild malaria	**Oral** therapy for infection acquired where **chloroquine resistance** has been reported	Atovaquone/proguanil *or* Artemether/ lumefantrine *or* [Quinine sulfate + doxycycline[b,c]] Primaquine phosphate should be administered *in addition to* one of the above	3 days 3 days 3–7 days 7 days 14 days	Mefloquine *or* [Chloroquine phosphate + doxycycline[b,l]] Primaquine phosphate should be administered *in addition to* one of the above	1 day 3 doses of 25 mg/kg over 48 hr 7 days 14 days	Artemether/lumefantrine is contraindicated during the first trimester; safety during the second and third trimester has not been established. It should not be used in patients with cardiac arrhythmias, bradycardia, severe cardiac disease, or prolonged QT interval, and it should not be given concomitantly with drugs that prolong the QT interval or are metabolized by CYP2D6. The longer course of quinine (7 days) should be used for patients who acquired infection in Southeast Asia. Mefloquine should not be used in pregnancy; it should not be given together with quinine or quinidine. Caution is required in treating patients with quinine or quinidine if they have received mefloquine as prophylaxis.

Continued

TABLE 1-6

RECOMMENDED TREATMENT FOR PARASITIC AND PROTOZOAL INFECTIONS (Continued)

Parasite/Where Infection Acquired	Host Category	Indication	Recommended Treatment	Duration	Alternative Treatment	Duration	Comments
Plasmodium vivax/ Tropical areas worldwide *(Continued)*							Primaquine is used to prevent relapse because of latent forms. Exclude G-6-PD deficiency before giving primaquine. Primaquine should not be used during pregnancy. **Consult CDC malaria hotline at 770-488-7788** Monday–Friday, 9:00 AM to 5:00 PM. Off-hours, weekends, and federal holidays, call 770-488-7100 and ask to have the malaria clinician on-call paged.
Plasmodium other than chloroquine-resistant *P. falciparum* and chloroquine-resistant *P. vivax*/Tropical areas worldwide	Uncomplicated or mild malaria	**Oral** therapy	Chloroquine phosphate	3 days	Hydroxychloroquine sulfate	3 days	Primaquine phosphate should be given (in addition to chloroquine phosphate or hydroxychloroquine sulfate) for 14 days if *Plasmodium ovale* or *P. vivax* is suspected.

							Consult CDC malaria hotline at 770-488-7788 Monday–Friday, 9:00 AM to 5:00 PM. Off-hours, weekends, and federal holidays, call 770-488-7100 and ask to have the malaria clinician on-call paged.
Plasmodium—all species in patients for whom parenteral therapy is warranted/ Tropical areas worldwide	Moderate, severe, or complicated malaria	**Parenteral** therapy	Quinidine gluconate[m] *or* Quinine dihydrochloride	Until oral therapy can be initiated Until oral therapy can be initiated. Reduce the dose by 30%–50% if >48 hr of IV therapy is required.	Artesunate[i] + [atovaquone/proguanil *or* doxycycline[b,c] *or* clindamycin *or* mefloquine]	5–7 days or until oral therapy can be initiated	Quinidine or quinine: Continuous monitoring of electrocardiogram, blood pressure, and serum glucose is recommended. Decrease or omit the loading dose for patients who have received mefloquine or quinine. Consider exchange transfusion for parasitemia >10%. Quinine is not available in the United States. Artesunate is not available in the United States except from the CDC through an investigational protocol in IV form.

Continued

TABLE 1-6

RECOMMENDED TREATMENT FOR PARASITIC AND PROTOZOAL INFECTIONS (Continued)

Parasite/Where Infection Acquired	Host Category	Indication	Recommended Treatment	Duration	Alternative Treatment	Duration	Comments
Plasmodium—all species in patients for whom parenteral therapy is warranted/Tropical areas worldwide *(Continued)*							**Consult CDC malaria hotline at 770-488-7788** Monday–Friday, 9:00 AM to 5:00 PM. Off-hours, weekends, and federal holidays, call 770-488-7100 and ask to have the malaria clinician on-call paged.
P. vivax and *P. ovale*/ Tropical areas worldwide	Previously infected	Prevention of relapse	Primaquine phosphate	Adults: 30 mg base/day for 14 days Children: 0.6 mg base/kg/day for 14 days			**Primaquine** should not be used during pregnancy. **Primaquine** can cause hemolysis, particularly in patients with G-6-PD deficiency. Relapses that occur despite this treatment should be treated with a second 14-day course of 30-mg base per day. **Consult CDC malaria hotline at 770-488-7788** Monday–Friday, 9:00 AM to 5:00 PM. Off-hours, weekends, and federal holidays, call 770-488-7100 and ask to have the malaria clinician on-call paged.

Pleistophora sp. (microsporidia)/ Not well defined	All	Disseminated microsporidiosis	Albendazole[b]		There is no known effective therapy for microsporidial infection. Albendazole may reduce symptoms. HIV+ patients may benefit from highly active antiretroviral therapy to improve their own immunity.
Pneumocystis jiroveci—see Table 1-4					
Sappinia diploidea/ Worldwide	All	Amebic meningoencephalitis	Azithromycin + pentamidine (IV) + itraconazole + flucytosine		This organism has been recently recognized as pathogenic. Successful treatment with this combined therapy has been reported. Surgical resection of CNS lesion may be required.
Schistosoma haematobium/ Africa, eastern Mediterranean	All		Praziquantel, 20 mg/kg/dose	2 doses in 1 day	Praziquantel does not kill developing worms; treatment given within 4–8 wk of exposure should be repeated 1–2 mo later.
Schistosoma japonicum/ China, Philippines, Indonesia	All		Praziquantel, 20 mg/kg/dose	3 doses in 1 day	Praziquantel does not kill developing worms; treatment given within 4–8 wk of exposure should be repeated 1–2 mo later.

Continued

TABLE 1-6

RECOMMENDED TREATMENT FOR PARASITIC AND PROTOZOAL INFECTIONS (Continued)

Parasite/Where Infection Acquired	Host Category	Indication	Recommended Treatment	Duration	Alternative Treatment	Duration	Comments
Schistosoma mansoni/ Africa, Caribbean, Venezuela, Brazil, Suriname, Arabian peninsula	All		Praziquantel 20 mg/kg/dose	1–2 doses in 1 day	Oxamniquine[i] 15 mg/kg PO once in adults; 20 mg/kg PO in 2 doses for children	One dose	Praziquantel does not kill developing worms; treatment given within 4–8 wk of exposure should be repeated 1–2 mo later. Oxamniquine dose should be increased in East Africa to 30 mg/kg, and in Egypt and South Africa to 30 mg/kg/day for 2 days. Oxamniquine is contraindicated in pregnancy.
Schistosoma mekongi/ Cambodia, Laos, Japan, Philippines, Central Indonesia	All		Praziquantel 20 mg/kg/dose	2–3 doses in 1 day			Praziquantel does not kill developing worms; treatment given within 4–8 wk of exposure should be repeated 1–2 mo later.

Strongyloides stercoralis/ Tropical and temperate climates worldwide	All		Ivermectin	1–2 days	Thiabendazole *or* Albendazole[b]	2 days 7 days	Prolonged treatment may be required in immunocompromised patients or in patients with disseminated disease. The recommended dose of thiabendazole may have to be reduced if toxicity (nausea, vomiting, diarrhea) occurs. Lower cure rates are reported with thiabendazole and albendazole treatment than with ivermectin.
Taenia saginata (beef tapeworm)/Worldwide	All	Diarrhea, abdominal pain, intestinal obstruction	Praziquantel[b]	1 dose	Niclosamide[i]	1 dose	Cobalamin injections and oral folic acid are indicated for individuals with evidence of vitamin B_{12} deficiency.
Taenia solium (pork tapeworm)		Diarrhea, abdominal pain, intestinal obstruction	Praziquantel[b]	1 dose	Niclosamide[i]	One dose	Cobalamin injections and oral folic acid are indicated for individuals with evidence of vitamin B_{12} deficiency.

Continued

TABLE 1-6

RECOMMENDED TREATMENT FOR PARASITIC AND PROTOZOAL INFECTIONS (Continued)

Parasite/Where Infection Acquired	Host Category	Indication	Recommended Treatment	Duration	Alternative Treatment	Duration	Comments
Taenia solium (pork tape worm) *(Continued)*		Cysticercosis	Albendazole (see Comment) *or* Praziquantel[b] (see Comment)	8–30 days 30 days			Usefulness of treatment with albendazole or praziquantel has not been demonstrated. Therapy may not be required for single cysts within brain parenchyma. Seizures should be treated with anticonvulsants. Surgery is indicated for obstructing cysts. Corticosteroids have been used in conjunction with surgery or in conjunction with albendazole or praziquantel to treat arachnoiditis, vasculitis, or cerebral edema. Neither albendazole nor praziquantel should be used to treat ocular or spinal cysts, even in conjunction with corticosteroids; an ophthalmologic examination should be performed before treating with these agents.

Toxocara canis; Toxocara catis/Worldwide	All	Visceral larva migrans	Albendazole[b] *or* Mebendazole[b]	5 days 5 days			Optimal duration of therapy is not known. Some experts treat as long as 20 days. Corticosteroids have been used to reduce inflammation when treating CNS or myocardial disease.
		Ocular larva migrans	Albendazole[b] *or* Mebendazole[b]	5 days 5 days			Antihelminthic treatment alone may not be effective. Additional treatment may include vitrectomy and corticosteroids.
Toxoplasma gondii/ Worldwide		Chorioretinitis	Pyrimethamine + [Sulfadiazine *or* Clindamycin[b]] + Leucovorin	3–6 wk 3–4 wk 3–4 doses With each dose of pyrimethamine	Trimethoprim-sulfamethoxazole[b]	3–4 doses	Adjunctive therapy with corticosteroids is recommended for macular involvement. Leucovorin is used to minimize pyrimethamine-associated hematologic toxicity.

Continued

TABLE 1-6

RECOMMENDED TREATMENT FOR PARASITIC AND PROTOZOAL INFECTIONS (Continued)

Parasite/Where Infection Acquired	Host Category	Indication	Recommended Treatment	Duration	Alternative Treatment	Duration	Comments
Toxoplasma gondii/ Worldwide *(Continued)*		CNS infection	Pyrimethamine + [Sulfadiazine *or* Clindamycin[b]] + Leucovorin	3–4 wk 3–4 wk 3–4 doses With each dose of pyrimethamine	Trimethoprim-sulfamethoxazole[b]	3–4 doses	Adjunctive therapy with corticosteroids is sometimes recommended. Repeated LPs may be necessary to manage intracranial increased pressure. HIV-infected individuals with encephalitis should receive lifelong therapy or until clinical disease is resolved and sustained (>6 mo) reconstitution has been achieved using antiretroviral therapy and CD4 T-lymphocyte percentage is >15% for >3 consecutive months. Leucovorin is used to minimize pyrimethamine-associated hematologic toxicity.
		Congenital infection	Pyrimethamine every 2–3 days + sulfadiazine daily + Leucovorin	1 yr 1 yr			Leucovorin is used to minimize pyrimethamine-associated hematologic toxicity. Appropriate duration of treatment is not known and consultation with a pediatric infectious diseases expert is recommended.

	Pregnant women	<18 wk gestation	Spiramycin	Duration of pregnancy if fetal infection is excluded		Spiramycin is the treatment of choice for primary infection in pregnancy if transmission to the fetus has not occurred. Spiramycin is not sold in the United States, but it can be obtained from Palo Alto Medical Foundation Toxoplasma Serology Laboratory (650-853-4828) or from the FDA (301-796-1600). If fetal infection is confirmed after the 17th wk of pregnancy, or if the mother acquires primary infection in the last trimester, pyrimethamine and sulfadiazine should be considered. Pyrimethamine is a potential teratogen, and it should not be used during the first trimester.

Continued

TABLE 1-6

RECOMMENDED TREATMENT FOR PARASITIC AND PROTOZOAL INFECTIONS (Continued)

Parasite/Where Infection Acquired	Host Category	Indication	Recommended Treatment	Duration	Alternative Treatment	Duration	Comments
Toxoplasma gondii/ Worldwide *(Continued)*		Fetal infection confirmed by amniocentesis after first trimester	Spiramycin + sulfadiazine + leucovorin	Until delivery			Spiramycin is not sold in the United States, but it can be obtained from Palo Alto Medical Foundation Toxoplasma Serology Laboratory (650-853-4828) or from the FDA (301-796-1600).
Trachipleistophora sp. (microsporidiosis)/ Not well defined	All	Disseminated microsporidiosis	Albendazole[b]				There is no known effective therapy for microsporidial infection. Albendazole may reduce symptoms. HIV+ patients may benefit from highly active antiretroviral therapy to improve their own immunity.
Trichinella spiralis/ Worldwide	All		Albendazole[b]	8–14 days	Mebendazole[b]	13 days	Corticosteroids help alleviate the inflammatory reaction and should be coadministered with mebendazole or albendazole when symptoms are severe.

Trichomonas vaginalis/ Worldwide	All		Metronidazole	2 g PO once (adults); 15 mg/kg/day in 3 doses PO × 7 days (children)	Tinidazole	2 g PO once (adults); 50 mg/kg PO once (children)	Sexual partners should be treated. Metronidazole-resistant strains should be treated with daily doses of 2–4 mg for 7–14 days (adults) or with high-dose tinidazole.
Trichostrongylus/ Worldwide	All		Pyrantel pamoate[b]	1 dose of 11 mg/kg base	Mebendazole[b] *or* Albendazole[b]	3 days 1 dose	
Trichuris trichiura (whipworm)/ Worldwide	All		Albendazole[b]	3 days	Mebendazole *or* Ivermectin	3 days 3 days	
Trypanosoma cruzi (Chagas' disease, American trypanosomiasis)/ Temperate, subtropical, tropical regions of the Americas and West Indies		Acute infection, indeterminate phase infection, congenital infection, reactivation associated with immunosuppression, transfusion-related infection	Benznidazole[i]	60–90 days	Nifurtimox[d]	90–120 days	Effectiveness of treatment of chronic infection has not been established. Negative side effects of benznidazole treatment are common and include rash, peripheral neuritis, anorexia, and hepatologic alterations. Prolonged treatment with Nifurtimax is associated with weakness, anorexia, nausea, vomiting, hepatitis, and peripheral and central nervous system symptoms.

Continued

TABLE 1-6

RECOMMENDED TREATMENT FOR PARASITIC AND PROTOZOAL INFECTIONS (Continued)

Parasite/Where Infection Acquired	Host Category	Indication	Recommended Treatment	Duration	Alternative Treatment	Duration	Comments
Trypanosoma brucei gambiense (sleeping sickness, West African trypanosomiasis)/ Western and Central Africa	All	Non-CNS infection	Pentamidine[b] (IM)	7 days	Suramin[d,i] (IV)	100–200 mg IV test dose followed by 1 gram daily on days 1, 3, 7, 14, and 21	Pediatric dose of Suramin is 20 mg/kg IV on days 1, 3, 7, 14, and 21.
		CNS involvement	Eflornithine[d] (400 mg/kg IV in 2 doses) *or* [Eflornithine[d] (400 mg/kg IV in 2 doses)+ nifurtimox] *or* melarsoprol[i]	14 days 7 days 10 days 10 days			Corticosteroids have been used to prevent encephalopathy. CSF should be repeated every 3–6 mo for 2 yr to detect possible relapse.
Trypanosoma brucei rhodesiense (East African trypanosomiasis, sleeping sickness)/Eastern Africa		Hemolymphatic stage	Suramin[d,i]	100–200 mg IV test dose followed by 1 gram daily on days 1, 3, 7, 14, and 21			Pediatric dose of Suramin is 20 mg/kg IV on days 1, 3, 7, 14, and 21.

		CNS involvement	Melarsoprol[k]	2–3.6 mg/kg/day for 3 days; after 7 days, 3.6 mg/kg/day for 3 days; repeat again after 7 days		Melarsoprol treatment may be initiated in small doses (18 mg) with progressive increase and/or preceded by treatment with suramin in debilitated patients. Corticosteroids have been used to prevent encephalopathy. CSF should be repeated every 3–6 mo for 2 yr to detect possible relapse.
Uncinaria stenocephala (cutaneous larva migrans)/ Worldwide	Symptomatic patient	Cutaneous larva migrans	Albendazole[b] *or* Ivermectin[b]	3 days 1–2 days		Disease is usually self-limited, lasting weeks to months without therapy.
Vittaforma corneae (microsporidiosis)/ Not well defined	All	Ocular microsporidiosis	Albendazole[b] + fumagillin[e] (eye drops)			There is no known effective therapy for microsporidial infection. Fumagillin is used to control microsporidial disease in honeybees, and fumagillin eye drops have been helpful in some HIV-infected patients. Albendazole may reduce symptoms. HIV+ patients may benefit from highly active antiretroviral therapy to improve their own immunity.

Continued

TABLE 1-6

RECOMMENDED TREATMENT FOR PARASITIC AND PROTOZOAL INFECTIONS (Continued)

Parasite/Where Infection Acquired	Host Category	Indication	Recommended Treatment	Duration	Alternative Treatment	Duration	Comments
Vittaforma corneae (microsporidiosis)/ Not well defined *(Continued)*	All	Disseminated microsporidiosis	Albendazole[b]				There is no known effective therapy for microsporidial infection. Albendazole may reduce symptoms. HIV+ patients may benefit from highly active antiretroviral therapy to improve their own immunity.
Wuchereria bancrofti (filariasis)/ Tropics worldwide		Tropical pulmonary eosinophilia	Diethylcarbamazine[d] (6 mg/kg/day in 3 doses)	12 days	Albendazole + [ivermectin *or* diethylcarbamazine]	1 dose 1 dose 1 dose	Antihistamines or corticosteroids may be required to decrease allergic reaction to microfilarial disintegration. Alternative therapy suppresses microfilaria but does not kill the adult forms.

ECTOPARASITES

Lice/Worldwide	All	*Pediculosis capitis* (head lice), *Pediculosis corporis* (body lice), *Pediculosis pubis* (pubic lice)	Malathion (0.5%, topical) *or* Permethrin (1% topical) *or* Pyrethrin with piperonyl butoxide (topical) *or* Ivermectin[b] (200 mcg/kg PO)	Apply twice, 7 days apart Twice, 7 days apart Twice, 7 days apart One dose (200 or 400 mcg/kg PO)			Malathion is contraindicated in children <2 yr of age. Petrolatum for pubic lice in eyelashes. Permethrin is not approved by the FDA for use in children <2 yr of age. Pyrethrins are contraindicated for people who are allergic to chrysanthemums or ragweed.
Sarcoptes scabiei (Scabies)/ Worldwide	Immunocompetent	Cutaneous infection	Permethrin (5% topical)	Apply twice, 7 days apart	Ivermectin[b] (200 mcg/kg PO) *or* Crotamiton (10% topical)	Twice, 7 days apart Overnight on days 1, 2, 3, 8	Permethrin or ivermectin treatment may have to be repeated in 10–14 days. Permethrin is not approved by the FDA for use in children <2 yr of age.
	Immunocompromised	Crusted scabies	Ivermectin[b] (200 mcg/kg PO) +/– a topical agent	Once			

A. Parasite/Protozoa Types by Category

1. **Filaria**
   a. *Brugia malayi*
   b. *Brugia timori*
   c. *Loa loa*
   d. *Mansonella ozzardi*
   e. *Mansonella perstans*
   f. *Mansonella streptocerca*
   g. *Onchocerca volvulus*
   h. *Wuchereria bancrofti*
2. **Flukes**
   a. *Capillaria philippinensis*
   b. *Clonorchis sinensis*
   c. *Fasciola buski*
   d. *Fasciola hepatica*
   e. *Heterophyes heterophyes*
   f. *Metagonimus yokogawai*
   g. *Metorchis conjunctus*
   h. *Nanophyetus salmincola*
   i. *Opisthorchis viverrini*
   j. *Paragonimus westermani*
3. **Hookworm**
   a. *Ancylostoma braziliense*
   b. *Ancylostoma caninum*
   c. *Ancylostoma duodenale*
   d. *Necator americanus*
   e. *Uncinaria stenocephala*
4. **Microsporidia**
   a. *Encephalitozoon hellem*
   b. *Encephalitozoon cuniculi*
   c. *Encephalitozoon (Septata) intestinalis*
   d. *Enterocytozoon bieneusi*
   e. *Pleistophora* sp.
   f. *Trachipleistophora* sp.
   g. *Vittaforma corneae*
5. **Tapeworms**
   a. *Diphyllobothrium latum*
   b. *Dipylidium caninum*
   c. *Hymenolepis nana*
   d. *Taenia saginata*
   e. *Taenia sol*

ACKNOWLEDGMENTS

We thank William G. Merz, PhD, for his help in the development of this guide to classification of pathogenic fungi.

Chapter 2

Recommended Empiric Antimicrobial Therapy for Selected Clinical Syndromes

Hiwot Hiruy, MD, Swathi Gowtham, MD, and Paul Sue, MD

TABLE 2-1

RECOMMENDED EMPIRIC ANTIMICROBIAL THERAPY FOR SELECTED CLINICAL SYNDROMES (for notes and abbreviations used in this table, see p. XV.)

Syndrome	Host Category	Common Treatable Pathogens	Preferred Treatment	Alternative Treatment	Comments
SYSTEMIC AND INTRAVASCULAR INFECTIONS					
Endocarditis	Native valve (including congenital heart disease)	Streptococci, especially Viridans streptococci group, *Streptococcus pneumoniae, staphylococci, enterococci*	[PCN *or* Ceftriaxone] + gentamicin *or* Oxacillin/nafcillin + gentamicin	Vancomycin + gentamicin	Antimicrobial therapy guided by blood culture results. Consider empiric vancomycin if culture results are not available. β-Lactams are highly preferable to vancomycin if organism is susceptible. Gentamicin at synergistic dosage for gram-positive organisms. Other less common organisms include HACEK group *(Haemophilus parainfluenzae, Haemophilus aphrophilus, Aggregatibacter actinomycetemcomitans, Cardiobacterium, Eikenella, Kingella), Bartonella, Coxiella burnetii, Chlamydia, Brucella, Nocardia, Mycobacterium* spp.
	Prosthetic valve	Coagulase-negative staphylococci, *Staphylococcus aureus,* enterococci, Viridans streptococci, gram-negative bacilli, diphtheroids	Vancomycin + gentamicin + rifampin		Surgical consultation. Antimicrobial therapy guided by blood culture results. β-Lactams are highly preferable to vancomycin if organism is susceptible. Gentamicin at synergistic dosage for gram-positive organisms. Other less common organisms include fungi such as *Candida* and *Aspergillus* spp.

	IV drug user	*S. aureus* (usually MRSA)	Vancomycin + gentamicin	Daptomycin	Daptomycin has been approved by the FDA for the treatment of right-sided endocarditis in adults only.
Intravascular catheter-related infection/bacteremia	Immunocompetent patient	*S. aureus*, coagulase-negative staphylococci, less likely enteric gram-negative rods, *Candida* spp.	Vancomycin +/– [PCS3 + AG]	Synercid* Daptomycin* +/– [aztreonam *or* FQ]	Strongly consider catheter removal, especially if clinical progression or severe illness. Consider gram-negative coverage, depending on patient risk factors and severity of illness. Add amphotericin B or fluconazole if suspicious of candidemia. Other less common organisms include *Corynebacterium*, *Bacillus* spp., *Propionibacterium*, *Enterococcus* spp.
	Immunocompromised patient	*S. aureus*, coagulase-negative staphylococci, gram-negative bacilli (especially *Pseudomonas* spp., Enterobacteriaceae), *Corynebacterium* spp.	Vancomycin + [pip/tazo *or* cefepime *or* ceftazidime] +/– AG	Vancomycin + [imipenem *or* meropenem]	Strongly consider catheter removal. Consider adding AG in patients who are critically ill, while awaiting culture results. Antibiotic lock therapy should be used in cases of catheter salvage. Strongly consider adding amphotericin B or fluconazole if suspicious of candidemia.

Continued

TABLE 2-1

RECOMMENDED EMPIRIC ANTIMICROBIAL THERAPY FOR SELECTED CLINICAL SYNDROMES (Continued)

Syndrome	Host Category	Common Treatable Pathogens	Preferred Treatment	Alternative Treatment	Comments
Myocarditis	Immunocompetent patient	*Borrelia* spp.	Supportive care If Lyme disease suspected, Ceftriaxone *or* Penicillin IV	If Lyme disease, doxycycline PO if mild/no symptoms and at least 8 yr	Viruses are most common cause of myocarditis (enteroviruses, adenovirus, CMV, influenza virus, parainfluenza virus, mumps virus, HIV). Less common organisms: *Rickettsia* spp., *Treponema pallidum, Trichinella, Trypanosoma* spp. Bacteria (especially *S. aureus, Neisseria meningitidis*) can cause myocardial abscesses and myocardial dysfunction but rarely cause myocarditis. Role of steroids and IVIg is controversial.
	Immunocompromised patient	*Borrelia* spp. and *Toxoplasma*	Same as above for immunocompetent patients		As above. Consider pyrimethamine plus sulfadiazine if toxoplasmosis is suspected.
Pericarditis (purulent)	All	*S. aureus, Streptococcus pneumoniae, N. meningitidis, H. influenzae,* Enterobacteriaceae, *Mycobacterium tuberculosis*	Vancomycin + PCS3	Severe PCN allergy: Vancomycin + [aztreonam *or* FQ]	Broad-spectrum antimicrobial therapy should be initiated empirically for suspected purulent pericarditis. Purulent effusion should be drained as soon as possible. Viral disease (enteroviruses) likely in nonpurulent pericarditis. Less common: fungal pathogens, other streptococci, anaerobic bacteria, *Rickettsia* spp., *Mycoplasma pneumoniae, Mycoplasma hominis, Ureaplasma urealyticum.*

Systemic febrile illness/ sepsis	Community-acquired infection, normal host	*S. pneumoniae*, *N. meningitidis*, *H. influenzae* type b, *S. aureus*, group A *Streptococcus*, *Salmonella*	Ceftriaxone +/– vancomycin	Carbapenem Severe PCN allergy: Vancomycin + aztreonam	Add vancomycin if critically ill patient, concern for staphylococcal infection, or if CNS involvement is likely. Consider doxycycline in tick-endemic areas or if petechial rash (*Ehrlichia, Rickettsia* spp.). In cases of shock, consider clindamycin for toxic shock syndrome. *H. influenzae* is rare in immunized individuals.
	Asplenia	*S. pneumoniae*, *Salmonella*, *N. meningitidis*, *H. influenzae* type b, *Capnocytophaga* spp., *Babesia* spp., *Erysipelothrix*	Ceftriaxone +/– vancomycin	Carbapenem Severe PCN allergy: Vancomycin + [aztreonam *or* FQ]	Add vancomycin if critically ill patient, concern for staphylococcal infection, or if CNS involvement is likely. Consider doxycycline in tick-infested areas or if petechial rash (*Ehrlichia, Rickettsia* spp). Add clindamycin and quinine if *Babesia* is a concern. In cases of shock, consider clindamycin for toxic shock syndrome.
	GU source	Gram-negative bacilli, enterococci	[Ampicillin + gentamicin] *or* Ceftriaxone	Pip/tazo *or* Ampicillin/ sulbactam *or* FQ	Some experts routinely add AG. Consider resistant organisms and broaden coverage for hosts with indwelling catheters, history of UTI, or other abnormalities of GU tract.
	Hospital-acquired infection	*S. pneumoniae*, *S. aureus*, other streptococci, gram-negative bacilli (especially *Pseudomonas aeruginosa*)	[Cefepime *or* Pip/tazo *or* Imipenem *or* Meropenem] +/– vancomycin	Severe PCN allergy: Vancomycin + [aztreonam *or* FQ]	Consider vancomycin if patient is critically ill, concern for central venous line site infection, or concern for *Staphylococcus*. Consider amphotericin if suspected fungal causative factor. In cases of shock, consider adding an AG.

2

Continued

TABLE 2-1

RECOMMENDED EMPIRIC ANTIMICROBIAL THERAPY FOR SELECTED CLINICAL SYNDROMES (Continued)

Syndrome	Host Category	Common Treatable Pathogens	Preferred Treatment	Alternative Treatment	Comments
Systemic febrile illness/ sepsis *(Continued)*	Intra-abdominal source or biliary source	*Enterococcus* spp., Enterobacteriaceae, *Bacteroides* spp. Other aerobic and anaerobic gram-negative bacilli. *Candida* spp. less common.	Ampicillin/sulbactam *or* [Ampicillin + gentamicin + metronidazole] *or* Pip/tazo *or* Tic/clav	Carbapenem Severe PCN allergy: Vancomycin + [aztreonam *or* FQ] + metronidazole	In cases of shock, add an AG (if not already part of the regimen).
	IV drug user	*S. aureus*	Oxacillin *or* Vancomycin	Linezolid *or* Synercid *or* Daptomycin	Empiric treatment depends on local antibiotic susceptibility patterns. β-Lactams are highly preferable to vancomycin if organism is susceptible.
	Neonate	GBS, *Escherichia coli, Listeria,* other enteric gram-negative bacilli (*Klebsiella, Enterobacter*), *S. aureus*	Ampicillin + gentamicin	Ampicillin + cefotaxime	Substitute cefotaxime for gentamicin if meningitis is a possibility or in cases of shock. Consider adding vancomycin or oxacillin if concern for *Staphylococcus* (neonatal intensive care unit patient or community-acquired MRSA). Consider testing for HSV and adding acyclovir if concern for HSV.

	Hospitalized neonate	GBS, *E. coli, Listeria,* other enteric gram-negative bacilli (*Klebsiella, Enterobacter*), *S. aureus,* coagulase-negative *Staphylococcus, H. influenzae, Enterococcus, Candida* spp.	Ampicillin + gentamicin +/– vancomycin	Ampicillin + cefotaxime	Substitute cefotaxime for gentamicin if meningitis cannot be excluded or depending on local antibiotic susceptibility patterns. Consider vancomycin if patient is critically ill, concern for central venous line site infection, or concern for *Staphylococcus.* Consider adding amphotericin B for *Candida.* Consider adding acyclovir if concern for HSV.
	Drug-induced neutropenia	Gram-negative bacilli (including *P. aeruginosa*), Viridans streptococci, *Staphylococcus* spp., *Candida* spp., other fungi	[Pip/tazo *or* cefepime *or* ceftazidime] +/– AG	[Imipenem *or* meropenem] +/– AG Severe PCN allergy: [Vancomycin + aztreonam] *or* FQ	Consider vancomycin if patient is critically ill, concern for central venous line site infection, or concern for MRSA. Consider adding AG while awaiting cultures in patients who are critically ill. If severe illness or no improvement with antibacterial therapy, add amphotericin B.
Toxic shock syndrome	All	*S. aureus,* GAS	Clindamycin + oxacillin +/– vancomycin	Vancomycin + clindamycin	Consider IVIg. Seek source. Consider adding vancomycin if concern for MRSA. β-Lactams are highly preferable to vancomycin in cases of GAS or MSSA.

Continued

2

TABLE 2-1

RECOMMENDED EMPIRIC ANTIMICROBIAL THERAPY FOR SELECTED CLINICAL SYNDROMES (Continued)

Syndrome	Host Category	Common Treatable Pathogens	Preferred Treatment	Alternative Treatment	Comments
OCULAR INFECTIONS					
Blepharitis	All		Warm compress and eyelid scrub		Unclear cause; may include *Staphylococcus* spp., seborrhea, meibomian gland dysfunction. Topical antistaphylococcal antimicrobials (e.g., tetracycline, erythromycin, bacitracin) sometimes used to decrease bacterial load on eyelids.
Conjunctivitis (bacterial)	Newborn (ophthalmia neonatorum)	Bacterial: *N. gonorrhoeae, C. trachomatis*	[Ceftriaxone *or* Cefotaxime] + [erythromycin *or* azithromycin]	[Ceftriaxone *or* Cefotaxime] + sulfonamide	Treat neonate for presumed systemic infection if *N. gonorrhoeae* is suspected: • Oral erythromycin in infants <6 wk old associated with increased risk for pyloric stenosis; risk from azithromycin not well studied. • Sulfonamide can be used beyond immediate neonatal period if intolerant of macrolides. • Cefotaxime is generally preferred over ceftriaxone in neonates because of the risk for exacerbating hyperbilirubinemia.

					Consider viral disease (HSV) and less common organisms: *Streptococcus* spp., *H. influenzae*, gram-negative bacilli. Chemical conjunctivitis less common because erythromycin is used as prophylaxis instead of silver nitrate. Consider ophthalmology evaluation. Treat mother and her partner(s) for cases of confirmed STI.
	Beyond newborn	Bacterial: *S. pneumoniae, H. influenzae, Moraxella, S. aureus*	Polymyxin B + trimethoprim drops	FQ drops	Consider viral disease (adenovirus). Topical therapy not necessary if giving systemic therapy for concomitant OM.
	Sexually active patient and/or associated with genital infection	*N. gonorrhoeae, C. trachomatis*	Ceftriaxone + doxycycline		Ophthalmic consultation and frequent irrigation if suspected *N. gonorrhoeae*. Treat partner(s) if confirmed STI.
Dacryocystitis	All	*S. pneumoniae, H. influenzae, S. aureus*, coagulase-negative Staphylococci, *Streptococcus pyogenes, P. aeruginosa*	Nafcillin/Oxacillin *or* Cephalexin *or* Clindamycin	Vancomycin	Consider ophthalmologic consultation to relieve obstruction and to obtain material for culture.

Continued

TABLE 2-1

RECOMMENDED EMPIRIC ANTIMICROBIAL THERAPY FOR SELECTED CLINICAL SYNDROMES (Continued)

Syndrome	Host Category	Common Treatable Pathogens	Preferred Treatment	Alternative Treatment	Comments
Endophthalmitis	Immunocompetent patient	Coagulase-negative staphylococci, *Bacillus* spp., *Propionibacterium acnes, S. pneumoniae, N. meningitidis,* gram-negative bacilli, *S. aureus*	[Ceftazidime] + vancomycin	Vancomycin + FQ	Obtain emergent ophthalmologic evaluation. *Bacillus* spp. and CoNS are the *most common cause of post-traumatic endophthalmitis.* *P. acnes* may cause chronic endophthalmitis after cataract surgery. Blood and vitreal cultures and stains should guide definitive therapy. Intravitreal administration of antibiotics essential in treatment of exogenous (traumatic) endophthalmitis. If history of trauma, consider antipseudomonal coverage.
	Immunosuppressed patient	See above bacterial, *Candida* spp., *Aspergillus* spp., *Listeria monocytogenes, Nocardia* spp.	[Ceftazidime *or* Cefepime] + vancomycin + amphotericin B	FQ + voriconazole	Obtain emergent ophthalmologic evaluation. Blood and vitreal cultures and stains should guide definitive therapy.

Keratitis	All	Viral: HSV1, HSV2; EBV, varicella-zoster virus, adenovirus, rubeola virus, rubella virus, mumps virus, measles virus, enteroviruses Bacterial: *S. aureus*, other *Staphylococcus* spp., *S. pneumoniae, S. pyogenes, C. trachomatis, Listeria, Moraxella catarrhalis,* gram-negative bacilli (especially *Pseudomonas*) Fungal: *Aspergillus* sp., *Fusarium* sp., *Candida* sp. Protozoal: *Acanthamoeba, Hartmannella*	Consider cephalosporin and AG drops pending further evaluation; for example, Cefazolin ophthalmic + AG ophthalmic	FQ ophthalmic	Obtain emergent ophthalmologic evaluation. Cultures and stains to guide therapy. Contact lens wearers at increased risk for *Pseudomonas.* In cases of epithelial HSV keratitis, consider vidarabine ointment or trifluridine drops pending on ophthalmologic evaluation.
Orbital cellulitis	Immunocompetent patient (secondary to sinusitis, trauma, or bacteremia)	Bacterial: *S. pneumoniae, H. influenzae, S. aureus, M. catarrhalis, S. pyogenes* (anaerobes, gram-negative bacilli)	[Vancomycin *or* Clindamycin] + PCS3 + metronidazole *or* [Ampicillin/sulbactam]	Severe PCN allergy: Vancomycin + [FQ *or* aztreonam] + metronidazole *or* Clindamycin + [FQ or aztreonam]	Consider vancomycin if concern for MRSA. β-Lactams are preferable to vancomycin if organism is susceptible. Recommend ophthalmologic consultation. Evaluate with CT scan for intracranial extension.
	Immunosuppressed patient	See above bacterial, especially *Pseudomonas* spp., other gram-negative bacilli	[Vancomycin *or* Clindamycin] + [pip/tazo *or* cefepime]	FQ PCN allergy: Vancomycin + [quinolone *or* aztreonam] + metronidazole	β-Lactams are preferable to vancomycin if organism is susceptible. Consider fungi (mucormycosis, *Rhizopus*) and presumptive antifungal therapy.

Continued

TABLE 2-1

RECOMMENDED EMPIRIC ANTIMICROBIAL THERAPY FOR SELECTED CLINICAL SYNDROMES (Continued)

Syndrome	Host Category	Common Treatable Pathogens	Preferred Treatment	Alternative Treatment	Comments
Preseptal cellulitis	Immunocompetent patient	*Streptococcus pneumoniae*, GAS, *S. aureus*, nontypeable *H. influenzae*, *M. catarrhalis*	Ampicillin/sulbactam *or* A/C *or* [PCS3 + clindamycin]	Cefuroxime *or* FQ	Consider adding vancomycin, TMP/SMX, or clindamycin if concern for MRSA. If suspected secondary to cutaneous trauma and not suspected to be associated with sinusitis, may choose narrow staphylococcal/streptococcal antibiotic (e.g., clindamycin).
	Immunosuppressed patient	*Streptococcus* spp., primarily GAS, *S. aureus*, nontypeable *H. influenzae*, *Moraxella*, anaerobes, *Pseudomonas* spp., fungi (*Candida*)	Pip/tazo + vancomycin	[Cefepime + clindamycin] *or* [Imipenem/ meropenem + vancomycin]	Consider adding antifungal.
Stye (hordeolum), external or internal	All	External and internal: *S. aureus*	Warm compress + [dicloxacillin *or* cephalexin *or* clindamycin]	A/C *or* TMP/SMX	Internal styes drain spontaneously; external styes usually do not drain spontaneously.

Dental abscess	All	Oral flora: often polymicrobial, including anaerobes	Clindamycin	A/C	Consider surgical drainage.
GENITOURINARY INFECTIONS					
Cervicitis/urethritis/ epididymitis (no pelvic inflammatory disease)	All	*C. trachomatis* *N. gonorrhoeae* Uncommon: *Trichomonas vaginalis*, HSV, *Mycoplasma genitalium, Ureaplasma urealyticum*	[Azithromycin × 1 dose *or* Doxycycline × 7 days] + Ceftriaxone × 1 dose	[Ceftriaxone *or* Cefixime *or* Spectinomycin[†] × 1 dose] + [azithromycin × 1 dose *or* doxycycline × 7 days]	Treatment for both chlamydial and gonorrheal infections should be given simultaneously because of the high rate of coinfection. Testing for other STIs and HIV should be offered. Sexual partners of patient with confirmed STIs should be examined and treated to avoid reinfection. FQ and OCS3 are no longer recommended for presumptive treatment of gonorrheal infection because of increasing resistance. If used, a test of cure is recommended.

Continued

TABLE 2-1

RECOMMENDED EMPIRIC ANTIMICROBIAL THERAPY FOR SELECTED CLINICAL SYNDROMES (Continued)

Syndrome	Host Category	Common Treatable Pathogens	Preferred Treatment	Alternative Treatment	Comments
Pelvic inflammatory disease	All	*N. gonorrhoeae*, *C. trachomatis*, streptococci, anaerobes (i.e., *Peptostreptococcus*, *Prevotella* sp., *Clostridia*) Gram-negative organisms: Enterobacteriaceae, *H. influenzae*	Outpatient: [Ceftriaxone IM *or* other PCS3 *or* cefoxitin IM/probenecid PO] + doxycycline +/– metronidazole Hospitalized patient: [(Cefoxitin *or* cefotetan) + (doxycycline × 14 days)] *or* [Clindamycin IV + gentamicin]	A/C + doxycycline *or* Ampicillin/ sulbactam + doxycycline	For hospitalized patients who improve clinically, parenteral therapy may be replaced after 24 hr. Continuing oral therapy: doxycycline plus clindamycin to complete 14 days. FQ are no longer recommended for presumptive treatment of gonorrheal infection because of increasing resistance.
UTI	Cystitis	Gram-negative organisms (i.e., *E. coli*, *Proteus*, Enterobacteriaceae), *Enterococcus* sp., *Staphylococcus saprophyticus* (postpubertal female patients)	TMP/SMX *or* Cefixime	Nitrofurantoin *or* OCS2 *or* OCS3	For cystitis, consider phenazopyridine (Pyridium) for comfort. *Note:* Urine may turn red.

Pyelonephritis, no urinary tract abnormalities (uncomplicated)	Gram-negative organisms (i.e., *E. coli*, *Proteus*, Enterobacteriaceae), *Enterococcus*	[Ampicillin + gentamicin] *or* Ceftriaxone	Cefixime *or* Ciprofloxacin for severe PCN allergy or resistant organism without other oral treatment options (≥1 yr old)	Therapy should be directed by culture results. Pyelonephritis without sepsis may be treated orally on an outpatient basis in selected patients.
Infants ≤3 mo	Same as above and group B *Streptococcus*	[Ampicillin + gentamicin] *or* Ceftriaxone	Cefixime *or* AG	Febrile infants with UTI should undergo renal and bladder ultrasonography (RBUS). VCUG is indicated if RBUS reveals findings suggestive of high-grade VUR, or in the case of recurrent febrile UTI.
Urinary tract abnormalities on prophylaxis	Same as above and resistant gram-negative organisms	Pip/tazo *or* Ceftazidime		Therapy should be directed by culture results, particularly for those on long-term prophylaxis where the flora may be altered.
Pregnant patient	Gram-negative organisms (i.e., *E. coli*, *Proteus*), *Enterococcus* sp., *S. saprophyticus*), group B *Streptococcus*	OCS2 *or* OCS3 *or* Nitrofurantoin	TMP/SMX	TMP/SMX should be avoided in the first trimester and must be discontinued 2 wk before estimated date of delivery because of risk for kernicterus in infant. Nitrofurantoin should be avoided in the first trimester if safe alternatives are available. FQ are contraindicated in pregnancy.

Continued

TABLE 2-1

RECOMMENDED EMPIRIC ANTIMICROBIAL THERAPY FOR SELECTED CLINICAL SYNDROMES (Continued)

Syndrome	Host Category	Common Treatable Pathogens	Preferred Treatment	Alternative Treatment	Comments
Renal abscess	All	*S. aureus*, gram-negative organisms (i.e., *E. coli, Proteus, Pseudomonas*), other gram-positive organisms (i.e., *Enterococcus* spp., *Streptococcus*), anaerobes	Oxacillin + gentamicin + [metronidazole *or* clindamycin]	Vancomycin + ceftriaxone	Therapy should be adjusted for abscess culture results because urine and blood cultures may not capture all pathogens. Renal abscess caused by hematogenous source is likely due to *S. aureus*; abscess secondary to UTI is more likely due to Enterobacteriaceae. Medical management initially, directed by clinical response; however, may need drainage if no resolution or obstruction.
Bacterial vaginosis	Nonpregnant patient	Usually polymicrobial, mostly associated with *Gardnerella vaginalis*, anaerobic bacteria	Metronidazole intravaginally *or* PO	Clindamycin vaginal cream or PO	Single-dose metronidazole not as effective as multiday course.
	Pregnant patient		Clindamycin PO *or* Metronidazole PO *or* intravaginally		Avoid clindamycin cream in pregnancy.
BONE, JOINT, AND SOFT TISSUE INFECTIONS					
Necrotizing fasciitis	All	*S. pyogenes* (GAS), *Clostridium perfringens* and other *Clostridium* spp., *Bacteroides* sp., *Prevotella* sp., gram-negative organisms, *S. aureus*	[(Nafcillin *or* oxacillin) + AG + clindamycin] *or* [Pip/tazo +/− clindamycin] *or* [Cefepime + clindamycin]	Carbapenem + clindamycin	Antibiotics are adjunctive; early surgical involvement crucial! If *S. aureus* concern, add vancomycin. Clindamycin may be superior adjunctive antibiotic for GAS because of toxin synthesis inhibition and inoculum effect.

Osteomyelitis, acute and chronic	All	*S. aureus* (MSSA/MRSA) GAS and *Streptococcus* spp., including GBS (neonates) Gram-negative organisms (e.g. *Kingella*)	Nafcillin *or* Oxacillin *or* Clindamycin	Vancomycin	Definitive therapy should be guided by biopsy and culture results when available. Biopsy/culture essential before broadening antibiotic coverage for inadequate response to initial empiric therapy. Vancomycin or clindamycin if MRSA prevalent, depending on local susceptibility trends. Rifampin has excellent bone penetration and can be good adjunctive therapy for gram-positives; it should never be used as monotherapy. Clindamycin alone is not effective treatment for *Kingella*.
	Immunocompromised patients and neonates	*Candida* sp. All pathogens listed for normal host, plus *Pseudomonas*	[Nafcillin *or* oxacillin *or* clindamycin] + [Ceftazidime *or* Cefepime *or* AP pen]	Vancomycin + [ceftazidime *or* cefepime *or* AP pen FQ]	
	Osteomyelitis of the foot (result of penetrating injury through sole of shoe)	*P. aeruginosa*	Ceftazidime *or* AP pen + AG		Remember: other pathogens, including mycobacteria and fungi, can cause osteomyelitis and should be considered particularly in unusual presentations or lack of clinical response. Initial treatment of penetrating wound to the foot should include antibiotics effective against *S. aureus*. If osteomyelitis develops, presumptive therapy should include treatment effective against *P. aeruginosa*.

Continued

TABLE 2-1

RECOMMENDED EMPIRIC ANTIMICROBIAL THERAPY FOR SELECTED CLINICAL SYNDROMES (Continued)

Syndrome	Host Category	Common Treatable Pathogens	Preferred Treatment	Alternative Treatment	Comments
Post–spinal fusion infection	All	*Staphylococcus* spp. (MSSA/MRSA/MRSE), *Streptococcus* spp., gram-negative organisms, particularly GI and GU pathogens	Vancomycin + pip/tazo		Although rod removal is usually optimal, it is often difficult or impossible. Deep-tissue cultures are essential for directed therapy. Consider adding rifampin to initial therapy if organism is susceptible for increased biofilm penetration; rifampin should never be used as monotherapy.
Pyomyositis	All	*S. aureus* (MSSA/MRSA), *Streptococcus* spp. (GAS), anaerobes	Nafcillin *or* Oxacillin *or* Cefazolin *or* Vancomycin *or* Clindamycin		Early surgical involvement crucial. Therapy should be guided by culture results. With increasing incidence of community-acquired MRSA, low threshold to choose vancomycin or clindamycin. Clindamycin or metronidazole should be part of presumptive therapy when infection is associated with trauma.
Spinal abscess	All	*Staphylococcus aureus* (MSSA/MRSA), *Streptococcus* spp.	Oxacillin *or* Nafcillin *or* Vancomycin *or* Clindamycin *or* Cefazolin		Debridement is an important component of therapy. Therapy should be guided by culture results when available. With increasing incidence of community-acquired MRSA, low threshold to choose vancomycin or clindamycin.

Arthritis, bacterial	Neonate	*S. aureus*, GBS, gram-negative bacilli	(Nafcillin *or* Oxacillin) + (Cefotaxime *or* Gentamicin)	Vancomycin + (cefotaxime *or* gentamicin)	Incision and drainage are important components of therapy.
	Child ≤5 yr old	*S. aureus*, group A *Streptococcus*, *S. pneumoniae*, *K. kingae*, *Haemophilus* spp., *Borrelia burgdorferi*	(Nafcillin *or* Oxacillin *or* Clindamycin) + cefotaxime	Vancomycin + cefotaxime	Therapy should be guided by gram-stained smear and culture results when available. Include clindamycin or vancomycin based on local prevalence and susceptibility patterns of MRSA. In Lyme-endemic areas, consider Borrelia and treatment with amoxicillin (<8 yr) or doxycycline. Persistent or recurrent arthritis due to *Borrelia* should be treated with ceftriaxone or IV penizillin or cefotaxime.
	Child >5 yr old	*S. aureus*, *Streptococcus* spp., *Borrelia burgdorferi*	Nafcillin *or* Oxacillin *or* Clindamycin	Vancomycin	Oral therapy may be appropriate once definite improvement is determined. In Lyme-endemic areas, consider Borrelia and treatment with ampicillin (<8 yr) or doxycycline.
	Adolescent	*S. aureus*, *Streptococcus* spp, must consider *N. gonorrhoeae*, *Borrelia burgdorferi*	[Nafcillin *or* Oxacillin *or* Clindamycin] + ceftriaxone	Vancomycin + (ceftriaxone *or* FQ)	In adolescents, ceftriaxone should be used when gonorrhea is a consideration. FQ should **not** be used for suspected gonococcal infection because of high resistance to FQ. Patients diagnosed with gonococcal arthritis should receive concurrent treatment for Chlamydia and undergo testing for other STIs including HIV and syphilis. In Lyme-endemic areas, consider Borrelia and treatment with doxycycline. Persistent or recurrent arthritis due to *Borrelia* should be treated with ceftriaxone or IV penizillin or cefotaxime.

Continued

TABLE 2-1

RECOMMENDED EMPIRIC ANTIMICROBIAL THERAPY FOR SELECTED CLINICAL SYNDROMES (Continued)

Syndrome	Host Category	Common Treatable Pathogens	Preferred Treatment	Alternative Treatment	Comments
Diskitis	All	*Staphylococcus* spp. (MSSA/MRSA), *Streptococcus* spp., *K. kingae,* gram-negative bacilli, *Mycobacterium* tuberculosis (Pott's disease)	Oxacillin *or* Nafcillin *or* Clindamycin	Vancomycin	Bedrest is considered essential. Therapy should be directed by clinical progress and recovered pathogen if culture performed. Add gram-negative coverage if gram-negative infection suspected. Consider TB with appropriate epidemiology.
Folliculitis, furuncles, carbuncles	All	*S. aureus* (MSSA/MRSA)	Warm compresses, incision, and drainage	Antistaphylococcal agent in more severe infections, that is, carbuncles: CFZ *or* Clindamycin *or* TMP/SMX *or* Dicloxacillin	With the increasing incidence of MRSA, clindamycin, TMP/SMX, or vancomycin may be preferred. With recurrent furuncles, boils, consider MRSA eradication with intranasal mupirocin and/or topical chlorhexidine. Incision, drainage, and culture are important in treatment and determination of definitive antibiotic therapy.
Erysipelas	All	*Streptococcus* spp., primarily GAS, *S. aureus*	Mild: Dicloxacillin *or* Cephalexin	Clindamycin *or* Macrolide	Occasionally, bacteremia may occur; blood cultures should be obtained. TMP/SMX not active against GAS.
			Severe: Parenteral penicillin therapy *or* Antistaphylococcal penicillin	Clindamycin *or* Vancomycin	

Cellulitis	Immunocompetent patient	*Streptococcus* spp., primarily GAS, *S. aureus*	Cephalexin *or* A/C *or* Clindamycin		Choose non–β-lactam option if MRSA is common. TMP/SMX not active against GAS.
	Immunocompromised patient, including diabetic individuals	*Streptococcus* spp., primarily GAS, *S. aureus, Pseudomonas*, fungi (*Candida*)	Clindamycin + ceftazidime) *or* (Pip/tazo + vancomycin)	Vancomycin + AG	For immunocompromised patients, consider presumptive therapy with amphotericin B, as well as antibacterials.
Hidradenitis suppurativa	All	*Staphylococcus* spp., anaerobes, *Pseudomonas*, gram-negative organisms	Clindamycin	Vancomycin	Adjust treatment based on culture results.
Ecthyma gangrenosum	Usually immunocompromised patients but can occur in immunocompetent patients	*P. aeruginosa, S. aureus*, other gram-negative organisms, fungal species (*Aspergillus*, Zygomycetes, *Candida* spp.)	(Ceftazidime + clindamycin) *or* Cefepime *or* Pip/tazo	Imipenem *or* Meropenem *or* FQ	Prompt initiation of therapy is critical. Sample for culture may be obtained by biopsy or by aspirating sample directly from the cellulitic region. Consider adding amphotericin B, particularly for patients with neutropenia.
LOWER RESPIRATORY TRACT INFECTIONS					
Aspiration pneumonia	All	Polymicrobial: oral anaerobes (*Bacteroides* sp., *Fusobacterium*), *Streptococcus* spp., *S. aureus, Klebsiella pneumoniae*	Clindamycin *or* BL/BLI	Imipenem *or* Meropenem	Adjust treatment based on culture results.
Lung abscess	All	Polymicrobial: oral anaerobes (*Bacteroides* sp., *Fusobacterium*), *Streptococcus* spp., *S. aureus, K. pneumoniae*	Clindamycin *or* BL/BLI	Imipenem *or* Meropenem	Consider vancomycin for MRSA coverage in severe disease; clindamycin efficacy will depend on local resistance patterns. Consider obtaining needle aspirate for culture.

Continued

TABLE 2-1

RECOMMENDED EMPIRIC ANTIMICROBIAL THERAPY FOR SELECTED CLINICAL SYNDROMES (Continued)

Syndrome	Host Category	Common Treatable Pathogens	Preferred Treatment	Alternative Treatment	Comments
Community-acquired pneumonia	Immunocompetent patient				
	Infant 4 wk to 3 mo old	Viruses most common; bacterial pathogens: *S. pneumoniae, C. trachomatis, Bordetella pertussis, S. aureus*	Afebrile, nonseptic—likely viral: most do not require treatment with an antibiotic. Consider Erythromycin *or* Azithromycin;		Erythromycin may increase the risk for pyloric stenosis in infants <6 wk old. Oseltamivir is not approved by FDA for infants <12 mo of age, but it can be used during influenza season when deemed necessary.
			Febrile, appears ill: Cefotaxime +/– oseltamivir	Consider adding vancomycin	
	Child 3 mo to 5 yr old	Viruses most common, *S. pneumoniae, Mycoplasma pneumoniae, Chlamydophila pneumoniae*, GAS, *S. aureus* (MRSA/MSSA)	Outpatient: Amoxicillin (high dose)	For severe penicillin allergy, consider Clindamycin *or* Azithromycin	Consider influenza antiviral therapy during influenza season.
			Inpatient: IV ampicillin *or* PCN +/– (clindamycin *or* vancomycin) +/– Oseltamivir	For severe penicillin allergy, [Clindamycin *or* Vancomycin] + azithromycin	Consider including clindamycin or vancomycin if there is pleural effusion, cavitary pneumonia, or more severe illness. Cefotaxime or ceftriaxone should be used rather than ampicillin/PCN for infants/children who are not fully immunized and in regions where local epidemiology of invasive pneumococcal strains documents high-level penicillin resistance.

				During influenza season, oseltamivir should be initiated early (within 48 hr). Note oseltamivir is approved by FDA for infants >12 mo old, but it can be used when deemed necessary in infants <12 mo old.
Child 5–15 yr old	Viruses most common, *S. pneumoniae*, *Mycoplasma, pneumoniae* *C. pneumoniae*, GAS, *S. aureus* (MRSA/MSSA), *M. tuberculosis*	Outpatient: Amoxicillin	Azithromycin +/– clindamycin	Consider influenza antiviral therapy during influenza season.
		Inpatient: IV ampicillin or PCN +/– [clindamycin *or* vancomycin] +/– azithromycin +/– oseltamivir (during influenza season)	For severe penicillin allergy, Azithromycin + [clindamycin *or* vancomycin] *or* Levofloxacin + [clindamycin *or* vancomycin]	Cefotaxime or ceftriaxone should be used rather than ampicillin/PCN for infants/children who are not fully immunized. Consider including clindamycin or vancomycin if there is pleural effusion, cavitary pneumonia, or more severe illness. Consider adding azithromycin if symptoms and epidemiology suggest atypical pneumonia. During influenza season, oseltamivir should be initiated early (within 48 hr).

Continued

2

TABLE 2-1

RECOMMENDED EMPIRIC ANTIMICROBIAL THERAPY FOR SELECTED CLINICAL SYNDROMES (Continued)

Syndrome	Host Category	Common Treatable Pathogens	Preferred Treatment	Alternative Treatment	Comments
Pneumonia	Immunocompromised patient, neutropenia, steroids, immunomodulators, graft-versus-host disease	Same as community-acquired pathogens; in addition, *P. aeruginosa*, other gram-negative organisms, *Aspergillus, Candida*	[Pip/tazo *or* cefepime] +/– AG +/– [Clindamycin or vancomycin] +/– Oseltamivir (during influenza season)	Imipenem *or* Meropenem	Send sputum for Gram stain and culture if possible. Therapy should be adjusted for culture data and clinical response. Low threshold for more definitive diagnostic procedures (i.e., bronchoscopy). Consider vancomycin or clindamycin with severe pneumonia and suspicion for MRSA. Also consider fungus, Pneumocystis, CMV, atypical mycobacteria, and other atypical bacteria, (e.g., *Nocardia*). During influenza season, oseltamivir should be initiated early (within 48 hr).
	Cystic fibrosis	*Pseudomonas* sp., *S. aureus*, other gram-negative organisms, especially *Burkholderia*	[Ceftazidime *or* Tic/clav *or* Cefepime] +/– AG +/– [clindamycin or vancomycin] +/– oseltamivir (during influenza season)	[Imipenem *or* Meropenem *or* FQ] +/– AG	Antimicrobials in conjunction with aggressive pulmonary toilet. Low threshold for adding additional antistaphylococcal coverage, particularly if no improvement. Culture results should be used to guide therapy. Also consider allergic bronchopulmonary aspergillosis, atypical mycobacteria. During influenza season, oseltamivir should be initiated early (within 48 hr).

HIV	*S. pneumoniae*, pathogens of community-acquired pneumonia; must also consider Pneumocystis, cryptococcosis, histoplasmosis, and tuberculosis based on CD4 count, antibiotic prophylaxis, and history.	(Ceftriaxone + azithromycin) +/– TMP/SMX +/– [clindamycin *or* vancomycin] +/– oseltamivir (during influenza season)	Severe penicillin allergy: (Vancomycin + AG) +/– TMP/SMX	Many experts would manage pneumonia in non–ill-appearing HIV-infected children receiving effective antiretroviral therapy and with preserved/restored CD4 counts in the same way as for children without HIV infection. TMP/SMX for PCP (CD4 <200 or <15%, especially with hypoxia). Induced sputum or BAL should be strongly considered, particularly in patients with CD4 <200 or 15%. Consider Pip/Tazo or cefepime for *Pseudomonas* if severe immunosuppression, damaged airways, and/or neutropenia. Consider adding clindamycin or vancomycin for MRSA coverage. During influenza season, oseltamivir should be initiated early (within 48 hr).
Neonates (<28 days old)	GBS, *Streptococcus* spp., *Listeria*, gram-negative organisms, particularly *E. coli, S. aureus,* HSV, CMV, enteroviruses	(Ampicillin + gentamicin) +/– cefotaxime		For neonates, consider adding vancomycin and acyclovir. Add cefotaxime if meningitis is a possible complication. Influenza antiviral therapy such as oseltamivir is not approved by FDA in <12-mo-old infants, but it can be used when it is deemed necessary during the influenza season.

Continued

2

TABLE 2-1

RECOMMENDED EMPIRIC ANTIMICROBIAL THERAPY FOR SELECTED CLINICAL SYNDROMES (Continued)

Syndrome	Host Category	Common Treatable Pathogens	Preferred Treatment	Alternative Treatment	Comments
Ventilator-associated pneumonia	All	Variable pathogens: *S. pneumoniae*, gram-negative bacilli (*Pseudomonas*, *Stenotrophomonas*, *Acinetobacter*, *Klebsiella*, etc.), *S. aureus*	Pip/tazo *or* Cefepime *or* Imipenem *or* Meropenem	Clindamycin + AG	Empiric therapy should be narrowed based on gram-stained smear and culture results promptly. Consider MRSA coverage. Ertapenem does not have antipseudomonal activity.
Bronchiolitis	All	Respiratory syncytial virus, parainfluenza virus, influenza virus, rhinovirus, human metapneumovirus	Supportive therapy		Infants <2 yr old with chronic lung disease, congestive heart disease, and/or prematurity (see AAP guidelines) should receive prophylactic RSV monoclonal antibody.
CENTRAL NERVOUS SYSTEM INFECTIONS					
Brain abscess	Previously healthy; complication of sinusitis (beyond neonatal period)	*Streptococcus* spp., gram-negative enterics, *Eikenella*, anaerobes, *S. pneumoniae*, *N. meningitidis*, *S. aureus*	Ceftriaxone + metronidazole +/− vancomycin	For patient with severe penicillin allergy, consider [Chloramphenicol *or* TMP/SMX] + metronidazole	Consider adding vancomycin (meningitic dose) for MRSA and penicillin/ceftriaxone non-susceptible *S. pneumoniae*. Surgical intervention may be required.

Immunocompromised patient	Consider *Listeria*, *Pseudomonas*, *Nocardia*, anaerobic bacteria, and fungi in addition to pathogens for community-acquired meningitis	(Ceftazidime *or* Cefepime) + vancomycin + metronidazole + ampicillin	For patient with severe penicillin allergy, consider Aztreonam + vancomycin + metronidazole	Consider amphotericin B if no response within 1 wk and organism unknown. Consider also *Toxoplasma* in patients with AIDS.
Complication of dental disease	Oral microflora (polymicrobial)	Penicillin (300,000 units/kg/day) + metronidazole	For patient with severe penicillin allergy, consider Vancomycin + metronidazole	Avoid clindamycin because of poor CNS penetration.
Postsurgery (neurosurgery, head trauma, CSF shunt–associated infection, cochlear implants)	Gram-negative organisms (including *Pseudomonas*) and *S. aureus*	(Ceftazidime *or* Cefepime) + vancomycin	Meropenem + vancomycin For patient with severe penicillin allergy, consider (Aztreonam *or* ciprofloxacin) + vancomycin	Add AG if gram-negative organisms seen on Gram stain.
Neonate	Group B *Streptococcus*, enteric gram-negative organisms (especially *Citrobacter* and *E. coli*), *Listeria*	Ampicillin + cefotaxime + AG		Attempt should be made to define specific pathogen. *Citrobacter* spp., *Enterobacter sakazakii*, and *Serratia marcescens* cause meningitis associated with brain abscesses.

Continued

TABLE 2-1

RECOMMENDED EMPIRIC ANTIMICROBIAL THERAPY FOR SELECTED CLINICAL SYNDROMES (Continued)

Syndrome	Host Category	Common Treatable Pathogens	Preferred Treatment	Alternative Treatment	Comments
Encephalitis	Previously healthy and beyond neonatal period	HSV, varicella-zoster virus	Acyclovir		Continue acyclovir until results from HSV PCR are available or alternate organism has been identified. Other causative factors include enteroviruses, arboviruses, including West Nile virus, EBV, cat-scratch disease (*Bartonella henselae*), Mycoplasma pneumoniae, rabies, Lyme disease (*Borrelia burgdorferi*), TB, malaria, and *Listeria* in immunocompromised patients. Autoimmune encephalitis due to antibodies against cell-surface proteins, such as NMDA, AMPA, and GABA(B) receptors is emerging as a common cause of encephalitis in children.
	Neonates	HSV	Acyclovir (60 mg/kg/day) in divided doses Q8 hr		For premature neonates, acyclovir dosage determined according to gestational age. Oral acyclovir suppressive therapy should be considered once patient completes IV therapy. Enteroviruses are most common cause.

Aseptic meningitis		*Borrelia burgdorferi*	Ceftriaxone *or* Cefotaxime	Doxycycline *or* Penicillin IV	Other causes of aseptic meningitis include viruses: enteroviruses, herpes viruses, lymphocytic choriomeningitis virus, arboviruses; fungi, TB, Mycoplasma pneumoniae; drugs: NSAIDs, sulfa antibiotics, immune globulins; cancer/systemic inflammatory diseases.
Bacterial meningitis (beyond neonatal period)	Community-acquired infection	*S. pneumoniae, N. meningitidis, H. influenzae* type b (rare in immunized populations)	(Ceftriaxone *or* Cefotaxime) + vancomycin (20 mg/kg/dose every 6–8 hr)	For patient with severe penicillin allergy, consider Chloramphenicol (instead of Ceftriaxone *or* Cefotaxime) + vancomycin	Benefit of dexamethasone with first dose (or 15–20 min prior) of antibiotics has been documented only for *H. influenzae* in children. Some experts also use for suspected pneumococcal infection. Vancomycin every 6 hr dosing preferred in children <12 yr old; levels should be monitored closely and dose adjusted accordingly. Prophylaxis of some close contacts is recommended for *N. meningitidis* and *H. influenzae* meningitis. See Chapter 8.
	Immunocompromised patient	In addition to community-acquired meningitis, consider *Listeria* and nonbacterial pathogens such as *Cryptococcus*	(Ceftriaxone *or* Cefotaxime) + ampicillin + vancomycin	(Cefepime *or* Meropenem) + TMP/SMX + vancomycin	Consider adding amphotericin B and flucytosine in patients with AIDS to treat *Cryptococcus.*

Continued

TABLE 2-1

RECOMMENDED EMPIRIC ANTIMICROBIAL THERAPY FOR SELECTED CLINICAL SYNDROMES (Continued)

Syndrome	Host Category	Common Treatable Pathogens	Preferred Treatment	Alternative Treatment	Comments
	Postsurgery (neurosurgery, head trauma, CSF shunt–associated infection, cochlear implants)	Consider *Pseudomonas* and staphylococci in addition to pathogens for community-acquired meningitis	(Ceftazidime *or* Cefepime) + vancomycin	Meropenem + vancomycin	
	Eosinophilic disease	*Angiostrongylus cantonensis*, *Baylisascaris procyonis*, *Gnathostoma spinigerum*, *Taenia solium*, noninfectious disorders (foreign body)	Identification of causative organism should be made before beginning antimicrobial; corticosteroids are beneficial in some cases		Although justified, examination of stool for ova and parasites may not be useful for all human neurotropic parasites. Neuroimaging may be useful for diagnosis. *A. cantonensis* is most common cause worldwide but not found in mainland United States; *B. procyonis* is found in the United States and is associated with exposure to raccoon feces; *G. spinigerum* is found in Southeast Asia in association with consumption of raw fish/poultry. Eosinophils also may be seen in CSF in meningitis due to *Toxoplasma*, *Cryptococcus*, and coccidioides.
	Neonatal	GBS, enteric gram-negative organisms (especially *E. coli*), *Listeria*	Ampicillin + cefotaxime (+ gentamicin if gram-negative organisms on Gram-stained smear)		In patients with diagnosis after prolonged hospitalization, consider coverage for *S. aureus*, enterococci, resistant enteric gram-negative organisms, and *Candida*.

GASTROINTESTINAL INFECTIONS

Intra-abdominal abscess	Community-acquired infection	Enteric gram-negative organisms, anaerobes, enterococci	(Ampicillin + gentamicin + metronidazole) *or* (Cefepime *or* Cefotaxime *or* ceftazidime) + metronidazole	Tic/clav *or* Pip/tazo *or* Imipenem *or* Meropenem For penicillin allergy: consider [Aztreonam + clindamycin] *or* (Ciprofloxacin + metronidazole)	Multiple organisms are usually involved. Surgical drainage may be required. Need to exclude complicated appendicitis; consider imaging, particularly in children <3 yr of age because they may present with atypical signs and symptoms. Ciprofloxacin for severe PCN allergy or resistant organism without other oral treatment options (≥1 yr old).
	Nosocomial infection	Above, + *Pseudomonas*	(Ceftazidime *or* cefepime) + metronidazole	Pip/tazo *or* Meropenem For penicillin allergy, consider (Aztreonam + clindamycin) *or* (Ciprofloxacin + metronidazole)	Surgical drainage may be required. Ciprofloxacin for severe PCN allergy or resistant organism without other oral treatment options (≥1 yr old).
	Perirectal infection	*S. aureus, S. pyogenes,* enteric gram-negative organisms and anaerobes	Clindamycin + gentamicin	BL/BLI +/– (clindamycin *or* vancomycin)	Surgical drainage important.

Continued

TABLE 2-1

RECOMMENDED EMPIRIC ANTIMICROBIAL THERAPY FOR SELECTED CLINICAL SYNDROMES (Continued)

Syndrome	Host Category	Common Treatable Pathogens	Preferred Treatment	Alternative Treatment	Comments
Intra-abdominal abscess *(Continued)*	Hepatic and/or splenic infection	*S. aureus*, *Brucella* spp., *Bartonella henselae*, gram-negative enterics, anaerobes	Clindamycin + (cefotaxime *or* ceftriaxone *or* cefepime *or* ceftazidime) + metronidazole	Pip/tazo *or* Imipenem *or* Meropenem	*Entamoeba histolytica* can cause liver abscess if intestinal organism migrates through bowel wall to portal circulation. If history and clinical findings suggest cat-scratch disease, azithromycin may shorten the course of illness. Consider CGD.
	Retroperitoneal infection	*S. aureus*, gram-negative enterics	Clindamycin + (cefotaxime *or* ceftriaxone *or* cefepime *or* ceftazidime)	Vancomycin instead of clindamycin	
Cholecystitis/cholangitis		Enteric gram-negative organisms, anaerobes, enterococci	Ampicillin + gentamicin + metronidazole	Tic/clav *or* Pip/tazo *or* Imipenem *or* Meropenem For penicillin allergy, consider Aztreonam + clindamycin	Drainage of obstructed biliary tract is an important component of therapy for severely ill patients.

Diarrhea	Antibiotic-associated infection	Perturbation of bowel flora, *Clostridium difficile*	Stop implicated antibiotic *C. difficile*–associated: oral Metronidazole (use IV drug only if oral drug cannot be administered)	Vancomycin PO *or* Metronidazole IV	Supportive care to maintain hydration status is important. Antimotility agents should be avoided. Limited data for Nitazoxanide. Fidamoxacin an option for adults, but no data for children. Some studies suggest that probiotics such as *Lactobacillus* are helpful in reducing antibiotic-associated diarrhea.
	Food- or water-borne disease	Bacterial (inflammatory): *E. coli, Salmonella, Shigella, Yersinia, Campylobacter*; parasitic: *Cryptosporidium, Giardia*	Antimicrobials are generally not recommended except for certain bacteria (*Shigella, Campylobacter*) and parasites (*Giardia*) Presumptive antimicrobial therapy for acute dysentery syndrome (blood and mucus in stool): cefixime *or* azithromycin	Ciprofloxacin *or* TMP/SMX *or* Ceftriaxone	Rehydration is the most important component of therapy. Some studies suggest that antimicrobial therapy increases the likelihood of hemolytic uremic syndrome in patients infected with enterohemorrhagic *E. coli.* Most common causes are not treatable: toxin-mediated (immediate-onset) *S. aureus, Bacillus cereus, C. perfringens*; viral: norovirus, rotavirus, astrovirus, enteric adenovirus; noninfectious causes (heavy metals, shellfish poisoning).
	Immunocompromised patient	In addition to above pathogens, *Listeria, Mycobacterium avium-intracellulare*, CMV, *Isospora, Cyclospora, Microsporidium*	Improve immune status; therapy should be guided by causative organism; no clear indication for empiric therapy; see specific organism		Specific laboratory testing and collection containers may be needed. Discuss with laboratory to ensure proper recovery.

2 *Continued*

TABLE 2-1

RECOMMENDED EMPIRIC ANTIMICROBIAL THERAPY FOR SELECTED CLINICAL SYNDROMES (Continued)

Syndrome	Host Category	Common Treatable Pathogens	Preferred Treatment	Alternative Treatment	Comments
Diarrhea *(Continued)*	Nosocomial infection	*C. difficile*	Stop implicated antibiotic, oral Metronidazole (use IV drug only if oral drug cannot be administered)	Vancomycin PO *or* Metronidazole IV	Most common causes are nontreatable: rotavirus, other viruses. There are limited data for Nitazoxamide to treat *C. difficile* in children. Fidamoxacin an option for adults but no data for children.
	Travel-associated infection	Traveler's diarrhea: enterotoxigenic *E. coli, Campylobacter, Salmonella, Shigella;* consider *Vibrio cholerae, E. histolytica* depending on epidemiology	Usually self-limited; may consider Azithromycin *or* Ciprofloxacin for traveler's diarrhea; see specific organism otherwise		Norovirus has been implicated in outbreaks on cruise ships.
Esophagitis	Almost all cases of infectious esophagitis occur in immunocompromised hosts	*C. albicans*, HSV, CMV	Fluconazole +/– Acyclovir IV	Amphotericin B *or* Caspofungin	Fluconazole if suspecting fungal organisms; acyclovir IV (if unable to take oral acyclovir or valacyclovir because of pain) if suspecting HSV. Infectious causes should prompt investigation for an immunologic disorder if seen in apparently immunocompetent host (i.e., HIV testing). Endoscopy, biopsy, and culture should be undertaken to determine specific pathogen and evaluate for noninfectious causes such as corrosive ingestion.

Necrotizing enterocolitis	Beyond neonatal period Immunocompromised patient: neutropenic host (typhilitis), AIDS, high-dose steroids, severe protein energy malnutrition	Enteric gram-negative organisms, anaerobes, enterococci; consider *Pseudomonas* in addition in hospitalized patients	(Ceftazidime *or* Cefepime) + metronidazole +/– ampicillin	Pip/tazo *or* Meropenem; For penicillin allergy, consider Aztreonam + clindamycin	Supportive management. Treat underlying disorder if possible; stop enteral feedings; surgical intervention may be required. Consider antifungal therapy if Gram stain or surgical specimen suggests fungal infection.
	Neonatal infection	Enteric gram-negative, streptococci, staphylococci, *Candida*	Ampicillin + gentamicin + metronidazole	Ampicillin + cefotaxime + metronidazole	Role of anaerobes is controversial. Adjust antibiotics if pathogen is recovered. Supportive management. Treat underlying disorder if possible; stop enteral feedings; surgical intervention may be required. Consider antifungal therapy if Gram stain or surgical specimen suggests fungal infection.
Peritonitis	Peritoneal dialysis–associated infection	Coagulase-negative staphylococci, *S. aureus,* gram-negative organisms, including *Pseudomonas, Candida*	(Ceftriaxone *or* Cefotaxime) + vancomycin		Therapy should be guided by appropriate cultures obtained before starting antimicrobials. Catheter removal may be necessary. Intraperitoneal therapy should be considered if the causative agent is known and use of the catheter is to be continued. Vancomycin, certain penicillins, cephalosporins, and AGs can be administered by this route.‡

Continued

TABLE 2-1

RECOMMENDED EMPIRIC ANTIMICROBIAL THERAPY FOR SELECTED CLINICAL SYNDROMES (Continued)

Syndrome	Host Category	Common Treatable Pathogens	Preferred Treatment	Alternative Treatment	Comments
Peritonitis *(Continued)*	Primary infection (spontaneous bacterial peritonitis)	*S. pneumoniae*, other streptococci, *S. aureus*, enteric gram-negative organisms	Ceftriaxone *or* Cefotaxime		Consider adding vancomycin for resistant *S. aureus* and *S. pneumoniae*. Tuberculosis should also be considered in the setting of appropriate epidemiology.
	Secondary infection (e.g., bowel perforation)	Enteric gram-negative organisms, anaerobes, *Enterococcus*; consider *Pseudomonas* in addition in hospitalized patients	[(Ampicillin + gentamicin) + (metronidazole *or* clindamycin)] *or* [(Ceftazidime *or* cefepime) + (metronidazole *or* clindamycin)]	Pip/tazo *or* Meropenem For penicillin allergy, consider Aztreonam + clindamycin	Surgical management is essential.
ODONTOGENIC INFECTIONS					
Gingivitis	Immunocompetent patients or patient with neutropenia	HSV	Acyclovir for HSV in immunocompromised host		Acyclovir may shorten the duration of symptoms but does not abort them. May be indicated in some healthy hosts with profound disease, hospitalized for, or at risk for, dehydration. Neutropenia and neutrophil defects may be associated with gingivitis. Only normal oral flora isolated.

Ludwig angina		Oral microflora (polymicrobial)	Ampicillin/sulbactam	For penicillin allergy, Clindamycin	Surgical drainage essential.
Periodontitis	Immunocompetent patient or patient with neutropenia	Oral microflora (polymicrobial)	A/C *or* Clindamycin		Neutropenia and neutrophil defects may be associated with gingivitis. Only normal oral flora isolated.
Stomatitis		HSV, aphthous stomatitis	Acyclovir	Famciclovir *or* Valacyclovir for adolescents	Acyclovir may be indicated in some healthy hosts with profound disease, hospitalized for, or at risk for, dehydration. Antimicrobials do not shorten the course of aphthous stomatitis.
Thrush		*C. albicans*	Nystatin topically	Fluconazole *or* Gentian violet *or* Clotrimazole	Mucosal candidiasis in >6 mo of age and in the absence of immunosuppressive or antimicrobial therapy should prompt investigation for immunologic disorder.
UPPER RESPIRATORY TRACT INFECTIONS					
OTITIS EXTERNA					
Malignant otitis externa	Generally immunosuppressed patient (AIDS, neutropenia, malignant tumor, or diabetes)	*Pseudomonas, Aspergillus*	Ceftazidime *or* cefepime; *or* ciprofloxacin-resistant organism without other oral treatment options (≥1 yr old). Consider amphotericin B if spread to soft tissues of face and scalp	Ciprofloxacian	Antimicrobials are adjunctive therapy; meticulous debridement and irrigation are essential. *Aspergillus* infection is associated with high mortality rate. Consider ciprofloxacin for resistant organism without other oral treatment options (≥1 yr old)

Continued

2

TABLE 2-1

RECOMMENDED EMPIRIC ANTIMICROBIAL THERAPY FOR SELECTED CLINICAL SYNDROMES (Continued)

Syndrome	Host Category	Common Treatable Pathogens	Preferred Treatment	Alternative Treatment	Comments
Swimmer's ear		*Pseudomonas,* gram-negative organisms, fungi (*Aspergillus niger, Candida*)	Local instillation of 2% vinegar or topical otic antibiotic drops (Ciprofloxacin *or* Polymyxin-neomycin)		Use analgesics for pain. For moderate to severe illness, use wick after removal of excessive debris from ear canal.
OTITIS MEDIA					
Acute otitis media		*S. pneumoniae, M. catarrhalis, H. influenzae* non-type b	Not severe <2 yr: Amoxicillin (80–90 mg/kg/day in 2 doses); observe if >6 mo and diagnosis not certain >2 yr: observe	For penicillin allergy, Cefdinir *or* Cefuroxime For severe penicillin allergy, Azithromycin If cannot take oral medications, Ceftriaxone	Use analgesics when pain present. "Observe" means deferring antimicrobials and then reevaluating at 48–72 hr. Failure to respond in 48–72 hr: if no therapy initially, start antimicrobial therapy; if amoxicillin used as initial therapy, switch to A/C. Treat for 10 days. Shorter course of 5–7 days acceptable for healthy children ≥6 yr old.
			Severe (moderate to severe otalgia or fever ≥39°C) A/C (80–90 mg/kg/day amoxicillin in 2 doses)	Cefuroxime *or* Cefdinir	Failure to respond in 48–72 hr: ceftriaxone. *or* Consider tympanocentesis and culture.
Chronic suppurative otitis media (see Chronic mastoiditis on p. 165)					
Otitis media with effusion		Viruses, prelude/sequela of acute otitis media	Symptomatic treatment		

PAROTITIS				
Acute infection	*S. aureus*, gram-negative organisms (neonate)	Clindamycin Neonates: Vancomycin + (AG or PCS3)	Nafcillin/oxacillin	Common causes include viruses: mumps, HIV, EBV, enteroviruses, etc. Surgical drainage and rehydration alone may be curative. Recurrent acute sialadenitis can occur once every few months to years; its pathogenesis is unknown; it usually resolves at adolescence.
Subacute/chronic infection		There is no indication for presumptive therapy without a clear diagnosis		Possible causative factors include mycobacteria, HIV, sarcoidosis, Sjögren syndrome, tumors.
INFECTIONS OF PHARYNX, LARYNX, AND TRACHEA				
Epiglottitis	*S. aureus, S. pyogenes, S. pneumoniae, H. influenzae* type b (rare in vaccinated populations)	(Cefotaxime *or* Ceftriaxone) + (clindamycin *or* vancomycin)		Artificial airway should be placed promptly in the operating room under controlled conditions. Frequent suctioning of airway is critical. Effective presumptive antistaphylococcal therapy should be determined based on local susceptibility patterns.
Laryngitis				Caused by a variety of respiratory viruses.
Lemierre syndrome (jugular vein septic phlebitis)	*Fusobacterium*, oral microflora	Metronidazole + (ceftriaxone *or* cefotaxime *or* cefuroxime)	(Pip/tazo *or* tic/clav) + (meropenem *or* imipenem)	May require surgical drainage. Some experts also recommend anticoagulation.

Continued

TABLE 2-1

RECOMMENDED EMPIRIC ANTIMICROBIAL THERAPY FOR SELECTED CLINICAL SYNDROMES (Continued)

Syndrome	Host Category	Common Treatable Pathogens	Preferred Treatment	Alternative Treatment	Comments
Parapharyngeal/ retropharyngeal/ peritonsillar abscess		*S. pyogenes,* other streptococci, *S. aureus,* oral microflora/anaerobes	Ampicillin/sulbactam *or* [(Ceftriaxone *or* Cefotaxime) + clindamycin]		Surgical drainage required. Close observation of the airway as artificial airway may be required.
Pharyngitis, exudative infection		*S. pyogenes* (GAS), group C and G streptococci, *Arcanobacterium haemolyticum, Mycoplasma*	For documented group A streptococcal infection, oral Penicillin V. (Amoxicillin is an acceptable alternative.)	For penicillin allergy, clindamycin *or* macrolides *or* cephalosporins	Other potential pathogens include *N. gonorrhoeae,* diphtheria, viruses, including EBV, influenza. For nonstreptococcal pharyngitis, therapy should be determined based on proven or suspected cause.
Vesicular pharyngitis/ stomatitis		Coxsackievirus, other enteroviruses, HSV	HSV infection: consider Acyclovir in immunocompromised host		Acyclovir may be indicated in some healthy hosts with profound disease, hospitalized for, or at risk for, dehydration.
Tracheitis	Normal host; community-acquired infection	Bacterial infection (*S. aureus,* group A *Streptococcus, Streptococcus pneumoniae*) may complicate viral infection (influenza virus, parainfluenza virus)	Bacterial: (Clindamycin *or* Nafcillin, *or* Oxacillin) + PCS3 Viral: Oseltamivir *or* Zanamivir	Vancomycin	Choice of antibacterial should be guided by local MRSA susceptibility patterns. Intubation and suctioning critical for bacterial tracheitis.

	Associated with tracheostomy or intubated trachea/ nosocomial	*Pseudomonas,* other gram-negative organisms, *S. aureus*	Cefepime	Pip/tazo *or* Meropenem For penicillin allergy, consider Aztreonam + clindamycin	Guide therapy based on culture data. Antimicrobials will only treat the acute episode but will not eradicate the organism if device present. Short course of antibiotics (5–7 days) is usually sufficient.
Sinusitis	Acute infection				
	Community-acquired infection	*S. pneumoniae, M. catarrhalis, H. influenzae* non-type b	Mild to moderate A/C (45–50 mg/kg/day amoxicillin). Consider high-dose amoxicillin (80–90 mg/kg/day) in areas of high (≥10%) non-susceptible *S. pneumoniae.*	For penicillin allergy, Cefpodoxime *or* Cefuroxime *or* Cefdinir *or* Azithromycin *or* RFQ	Failure to respond in 48–72 hr: high-dose A/C. Failure to respond in 48–72 hr: imaging and/or sinus drainage. Alternatively, a trial with IV cefotaxime or ceftriaxone may be used. Treat sinusitis for at least 10–14 days.
	Immunocompromised patient (neutropenia, diabetes, AIDS, deferoxamine therapy)	*S. aureus, Pseudomonas,* gram-negative organisms, anaerobes, *Rhizopus, Mucor, Aspergillus*	(Cefepime *or* Pip/tazo) + amphotericin B	High-dose liposomal Amphotericin B may be more efficacious	Surgical intervention required. *Rhizopus, Mucor* should be considered in patients on long courses of voriconazole.

2

TABLE 2-1

RECOMMENDED EMPIRIC ANTIMICROBIAL THERAPY FOR SELECTED CLINICAL SYNDROMES (Continued)

Syndrome	Host Category	Common Treatable Pathogens	Preferred Treatment	Alternative Treatment	Comments
Sinusitis *(Continued)*	Nosocomial (especially with nasal tubes)	*Pseudomonas*, gram-negative organisms, *S. aureus*, polymicrobial	Cefepime	Pip/tazo *or* Meropenem For penicillin allergy, consider Aztreonam + clindamycin	Remove nasal tube. Guide therapy based on culture data.
	Chronic infection	*S. pneumoniae*, *M. catarrhalis*, *H. influenzae* non-type B, *S. aureus*, anaerobes	A/C (80–90 mg/kg/day) +/– clindamycin (anaerobic coverage, MRSA, PCN allergy)	(Ceftriaxone *or* Cefotaxime) +/– (clindamycin *or* vancomycin) *or* Metronidazole + (cefuroxime, *or* cefpodoxime *or* cefdinir)	Consider culture to guide therapy. Continue antibiotic therapy for 14–21 days. Underlying disorders (anatomic defects, allergic rhinitis, cystic fibrosis, immunodeficiency, ciliary dyskinesia) should be ruled out.

Mastoiditis	Acute infection	*S. pneumoniae, S. pyogenes, S. aureus*	Vancomycin empirically *or* Clindamycin		Surgical management required. Definitive therapy should be guided by culture obtained at surgery. Add antipseudomonal agent if prior history of antibiotic exposure with prior ear infections.
	Chronic (chronic suppurative otitis media)	*Pseudomonas,* gram-negative organisms, *S. aureus*	Ofloxacin otic drops	Ceftazidime *or* Cefepime	Daily suctioning of the external canal (aural toilet) is an important part of therapy. Consider addition of ceftazidime or cefepime in patients at risk for resistant organisms and/or who have not responded to topical therapy.
Cervical lymphadenitis	Acute infection	*S. aureus, S. pyogenes;* consider GBS in neonates	A/C *or* Cephalexin *or* Dicloxacillin *or* Clindamycin (if MRSA prevalent)	For penicillin allergy, Cefdinir *or* Cefuroxime For severe penicillin allergy, Vancomycin	Bacteria usually cause unilateral or bilateral lymphadenitis, whereas viruses (EBV, rubella virus, adenovirus) cause bilateral lymphadenitis (lymphadenopathy). Neonates should be treated with parenteral antibiotics. Kawasaki disease presents with nonsuppurative, unilateral cervical lymphadenopathy. Surgical drainage may be required in some cases.

2

Chapter 3

Drug Dosing in Special Circumstances

Angela M. Helder, PharmD, BCPS, Elizabeth A. Sinclair, PharmD, BCPS, and Carlton K. K. Lee, PharmD, MPH

I. GENERAL PEDIATRIC DRUG DOSING

A. Body Mass Calculation

The most common method of individualized pediatric drug dosing is body mass dosing (mg/kg). Conversion from pounds (lb) to metric kilograms (kg) is as follows:

$$\text{Wt(kg)} = \frac{\text{Wt(lb)}}{2.2}$$

B. Body Surface Area Calculation

Certain antimicrobial agents (e.g., acyclovir and cotrimoxazole) require body surface area (BSA) dosing. It has been suggested that drugs that are distributed extensively into extracellular water (ECW) should be dosed by surface area (SA) because ECW and total body water are better paralleled by SA than by body weight. The following nomogram or Mosteller formula can be used in children.

1. **Nomogram:** SA is determined by drawing a straight line that connects the patient's height and weight. The intersection of the straight line on the SA column reflects the value. If the patient is roughly of average size, SA can be determined by weight alone as indicated in the second column (Fig. 3-1).
2. Alternative Mosteller formula:*

$$\text{BSA}(\text{m}^2) = \sqrt{\frac{\text{Ht(cm)} \times \text{Wt(kg)}}{3600}}$$

*Equation from Mosteller RD: Simplified calculation of body surface area. *N Engl J Med.* 1987;317(17):1098.

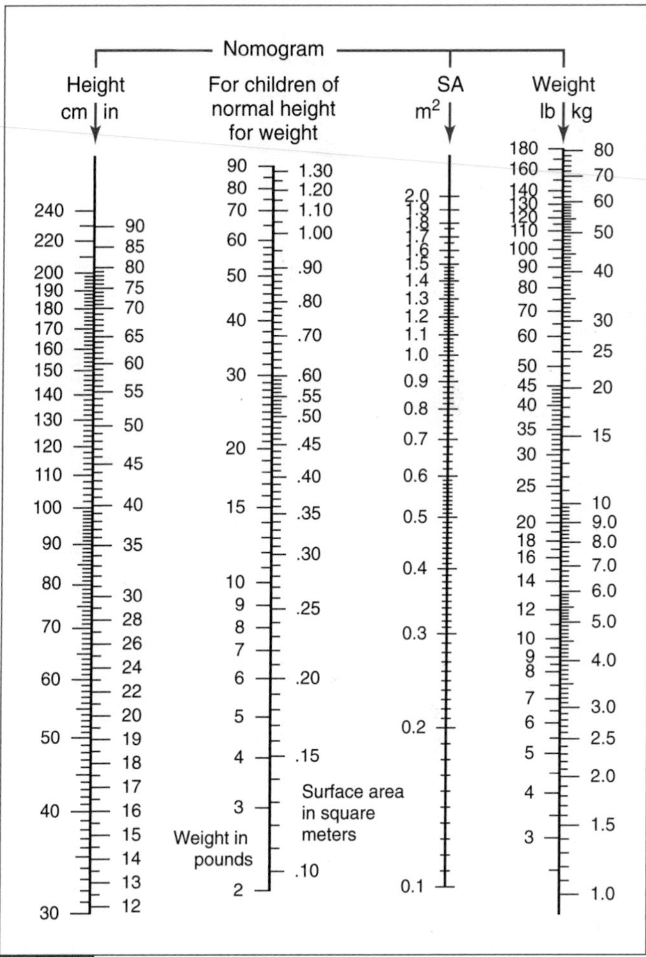

FIGURE 3-1

Surface area estimation: pocket calculator versus nomogram. *(Data from Briars GL, Bailey BJ. Surface area estimation: Pocket calculator v nomogram. Arch Dis Child. 1994;70:246–247.)*

II. DEVELOPMENTAL DOSING CONSIDERATIONS (DEVELOPMENTAL PHARMACOLOGY) (TABLE 3-1)

TABLE 3-1

AGE-DEPENDENT PHYSIOLOGIC VARIABLES INFLUENCING DRUG DISPOSITION IN CHILDREN (for notes and abbreviations used in this table, see p. xvi.)

Disposition Parameter	Physiologic Variable vs. Adult	Age When Adult Level Achieved	Pharmacokinetic Result	Example Drug
ABSORPTION				
Perioral pH	↑ Gastric pH (lower acid output)	3 mo	↑ Bioavailability of basic drugs ↓ Bioavailability of acidic drugs	Penicillin
GI motility	↓ Gastric and intestinal motility (gastric emptying time is 6–8 hr at birth)	6–8 mo	Unpredictable bioavailability and prolonged time to peak concentration	
GI contents	↓ Bile acids and pancreatic enzymes	~1 yr	↓ Bioavailability of fat-soluble drugs	
Intramuscular	↓ Vascular perfusion	?		
Percutaneous	↑ Absorption	4-mo epidermal layer with ↑ BSA/weight ratio with neonates	↑ Absorption	Lindane (Kwell) seizures, contraindicated
DISTRIBUTION				
% Body water	↑ Total body water ↑ Extracellular body water, rapid changes in first year	~12 yr	↑ Volume of distribution of water-soluble drugs	Aminoglycosides
% Fat	Full-term birth at 12%–16%, ↑ at 5–10 yr of age followed by a ↓	~17 yr		
Plasma proteins	↓ Total protein, albumin, and α-1 acid glycoprotein	Gradual changes over the first year	↑ Volume of distribution and free drug concentration of protein-bound drugs	Nafcillin, ampicillin
	↑ Unconjugated bilirubin and free fatty acids	Gradual changes over the first year	Potential displacement of bilirubin with highly protein-bound drugs	Sulfamethoxazole, ceftriaxone
Blood–brain barrier	Immature barrier caused by incomplete myelination	?	↑ CNS penetration	Aminoglycosides

METABOLISM				
CYP-450 ENZYME				
1A2 isoform	Lower at birth	4 mo; may exceed adult levels before decreasing to adult levels at puberty	Altered drug clearance; maturation dependent	
2C9 isoform*	Lower at birth	6 mo; exceeds adult levels at 3–10 yr before decreasing to adult levels after puberty	Altered drug clearance; maturation dependent	
2C19 isoform*	Lower at birth; 50% of adult at 1 mo to 10 yr	?; infant levels may exceed adults	Altered drug clearance; maturation dependent	Voriconazole
2D6 isoform*	Lower at birth; 50% of adult at 1 mo	3–5 yr; pharmacogenomics effects > ontogeny	Altered drug clearance; maturation dependent	
2E1 isoform	Lower at birth	?	Altered drug clearance; maturation dependent	Isoniazid
3A4 isoform*,†	Lower at birth; 30%–40% of adult at 1 mo	6 mo; may exceed adult levels at 1–4 mo before decreasing to adult levels after puberty	Altered drug clearance; maturation dependent	Erythromycin, protease inhibitors
Glucuronidation*	Lower at birth	6–24 mo; isoform specific (≥10 different isoforms)	↓ Glucuronide metabolite	Chloramphenicol, zidovudine
Sulphation*	At adult level			
N-acetyltransferase*	Lower	3–4 yr	Altered drug clearance; maturation and genetic dependence	Sulfamethoxazole, isoniazid
ELIMINATION				
Glomerular filtration	Lower at birth, especially if preterm	3–6 mo	↑ Elimination $T_{1/2}$	Aminoglycosides
Tubular secretion	Lower at birth	7 mo–1 yr	↑ Elimination $T_{1/2}$	Penicillins, sulfonamides

Modified from Misap RL, Hill MR, Szelfler SL. Special pharmacokinetic considerations in children. In Evans WE, editor: *Applied Pharmacokinetics,* ed 3, Spokane, Wash, 1992, Applied Therapeutics; and Blake MJ, Castro L, Leeder SJ, et al. Ontogeny on drug metabolizing enzymes in the neonate. *Semin Fetal Neonatal Med* 10:123–138, 2005.

III. DRUG DOSING IN RENAL INSUFFICIENCY

Many drugs are excreted by the kidneys and may require dosage adjustments with renal insufficiency. Age-specific normal values of glomerular filtration rates (GFRs) are listed in Table 3-2. See section III.B.3 and Table 3-3 for information on antimicrobials requiring dosage adjustment in renal insufficiency.

A. Glomerular Filtration Rate Estimation Methods

Calculations using either the Cockroft and Gault method or the Jelliffe method are designed specifically for adults and should not be used in pediatrics. The creatinine clearance rate (CrCl) is used clinically as a substitute for actual measuring of the GFR.

1. **Urinary creatinine method:** The urinary creatinine method estimates the GFR.

   The CrCl actually measures the theoretical volume of plasma cleared of creatinine in a finite period of time (mL/min). Although creatinine clearance is used to estimate GFR, it usually overestimates GFR (especially when GFR is low) because some creatinine is secreted by the renal tubules. The CrCl is usually inaccurate in children with obstructive uropathy or problems with bladder emptying.

$$\text{Formula*: } CrCl = \frac{Cr_u \times V}{Cr_p} \times \frac{1.73}{BSA}$$

   where

   CrCl = creatinine clearance (mL/min/1.73 m^2),
   Cr_u = urine creatinine concentration (mg/dL),
   V = volume of urine collected divided by duration of collection (mL/min),
   Cr_p = plasma creatinine (mg/dL), may use average of two levels, and
   BSA = body surface area measured in meters squared.

2. **Serum creatinine methods:** Serum creatinine methods are used to estimate creatinine clearance without the need for urine collection. Creatinine clearance is used clinically as a substitute for actual measuring of the GFR. The proper GFR estimation formula/method is dependent on the type of serum creatinine assay used to measure serum creatinine. The original Schwartz method and more recent Bedside Schwartz method were developed by using the alkaline picrate (Jaffe) and isotope dilution mass spectrometry (IDMS)–traceable serum creatinine assay methods, respectively. Use of the original Schwartz method with the more specific IDMS-traceable serum creatinine assay is known to overestimate GFR inversely

*Equation from Cohen ML, Rifkind D. *The Pediatric Abacus: Review of Clinical Formulas and How to Use Them.* London: Informa Healthcare; 2002.

TABLE 3-2

NORMAL VALUES OF GLOMERULAR FILTRATION RATE

Age	Mean Glomerular Filtration Rate (mL/min/1.73 m^2)	Range (mL/min/1.73 m^2)
NEONATES <34 WK GESTATIONAL AGE		
2–8 days	11	11–15
4–28 days	20	15–28
30–90 days	50	40–65
NEONATES ≥34 WK GESTATIONAL AGE		
2–8 days	39	17–60
4–28 days	47	26–68
30–90 days	58	30–86
1–6 mo	77	39–114
6–12 mo	103	49–157
12–19 mo	127	62–191
2 yr to adult	127	89–165

Data from Holliday MA, Barratt TM, Avner ED, editors: *Pediatric nephrology,* ed 3, Baltimore, Md, 1994, Williams & Wilkins.

proportional to the level of renal function and has been reported in pediatric patients with bone marrow transplant.[1–4] Check with your clinical laboratory to see which serum assay is in use at your institution.

Independent of serum creatinine assay method used, the following conditions may contribute to inaccurate GFR estimations[5]:

- Underestimate renal function (increase creatinine production): African American patients, muscular body types, and excessive ingestion of cooked meats (protein)
- Overestimate renal function (decrease creatinine production): increased age, female patients, Asian patients, amputees, malnutrition, inflammation, cancer, cardiovascular diseases, neuromuscular diseases, and vegetarian diet

a. Alkaline picrate (Jaffe) serum creatinine assay (original Schwartz method)[2]:

$$\mathrm{CrCl} = \frac{k \times \mathrm{L}}{\mathrm{S_{cr}}}$$

where

CrCl is measured in mL/min/1.73 m^2,

k = constant (see the following list),

L = body length (cm),

S_{cr} = serum creatinine concentration (mg/dL); measured by alkaline picrate (Jaffe) method.

Continued on page 185

TABLE 3-3

ANTIMICROBIALS REQUIRING ADJUSTMENTS IN RENAL FAILURE[6–10] (for notes and abbreviations used in this table, see p. xvi.)

	Adjustments in Renal Failure							
	Pharmacokinetics				Creatinine Clearance (mL/min)			
Drug	**Route of Excretion***	**Normal T1/2 (hr)**	**Normal Dose Interval**	**Method**	**Mild (>50)**	**Moderate (10–50)**	**Severe (<10)**	**Supplemental Dose for Dialysis**
Acyclovir (IV)	Renal	2–4	Q8 hr	DI	Q8 hr	Q12 hr (CrCl 25–50) Q24 hr (CrCl 10–25)	50% and Q24 hr	Y (He) N (P)
Adefovir (PO)	Renal	7.5	Q24 hr	I	Q24 hr	Q48 hr (CrCl 30–49) Q72 hr (CrCl 10–29)	Q72 hr	N (He, P)
Amantadine	Renal	10–28	Q12–24 hr	I	Q12–24 hr	Q24 hr (CrCl 30–50) Q48 hr (CrCl 15–29)	Q7 days (CrCl <15)	N (He, P)
Amikacin[†]	Renal	1.5–3	Q8–12 hr	I	Q8–12 hr	Give usual initial dose × 1 and monitor levels	Give usual initial dose × 1 and monitor levels	Y (He, P)
Amoxicillin	Renal	1–3.7	Q8–12 hr	I	Q8–12 hr	Q12 hr (CrCl 10–30)	Q24 hr	Y (He)
Amoxicillin-clavulanate	Renal	1	Q8–12 hr	I	Q8–12 hr	Q12 hr (CrCl 10–30)	Q24 hr	Y (He)
Amphotericin B	Renal (40% over 7 days)	Initial: 15–48 hr Terminal: 15 days	Q24 hr	D, I	Dosage adjustments are unnecessary with preexisting renal impairment; if decreased renal function is due to amphotericin B, the daily dose can be decreased by 50% or the dose given every other day.			N (He, P)
Amphotericin B, cholesteryl sulfate (Amphotec)		28–29	Q24 hr		No guidelines established			N (He, P)

Amphotericin B, lipid complex (Abelcet)	Renal 1%	173	Q24 hr		No guidelines established			N (He, P)
Amphotericin B, liposomal (AmBisome)	Renal ≤10%	100–153	Q24 hr		No guidelines established			N (He, P)
Ampicillin	Renal	1–4	Q6 hr	I	Q6 hr	Q8–12 hr (CrCl 10–29)	Q12 hr	Y (He)
Ampicillin/sulbactam	Renal	1–1.8	Q4–6 hr	I	Q4–6 hr	Q12 hr (CrCl 15–29)	Q24 hr (CrCl <15)	Y (He)
Aztreonam	Renal (hepatic)	1.3–2.2	Q6–12 hr	D	100%	50% (CrCl 10–30)	25%	Y (He)
Cefaclor	Renal	0.5–1	Q8–12 hr	D	100%	100%	50%	Y (He)
Cefadroxil	Renal	1–2	Q12 hr	I	Q12 hr	Q24 hr (CrCl 10–25)	Q36 hr	Y (He, P)
Cefazolin **NOTE:** Give initial loading dose, then adjust subsequent doses for renal function.	Renal	1.5–2.5	Q6–8 hr	DI	60% Q12 hr (CrCl 40–70)	25% Q12 hr (CrCl 20–40)	10% Q24 hr (CrCl <20)	Y (He)
Cefdinir	Renal	1.1–2.3	Q12–24 hr	DI	Q12–24 hr	7 mg/kg/dose Q24 hr [max dose 300 mg (CrCl <30)]	7 mg/kg/dose Q24 hr (maximum dose 300 mg)	Y (He)
Cefditoren pivoxil	Renal	1.2–2	Q12 hr	DI	100%	200 mg Q12 hr (maximum) (CrCl 30–49) 200 mg Q24 hr (maximum) (CrCl <30)	200 mg Q24 hr (maximum)	?

Continued

TABLE 3-3

ANTIMICROBIALS REQUIRING ADJUSTMENTS IN RENAL FAILURE (Continued)

	Adjustments in Renal Failure							
	Pharmacokinetics				Creatinine Clearance (mL/min)			
Drug	Route of Excretion*	Normal T1/2 (hr)	Normal Dose Interval	Method	Mild (>50)	Moderate (10–50)	Severe (<10)	Supplemental Dose for Dialysis
Cefepime	Renal	1.8–2	Q8–12 hr	DI	*Q12 hr regimens:* 100% and Q24 hr (CrCl 30–60) *Q8 hr regimens:* 100% and Q12 hr (CrCl 30–60)	50%–100% and Q24 hr (CrCl 11–29) 100% and Q24 hr (CrCl 11–29)	25%–50% and Q24 hr 50% and Q24 hr	Y (He)
Cefixime	Renal (hepatic)	3–4	Q12–24 hr	D	100%	75% (CrCl 21–60) 50% (CrCl <20)	50%	Y (He)
Cefotaxime	Renal	1–3.5	Q4–12 hr	I	Normal interval	Q8–12 hr (CrCl 30–50) Q12 hr (CrCl 10–29)	Q24 hr	Y (He)
Cefotetan	Renal (hepatic)	3.5	Q12 hr	I	Q12 hr	Q24 hr (CrCl 10–30)	Q48 hr	Y (He)
Cefoxitin	Renal	0.75–1.5	Q4–8 hr	I	Normal interval	Q8–12 hr (CrCl 30–50) Q12–24 hr (CrCl 10–30)	Q24–48 hr	Y (He)
Cefpodoxime proxetil	Renal	2.2	Q12 hr	I	Q12 hr	Q24 hr (CrCl <30)	Q24 hr	Y (He) N (P)
Cefprozil	Renal	1.3	Q12–24 hr	D	100%	50% (CrCl <30)	50%	Y (He)
Ceftazidime	Renal	1–2	Q8–12 hr	I	Q8–12 hr	Q12 hr (CrCl 30–50) Q24 hr (CrCl 10–30)	Q24–48 hr	Y (He)
Ceftibuten	Renal	1.5–2.5	Q24 hr	D	100%	50% (CrCl 30–49)	25% (CrCl 5–29)	Y (He)
Cefuroxime (IV)	Renal	1.6–2.2	Q8–12 hr	I	Q8–12 hr	Q12 hr (CrCl 10–20)	Q24 hr	Y (He)

Cephalexin	Renal	0.5–1.2	Q6 hr	I	Q6 hr	Q8–12 hr	Q12–24 hr	Y (He)
Cephapirin	Renal	0.6–0.8	Q4–6 hr	I	Q6 hr	Q6–8 hr	Q12 hr	Y (He)
Chloroquine hydrochloride/ phosphate	Renal	6–60 days	Q24 hr	D	100%	100%	50%	?
Ciprofloxacin	Renal (hepatic)	1.2–5	Q8–12 hr	D, I	100%	50–75% or Q18 hr (CrCl <30)	50% or Q24 hr	Y (He, P)
Clarithromycin	Renal/hepatic	3–7	Q12 hr	DI	No change	50% and Q12 hr (CrCl <30)	50% and Q24 hr	Y (He)
Colistimethate sodium	Renal	1.6–4	Q6–12 hr	DI	No change	See package insert	See package insert	Y (He)
Cycloserine	Renal	10–25	Q12 hr	I	100%	Q24 hr	Q36–48 hr	N (He)
Daptomycin	Renal	7–11	Q24 hr	I	100%	Q48 hr (CrCl <30)	Q48 hr	Y (He, P)
Didanosine	Renal	1.3–1.5	Q12 hr	DI	Patients <60 kg: CrCl 30–59 = 75 mg Q12 hr or 150 mg Q24 hr (oral solution) or 125 mg once daily (delayed-release capsule) CrCl 10–29 = 100 mg Q24 hr or 125 mg once daily (delayed-release capsule) CrCl <10 = 75 mg Q24 hr (oral solution) or use alternative formulation (delayed-release capsule) Patients ≥60 kg: CrCl 30–59 = 100 mg Q12 hr or 200 mg Q24 hr (oral solution) or 200 mg once daily (delayed-release capsule) CrCl 10–29 = 150 mg Q24 hr (oral solution) or 125 mg once daily (delayed-release capsule) CrCl <10 = 100 mg Q24 hr (oral solution) or 125 mg once daily (delayed-release capsule)			N (He, P)

Continued

TABLE 3-3

ANTIMICROBIALS REQUIRING ADJUSTMENTS IN RENAL FAILURE (Continued)

	Adjustments in Renal Failure							
	Pharmacokinetics				Creatinine Clearance (mL/min)			
Drug	**Route of Excretion***	**Normal T1/2 (hr)**	**Normal Dose Interval**	**Method**	**Mild (>50)**	**Moderate (10–50)**	**Severe (<10)**	**Supplemental Dose for Dialysis**
Doripenem	Renal	1	Q8 hr	DI	100%	50% (CrCl 30–50) 50% and Q12 hr (CrCl 10–30)	No recommendation available	?
Emtricitabine	Renal	10	Q24 hr	D, I	CrCl 30–49 = Q48 hr (capsule) or 50% (solution) CrCl 15–29 = Q72 hr (capsule) or 33.3% (solution) CrCl <15 = Q96 hr (capsule) or 25% (solution)			Y (He)
Entecavir	Renal	129–148	Q24 hr	DI	100%	50% or Q48 hr (CrCl 30–49) 30% or Q72 hr (CrCl 10–29)	10% or Q7 days	Y (He, P)
Ertapenem	Renal (hepatic)	4	Q12–24 hr	D	100%	50% (CrCl <30)	50%	Y (He)
Erythromycin	Hepatic (renal)	1.5–2	Q6–8 hr	D	100%	100%	50%–75%	N (He, P)
Ethambutol	Renal (hepatic)	2.5–3.6	Q24 hr	I	Q24 hr	Q24–36 hr	Q48 hr	Y (He)
Ethionamide	Renal	1.85–3	Q8–12 hr	D	100%	100%	50%	N (He, P)

Famciclovir	Renal (hepatic)	2–3	500 mg Q8 hr	DI	500 mg Q12 hr (CrCl 40–59)	500 mg Q24 hr (CrCl 20–39)	250 mg Q48 hr (CrCl <20)	Y (He)
Fluconazole[†]	Renal	19–25	Q24 hr	D	100%	50% (CrCl <50)	50%	Y (He)
Flucytosine[†]	Renal	3–8	Q6 hr	I	Q6 hr	Q12 hr (CrCl 20–40) Q24 hr (CrCl 10–20)	Q24–48 hr	Y (He, P)
Foscarnet	Renal	3–4.5	Q8–12 hr	D		See package insert		Y (He)
Ganciclovir	Renal	2.5–3.6	IV: Q12 hr	DI	Induction (IV): 50% and Q12 hr (CrCl 50–69) Maintenance (IV): 50% and Q24 hr (CrCl 50–69)	50% and Q24 hr (CrCl 25–49) 25% and Q24 hr (CrCl 10–24) Maintenance: 25% and Q24 hr (CrCl 25–49) 12.5% and Q24 hr (CrCl 10–24)	25% post-HD Maintenance: 12.5% post-HD	Y (He) N (P)
Gemifloxacin	Hepatic (renal)	4–12	Q24 hr	D	100%	50% (CrCl <40)	50%	Y (He, P)
Gentamicin[†,‡]	Renal	1.5–3	Q8–12 hr	I	Q8–12 hr	Give usual initial dose × 1 and monitor levels	Give usual initial dose × 1 and monitor levels	Y (He, P)
Imipenem/cilastatin	Renal	1–1.4	Q6–8 hr	DI	50% and Q6 hr (CrCl 41–70)	37% and Q8 hr (CrCl 21–40) 25% and Q12 hr (CrCl 6–20)	Avoid unless HD (CrCl <5)	Y (He)

Continued

TABLE 3-3

ANTIMICROBIALS REQUIRING ADJUSTMENTS IN RENAL FAILURE (Continued)

	Adjustments in Renal Failure							
	Pharmacokinetics				Creatinine Clearance (mL/min)			
Drug	**Route of Excretion***	**Normal T1/2 (hr)**	**Normal Dose Interval**	**Method**	**Mild (>50)**	**Moderate (10–50)**	**Severe (<10)**	**Supplemental Dose for Dialysis**
Kanamycin	Renal	2–3	Q8 hr	DI	Q12–24 hr	Q24–72 hr; monitor levels	Q48–72 hr; monitor levels	Y (He, P)
Lamivudine[§] **NOTE:** First dose at 100% for CrCl 5–29 and 33% for CrCl <5.	Renal	1.7–2.5	Q12 hr	DI	100%	100% and Q24 hr (CrCl 30–49) 66% and Q24 hr (CrCl 15–29)	33% and Q24 hr (CrCl 5–14) 17% and Q24 hr (CrCl <5)	N (He, P)
Levofloxacin	Renal (hepatic)	6–8	Q12–24 hr	DI	500 mg Q24 hr regimen: 100% 750 mg Q24 hr regimen: 100% 250 mg Q24 hr regimen: 100%	50% (CrCl 20–49) 100% and Q48 hr (CrCl 20–49) 100% (CrCl ≥20)	50% and Q48 hr (CrCl ≤19) 66% Q48 hr (CrCl ≤19) Give 750 mg for initial dose 100% Q48 hr (CrCl ≤19)	N (He, P)

Maraviroc	Hepatic	14–18	Q12 hr	D	100%	Regimen containing strong CYP 3A4 inhibitor or inducer: drug not recommended (CrCl <30). Regimen containing tipranavir/ritonavir, nevirapine, raltegravir, all NRTIs, and enfuvirtide: 50% if signs of postural hypotension is present (CrCl <30)	Regimen containing strong CYP 3A4 inhibitor or inducer: drug not recommended. Regimen containing tipranavir/ritonavir, nevirapine, raltegravir, all NRTIs, and enfuvirtide: 50% if signs of postural hypotension are present	N (He)
Meropenem	Renal	1–1.5	Q8 hr	DI	100% and Q8 hr	100% and Q12 hr (CrCl 26–50) 50% and Q12 hr (CrCl 10–25)	50% and Q24 hr	Y (He)
Methenamine	Renal	4.3	Q6–12 hr		100%	Avoid use (CrCl <50)		N (He, P)
Metronidazole	Hepatic (renal)	6–12	Q6–12 hr	D	100%	100%	50%	Y (He, P)

Continued

3

TABLE 3-3

ANTIMICROBIALS REQUIRING ADJUSTMENTS IN RENAL FAILURE (Continued)

	Adjustments in Renal Failure							
	Pharmacokinetics				Creatinine Clearance (mL/min)			
Drug	**Route of Excretion***	**Normal T1/2 (hr)**	**Normal Dose Interval**	**Method**	**Mild (>50)**	**Moderate (10–50)**	**Severe (<10)**	**Supplemental Dose for Dialysis**
Nafcillin	Renal (hepatic)	0.5–1	Q4–12 hr	D	100%	100%	50% (in patients with both severe renal and hepatic impairment)	N (He, P)
Neomycin	Renal	3	Q4–8 hr	I	Q6 hr	Q12–18 hr	Q18–24 hr	Y (He)
Norfloxacin	Hepatic (renal)	3–4	Q12 hr	I	Q12 hr	Q24 hr (CrCl <30)	Q24 hr	?
Ofloxacin	Renal	5–7.5	Q12 hr	DI	Q12 hr	Q24 hr (CrCl 20–50)	50% and Q24 hr (CrCl <20)	Y (He) N (P)
Oseltamivir	Renal	1–10	Q12–24 hr	I	Normal	Treatment: Q24 hr (CrCl 10–30) Prophylaxis: Q48 hr (CrCl 10–30)	No data for treatment and prophylaxis	Y (He)
Oxacillin	Renal (hepatic)	23–45 min	Q4–12 hr	D	100%	100%	Use lower range of normal dose	N (He, P)
Penicillin G	Renal (hepatic)	20–50 min	Q4–6 hr	D	100%	75%	20%–50%	Y (He)
Penicillin VK (PO)	Renal (hepatic)	30–40 min	Q6–8 hr	I	Q6 hr	Q6 hr	Q8 hr	Y (He)

Pentamidine	Renal	6.4–9	Q24 hr	I	Q24 hr	Q36 hr (CrCl 10–30)	Q48 hr	N (He, P)
Phenazopyridine	Renal (hepatic)	?	TID-QID × 2 days	I	Q8–16 hr (CrCl 50–80)	**Avoid**	**Avoid**	N/A
Piperacillin	Renal (hepatic)	0.5–1.5	Q4–6 hr	I	Q4–6 hr	Q8 hr (CrCl 20–40)	Q12 hr (CrCl <20)	Y (He)
Piperacillin/ tazobactam	Renal (hepatic)	Piperacillin: 0.5–1.5 Tazobactam: 0.7–1.6	Q6–8 hr	DI	100% and Q6–8 hr	70% and Q6 hr (CrCl 20–40)	70% and Q8 hr (CrCl <20)	Y (He)
Pyrazinamide	Renal	9–23	Q12–24 hr	D	100%	100%	50% and Q24 hr	Y (He, P)
Quinidine	Renal	2.5–8	Q4–6 hr	D	100%	100%	75%	Y (He)
Quinine	Renal	6–14	Q8 hr	I	Q8 hr	Q8–12 hr	Q24 hr	?
Ribavirin (PO)	Hepatic	24–36	Q12 hr	DI	Q12 hr	**Avoid**	**Avoid**	
Rifabutin	Renal (hepatic)	36–45	Q12–24 hr	D	100%	50% (CrCl <30)	50%	?
Rifampin	Hepatic (renal)	1.5–5	Q12–24 hr	D	100%	50%–100%	50%	N (He) Y (P)
Rimantadine	Renal	19.8–36.5	Q12–24 hr	I	Q12 hr	Q24 hr (CrCl <30)	Q24 hr	N (He)
Stavudine	Renal	0.9–1.6	Q12 hr	DI	100% and Q12 hr	50% and Q12 hr (CrCl 26–50) 50% and Q24 hr (CrCl 10–25)		Y (He)
Streptomycin	Renal	2.5	Q24 hr	DI	50% and Q24 hr (CrCl 50–80)	50% and Q24–72 hr	50% and Q72–96 hr	Y (He)
Sulfamethoxazole/ Trimethoprim	Sulfamethoxazole: hepatic (renal) Trimethoprim: renal (hepatic)	Sulfamethoxazole: 9–12 Trimethoprim: 6–11	Q12 hr	D	100%	50% (CrCl 15–30)	(CrCl <15)	Y (He)

Continued

TABLE 3-3

ANTIMICROBIALS REQUIRING ADJUSTMENTS IN RENAL FAILURE (Continued)

	Adjustments in Renal Failure							
	Pharmacokinetics				Creatinine Clearance (mL/min)			
Drug	**Route of Excretion***	**Normal T1/2 (hr)**	**Normal Dose Interval**	**Method**	**Mild (>50)**	**Moderate (10–50)**	**Severe (<10)**	**Supplemental Dose for Dialysis**
Sulfisoxazole	Renal	4–8	Q6–12 hr	I	Q6 hr	Q8–12 hr	Q12–24 hr	Y (He, P)
Telbivudine	Renal	40–49	Q24 hr	I	Q24 hr	Q48 hr (CrCl 30–49)	Q72 hr (CrCl <30)	Y (He)
Telavancin	Renal	6.6–9.9	Q24 hr	D, I	100% Q24 hr	75% and Q24 hr (CrCl 30–50) 100% and Q48 hr (CrCl 10–29)	No recommendation available	?
Telithromycin	Renal	10–13	Q24 hr	D	100%	75% (CrCl <30) 50% (CrCl <30 with hepatic impairment)	75% (50% if comorbid hepatic impairment)	Y (He)
Tenofovir	Renal	4–8	Q24 hr	I	Q24 hr	Q48 hr (CrCl 30–49) Q72–96 hr (CrCl 10–29)	No data	Y (He)
Tetracycline	Renal (hepatic)	8–10	Q6 hr	I	Q8–12 hr (CrCl 50–80)	Q12–24 hr	Q24 hr	N (He, P)
Ticarcillin¶	Renal	0.9–1.3	Q4–6 hr	I	Q4–6 hr	Q8 hr (CrCl 10–30)	Q12 hr	Y (He)

Ticarcillin-clavulanate[¶]	Renal	Ticarcillin: 0.9–1.3 Clavulanate: 1–1.5	Q4–6 hr	I	Q4–6 hr	Q8 hr (CrCl 10–30)	Q12 hr (Q24 hr if comorbid hepatic impairment)	Y (He)
Trimethoprim	Renal	8–10	Q6–24 hr	D	100%	50% (CrCl 15–30)	Avoid use (CrCl <15)	Y (He, P)
Tobramycin[†,‡]	Renal	1.5–3	Q8–12 hr	I	Q8–12 hr	Give usual initial dose × 1 and monitor levels	Give usual initial dose × 1 and monitor levels	Y (He, P)
Valacyclovir	Hepatic	2.5–3.6	Q8–24 hr	DI	Herpes zoster: 100% and Q8 hr	100% and Q12 hr (CrCl 30–49) 100% and Q24 hr (CrCl 10–29)	50% and Q24 hr	Y (He) N (P)
					Genital herpes (initial): 100% and Q12 hr	100% and Q24 hr (CrCl 10–29)	50% and Q24 hr	
					Genital herpes (recurrent): 100% and Q12 hr	100% and Q24 hr (CrCl <30)	100% and Q24 hr	
					Genital herpes (suppressive): 100% and Q24 hr	50% and Q24 hr or 100% and Q48 hr (CrCl 10–29)	50% and Q24 hr or 100% and Q48 hr	

Continued

TABLE 3-3

ANTIMICROBIALS REQUIRING ADJUSTMENTS IN RENAL FAILURE (Continued)

	Adjustments in Renal Failure							
	Pharmacokinetics				Creatinine Clearance (mL/min)			
Drug	Route of Excretion*	Normal T1/2 (hr)	Normal Dose Interval	Method	Mild (>50)	Moderate (10–50)	Severe (<10)	Supplemental Dose for Dialysis
Valganciclovir (PO)	Renal	0.4–0.6	Q12–24 hr	DI	Induction (PO): 50% and Q12 hr (CrCl 40–59)	50% and Q24 hr (CrCl 25–39) 50% and Q48 hr (CrCl 10–24)	Not recommended	
					Maintenance (PO): 50% and Q24 hr (CrCl 40–59)	50% and Q48 hr (CrCl 25–39) 50% and 2×/wk (CrCl 10–24)	Not recommended	
Vancomycin†	Renal	2.2–8	Q6–12 hr	I	Q6–12 hr	Give usual initial dose × 1 and monitor levels	Give usual initial dose × 1 and monitor levels	Y/N (He)* N (P)
Zalcitabine	Renal	1–3	Q8 hr	I	Q8 hr	Q12 hr (CrCl 10–40)	Q24 hr	Y (He)

Continued from page 171

Note that k values vary with body size and sex:

Age	k Value
Preterm infants up to 1 yr	0.33
Full-term infants up to 1 yr	0.45
Children (2–12 yr) and adolescent girls (13–21 yr)	0.55
Adolescent boys (13–21 yr)	0.70

b. IDMS-traceable method serum creatinine assay (Bedside Schwartz method) for children 1 to 17 years old[4]:

$$CrCl = \frac{0.413 \times L}{S_{cr}}$$

where CrCl is measured in mL/min/1.73 m^2, L represents body length (cm), and S_{cr} (mg/dL) is measured by IDMS-traceable method.

3. **Glomerular function determined by nuclear medicine scans:** Renal clearance of exogenous radioactive chemicals such as ^{125}I-iothalamate and ^{54}Cr-EDTA has been used to determine glomerular function.

B. Dose Adjustment Methods for Antimicrobial Agents

1. **Maintenance dose:** In patients with renal insufficiency, the dose may be adjusted using the following methods:
   a. Interval extension (I): Lengthen the intervals between individual doses, keeping the dose size normal. For this method, the suggested interval is shown in Table 3-3.
   b. Dose reduction (D): Reduce the amount of the individual doses, keeping the interval between the doses normal. This method is particularly recommended for drugs with which a relatively constant blood level is desired. For this method, the percentage of the usual dose is shown in Table 3-3.
   c. Interval extension and dose reduction (DI): Lengthen the interval and reduce the dose.
   d. Interval extension or dose reduction (D, I): In some instances, either the dose *or* the interval can be changed.

   NOTE: These dose adjustments are for infants beyond the neonatal period. These dose modifications are only approximations. Each patient must be monitored closely for signs of drug toxicity, and serum levels must be measured when available. Drug dose and interval should be monitored accordingly.
2. **Dialysis:** The quantitative effects of hemodialysis (He) and peritoneal dialysis (P) on drug removal are shown. "Y" indicates the need for a supplemental dose with dialysis. "N" indicates no need for adjustment. The designation "No" does not preclude the use of dialysis or hemoperfusion for drug overdose (see Table 3-3).

C. Dosing in Continuous Renal Replacement Therapy

The clearance/elimination of certain medications may be affected by continuous renal replacement therapies (CRRT) such as continuous venovenous hemofiltration, continuous arteriovenous hemofiltration, continuous arteriovenous hemodialysis, continuous venovenous hemodialysis, and continuous venovenous hemodiafiltration.

1. **Factors that influence drug removal with CRRT**

a. Drug's physiochemical characteristics favoring removal by convection or diffusion
   (1) Small molecular weight
   (2) Low protein binding
   (3) Negatively charged (anionic)
   (4) Small volume of distribution
   (5) High water solubility/low lipid solubility

b. Technical features of dialysis circuit components and procedure favoring drug removal
   (1) Filter properties: larger membrane pore size
   (2) Increasing blood/dialysate flow rates
   (3) Increasing ultrafiltration rates

2. **Optimal approach to administering drugs to pediatric patients receiving CRRT:** The optimal approach to administering drugs to pediatric patients receiving CRRT is based on the properties of the drug, specific characteristics of the dialysis system, interactions between the drug and CRRT system that yield the sieving coefficient, and the drug clearance by the CRRT modality chosen.
3. Data regarding drug removal by CRRT are currently limited in both children and adults.
4. **Antimicrobials that require adjustment with CRRT** (Tables 3-4 and 3-5)[7–9,11–15]

TABLE 3-4

EMPIRIC DOSING RECOMMENDATIONS OF ANTIMICROBIALS KNOWN TO BE AFFECTED BY CONTINUOUS RENAL REPLACEMENT THERAPIES[9,11–15]

		Dosages for CAVH/CVVH and CAVHD/CVVHD	
Drug	**Usual Dosage**	**<1500 mL/m²/hr**	**≥1500 mL/m²/hr**
Acyclovir	5–10 mg/kg IV Q8 hr or 250–500 mg/m² IV Q8 hr	3.75–7.5 mg/kg IV Q24 hr or 175–350 mg/m² IV Q24 hr	5–10 mg/kg IV Q24 hr or 250–500 mg/m² IV Q24 hr
Amikacin	5–7.5 mg/kg IV Q8 hr; monitor levels to optimize safety and efficacy	Required dosages are highly variable; 5–7.5 mg/kg IV once, then measure levels to identify appropriate regimen	Required dosages are highly variable; 5–7.5 mg/kg IV once, then measure levels to identify appropriate regimen
Ampicillin	25–50 mg/kg IV Q6 hr CNS infections: 50–100 mg/kg IV Q6 hr Maximum: 12 g/24 hr	25–50 mg/kg IV Q8–12 hr CNS infections: 50–100 mg/kg IV Q8–12 hr	25–50 mg/kg IV Q6–8 hr CNS infections: 50–100 mg/kg IV Q6–8 hr
Cefepime	50 mg/kg IV Q8–12 hr Maximum: 6 g/24 hr	25–50 mg/kg IV Q12–18 hr	25–50 mg/kg IV Q12 hr
Cefotaxime	25–50 mg/kg IV Q6–8 hr CNS infections: 75 mg/kg IV Q6 hr Maximum: 12 g/24 hr	25–50 mg/kg IV Q8–12 hr CNS infections: 75 mg/kg IV Q8–12 hr	25–50 mg/kg IV Q8 hr CNS infections: 75 mg/kg IV Q8 hr
Cefotetan	20–40 mg/kg IV Q12 hr Maximum: 6 g/24 hr	10–20 mg/kg IV Q12–24 hr	10–25 mg/kg IV Q12 hr
Cefoxitin	20–40 mg/kg IV Q6 hr	20–40 mg/kg IV Q18 hr	20–40 mg/kg IV Q12 hr
Ceftazidime	30–50 mg/kg IV Q8 hr	15–35 mg/kg IV Q12 hr	15–50 mg/kg IV Q12 hr
Ceftriaxone	25–50 mg/kg IV Q12 hr Maximum: 4 g/24 hr	25–50 mg/kg IV Q12–24 hr Maximum: 4 g/24 hr	25–50 mg/kg IV Q12 hr Maximum: 4 g/24 hr
Cefuroxime sodium	25–50 mg/kg IV Q8 hr Maximum: 6 g/24 hr	25–50 mg/kg IV Q12–18 hr	25–50 mg/kg IV Q12 hr
Ciprofloxacin	5–10 mg/kg IV Q12 hr Maximum: 800 mg/24 hr CF: 10 mg/kg IV Q8 hr Maximum (CF): 1.2 g/24 hr	2.5–5 mg/kg IV Q12 hr Maximum: 400 mg/24 hr CF: 5 mg/kg IV Q8 hr Maximum (CF): 600 mg/24 hr	3.75–7.5 mg/kg IV Q12 hr Maximum: 600 mg/24 hr CF: 7.5 mg/kg IV Q8 hr Maximum (CF): 900 mg/24 hr
Fluconazole	6–10 mg/kg IV/PO loading; 3–12 mg/kg IV/PO Q24 hr	6–10 mg/kg IV/PO loading, then 3–12 mg/kg IV/PO Q24 hr	6–10 mg/kg IV/PO loading, then 6–12 mg/kg IV/PO Q24 hr
Flucytosine	25–37.5 mg/kg PO Q6 hr	25–37.5 mg/kg PO Q12–18 hr	25–37.5 mg/kg PO Q8–12 hr

Continued

TABLE 3-4

EMPIRIC DOSING RECOMMENDATIONS OF ANTIMICROBIALS KNOWN TO BE AFFECTED BY CONTINUOUS RENAL REPLACEMENT THERAPIES (Continued)

		Dosages for CAVH/CVVH and CAVHD/CVVHD	
Drug	**Usual Dosage**	**<1500 mL/m²/hr**	**≥1500 mL/m²/hr**
Ganciclovir	Induction: (CrCl >70) 5 mg/kg IV Q12 hr, (CrCl 50–69) 2.5 mg/kg IV Q12 hr Maintenance: (CrCl >70) 2.5 mg/kg IV Q12 hr, (CrCl 50–69) 1.25 mg/kg IV Q12 hr	Induction: 1.25–2.5 mg/kg IV Q24 hr Maintenance: 0.625–1.25 mg/kg IV Q24 hr	Induction: 2.5–3.75 mg/kg IV Q24 hr Maintenance: 1.25–2.5 mg/kg IV Q24 hr
Gentamicin	2–3 mg/kg IV Q8 hr; monitor levels to optimize safety and efficacy	Required dosages are highly variable; 2–3 mg/kg IV once, then measure levels to identify appropriate regimen	Required dosages are highly variable; 2–3 mg/kg IV once, then measure levels to identify appropriate regimen
Imipenem-cilastatin	33 mg/kg IV Q8 hr or 25 mg/kg IV Q6 hr Maximum: 4 g/24 hr	15–20 mg/kg IV Q12 hr	20–25 mg/kg IV Q8–12 hr
Itraconazole	3–5 mg/kg PO Q12–24 hr	3–5 mg/kg PO Q12–24 hr	3–5 mg/kg PO Q12–24 hr
Linezolid	10 mg/kg IV/PO Q8 hr (<3 mo of age) or Q12 hr (≥3 mo of age) Maximum: 1200 mg/24 hr	10 mg/kg IV/PO Q8 hr (<3 mo of age) or Q12 hr (≥3 mo of age) Maximum: 1200 mg/24 hr	10 mg/kg IV/PO Q8 hr (<3 mo of age) or Q12 hr (≥3 mo of age) Maximum: 1200 mg/24 hr
Meropenem	20 mg/kg IV Q8 hr CNS infection: 40 mg/kg IV Q8 hr Maximum: 6 g/24 hr	10–20 mg/kg IV Q12 hr	20–40 mg/kg IV Q12 hr
Metronidazole	5–17 mg/kg IV/PO Q8 hr Maximum: 4 g/24 hr	5–17 mg/kg IV/PO Q8 hr Maximum: 4 g/24 hr	5–17 mg/kg IV/PO Q8 hr Maximum: 4 g/24 hr
Oxacillin	25–33 mg/kg IV Q4–6 hr Maximum: 12 g/24 hr	25–33 mg/kg IV Q6 hr	25–33 mg/kg IV Q6 hr
Piperacillin	50–75 mg/kg IV Q6 hr CF: 85–150 mg/kg IV Q6 hr Maximum: 24 g/24 hr	50–75 mg/kg IV Q8–12 hr CF: 85–150 mg/kg IV Q8–12 hr	50–75 mg/kg IV Q6–8 hr CF: 85–150 mg/kg IV Q6–8 hr
Piperacillin-tazobactam	100 mg/kg IV Q6–8 hr Maximum: 24 g piperacillin/24 hr	70 mg/kg IV Q6–8 hr	70–100 mg/kg IV Q6–8 hr
Sulfamethoxazole-trimethoprim	3–5 mg/kg IV/PO Q12 hr PCP: 5 mg/kg IV/PO Q6 hr	3–5 mg/kg IV/PO Q18 hr PCP: 5 mg/kg IV/PO Q8 hr	4–5 mg/kg IV/PO Q18 hr PCP: 5 mg/kg IV/PO Q8 hr

TABLE 3-4

EMPIRIC DOSING RECOMMENDATIONS OF ANTIMICROBIALS KNOWN TO BE AFFECTED BY CONTINUOUS RENAL REPLACEMENT THERAPIES (Continued)

Drug	Usual Dosage	Dosages for CAVH/CVVH and CAVHD/CVVHD	
		<1500 mL/m²/hr	≥1500 mL/m²/hr
Ticarcillin	50–75 mg/kg IV Q6 hr CF: 75–150 mg/kg IV Q6 hr Maximum: 24 g/24 hr	50–75 mg/kg IV Q8–12 hr CF: 75–150 mg/kg IV Q8–12 hr	50–75 mg/kg IV Q6–8 hr CF: 75–150 mg/kg IV Q6–8 hr
Ticarcillin-clavulanate	50–75 mg/kg IV Q6 hr CF: 75–150 mg/kg IV Q6 hr Maximum: 24 g ticarcillin/24 hr	50–75 mg/kg IV Q8–12 hr CF: 75–150 mg/kg IV Q8–12 hr	50–75 mg/kg IV Q6–8 hr CF: 75–150 mg/kg IV Q6–8 hr
Tobramycin	2–3 mg/kg IV Q8 hr; monitor levels to optimize safety and efficacy	Required dosages are highly variable; 2–3 mg/kg IV once, then measure levels to identify appropriate regimen	Required dosages are highly variable; 2–3 mg/kg IV once, then measure levels to identify appropriate regimen
Vancomycin	10–20 mg/kg IV Q6–8 hr Dose and interval dependent on indication and age, respectively; titrate dosing to desired goal trough levels Maximum single dose: 2 g	Required dosages are highly variable; 10–15 mg/kg IV once, then measure levels to identify appropriate regimen	Required dosages are highly variable; 10–15 mg/kg IV once, then measure levels to identify appropriate regimen

Adapted from Veltri MA, Neu AM, Fivush BA, et al: Drug dosing during intermittent hemodialysis and continuous renal replacement therapy: special considerations in pediatric patients. *Pediatr Drugs* 6(1):45–65, 2004.

CAVH, Continuous arteriovenous hemodialysis; *CAVHD,* continuous arteriovenous hemodialysis, *CF,* cystic fibrosis; *CrCl,* creatinine clearance rate; *CNS,* central nervous syndrome; *CVVH,* continuous venovenous hemofiltration; *CVVHD,* continuous venovenous hemodialysis; *IV,* intravenous; *PCP,* Pneumocystis pneumonia; *PO,* by mouth.

IV. DRUG DOSING IN HEPATIC INSUFFICIENCY

A. Child–Pugh Score[16,17]

The Child–Pugh score (also known as the Child–Turcotte–Pugh score) is used to assess the prognosis of chronic liver disease, mainly cirrhosis (Table 3-6).

B. PHARMACOKINETIC CHANGES IN HEPATIC INSUFFICIENCY[18]

1. **Pharmacokinetics are usually mildly altered in liver diseases without cirrhosis.**
2. **Cirrhosis and cholestasis may cause pharmacokinetic changes that necessitate dose adjustments.**
3. **Common pharmacokinetic alterations:**

TABLE 3-5

ADDITIONAL EMPIRIC DOSING RECOMMENDATIONS OF ANTIMICROBIALS WITH CONTINUOUS RENAL REPLACEMENT THERAPIES FROM ADULT REFERENCES[7–9]

Drug	Usual Pediatric Dosage	Dosages for Continuous Renal Replacement Therapies (from adult recommendations)
Capreomycin	<15 yr and ≤40 kg: 15–30 mg/kg/24 hr IV for 2–4 mo, followed by 15–30 mg/kg IV twice weekly	5 mg/kg IV Q24 hr
Ceftibuten	<12 yr: 9 mg/kg PO Q24 hr (maximum dose 400 mg) ≥12 yr: 400 mg PO Q24 hr	Reduce dose by 25%–50%
Cycloserine	10–20 mg/kg/24 hr PO divided Q12 hr (maximum dose of 1000 mg/24 hr)	Administer Q24 hr
Daptomycin	Children 2–6 yr: 8–10 mg/kg IV Q24 hr Children ≥6 yr and <12 yr: 7 mg/kg IV Q24 hr Children ≥12 yr and adolescents: 6–10 mg/kg IV Q24 hr	Suggested adjustments include 8 mg/kg Q48 hr or 4–6 mg/kg Q24 hr Monitor levels
Foscarnet	CMV maintenance: 90–120 mg/kg/dose IV Q24 hr	60–80 mg/kg/dose IV Q48 hr
Kanamycin	15–30 mg/kg/day divided Q8–12 hr	30%–70% of dose Q12 hr Monitor levels
Lamivudine	4 mg/kg/dose PO Q12 hr (maximum dose: 150 mg Q12 hr)	4 mg/kg/dose Q24 hr
Penicillin G preparations: aqueous potassium and sodium	100,000–400,000 units/kg/24 hr IV divided Q4–6 hr	75% of normal dose Q6 hr
Ofloxacin	15 mg/kg/day IV divide Q12 hr	7.5 mg/kg IV Q24 hr
Quinine	10 mg/kg IV Q8 hr	10 mg/kg PO Q8–12 hr
Stavudine	<30 kg: 1 mg/kg PO Q12 hr 30–59 kg: 30 mg PO Q12 hr ≥60 kg: 40 mg PO Q12 hr	Reduce dose by 50%
Streptomycin	20–40 mg/kg IM Q24 hr	7.5 mg/kg IM Q24–72 hr Monitor levels

CMV, Cytomegalovirus; *IM,* intramuscular; *IV,* intravenous; *PO,* oral.

a. Decreased "first-pass effect" resulting in increased bioavailability of some medications
b. Decreased plasma protein binding because of reduced synthesis of albumin and α_1-acid glycoprotein, inhibition of protein binding caused by accumulation of endogenous compounds, and qualitative changes in plasma proteins
c. Increased volume of distribution of hydrophilic drugs with ascites

TABLE 3-6

CHILD–PUGH SCORE (ALSO KNOWN AS THE CHILD–TURCOTTE–PUGH SCORE)

Clinical and Biochemical Measurements	**Points Scored for Increasing Abnormality** 1	2	3
Hepatic encephalopathy (grade)	None	Grades I–II	Grades III–IV
Ascites	Absent	Mild (suppressed with medication)	Moderate (refractory)
Total bilirubin (mg/dL)	<2.0	2.0–3.0	>3.0
Serum albumin (g/dL)	>3.5	2.8–3.5	<2.8
INR	<1.70	1.71–2.20	>2.20
or	or	or	or
prothrombin time (seconds prolonged)	<4	4–6	>6
Points	**Child–Pugh Class**	**1-Yr Survival**	**2-Yr Survival**
INTERPRETATION			
5–6	A	100%	85%
7–9	B	81%	57%
10–15	C	45%	35%

d. Decreased metabolism by CYP450 enzyme system
   (1) Early hepatic disease CYP2C19 activity is reduced, whereas activity of other isoforms is almost normal.
   (2) In end-stage liver disease, clearance by all isoforms is reduced.
e. Conjugation reactions are less affected by cirrhosis than CYP450 reactions, but can also be impaired
f. Patients with cholestasis can have accumulation of drugs and metabolites that undergo significant biliary excretion
g. Hepatorenal syndrome leads to reduced renal excretion of medications

C. Drugs That Require Attention in Hepatic Insufficiency[19–22]

Drugs that require attention in patients with hepatic insufficiency may need to be dose adjusted, discontinued, or used with caution (Table 3-7).

TABLE 3-7

HEPATIC DOSAGE ADJUSTMENT[19–22]

	Use with Caution	Contraindicated	Hepatic Adjustment/Comments
Abacavir sulfate	+	Contraindicated in patients with moderate or severe hepatic impairment	Child–Pugh class A: 200 mg twice daily (oral solution is recommended)
Adefovir	+		
Albendazole	+		
Amantadine	+		
Amoxicillin with clavulanic acid		Contraindicated in patients with history of amoxicillin/clavulanic acid–associated cholestatic jaundice or hepatic impairment	
Amprenavir	+	Contraindicated in patients with hepatic failure	Dose recommendations not available for children. Adults: Capsules: Child–Pugh score 5–8: 450 mg twice daily Child–Pugh score 9–12: 300 mg twice daily Solution: Child–Pugh score 5–8: 513 mg (34 mL) twice daily Child–Pugh score 9–12: 342 mg (23 mL) twice daily
Anidulafungin (Eraxis)	+		
Artemether + lumefantrine	+		No specific dose adjustments in mild to moderate hepatic impairment; use with caution in severe impairment as safety and efficacy have not been established

Artesunate	+	
Atazanavir	+	Adolescents ≥16 yr and adults: Child–Pugh class B and no prior virologic failure: reduce dose to 300 mg once daily Child–Pugh class C: do not use Patients with hepatitis B or C and markedly elevated transaminases before therapy are at risk for hepatic decompensation; monitor closely Combination therapy with ritonavir is not recommended in patients with hepatic impairment
Atovaquone + proguanil (Malarone)		No adjustment needed in mild to moderate impairment; no data are available for patients with severe hepatic impairment
Azithromycin	+	
Boceprevir	+	No adjustment required for any severity of impairment
Caspofungin	+	Child–Pugh class A: no dosage adjustment necessary Child–Pugh class B: Children: decrease daily dose by 30% Adults: 70 mg loading dose, then 35 mg daily Child–Pugh class C: not recommended
Cefazolin	+	

Continued

TABLE 3-7

HEPATIC DOSAGE ADJUSTMENT (Continued)

	Use with Caution	Contraindicated	Hepatic Adjustment/Comments
Cefditoren	+		Use may be associated with increased INR; no adjustment required in mild to moderate impairment; no specific recommendations for severe impairment
Cefoxitin	+		
Ceftriaxone	+		Do not exceed 2 g/day in patients with concurrent hepatic and renal dysfunction
Cefuroxime (IV/IM)/Cefuroxime axetil	+		Use may be associated with increased INR
Chloramphenicol	+		Dose reduction should be based on serum chloramphenicol concentrations
Chloroquine HCl/Phosphate	+		
Clarithromycin	+		Dose adjustment not required in patients with normal renal function
Clindamycin	+		
Daptomycin	+		Dose adjustment not required in Child–Pugh class A and B; use has not been evaluated in Child–Pugh class C
Darunavir	+	Canadian labeling contraindicated use in Child–Pugh score 10–15	Dose adjustment not required in Child–Pugh class A and B; use is not recommended in Child–Pugh class C
Delavirdine	+		
Demeclocycline	+	Avoid use in hepatic impairment	

Didanosine	+		Dose adjustment not required; monitor closely as patients with hepatic impairment may be at increased risk for toxicity
Doxycycline	+	Avoid use in hepatic impairment	
Efavirenz	+		Adults: Child–Pugh class A: no dosage adjustment recommended Child–Pugh class B and C: use not recommended
Emtricitabine	+		
Entecavir	+		
Erythromycin ethylsuccinate + acetylsulfisoxazole	+	Contraindicated in patients with liver dysfunction	
Erythromycin preparations	+		
Ethambutol HCl	+		
Ethionamide (Trecator SC)	+	Contraindicated in patients with severe hepatic impairment	
Famciclovir	+		Child–Pugh class A and B: no dose adjustment necessary Child–Pugh class C: conversion of famciclovir to active metabolite may be decreased, affecting efficacy
Fluconazole	+		
Flucytosine	+		

Continued

3

TABLE 3-7

HEPATIC DOSAGE ADJUSTMENT (Continued)

	Use with Caution	Contraindicated	Hepatic Adjustment/Comments
Fosamprenavir	+		Adults: unboosted regimens: Child–Pugh class A and B: 700 mg twice daily Child–Pugh class C: 350 mg twice daily Regimens boosted with 100 mg ritonavir once daily: Child–Pugh class A: 700 mg twice daily Child–Pugh class B: 450 mg twice daily Child–Pugh class C: 300 mg twice daily
Griseofulvin	+	Contraindicated in patients with severe liver disease	
Hydroxychloroquine	+	–	Children: daily doses >6–6.5 mg/kg/day may be associated with increased retinal toxicity in patients with abnormal hepatic or renal function
Indinavir	+	–	Adults: Mild to moderate hepatic impairment: 600 mg Q8 hr Severe impairment: no dosing information available
Iodoquinol	+	Contraindicated in patients with hepatic impairment	
Isoniazid	+	Contraindicated in patients with acute liver disease and/or previous history of hepatic damage during INH therapy	Risk for hepatitis and hepatotoxicity increases with age; daily ethanol consumption may also increase risk
Itraconazole	+		

Ketoconazole	+		
Lamivudine	+		
Linezolid	+		Child–Pugh class A and B: no dose adjustment necessary Child–Pugh class C: has not been adequately evaluated
Lopinavir/Ritonavir	+		Mild to moderate hepatic impairment: lopinavir area under the curve may be increased ~30%; use with caution Severe impairment: dosing information not available
Maraviroc	+		Mild to moderate hepatic impairment: dose adjustments not recommended; use with caution Moderate impairment with concomitant strong CYP3A4 inhibitor: use caution; monitor closely for adverse events Severe impairment: population has not been studied
Mefloquine HCl	+		Half life may be prolonged and plasma levels may be higher; specific dose adjustments not available
Melarsoprol	+		
Methenamine mandelate/ Methenamine hippurate	+	Contraindicated in patients with severe hepatic impairment	
Metronidazole	+		Decrease dose by 50%–67%

Continued

TABLE 3-7

HEPATIC DOSAGE ADJUSTMENT (Continued)

	Use with Caution	Contraindicated	Hepatic Adjustment/Comments
Micafungin	+		No adjustment needed in mild to moderate impairment; no data are available for patients with severe hepatic impairment
Minocycline	+		
Moxifloxacin	+		No dose adjustment required in mild, moderate, or severe hepatic impairment; hepatic impairment may increase risk for QT prolongation
Nafcillin	+		In patients with concomitant hepatic and renal dysfunction, reduce dose by 50%
Nelfinavir	+		Child–Pugh class A: no dose adjustment necessary Child–Pugh class B and C: not recommended
Nevirapine	+	Contraindicated in Child–Pugh class B and C	
Nitazoxinide	+		
Nifurtimox	+		Specific dosing recommendations are not available
Ofloxacin	+		Severe impairment: maximum dosage 400 mg/day
Para-aminosalicylic acid	+		
Pentamidine	+		
Phenazopyridine	+	Contraindicated in patients with liver disease	

Posaconazole	+		
Praziquantel	+		Use with caution in Child–Pugh class B and C; higher and prolonged serum concentrations may occur; no specific dose adjustments available
Pyrantel pamoate	+		
Pyrazinamide	+	Contraindicated in patients with severe hepatic damage	
Pyrimethamine + sulfadoxine	+	Repeated prophylaxis is contraindicated in patients with hepatic failure	
Quinidine gluconate	+		Dose decrease recommended, but no specific recommendations are available
Quinine sulfate	+		No dose adjustment required in Child–Pugh class A and B; data not available for Child–Pugh class C
Quinupristin with dalfopristin	+		Dosage adjustment may be necessary; no specific recommendations are available
Ribavirin	+	Contraindicated in patients with autoimmune hepatitis and in Child–Pugh class B and C	Discontinue therapy if hepatic decompensation is observed (Child–Pugh score ≥6)
Rifabutin	+		Discontinue therapy if AST >3 × ULN, ALT ≥5 × ULN, regardless of symptoms, or if significant bilirubin or alkaline phosphatase elevations occur
Rifampin	+		
Rifapentine	+		Administer only when absolutely necessary; monitor liver function every 2–4 wk and discontinue treatment if liver function worsens

Continued

TABLE 3-7

HEPATIC DOSAGE ADJUSTMENT (Continued)

	Use with Caution	Contraindicated	Hepatic Adjustment/Comments
Rifaximin	+		Use with caution in Child–Pugh class C
Rilpivirine			Child–Pugh class A and B, no dose adjustment necessary; Child–Pugh class C has not been studied
Rimantadine	+		Severe dysfunction: adults 100 mg/day
Ritonavir	+		Mild to moderate hepatic impairment: no adjustment recommended; lower ritonavir concentrations have been reported in patients with moderate hepatic impairment Severe hepatic impairment: use with caution
Saquinovir	+	Contraindicated in patients with severe hepatic impairment	
Stavudine	+		
Stibogluconate	+		
Sulfadiazine	+		
Sulfamethoxazole/trimethoprim	+		
Sulfisoxazole	+		
Suramin	+		Highly protein bound, patients with severe hepatic dysfunction resulting in hypoalbuminemia may experience toxicity because of increased free fraction of the drug; specific dosage adjustments are not available

Telaprevir	+	Child–Pugh class A: no dose adjustment necessary Child–Pugh class B and C: use not recommended; has not been studied
Telithromycin	+	Dose adjustment only required with concomitant severe renal impairment
Tenctovir disproxil furnarate	+	
Terbinafine	+	Clearance is decreased by ~50% with hepatic cirrhosis; use is not recommended
Tetracycline	+	Avoid when possible; may increase endogenous nitrogen load; do not exceed 1 g/day in patients with hepatic impairment
Thalidomide	+	
Thiabendazole	+	
Ticarcillin	+	Adults: patients with hepatic impairment and CrCl <10 mL/min administer 2 g Q24 hr
Ticarcillin with clavulanate	+	Adults: patients with hepatic impairment and CrCl <10 mL/min administer 2 g ticarcillin component Q24 hr
Tigecycline	+	Mild-to-moderate hepatic disease: no dosage adjustment required Severe hepatic impairment (Child–Pugh class C): initial dose of 100 mg should be followed with 25 mg Q12 hr

Continued

TABLE 3-7

HEPATIC DOSAGE ADJUSTMENT (Continued)

	Use with Caution	Contraindicated	Hepatic Adjustment/Comments
Tinidazole	+		
Tipronavir	+	Contraindicated in Child–Pugh class B and C	Child–Pugh class A: no dose adjustment necessary
Trimethoprim	+		
Trimetrexate glucuronate	+		Dose adjustment may be needed with hepatic impairment; no specific dosage recommendations exist; if transaminases or alkaline phosphatase levels increase above 5 × ULN, therapy should be interrupted
Voriconazole	+		Child–Pugh class A and B: use standard loading dose; decrease maintenance dose by 50% Child–Pugh class C: not recommended unless benefit outweighs risk
Zalcitabine	+		Use with caution; if liver enzymes exceed 5 × ULN, therapy interruption is recommended
Zidovudine	+		Hematologic toxicity risk may be increased. No specific dosage adjustments are available; monitor closely for toxicity

+, Use with caution in the presence of hepatic impairment; *IM,* intramuscular; *INR,* international normalized ratio; *IV,* intravenous.

V. DRUG DOSING IN OBESITY

A. Determining Appropriate Dosage Regimens for Antimicrobials

The most appropriate dosage regimens for antimicrobials in overweight and obese individuals are often unknown; data are especially limited in pediatrics. Body mass index (BMI) is used to define overweight and obesity because it correlates well with more accurate measures of body adiposity and is derived from easily obtainable weight and height data.

$$BMI = weight\ (kg)/[height\ (m)]^2$$

BMI between 85th and 95th percentile for age and sex is considered overweight, and BMI at or above the 95th percentile is considered obese. Figures 3-2 and 3-3 illustrate the BMI percentiles for children 2 to 20 years old. For infants younger than 2 years, weight-for-length percentile above the 95th percentile for age is considered overweight. Figures 3-4 and 3-5 illustrate the weight-for-length percentiles for children from birth to 36 months. Additional growth chart information can be found at the Centers for Disease Control and Prevention (CDC) website (www.cdc.gov/growthcharts) (see Figs. 3-2 through 3-7).

B. Ideal Body Weight Characterization in Children[23]

Adult methods to estimate ideal body weight (IBW) are unsuitable for pediatric use. Various methods have been used to calculate IBW for pediatric patients, but there is no consensus on the correct method for IBW calculation. Three commonly used methods, McLaren, Moore, and BMI, are presented below. Growth charts are required for calculation. There is extremely good correlation among the three methods for patients up to age 18 years who are at the 50th percentile for height. Discrepancies among the methods are greatest at heights farthest from the 50th percentile and at older ages. The BMI method is preferred for children who are too tall for the McLaren method because using the Moore method in these children may overestimate IBW.

1. **McLaren method:** Using stature-for-age and weight-for-age percentiles chart (see Figs. 3-6 and 3-7):
   a. Plot the child's stature-for-age.
   b. Draw a horizontal line from child's stature-for-age to the 50th percentile stature-for-age line.
   c. Extend a vertical line from the point on the stature-for-age line to the 50th percentile weight-for-age line.
   d. This point is the IBW.
2. **Moore method:** Using stature-for-age and weight-for-age percentiles chart (see Figs. 3-6 and 3-7):
   a. Determine the child's stature-for-age percentile.
   b. Find the weight-for-age that is the same percentile as the patient's stature-for-age.
   c. This is the IBW.

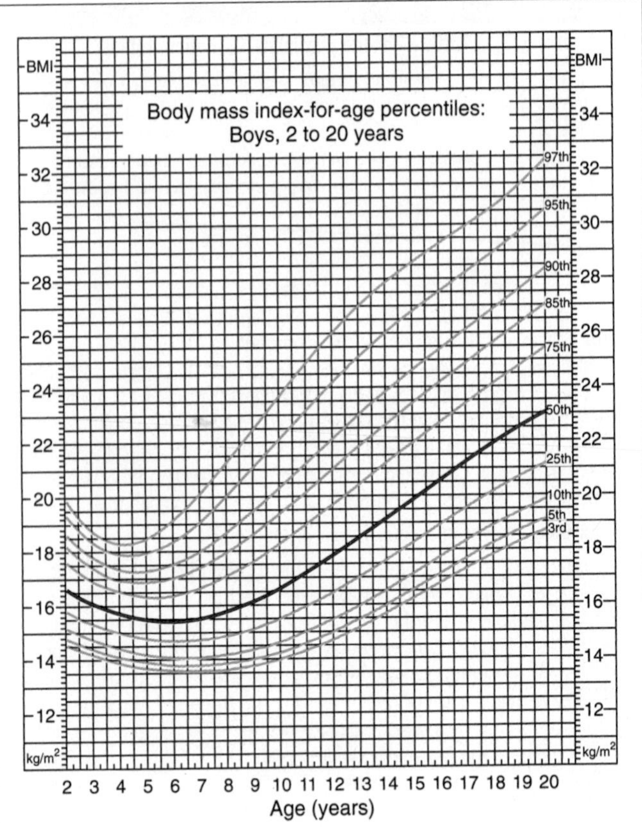

FIGURE 3-2

Body mass index for boys 2 to 20 years old. *(Developed by the National Center for Health Statistics in collaboration with the National Center for Chronic Disease Prevention and Health Promotion, 2000.* http://www.cdc.gov/growthcharts/clinical_charts.htm*)*

3. **BMI method:** Using BMI chart (see Figs. 3-2 and 3-3):
   a. Determine 50th percentile BMI for child's age and sex.
   b. IBW = [BMI at the 50th percentile for child's age × (child's height in m)^2].

C. Antimicrobial Dosing in Obesity

Table 3-8 summarizes known antimicrobial dosage modifications for obese patients. Data are quite limited, and recommendations are often

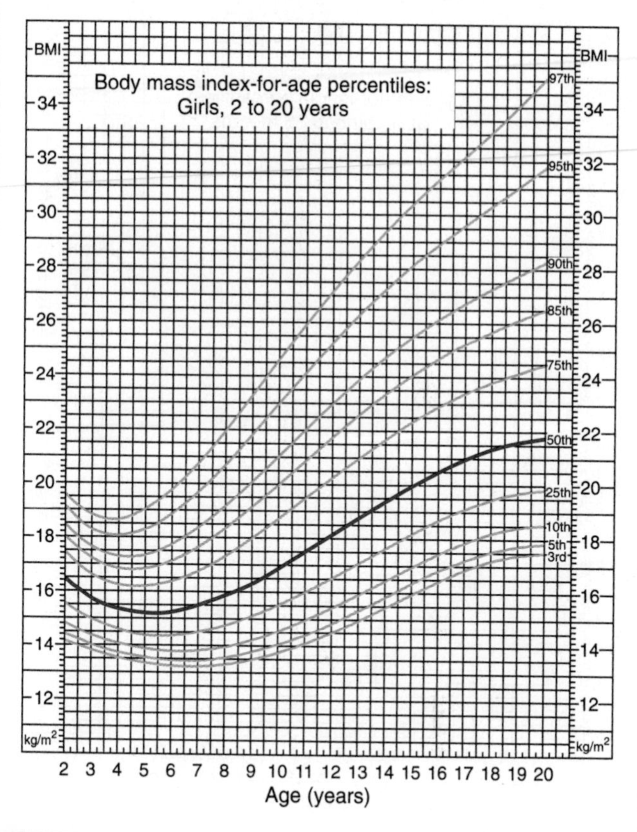

FIGURE 3-3

Body mass index for girls 2 to 20 years old. *(Developed by the National Center for Health Statistics in collaboration with the National Center for Chronic Disease Prevention and Health Promotion, 2000.* http://www.cdc.gov/growthcharts/clinical_charts.htm)

based on adult studies. Drug-specific adjusted body weight (ABW) may be calculated for determining the obese patient's individualized dosage. Required elements include the patient's actual or total body weight and determination of their IBW.

For example, to calculate the gentamicin dosage (2.5 mg/kg/dose intravenously [IV] Q8 hr) for an obese 8-year-old with a total body weight of 40 kg and IBW of 25 kg, use a correction factor of 0.4 to determine the ABW.

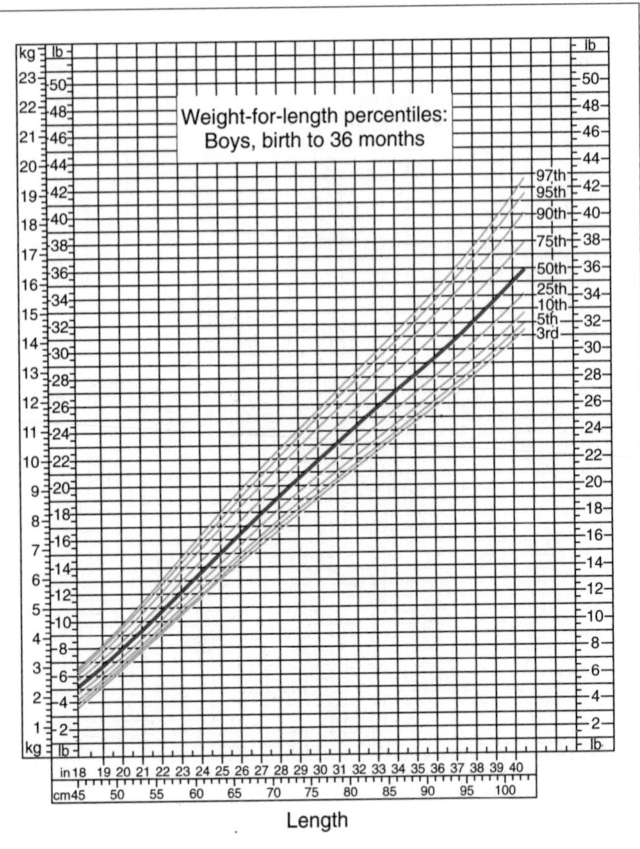

FIGURE 3-4

Weight-for-length percentiles for boys, from birth to 36 months. *(Developed by the National Center for Health Statistics in collaboration with the National Center for Chronic Disease Prevention and Health Promotion, 2000.* http://www.cdc.gov/growthcharts/clinical_charts.htm*)*

1. **Determine the ABW:**

$$ABW = 25\,kg + 0.4\,(40\,kg - 25\,kg) = 31\,kg$$

2. **Calculate dosage with ABW:**

Gentamicin: [2.5 mg/kg/dose × 31 kg] IV q8 hr or 77.5 mg IV q8 hr

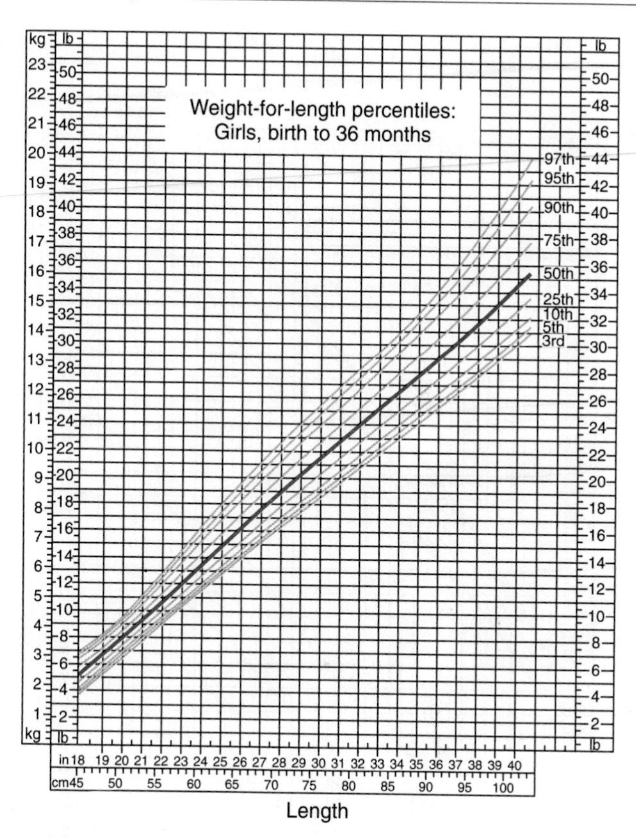

FIGURE 3-5

Weight-for-length percentiles for girls, from birth to 36 months. *(Developed by the National Center for Health Statistics in collaboration with the National Center for Chronic Disease Prevention and Health Promotion, 2000.* http://www.cdc.gov/growthcharts/clinical_charts.htm*)*

3

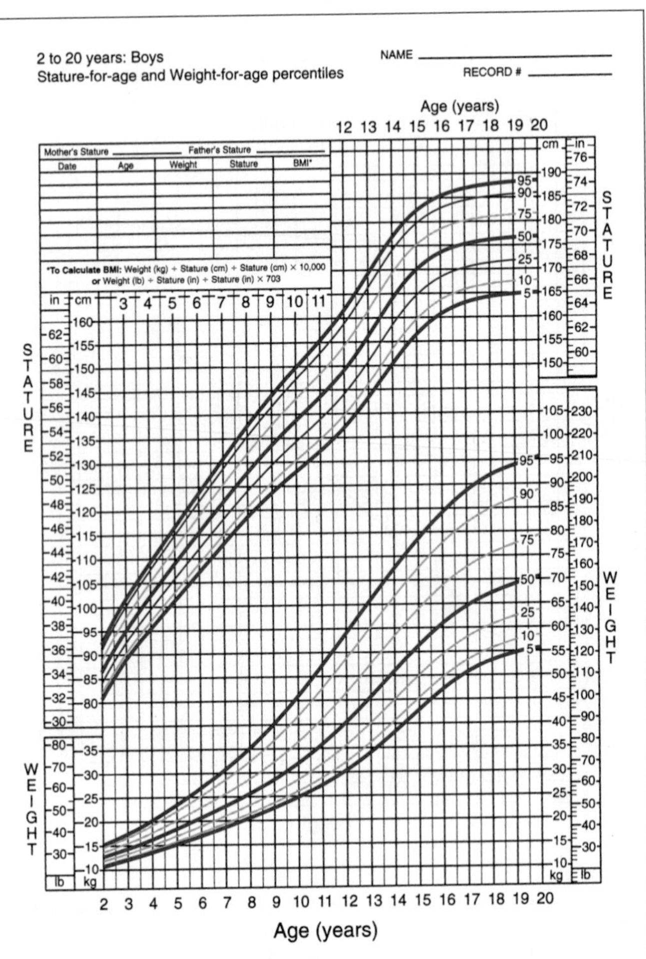

FIGURE 3-6

Stature-for-age and weight-for-age percentiles for boys, from 2 to 20 years. *(Developed by the National Center for Health Statistics in collaboration with the National Center for Chronic Disease Prevention and Health Promotion, 2000. http://www.cdc.gov/growthcharts/clinical_charts.htm)*

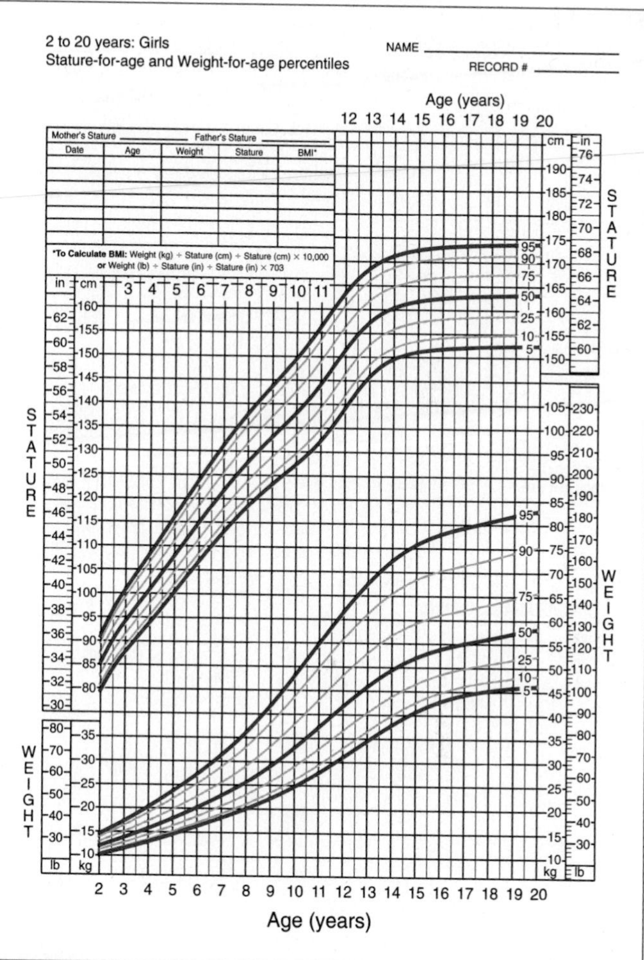

FIGURE 3-7

Stature-for-age and weight-for-age percentiles for girls, from 2 to 20 years. *(Developed by the National Center for Health Statistics in collaboration with the National Center for Chronic Disease Prevention and Health Promotion, 2000.* http://www.cdc.gov/growthcharts/clinical_charts.htm*)*

TABLE 3-8

ANTIMICROBIAL DOSING IN OBESITY

Antimicrobial Agent	Recommended Weight Used for Dose Calculation
AMINOGLYCOSIDES[24]	
Amikacin Gentamicin Tobramycin	Initial doses should be based on Vd using ABW with correction factor of 0.4 (ABW = IBW + 0.4 [TBW − IBW]). Final dosage adjustments should be based on serum concentrations.
β-LACTAMS/PENICILLINS	
Little information is available on penicillins in obesity. May consider empiric dosing based on the water content of fat using 0.3 as correction factor, although no clinical data support this[25] (ABW = IBW + 0.3 [TBW − IBW]).	
Ampicillin[25]	Empiric dose adjustment for obesity not recommended.
Ampicillin-sulbactam	No information available on dosing in obesity.
Nafcillin[25]	A case report showed increased volume of distribution in an obese adult; the report suggested adult-sized patients may require higher doses such as 3 g Q6 hr, but no conclusive data are available.
Penicillin G	No information available on dosing in obesity.
Piperacillin-tazobactam[26,27]	Two adult case reports demonstrate that normal adult maximum dose may not adequately achieve desired pharmacodynamic properties because of increased volume of distribution. Conclusive data for an optimal regimen are not available.
Ticarcillin-clavulanate	No information available on dosing in obesity.
β-LACTAMS/CEPHALOSPORINS	
Little information is available on cephalosporins in obesity. May consider empiric dosing based on the water content of fat using 0.3 as correction factor, although no clinical data support this[25] (ABW = IBW + 0.3 [TBW − IBW]). In obese adult-sized patients with severe infections, it may be considered to adjust dose to body surface area.[28]	
Cefazolin[29,30]	Dose on TBW. When using adult dosing ranges, dose at the upper end of the therapeutic range.
Cefepime[31]	Doses up to 2 g Q8 hr may be needed.
Cefotaxime[25]	Empiric dose adjustment for obesity not recommended for adult patients.
Cefotetan	No information available on dosing in obesity.
Ceftazidime	No information available on dosing in obesity.
Ceftriaxone	No information available on dosing in obesity.
Cefuroxime	No information available on dosing in obesity.
β-LACTAMS/CARBAPENEMS	
Ertapenem[28]	Doses >1 g may be needed for bacteria with MIC >0.25 mcg/mL.
Meropenem[30]	No dose adjustment recommended.
Imipenem-cilastatin	Base dose on Cl_{Cr}.

TABLE 3-8

ANTIMICROBIAL DOSING IN OBESITY (Continued)

Antimicrobial Agent	Recommended Weight Used for Dose Calculation
FLUOROQUINOLONES	
Ciprofloxacin[30,32]	Use of ABW with correction factor of 0.45 achieved plasma levels similar to nonobese patients dosed on TBW (ABW = IBW + 0.45 [TBW – IBW]). Penetration into skeletal muscle and subcutaneous adipose tissue is decreased in obese patients; thus, dosing on TBW may be needed to achieve adequate interstitial levels, despite increased plasma levels.
Levofloxacin[33]	Limited adult data show patients with normal renal function may be underexposed at traditional adult doses. Consider dose adjustments in obese patients with good renal function or worrisome pathogens.
Moxifloxacin[34]	Dose adjustment for obesity is not necessary.
MACROLIDES	
Azithromycin	No information is available on dosing in obesity.
Erythromycin[25]	Base dose on IBW.
MISCELLANEOUS	
Acyclovir[25]	Base dose on IBW.
Amphotericin B[25]	Base dose on TBW.
Aztreonam[35]	Use dose at upper end of dosage range for treating serious infections.
Clindamycin	No information is available on dosing in obesity.
Daptomycin[30]	Base dose on TBW, assessing for accumulation and skeletal muscle toxicity in patients with CrCl <30 mL/min/1.73 m^2.
Doxycycline	No information is available on dosing in obesity.
Fluconazole[25]	Doses >400 mg may be necessary in obese adolescents and adults, but optimal dosing is not known.
Flucytosine[30]	Base dose on IBW.
Linezolid[30]	Dose adjustment for obesity is not necessary.
Metronidazole	No information is available on dosing in obesity.
Micafungin[36]	Clearance in liters per hour increases as TBW increases, making the need for increased dosing likely, but optimal dosing is not known.
Oseltamivir[37,38]	Dose adjustment for obesity is not necessary.
Sulfamethoxazole-trimethoprim	No information is available on dosing in obesity.
Sulfisoxazole[30]	Dose adjustment for obesity is not necessary.
Tigecycline	No information is available on dosing in obesity.
Quinupristin-dalfopristin[30]	Base dose on TBW.
Vancomycin[39]	Base dose on TBW.
Voriconazole[40]	Oral: normal adult maximums may be observed. Increases based on TBW are not necessary. Intravenous: no information is available on dosing in obesity.

ABW, Adjusted body weight (kg); *ClCr*, creatinine clearance (mL/min/1.73m^2); *CrCl*, creatine clearance; *IBW*, ideal body wieght (kg); *MIC*, minimum inhibitory concentration; *TBW*, total or actual body weight (kg); *Vd* volume of distribution (L/kg).

VI. ANTIMICROBIAL TISSUE DISTRIBUTION BY KEY ORGAN SYSTEMS (TABLE 3-9)

TABLE 3-9

ANTIMICROBIAL TISSUE DISTRIBUTION BY KEY ORGAN SYSTEMS[7,10,41–43]

	Peak Serum Level (mcg/mL)	CNS	CSF Level Potentially Therapeutic	Bone	Ocular	Bile	Pulmonary	Other
Abacavir sulfate	3.3	CSF, 18%–33%						
Acyclovir	PO: 0.83–1.6 IV: 9.8–22.9	CSF, good, 13%–52%	Yes		AQUEOUS HUMOR, extensive	LIVER, good	LUNG, significant	TISSUES, significant (kidney, muscle, spleen, vaginal mucosa, heart tissue)
Albendazole	0.24–2.96	CSF, 43%						CYST FLUID, good, 13%–22%
Amantadine		CSF, 75%						
Amikacin		CSF, 10%–20%; up to 50% with inflamed meninges	No; intrathecal: 5–10 mg	BONE, therapeutic	AQUEOUS HUMOR, poor	BILE, low	BRONCHIAL SECRETIONS, 20% SPUTUM, 24.5%–43%	BODY FLUIDS, excellent BLISTER FLUID, 48% FAT AND MUSCLE, poor KIDNEY, excellent PERITONEAL FLUID, 39% SYNOVIAL FLUID, excellent TEARS, poor

Amoxicillin	5–10	CSF, 13%–14% with inflamed meninges	Yes			BILIARY, GALLBLADDER, and LIVER, concentrations exceed MIC for most bacteria	BRONCHIAL FLUID AND SPUTUM, 3.8%–7.2% LUNG AND PLEURAL FLUID, concentrations exceed MIC for most bacteria	MIDDLE EAR FLUID, >2 mcg/mL
Amoxicillin with clavulanic acid	Adults: 3.3–17/1–2 Pediatrics: 15.7/1.7	CSF, amoxicillin, 5%; clavulanic acid, 0%–8.4%		BONE, adequate			MUCOSA, 200% amoxicillin, 118% clavulanic acid LUNG AND PLEURAL FLUID	TONSILLAR TISSUE, 23% amoxicillin, 8% clavulanic acid MIDDLE-EAR EFFUSIONS, excellent
Amphotericin B	0.5–2	CSF, <2.5%			AQUEOUS HUMOR, ~67%		PLEURAL FLUID, ~67%	PERITONEAL FLUID, ~67% SYNOVIAL FLUID, ~67%
Amphotericin B cholesteryl sulfate	2.9	<1%						
Amphotericin B lipid complex	1.7	<1%				LIVER, high	LUNG, high	SPLEEN, high
Amphotericin B, liposomal	12.2–83	<1%				LIVER, 14%–22%	LUNG, <1%	SPLEEN, <6% HEART AND KIDNEY, <1%

Continued

3

TABLE 3-9

ANTIMICROBIAL TISSUE DISTRIBUTION BY KEY ORGAN SYSTEMS (Continued)

	Peak Serum Level (mcg/mL)	CNS	CSF Level Potentially Therapeutic	Bone	Ocular	Bile	Pulmonary	Other
Ampicillin	47	CSF, 13%–14% with inflamed meninges	Yes	BONE, 4.5%–15.4%	AQUEOUS HUMOR, adequate	Therapeutic concentrations not obtained with obstructive biliary tract disease	BRONCHIAL SECRETIONS, 3.2%–5.2%	KIDNEY, 50%–80%
Ampicillin with sulbactam	Adults: 50–120/30–60 Neonates: 86.3/110.2	CSF, 30%		BONE, ampicillin, 8%–25%; sulbactam, 18%–42%			BRONCHIAL SECRETIONS, ampicillin 6%, sulbactam 8%	PERITONEAL FLUID, ampicillin 92%, sulbactam 96%
Anidulafungin	Adults: 4.2–7.2 Pediatrics: 3.32–7.57	0	No					
Atazanavir	3.2–5.2	CSF, low						
Azithromycin	0.3–3.6					BILE, high	BRONCHIAL SECRETIONS, high and persistent SPUTUM, excellent	BLISTER FLUID, 74% EAR, excellent LYMPH, good TISSUES, excellent

Aztreonam	54–255	CSF, therapeutic with inflamed meninges	+/–	BONE, therapeutic	AQUEOUS HUMOR, therapeutic	BILE, therapeutic LIVER, therapeutic	BRONCHIAL SECRETIONS, therapeutic LUNG, therapeutic PLEURAL FLUID, therapeutic	BLISTER FLUID, therapeutic FAT, therapeutic GALL BLADDER, therapeutic KIDNEY, therapeutic LARGE INTESTINE, therapeutic PERICARDIAL FLUID, therapeutic PERITONEAL FLUID, therapeutic MUSCLE, therapeutic SKIN, therapeutic SYNOVIAL FLUID, therapeutic
Capreomycin	20–47		No					
Caspofungin	Adults: 6.6–20.9 Pediatrics: 11.9–20.9	CSF, 6%	No			LIVER, 1600%	LUNG, ~100%	TISSUES, 92% KIDNEYS, 300% HEART, 30% SMALL INTESTINE AND SPLEEN, ~100% LARGE INTESTINE, ~100%
Cefaclor	5–15					BILE, >60%		

Continued

TABLE 3-9

ANTIMICROBIAL TISSUE DISTRIBUTION BY KEY ORGAN SYSTEMS (Continued)

	Peak Serum Level (mcg/mL)	CNS	CSF Level Potentially Therapeutic	Bone	Ocular	Bile	Pulmonary	Other
Cefadroxil	Adults: 10–35 Pediatrics: 13.7					BILE, 22%		
Cefazolin	185	CSF, minimal	No	BONE, well, especially with inflamed bone		BILE, adequate	BRONCHIAL SECRETIONS, 32%	SYNOVIAL FLUID, adequate
Cefdinir	Adults: 1.6–2.87 Pediatrics: 2.2–3.86						BRONCHIAL MUCOSA, 15%–48%	MAXILLARY SINUS, 65% SKIN, 33% SPUTUM, 1.6%–1.9% MIDDLE-EAR FLUID, BLISTER FLUID, AND TONSILS, 15%–48%
Cefditoren	Adults: 2.5–4.6 Pediatrics: 1.2–2.6					GALLBLADDER, BILE, AND LIVER, high		

Cefepime	17.5–137	CSF, 10%	Yes		AQUEOUS HUMOR, temporarily therapeutic	BILE, therapeutic GALLBLADDER, therapeutic	BRONCHIAL MUCOSA, therapeutic	APPENDIX TISSUE, therapeutic BLISTER FLUID, therapeutic PERITONEAL FLUID, therapeutic SPUTUM, therapeutic URINE, therapeutic
Cefixime	1.9–7.7					BILE, 800%		SPUTUM, 2%–10%
Cefotaxime	3–214	CSF, 10%	Yes	BONE, good	AQUEOUS HUMOR, 0.16–2.3 mcg/mL	BILE, 15%–75%		TISSUES, good SPUTUM, 0.55%–8.5% SKIN, high
Cefotetan	126–158	CSF, 80%–360%				BILE, 2–21 times higher than concurrent serum concentrations		PELVIC GENITAL ORGANS, adequate
Cefoxitin	48.9–114.9	CSF, minimal penetration	+/–		AQUEOUS HUMOR, fair	BILE, 280%		PERITONEAL FLUID, 86%

Continued

TABLE 3-9

ANTIMICROBIAL TISSUE DISTRIBUTION BY KEY ORGAN SYSTEMS (Continued)

	Peak Serum Level (mcg/mL)	CNS	CSF Level Potentially Therapeutic	Bone	Ocular	Bile	Pulmonary	Other
Cefpodoxime proxetil	1.5–4.5					BILE, 115%	PLEURAL FLUID, fluid to plasma ratios were 0.24–1.07 PULMONARY TISSUE, rapid and extensive penetration, 0.53–0.78	BLISTER FLUID, 70% PROSTATIC FLUID, media plasma to prostatic fluid ratio was 0.1 TONSILS, moderate
Cefprozil	6–18							BLISTER FLUID, 50% MIDDLE EAR, good TONSILS, 37%–47%
Ceftaroline	21.3							Animal data indicate the drug is distributed into the kidneys, lungs, and skin
Ceftazidime	42–170	CSF, 20%–40% INTRACRANIAL ABSCESS, therapeutic	Yes			BILE, 13%–54%		

Ceftibuten	Adults: 15 Pediatrics: 5–19						BRONCHIAL SECRETIONS, 30% BRONCHOALVEOLAR LAVAGE FLUID, 81% LUNG TISSUE, 39%	BLISTER FLUID, 85%–132% NASAL SECRETIONS, 47% TRACHEAL SECRETIONS, 50%
Ceftriaxone	Adults: 82–257 Pediatrics: 216–275	CSF, 1%–32%	Yes	CANCELLOUS BONE, good STERNAL BONE, therapeutic	AQUEOUS HUMOR, low	BILE, 200%–500%	BRONCHIAL TISSUE, good	
Cefuroxime (IV/IM)	50–100	CSF, 17%–88%, therapeutic with inflamed meninges	Therapeutic with inflamed meninges	BONE, therapeutic	AQUEOUS HUMOR, therapeutic	BILE, therapeutic	BRONCHIAL SECRETIONS, therapeutic	PLEURAL FLUID, therapeutic JOINT FLUID, therapeutic
Cefuroxime axetil (PO)	2.1–13.6						BRONCHIAL SECRETIONS, therapeutic	
Cephalexin	9–32			JOINTS, therapeutic		BILE, 1%		SPUTUM, 4%–6%
Cephapirin	9–17			BONE, therapeutic				
Chloramphenicol	10–20	CSF, 45%–89%	Yes			LIVER, high		KIDNEY, high

Continued

3

TABLE 3-9

ANTIMICROBIAL TISSUE DISTRIBUTION BY KEY ORGAN SYSTEMS (Continued)

	Peak Serum Level (mcg/mL)	CNS	CSF Level Potentially Therapeutic	Bone	Ocular	Bile	Pulmonary	Other
Chloroquine HCL/ phosphate	0.125–0.15					LIVER, 200–700 times higher than plasma concentration	LUNG, 200–700 times higher than plasma concentration	SALIVA, 53% BRAIN, 10–30 times higher than plasma concentration KIDNEY, 200–700 times higher than plasma concentration
Cidofovir	26–43 (with probenecid)	Does not significantly cross into the CSF	No					
Ciprofloxacin	0.93–5.4	CSF, 26% (IV administration)	Inadequate for *Streptococcus* species		AQUEOUS HUMOR, fair (23%)	BILE, 2800%–4500% LIVER, good	LUNG, excellent (70%–170%)	BLISTER FLUID, good GALLBLADDER, good PERITONEAL, good (95%) SYNOVIAL FLUID, good (93%–647%) SPUTUM, good (22.7%–46.9%) TONSILS, excellent GYNECOLOGIC TISSUES, excellent

Clarithromycin	Adult: 1–4 Pediatric: 3–7	CSF, minimal				BILE, 7000%	LUNG, excellent	GASTRIC TISSUE, excellent MIDDLE-EAR EFFUSION, good SPUTUM, good TONSILS, excellent
Clindamycin	IV: 2.6–29 (adults); 8–10 (pediatrics) PO: 1.9–2.9 (adults); 1.29–2.44 (pediatrics)	CSF, poor even with inflamed meninges	No	BONE, therapeutic		BILIARY EXCRETION, 250%–300%	BRONCHIAL SECRETIONS, 35%–117%	TISSUES (HEAD and NECK), therapeutic
Clofazimine						BILE, LIVER, AND GALLBLADDER, excellent		
Cloxacillin	Adults: 7.5–15 Pediatrics: 28–80	CSF, poor			AQUEOUS HUMOR, poor	BILE, therapeutic	PLEURAL FLUID, therapeutic	ASCITES, poor SALIVA, poor SYNOVIAL FLUID, good
Colistimethate sodium	5–7.5	CSF, poor	No			BILIARY EXCRETION, 0%		

Continued

TABLE 3-9

ANTIMICROBIAL TISSUE DISTRIBUTION BY KEY ORGAN SYSTEMS (Continued)

	Peak Serum Level (mcg/mL)	CNS	CSF Level Potentially Therapeutic	Bone	Ocular	Bile	Pulmonary	Other
Cycloserine	20–30	CSF, 80%–100% (with inflamed meninges); 50%–80% (with uninflamed meninges)						TISSUES AND FLUIDS, widely distributed
Dapsone	1.1	CSF, good				LIVER, excellent	LUNG, good	
Delavirdine	0.91–45.66	CSF, very low, 0.4%						SALIVA, 6%
Demeclocycline	0.9–1.7	CSF, low						SKIN, well TISSUE, well
Dicloxacillin sodium	Adults: 10–18 Pediatrics: 12–40	CSF, minimal		BONE, 15%–72%				SYNOVIAL FLUID, 70%
Didanosine (IV not available in the United States)		CSF, 12%–85% (IV administration)	?					
Diethylcarbamazine		CSF, crosses the BBB						
Doripenem	16.4–29.6					BILE AND GALLBLADDER, excellent		PERITONEAL AND RETROPERITONEAL FLUIDS, AND URINE, excellent

Doxycycline	1.5–2.1	CSF, 26%	No	BONE, good	AQUEOUS HUMOR, good	BILE, 200%–3200%	BRONCHIAL SECRETIONS, good (16%) LUNG TISSUE, good	GYNECOLOGIC TISSUES, good
Efavirenz	9.2–16.6 mcmol	CSF, limited, 0.26%–1.19%						
Emtricitabine	1.1–2.5							SALIVA, excellent
Enfuvirtide	3.09–6.09	CSF, not measurable						
Ertapenem	155					BILE, 10%		
Erythromycin ethylsuccinate and acetylsulfisoxazole	127–211	CSF, variable					LUNG TISSUE, good	MIDDLE EAR, fair BODY FLUIDS, good TONSILS, good
Erythromycin preparations	0.3–2	CSF, limited	No				LUNG TISSUE, excellent	MIDDLE-EAR FLUID, excellent SINUS SECRETIONS, good SPUTUM, good TONSILS, excellent
Ethambutol HCl	2–5	CSF, 20%–80%	Yes with inflamed meninges				LUNG, good	KIDNEY, good
Ethionamide	2.16	CSF, significant concentrations						
Etravirine	0.002–4.852	CSF, good						

Continued

TABLE 3-9

ANTIMICROBIAL TISSUE DISTRIBUTION BY KEY ORGAN SYSTEMS (Continued)

	Peak Serum Level (mcg/mL)	CNS	CSF Level Potentially Therapeutic	Bone	Ocular	Bile	Pulmonary	Other
Fidaxomicin	0.002–0.179							FECES, extensive
Fluconazole	Adults: 4.12–8.1 Pediatrics: 2.9–14.1	CSF, 50%–90% (inflamed and normal meninges)	Yes				LUNG, good	BLISTER FLUID, 200% SALIVA, 100% URINE, 1000%
Flucytosine	30–40	CSF, 60%–100%	Yes		AQUEOUS HUMOR, high	LIVER, concentration equal to serum	LUNG, concentration equal to serum	HEART AND KIDNEY, concentration equal to serum
Fosamprenavir	4.06–8.68	CSF, 1.2% of serum concentration						
Foscarnet	155	CSF, 13%–103%		BONE, 3%–28%				
Fosfomycin	17–35.1	CSF, poor					BRONCHIAL SECRETIONS, 3.5%	
Ganciclovir	Adults: 7.25–10.4 Pediatrics: 6.6–7.9	CSF, 24%–70%	Yes		AQUEOUS HUMOR, poor to good	LIVER, 92%	LUNG, 99%	
Gentamicin		CSF, limited (0%–30%)	No; intrathecal: 5–10 mg	BONE, limited	AQUEOUS HUMOR, poor (4%–9%)	BILE, low (10%–60%)	BRONCHIAL TREE, limited (14%)	SALIVA, variable SYNOVIAL FLUID, good UROGENITAL TISSUE, good

Griseofulvin	0.5–2							SKIN, therapeutic HAIR AND NAILS, therapeutic
Imipenem-Cilastatin	40–60	CSF, 8.5%	Yes (concern for seizure potential)	BONE, dry weight bone concentrations 0.4–5.4 mcg/g		BILE, minimal	BRONCHIAL SECRETIONS, 6.7%	ASCITIC FLUID, exceeds MIC-90 for most organisms that cause peritonitis PANCREATIC SECRETIONS, exceeded MIC values for many organisms associated with pancreatic infections PERICARDIUM, 10-fold over the MIC for a majority of pathogens PERITONEAL FLUID, ~73%
Indinavir	12.6 mcM	CSF, 5%–9%						
Isoniazid	1–5	CSF, 90%–100%	Yes					SALIVA, 81% SYNOVIAL FLUID, 87.5%–133.3% TISSUES, similar to serum levels

Continued

3

TABLE 3-9

ANTIMICROBIAL TISSUE DISTRIBUTION BY KEY ORGAN SYSTEMS (Continued)

	Peak Serum Level (mcg/mL)	CNS	CSF Level Potentially Therapeutic	Bone	Ocular	Bile	Pulmonary	Other
Itraconazole	0.5–1.1	CSF, 0%, limited efficacy has been demonstrated in the treatment of cryptococcal and coccidioidal meningitis (penetration into the meninges as opposed to CSF levels)		BONE, excellent		LIVER, excellent	BRONCHIAL FLUID, excellent	TISSUES, excellent (skin, adipose tissue, endometrium, pus) NAIL, excellent
Ivermectin	0.05–0.08							LIVER AND ADIPOSE TISSUE, concentrated
Kanamycin		CSF, 0%–30%	No; intrathecal: 5–10 mg			BILE, 10%–60%	PLEURAL FLUID, excellent	ASCITIC FLUID, excellent SYNOVIAL FLUID, excellent
Ketoconazole	0.8	CSF, negligible						TISSUES, widely distributed

Lamivudine	1.5	CSF, 6%–11%	No data			
Levofloxacin	5.7–6.2	CSF, 30%–50%		AQUEOUS HUMOR, good	LUNG TISSUE, 200%–500%	BLISTER FLUID, extensive (100%) TISSUES, good to excellent (prostate and gynecologic tissues, semen, maxillary sinus mucosa, tonsils, and salivary glands)
Linezolid	IV: 12.9–15.1 (adults); 11–16.7 (pediatrics)	CSF, variable (pediatrics); excellent (adults)	Yes		PLEURAL FLUID, >4 mcg/mL	PANCREAS, 11–31.6 mcg/mL
Lopinavir/Ritonavir	8.1–15.5 (adults); 2.48–13.3 (pediatrics)	CSF, 0.225%	No			
Maraviroc	0.266–0.618	CSF, 1%–10%	No			
Mebendazole	0.02–0.5	CSF, 8.6 mcg/L				TISSUES, detected in liver, kidney, fat, muscle, and spleen
Mefloquine HCl	0.56–1.8	CSF, excellent, >1000 ng/mL				

Continued

TABLE 3-9

ANTIMICROBIAL TISSUE DISTRIBUTION BY KEY ORGAN SYSTEMS (Continued)

	Peak Serum Level (mcg/mL)	CNS	CSF Level Potentially Therapeutic	Bone	Ocular	Bile	Pulmonary	Other
Melarsoprol	4.7–6.7	CSF, low and variable						
Meropenem	14–58	CSF, 21%	Yes			BILE, high	BRONCHIAL MUCOSA, 4.5 mcg/mL BRONCHIAL SECRETIONS, high	BLISTER, 85% meropenem achieves concentrations that match or exceed those required to inhibit most susceptible bacteria in most body fluids and tissues
Metronidazole	IV: 18–25 PO: 6–40	CSF, ~100% (with inflamed meninges); 43% (with uninflamed meninges)				BILE, significant	BRONCHIAL SECRETIONS, ~100%	ABSCESSES, significant SALIVA, ~100%
Micafungin	Adults: 5.1–16.4 Pediatrics: 15.6–37.6	CSF, 0%	No					BONE ESCHAR, 2.2–6.4 times higher than plasma concentration

Miconazole		CSF, poor						TISSUE, widely distributed
Minocycline	2.62–6.63	CSF, limited (>doxycycline)		SYNOVIAL FLUID, limited	AQUEOUS HUMOR, good, 50%	BILE, 200%–3200%		GINGIVAL FLUID, excellent SALIVA/TEARS, good SINUS SECRETIONS, limited
Moxifloxacin	3.4–7.4	CSF, good penetration					BRONCHIAL MUCOSA, good	ABDOMINAL TISSUE AND FLUIDS, good SALIVA, exceeds plasma levels BLISTER FLUID, 200%
Nafcillin	30	CSF, good (>oxacillin, cloxacillin, dicloxacillin)	Yes, with high-dose IV therapy	SYNOVIAL FLUID, good	AQUEOUS HUMOR, negligible	BILE, >100%		PLEURAL FLUID, good
Nelfinavir	3–4	CSF, undetectable						
Neomycin sulfate	1–4							KIDNEY, good INNER EAR, good TISSUES, good
Nevirapine	0.9–3.6	CSF, present (45%)						
Nitrofurantoin								URINE, therapeutic

Continued

3

TABLE 3-9

ANTIMICROBIAL TISSUE DISTRIBUTION BY KEY ORGAN SYSTEMS (Continued)

	Peak Serum Level (mcg/mL)	CNS	CSF Level Potentially Therapeutic	Bone	Ocular	Bile	Pulmonary	Other
Norfloxacin	0.75–3.9					BILE, good GALLBLADDER, good		BLISTER FLUID, good PROSTATE, excellent TISSUE, good URINE, excellent
Ofloxacin	1.96–7.17	CSF, limited, 50% (with inflamed meninges)		BONE, limited, 25%	AQUEOUS HUMOR, excellent	BILE, excellent GALLBLADDER, excellent	BRONCHIAL SECRETIONS, good LUNG, excellent	ASCITIC FLUID, 80% BLISTER FLUID, good MIDDLE-EAR MUCOSA, excellent SALIVA, limited SPUTUM, excellent (71.6%–86%) TONSILS, good PLEURAL FLUID, good
Oseltamivir phosphate	0.065–0.348 (carboxylate)						LUNG, good to excellent	
Oxacillin	52–63	CSF, poor (>oxacillin, cloxacillin, dicloxacillin)	Yes, with high-dose IV therapy	BONE, generally not therapeutic	AQUEOUS HUMOR, poor	BILE, good	PLEURAL FLUID, good	ASCITES, poor

Para-aminosalicylic acid		CSF, low concentrations, does not cross the BBB unless meninges are inflamed			LIVER, high concentrations	LUNG, high concentrations	KIDNEYS, high concentrations
Penicillin G preparations—aqueous potassium and sodium	20	CSF, 5%–10%, poor, even with inflamed meninges	Yes for Pen-sens. *Streptococcus pneumoniae*	BONE, sufficient	BILE, 500%		FRACTURE HEMATOMA, sufficient SEPTIC JOINT EFFUSIONS, sufficient SYNOVIAL FLUID, variable
Penicillin G preparations—benzathine	0.15	CSF, minimal	No				
Penicillin G preparations—procaine		CSF, minimal, up to 4.5%, oral probenecid enhances penetration into the CSF resulting in sufficient treponemicidal concentrations (0.018 mcg/mL)					SYNOVIAL FLUID, well

Continued

3

TABLE 3-9

ANTIMICROBIAL TISSUE DISTRIBUTION BY KEY ORGAN SYSTEMS (Continued)

	Peak Serum Level (mcg/mL)	CNS	CSF Level Potentially Therapeutic	Bone	Ocular	Bile	Pulmonary	Other
Penicillin V potassium	4.9–6.3	CSF, minimal	No			BILE, low	PLEURAL FLUID, good	ASCITIC FLUID, good SYNOVIAL FLUID, good MIDDLE-EAR CONCENTRATIONS, 2.1–6.3 mcg/mL PERICARDIAL FLUID, good SALIVA, minimal
Pentamidine isethionate	IV: 0.3–1.4 Inhalation: 0.018–0.021					LIVER, extensive	BRONCHOALVEOLAR LAVAGE FLUID, 23.2 ng/mL	TISSUES, extensive (spleen, kidney, adrenals)
Piperacillin	305–775	CSF, good after continuous infusions		BONE, widely distributed		BILE, excellent		ADIPOSE TISSUE, excellent GALLBLADDER TISSUE, excellent SKELETAL MUSCLE, excellent HEART, widely distributed SPUTUM, 6%–22%

Piperacillin with tazobactam	76.5–139.9/ 13.9–29.5	CSF, low (when meninges are not inflamed)		BONE, well CANCELLOUS BONE, piperacillin 23%, tazobactam 26% CORTICAL BONE, piperacillin 18%, tazobactam 22%	BILE, well	LUNG TISSUE, well (92%)	BLISTER FLUID, 35%–42%
Posaconazole (Noxafil)	0.9–2		Yes				
Praziquantel	1	CSF, 14%–24%					
Pyrazinamide	Adults: 30–50 Pediatrics: 25.5–35	CSF, 100%	Yes		LIVER, adequate	LUNG, adequate	TISSUES, adequate penetration
Pyrimethamine + sulfadoxine	0.13–0.4/ 51–76						EXTRAVASCULAR FLUID, sulfadoxine penetrates well TISSUE, sulfadoxine not widely distributed
Quinidine gluconate	9.4	CSF, 7%–17%			LIVER, high		

Continued

3

TABLE 3-9

ANTIMICROBIAL TISSUE DISTRIBUTION BY KEY ORGAN SYSTEMS (Continued)

	Peak Serum Level (mcg/mL)	CNS	CSF Level Potentially Therapeutic	Bone	Ocular	Bile	Pulmonary	Other
Quinine sulfate	Adults: 3.2–8.4 Pediatrics: 3.4–7.5	CSF, poor (2%–7%)						RED BLOOD CELLS, 30%–50%
Quinupristin with dalfopristin	1–2/5–6							TISSUES, good, 83%
Raltegravir	2.2–6.5	CSF exceeded 50% inhibitory concentration for wild-type HIV by 4.5-fold						
Ribavirin	Inhalation: 0.44–1.55 mcmol PO: 3.68 (adults); 3.27 (pediatrics)						TRACHEAL SECRETIONS, excellent (>100× the MIC for RSV after 8 hr of aerosolized therapy)	RED BLOOD CELLS, may exceed serum level by 50-fold
Rifabutin							LUNG, lung-to-plasma ratio, 6.5:1	

Rifampin	Adults: 9–17.5 (IV)/4–32 (PO) Pediatrics: 11.7–41.5 (IV)/3.5–15 (PO)	CSF, 7%–56%	Yes	BONE, 3.9%–47%		BILE, high LIVER, excellent	LUNG, therapeutic BRONCHIAL MUCUS, 41.5%	ABSCESSES, 2.4–5 mcg/mL SALIVA, therapeutic in two thirds of patients SPUTUM, 1–3 mcg/mL STOMACH WALL, excellent ASCITIC FLUID, excellent
Rimantadine	0.1–0.57							NASAL MUCUS, 173%
Ritonavir	5–11.2	CSF, 0.1%–0.5%						
Saquinavir		CSF, 0.1%–0.2%; combination therapy, <2.5 ng/mL; with NRTI, 167 ng/mL; dual PI, 1094 ng/mL	No					
Stavudine	0.39–0.68	CSF, 16%–59%						
Streptomycin sulfate	25–50	CSF, poor	No; intrathecal: 5–10 mg		AQUEOUS HUMOR, good (subconjunctival administration)	BILE, 33%	BRONCHIAL SECRETIONS, 24% PLEURAL FLUID, 33%	ASCITIC FLUID, excellent

Continued

TABLE 3-9

ANTIMICROBIAL TISSUE DISTRIBUTION BY KEY ORGAN SYSTEMS (Continued)

	Peak Serum Level (mcg/mL)	CNS	CSF Level Potentially Therapeutic	Bone	Ocular	Bile	Pulmonary	Other
Sulfadiazine	60	CSF, 40%–60%						LYMPH, limited GALLBLADDER, limited
Sulfamethoxazole + trimethoprim	IV: 46.3/3.4 PO: 30–50/0.9–1.9	CSF, 40%–50%			AQUEOUS HUMOR, widely distributed	BILE, widely distributed		SPUTUM, widely distributed MIDDLE EAR, 20%/75%
Sulfisoxazole	50–100	CSF, 94 mcg/mL						
Suramin	127–211	CSF, extremely poor						TISSUES, ~100% (except brain) KIDNEY, ~200%
Telavancin	74.7–213							SKIN BLISTER FLUID, 40%
Telithromycin	1.9–2.9						BRONCHOPULMONARY TISSUE, extensive	WHITE BLOOD CELLS, 40 times higher than plasma SALIVA, exceeds plasma values
Tenofovir disoproxil fumarate	0.3–0.4	CSF, poor						LYMPHOCYTES, extensive SALIVA, poor

Terbinafine	1							TISSUES, extensive (adipose tissue, skin, nails)
Tetracycline HCl	1.5–2.2	BRAIN, good CSF, limited	No	BONE AND JOINTS, good		BILE, excellent	BRONCHIAL SECRETIONS, limited, 10%	TISSUES, good (skin, fat) PERIODONTAL TISSUE, excellent
Thiabendazole		CSF, 1.8 mcg/mL						
Ticarcillin	18–35	CSF, poor				BILE, good	PLEURAL FLUID, good	TISSUES, good
Ticarcillin with clavulanate	Adults: 330/8 Neonates: 278.7/8.4	CSF, poor and variable ticarcillin, 1.09–34.79 mg/L; clavulanic acid, 0.14–2.69 mg/L		BONE, adequate		BILE, ticarcillin, good; clavulanic acid, 42.8%	PLEURAL FLUID, adequate	BLISTER FLUID, ticarcillin, 58%; clavulanic acid, 77% LYMPH FLUID, excellent
Tigecycline	0.63–1.45		No	BONE, 35% SYNOVIAL FLUID, 585		BILE, 138%	LUNG, 8.6-fold higher than serum	COLON, 2.1-fold higher than serum GALLBLADDER, 38-fold higher than serum
Tinidazole	IV: 12.6–35.2 PO: 40–60				AQUEOUS HUMOR, 47%	BILE, widely distributed		SKIN, similar to plasma TISSUES, widely distributed (muscle, fat, appendix)

Continued

TABLE 3-9

ANTIMICROBIAL TISSUE DISTRIBUTION BY KEY ORGAN SYSTEMS (Continued)

	Peak Serum Level (mcg/mL)	CNS	CSF Level Potentially Therapeutic	Bone	Ocular	Bile	Pulmonary	Other
Tobramycin		CSF, 0%–30%	No; intrathecal: 5–10 mg	SYNOVIAL FLUID, excellent, >50%	AQUEOUS HUMOR, good (subconjunctival injection)	BILE, 10%–60%	BRONCHIAL SECRETIONS, good INTERSTITIAL FLUID, good	KIDNEY, good PERICARDIAL FLUID, good PERITONEAL FLUID, excellent, 15%–183% TEARS, limited
Trimethoprim	1.2–3.2			BONE, does not penetrate compact bone	AQUEOUS HUMOR, good though less than plasma	BILE, good though less than plasma	BRONCHIAL SECRETIONS, tissue-to-plasma ratio, 2:1	BLISTER FLUID, 76%–141% SALIVA, saliva to serum ration, 2:1
Trimetrexate	IV: 12 mcmol/L PO: 3 mcg/L	CSF, poor, 1%–4%					LUNG, good	
Valacyclovir	Adults: 4.3–5.6 Pediatrics: 2.6–5.9	CSF, 3.5–7.8 mcmol/L						

Vancomycin	30–60	CSF, 7%–14%, increased with meningitis	Need high doses		BILE, 50%	PLEURAL FLUID, well	BODY FLUIDS, well (pericardial, ascitic, synovial, urine, peritoneal)
Voriconazole	Adults: 2–3 Pediatrics: 3–11.4 (IV)/1.2–3 (PO)	CSF, 68%–100%	Yes			PLEURAL FLUID, 45.2%–64.5%	
Zalcitabine	0–0.2 mcmol/L	CSF, 9%–37%	Yes				
Zanamivir	0.017–0.142						SPUTUM, 47–1336 ng/mL (inhaled); no antiviral activity with systemic administration
Zidovudine	0.4–0.68	CSF, 50%–70%	Yes				FETAL BLOOD, 100% maternal blood

+/–, Yes in some studies, no in others; *BBB,* blood–brain barrier; *CNS,* central nervous system; *CSF,* cerebrospinal fluid; *IM,* intramuscular; *IV,* intravenous; *MIC,* minimum inhibitory concentration; *NRTI,* nucleoside reverse transcriptase inhibitor; *PI,* protease inhibitor.

REFERENCES

1. Jacobson P, West N, Hutchinson RJ. Predictive ability of creatinine clearance estimate models in pediatric bone marrow transplant patients. *Bone Marrow Transplant.* 1997;19:481-485.
2. Schwartz GJ, Brion LP, Spitzer A. The use of plasma creatinine concentration for estimating glomerular filtration rate in infants, children, and adolescents. *Pediatr Clin North Am.* 1987;34:571-590.
3. Seikaly MG, Browne R, Gajaj G, et al. Limitations of body length/serum creatinine ratio as an estimate of glomerular filtration in children. *Pediatr Nephrol.* 1996;10:709-711.
4. Schwartz GJ, Munoz A, Schneider MF, et al. New equations to estimate GFR in children with CKD. *J Am Soc Nephrol.* 2009;20(3):629-637.
5. Stevens LA, Coresh J, Greene T, et al. Assessing kidney function—measured and estimated glomerular filtration rate. *N Engl J Med.* 2006;354(23):2473-2483.
6. Lexi-Comp Online, Pediatric and Neonatal Lexi-Drugs. Hudson, Ohio, Lexi-Comp. Accessed October 5, 2012.
7. Micromedex Healthcare Series [intranet database], version 5.1. Greenwood Village, Colo., Thomson Reuters (Healthcare). Accessed October 5, 2012.
8. Lexi-Comp Online, Lexi-Drugs Online [intranet database]. Hudson, Ohio, Lexi-Comp. Accessed September 14, 2012.
9. Aronoff GR, Bennett WM, Berns JS, et al. *Drug Prescribing in Renal Failure.* 5th ed. Philadelphia, Pa.: American College of Physicians; 2007:39.
10. Lexi-Comp Online, AHFS DI [intranet database], Hudson, Ohio, Lexi-Comp. Accessed October 5, 2012.
11. Hudson JQ. Drug disposition in patients receiving continuous renal replacement therapies. *J Pediatr Pharmacol Ther.* 2001;6:15-39.
12. Joy MS, Matzke GR, Armstrong DK, et al. A primer on continuous renal replacement therapy for critically ill patients. *Ann Pharmacother.* 1998;32:362-375.
13. Mouser JF, Thompson JB. Drugs removed by renal replacement therapies. *J Pediatr Pharmacol Ther.* 2001;6:79-87.
14. Veltri MA, Neu AM, Fivush BA, et al. Drug dosing during intermittent hemodialysis and continuous renal replacement therapy: Special considerations in pediatric patients. *Pediatr Drugs.* 2004;6(1):45-65.
15. Johns Hopkins Children's Center. Guidelines for Vancomycin Dosing and Therapeutic Drug Monitoring in Neonatal and Pediatric Patients. January 27, 2012.
16. Pugh RNH, Murray-Lyon IM, Dawson JL, et al. Transection of the oesophagus for bleeding oesophageal varices. *Br J Surg.* 1973;60:646-649.
17. Lucey MR, Brow KA, Everson GJ, et al. Minimal criteria for placement of adults on the liver transplant waiting list: A report of a national conference organized by the American Society of Transplant Physicians and the American Association for the Study of Liver Diseases. *Liver Transplant Surg.* 1997;3:628-637.
18. Verbeeck RK. Pharmacokinetics and dosage adjustment in patients with hepatic dysfunction. *Eur J Clin Pharmacol.* 2008;64:1147-1161.
19. Lexi-Drugs (website). Hudson, Ohio, Lexi Comp, 1978–2012: www.crlonline.com. Accessed July 12, 2012.

20. Drugdex System (website). Greenwood Village, Colo., Thomson Reuters (Healthcare), 1974–2012: http://www.thomsonhc.com. Accessed July 12, 2012.
21. AHFS Drug Information (website). Bethesda, Md., American Society of Health-System Pharmacists, 1959–2012: www.ahfsdruginformation.com. Accessed July 12, 2012.
22. Pediatric and Neonatal Lexi-Drugs (website). Hudson, Ohio, Lexi Comp, 1978–2012: www.crlonline.com. Accessed July 12, 2012.
23. Phillips S, Edlbeck A, Kirby M, Goday P. Ideal body weight in children. *Nutr Clin Pract.* 2007;22:240-245.
24. Bearden DT, Rodvold KA. Dosage adjustments for antibacterials in obese patients. *Clin Pharmacokinet.* 2000;38:415-426.
25. Wurtz R, Itokazu G, Rodvold K. Antimicrobial dosing in obese patients. *Clin Infect Dis.* 1997;25:112-118.
26. Newman D, Scheetz MH, Adeyemi OA, et al. Serum piperacillin/tazobactam pharmacokinetics in a morbidly obese individual. *Ann Pharmacother.* 2007;41:1734-1739.
27. Deman H, Verhaegen J, Willems L, Spriet I. Dosing of piperacillin/tazobactam in a morbidly obese patient. *J Antimicrob Chemother.* 2012;67:782-783.
28. Medico CJ, Walsh P. Pharmacotherapy in the critically ill obese patient. *Crit Care Clin.* 2010;26:679-688.
29. Kendrick JG, Carr RR, Ensom MHH. Pharmacokinetics and drug dosing in obese children. *J Pediatr Pharmacol Ther.* 2010;15:94-109.
30. Pai M, Bearden DT. Antimicrobial dosing consideration in obese adult patients: Insights from the Society of Infectious Diseases Pharmacists. *Pharmacotherapy.* 2007;27(8):1081-1091.
31. Rich BS, Keel R, Ho VP, et al. Cefepime dosing in the morbidly obese patient population. *Obes Surg.* 2012;22:465-471.
32. Hollenstein UM, Brunner M, Schmid R, Müller M. Soft tissue concentrations of ciprofloxacin in obese and lean subjects following weight-adjusted dosing. *Int J Obes.* 2001;25:3354-3358.
33. Cook AM, Martin C, Adams VR, Morehead RS. Pharmacokinetics of intravenous levofloxacin administered at 750 milligrams in obese adults. *Antimicrob Agents Chemother.* 2011;55:3240-3243.
34. Kees MG, Weber S, Kees F, Horbach T. Pharmacokinetics of moxifloxacin in plasma and tissue of morbidly obese patients. *J Antimicrob Chemother.* 2011;66:2230-2235.
35. Erstad BL. Dosing of medications in morbidly obese patients in the intensive care unit setting. *Intensive Care Med.* 2004;30:18-32.
36. Hall RG, Swancutt MA, Gumbo T. Fractal geometry and the pharmacometrics of micafungin in overweight, obese, and extremely obese people. *Antimicrob Agents Chemother.* 2011;55:5107-5112.
37. Pai MP, Lodise TP. Oseltamivir and oxeltamivir carboxylate pharmacokinetics in obese adults: Dose modification for weight is not necessary. *Antimicrob Agents Chemother.* 2011;55:5640-5645.
38. Thorne-Humphrey LM, Goralski KB, Slayter KL, et al. Oseltamivir pharmacokinetics in morbid obesity (OPTIMO trial). *J Antimicrob Chemother.* 2011;66:2083-2091.
39. Moffett BS, Kim S, Edwards MS. Vancomycin dosing in obese pediatric patients. *Clin Pediatr.* 2011;50:442-446.

3

40. Pai MP, Lodise TP. Steady-state plasma pharmacokinetics of oral voriconazole in obese adults. *Antimicrob Agents Chemother.* 2011;55:2601-2605.
41. Gilbert DN, Moellering RC, Eliopoulis GM, et al. *The Sanford Guide to Antimicrobial Therapy 2012.* 42th ed. Sperryville, Va.: Therapy; 2012.
42. Lustar I, McCracken G, Friedland I. Antibiotic pharmacodynamics in cerebrospinal fluid. *Clin Infect Dis.* 1998;27:1117-1129.
43. Kethireddy S, Andes D. CNS pharmacokinetics of antifungal agents. *Expert Opin Drug Metab Toxicol.* 2007;3(4):573-581.

Chapter 4

Mechanisms of Action and Routes of Administration of Antimicrobial Agents

Karen C. Carroll, MD

TABLE 4-1

MECHANISMS OF ACTION AND ROUTES OF ADMINISTRATION OF ANTIMICROBIAL AGENTS

			Routes of Administration				
Class	**Mechanism of Action**	**Antibacterial**	**PO**	**IM**	**IV**	**T**	**INHAL**
ANTIBACTERIAL							
Aminoglycoside	Protein synthesis inhibition caused by high-avidity binding of mRNA and interference with mRNA translation and translocation	Amikacin		X	X		
		Gentamicin		X	X	X	
		Kanamycin		X	X		
		Neomycin				X	
		Paromomycin	X				
		Spectinomycin		X	X		
		Streptomycin		X	X		
		Tobramycin		X	X		X
β-Lactam/β-lactamase inhibitor	Inhibition of cell-wall synthesis by inactivation of various penicillin-binding proteins (PBPs) class A β-lactamase inhibitors	Amoxicillin/Clavulanic acid	X				
		Ampicillin/Sulbactam			X		
		Piperacillin/Tazobactam			X		
		Ticarcillin/Clavulanate			X		
β-Lactam/Carbapenem/Carbacephem	Inhibition of cell-wall synthesis by inactivation of most high-molecular-weight PBPs	Doripenem			X		
		Ertapenem		X	X		
		Imipenem/Cilastatin			X		
		Meropenem			X		
	β-lactamase stable	Loracarbef	X		X		
β-Lactam/Cephalosporin I	Inhibits cell-wall synthesis by binding to PBPs	Cefadroxil	X				
		Cefazolin		X	X		
		Cephalexin	X				
β-Lactam/Cephem/Cephalosporin II	Inhibits cell-wall synthesis by binding to PBPs	Cefaclor	X	X			
		Cefprozil	X				
		Cefuroxime		X	X		
β-Lactam/Cephalosporin III	Inhibits cell-wall synthesis by binding to PBPs	Cefdinir	X				
		Cefditoren	X				
		Cefixime	X				
		Cefotaxime		X	X		
		Cefpodoxime	X				
		Ceftazidime		X	X		
		Ceftibuten	X				
		Ceftizoxime		X	X		
		Ceftriaxone		X	X		
β-Lactam/Cephalosporin IV	Inhibits cell-wall synthesis by binding to PBPs	Cefepime		X	X		
		Ceftaroline*			X		
β-Lactam/Cephamycin	Inhibits cell-wall synthesis by binding to PBPs	Cefotetan		X	X		
		Cefoxitin		X	X		

TABLE 4-1

MECHANISMS OF ACTION AND ROUTES OF ADMINISTRATION OF ANTIMICROBIAL AGENTS (Continued)

Class	Mechanism of Action	Antibacterial	Routes of Administration				
			PO	IM	IV	T	INHAL
β-Lactam/ Penicillin	Inhibits cell-wall synthesis by binding to PBPs	Amoxicillin	X				
		Ampicillin	X	X	X		
		Penicillin G	X	X	X		
		Penicillin V	X				
β-Lactam/ Penicillinase stable penicillin	Inhibits cell-wall synthesis by binding to PBPs	Cloxacillin	X				
		Dicloxacillin	X				
		Nafcillin			X		
		Oxacillin		X	X		
β-Lactam/ Monobactam	Inhibition of cell-wall synthesis by binding to PBPs	Aztreonam		X	X		X
Fluoroquinolone	Inhibits bacterial DNA synthesis by inhibiting DNA gyrase and topoisomerase IV	Norfloxacin	X				
		Ofloxacin	X	X	X	X	
		Ciprofloxacin	X		X	X[†]	
		Gemifloxacin	X		X		
		Levofloxacin	X		X		
		Moxifloxacin	X			X	
Macrolide	Inhibits protein synthesis by binding to 23S rRNA preventing peptide chain elongation	Azithromycin	X		X		
		Clarithromycin	X				
		Erythromycin	X		X	X	
Macrocyclic antibiotic with 18-membered core	Inhibits RNA synthesis by binding to and inhibiting DNA-dependent RNA polymerase	Fidaxomicin	X				
Sulfonamide	Interferes with folic acid/folate synthesis by inhibiting incorporation of para-aminobenzoic acid	Sulfacetamide	X		X		
		Sulfadiazine	X		X		
		Sulfisoxazole	X		X		
Trimethoprim	Interferes with folic acid synthesis by inhibiting dihydrofolate reductase	Trimethoprim	X				
Trimethoprim/ Sulfamethoxazole	Folic acid synthesis inhibition	Co-trimoxazole (trimethoprim/ sulfamethoxazole)	X		X		
Lipopeptide	Disrupts bacterial cell membrane through calcium-dependent binding resulting in loss of intracellular potassium	Daptomycin			X		

Continued

TABLE 4-1

MECHANISMS OF ACTION AND ROUTES OF ADMINISTRATION OF ANTIMICROBIAL AGENTS (Continued)

			Routes of Administration				
Class	**Mechanism of Action**	**Antibacterial**	**PO**	**IM**	**IV**	**T**	**INHAL**
Polymyxins	Disrupt bacterial cell membranes by interacting with phospholipids	Polymyxin B			X	X	
		Colistin (Polymyxin E)			X	X	X
Tetracycline	Inhibits protein synthesis by binding to 30S rRNA subunit	Doxycycline	X		X		
		Minocycline	X		X		
		Tetracycline	X		X		
Glycylcycline	Inhibits protein synthesis by binding to 30S rRNA subunit	Tigecycline			X		
Phenicol	Inhibits protein synthesis by reversibly binding to the larger 50S subunit of the 70S ribosome	Chloramphenicol	X		X	X	
Lincosamide	Inhibits protein synthesis by binding to 50S ribosomal subunit	Clindamycin	X	X	X		
Streptogramins	Inhibit elongation stage of protein synthesis by binding to 50S ribosomal subunit	Quinupristin/ Dalfopristin			X		
Oxazolidinone	Inhibits earliest steps of bacterial protein synthesis by binding to 50S ribosomal unit at the interface with the 30S subunit	Linezolid	X		X		
Glycopeptide	Inhibits late stages of cell-wall synthesis in bacteria	Vancomycin	X		X	X	
		Teicoplanin	X	X	X		
Fosfomycin	Inhibits peptide synthesis	Fosfomycin	X				
Nitrofuran	Inhibits bacterial aerobic energy metabolism and synthesis; damages bacterial DNA	Nitrofurantoin	X				
Nitroimidazoles	DNA damage	Metronidazole	X		X	X	
Rifamycins	Inhibit RNA synthesis by inhibiting β subunit of DNA-dependent RNA polymerase	Rifampin	X		X		
		Rifaximin	X				

TABLE 4-1

MECHANISMS OF ACTION AND ROUTES OF ADMINISTRATION OF ANTIMICROBIAL AGENTS (Continued)

Class	Mechanism of Action	Antibacterial	Routes of Administration				
			PO	IM	IV	T	INHAL
Pseudomonic acid	Inhibits RNA and protein synthesis by binding to isoleucyl-tRNA synthetase	Mupirocin				X	
Cyclic peptides	Inhibit cell-wall synthesis	Bacitracin				X	
ANTIMYCOBACTERIAL							
Isonicotinic acid derivative	Inhibition of cell-wall mycolic acid synthesis; also inhibits catalase-peroxidase enzyme	Isoniazid	X	X	X		
		Ethionamide	X				
Rifamycins	Inhibit RNA synthesis by inhibiting β subunit of DNA-dependent RNA polymerase	Rifampin	X		X		
		Rifabutin	X				
		Rifapentine	X				
Ethambutol	Inhibits cell-wall (arabinogalactan) biosynthesis	Ethambutol	X				
Salicylic acid	Inhibits folate synthesis	*p*-Aminosalicylic acid	X				
Pyrazine analogue of nicotinamide	Membrane potential/ proton motive force	Pyrazinamide	X				
Basic polypeptide	Inhibits protein synthesis	Capreomycin		X	X		
Sulfone	Inhibits folate synthesis	Dapsone	X				
Phenazine dye	Not entirely known; may chelate iron	Clofazimine	X				
ANTIFUNGAL							
Polyenes	Disrupt fungal membrane; binds to ergosterol	Amphotericin B/ Amphotericin B lipid formulations			X	X	X
		Nystatin	X			X	
Antimetabolite	Inhibits DNA synthesis	5-Fluorocytosine (Flucytosine)	X			X	
Imidazoles	Disrupt membrane (ergosterol) biosynthesis	Ketoconazole	X			X	
		Clotrimazole	X			X	
		Miconazole	X			X	
Triazoles	Disrupt membrane (ergosterol) biosynthesis	Fluconazole	X		X		
		Itraconazole	X				
		Terconazole				X[‡]	
		Voriconazole	X		X		
		Posaconazole	X				

Continued

TABLE 4-1

MECHANISMS OF ACTION AND ROUTES OF ADMINISTRATION OF ANTIMICROBIAL AGENTS (Continued)

			Routes of Administration				
Class	**Mechanism of Action**	**Antibacterial**	**PO**	**IM**	**IV**	**T**	**INHAL**
Echinocandins	Inhibit cell-wall (1, 3-β-D-glucan) synthesis	Caspofungin			X		
		Anidulafungin			X		
		Micafungin			X		
Griseofulvin	Inhibits mitosis and microtubules	Griseofulvin	X			X	
Allylamine	Inhibits ergosterol biosynthesis	Terbinafine	X			X	
ANTIVIRAL							
Antiherpes virus	Inhibits viral DNA synthesis	Vidarabine			X	X†	
		Acyclovir	X			X	
		Valacyclovir	X		X		
		Cidofovir			X		
		Famciclovir	X				
		Idoxuridine				X†	
		Penciclovir				X	
		Trifluridine				X†	
		Valganciclovir	X		X		
		Ganciclovir				X†	
Pyrophosphate analogue	Blocks pyrophosphate exchange on viral DNA polymerase	Foscarnet			X		
Synthetic thymidine nucleoside analogue	Inhibits HBV DNA polymerase (but not HIV)	Telbivudine	X				
Antiretroviral nucleoside/ nucleotide analogues	Inhibit of reverse transcriptase	Zidovudine	X		X		
		Stavudine	X				
		Didanosine	X				
		Zalcitabine	X				
		Lamivudine	X				
		Emtricitabine	X				
		Abacavir	X				
		Tenofovir	X				
Antiretroviral	Non-nucleoside reverse transcriptase inhibition	Nevirapine	X				
		Efavirenz	X				
		Delavirdine	X				
		Etravirine	X				

*Unique among β-lactams; binds to PBP2a, so it has methicillin-resistant Staphylococcus aureus activity.

†Ophthalmic drops or retinal administration.

‡Vaginal cream.

HBV, hepatitis B virus; *IM*, intramuscular; *INHAL*, inhalation; *IV*, intravenous; *mRNA*, messenger RNA; *PBP*, penicillin-binding protein; *PO*, by mouth; *rRNA*, ribosomal RNA; *T*, topical; *tRNA*, transfer RNA.

TABLE 4-1

MECHANISMS OF ACTION AND ROUTES OF ADMINISTRATION OF ANTIMICROBIAL AGENTS (Continued)

			Routes of Administration				
Class	**Mechanism of Action**	**Antibacterial**	**PO**	**IM**	**IV**	**T**	**INHAL**
Antiretroviral	HIV protease inhibitors	Saquinavir	X				
		Indinavir	X				
		Ritonavir	X				
		Nelfinavir	X				
		Lopinavir/ritonavir	X				
		Atazanavir	X				
		Fosamprenavir	X				
		Tipranavir	X				
		Darunavir	X				
Antiretroviral	HIV entry inhibitors	Enfuvirtide		X			
		Maraviroc	X				
Antiretroviral	Integrase strand transfer inhibitors	Raltegravir	X				
Tricyclic amines	Inhibit M protein ion channel function and inhibit hemagglutinin formation of influenza A viruses	Amantadine	X				
		Rimantadine	X				
Nucleoside analogue	Interferes with capping and elongation of mRNA	Ribavirin	X		X		X
		Adefovir	X		X		
Neuraminidase inhibitors	Inhibit influenza virus neuraminidase activity	Oseltamivir	X				
		Peramivir			X		
		Zanamivir					X
Cytidine analogue	Selective inhibitor of HIV-1, HIV-2, and HBV	Emtricitabine	X				
Protease inhibitor (non-HIV)	Inhibits hepatitis C viral serine protease	Telaprevir	X				
ANTIPARASITIC							
Benzimidazoles	Inhibition of tubulin polymerization, cytoskeletal disruption	Albendazole	X				
		Mebendazole	X				
		Thiabendazole	X				
Nitroimidazoles	Production of free radicals that damage DNA	Metronidazole	X		X	X[‡]	
		Tinidazole	X				
Avermectins	Hyperpolarization of susceptible cell membranes	Ivermectin	X				
Piperazine derivative	Alteration of the surface membrane of microfilariae	Diethylcarbamazine	X				
Emetine derivative	Inhibits protein synthesis by blocking peptide elongation	Dehydroemetine		X	X		

Continued

TABLE 4-1

MECHANISMS OF ACTION AND ROUTES OF ADMINISTRATION OF ANTIMICROBIAL AGENTS (Continued)

			Routes of Administration				
Class	**Mechanism of Action**	**Antibacterial**	**PO**	**IM**	**IV**	**T**	**INHAL**
4-Aminoquinoline	Nonenzymatic inhibition of heme polymerization	Chloroquine	X	X			
		Hydroxychloroquine	X				
8-Aminoquinoline	Inhibition of parasitic mitochondrial enzymes	Primaquine	X				
Aminoalcohols	Mechanism unknown	Halofantrine	X				
		Lumefantrine/ artemether	X				
Cinchona alkaloids	Interfere with hemoglobin digestion, inhibition of nucleic acid, and protein synthesis	Quinine	X		X		
Synthetic quinolines	Interfere with hemoglobin metabolism	Mefloquine	X				
Artemisinin derivatives	Damage of parasite organelles through oxidation by free radicals	Artemisinin	X				
		Artesunate	X	X	X		
		Artemether	X	X			
Folate antagonists	Inhibits plasmodial dihydrofolate reductase	Pyrimethamine/ Sulfadoxine	X				
		Proguanil (administered with atovaquone)	X				
Combination agent	Inhibition of electron transport, blocking nucleic synthesis Synergistic loss of mitochondrial membrane potential	Atovaquone/ proguanil	X				
Acetanilide	Unknown	Diloxanide furoate	X				
Aromatic diamidine	Inhibition of dihydrofolate reductase, glycolysis, and DNA, RNA, and protein synthesis	Pentamidine isethionate		X	X	X	
Antimonials	Inhibit parasite energy processes	Sodium stibogluconate		X	X		
		Meglumine antimoniate		X	X		
Organic arsenical	Inhibits several key parasite enzymes	Melarsoprol			X		

TABLE 4-1

MECHANISMS OF ACTION AND ROUTES OF ADMINISTRATION OF ANTIMICROBIAL AGENTS (Continued)

Class	Mechanism of Action	Antibacterial	Routes of Administration				
			PO	IM	IV	T	INHAL
Fluorinated analogue of ornithine	Interferes with polyamine synthesis	Eflornithine			X		
Oxazolidinone	Damages cellular components	Furazolidone	X				
Hydroxybenzamide (Teniacide)	Inhibits oxidative phosphorylation in mitochondria of tapeworms	Niclosamide	X				
Nitrofuran derivative	Compound is reduced to a variety of cytotoxic molecules	Nifurtimox	X				
Nitrobenzamide	Interferes with anaerobic energy metabolism	Nitazoxanide	X				
Cyclic pyrazino isoquinoline antihelmintic	Interferes with parasite metabolism and disrupts parasite integument	Praziquantel	X				

Chapter 5

Mechanisms of Drug Resistance

Karen C. Carroll, MD

I. COMMON MECHANISMS OF MICROBIAL RESISTANCE

TABLE 5-1

COMMON MECHANISMS OF MICROBIAL RESISTANCE

Resistance Category	Antibiotics	Specific Mechanism
Enzymatic modification or nonactivation of the antimicrobial agent	β-Lactams	β-Lactamases
	Aminoglycosides	Aminoglycoside-inactivating (acetylases, phosphorylases, adenylases) enzymes
	Chloramphenicol	Chloramphenicol acetyltransferases
	Macrolides	Macrolide esterases/phosphorylases
	Lincosamides/Streptogramins	Adenylases/Acetylases
	5-Fluorocytosine	Mutation in cytosine deaminase
	Metronidazole	Decrease in activation by pyruvate/ferredoxin oxidoreductase system
	Fluoroquinolone	Bifunctional enzymes that acetylate quinolones (specifically ciprofloxacin) and aminoglycosides
	Tetracycline	TetX hydrolysis of tetracyclines including tigecycline
Alteration of target site	β-Lactams	Structural change in PBPs or importation of new PBP
	Aminoglycosides	Methylation of 16S rRNA
	Macrolides	Methylation of rRNA (macrolide, lincosamide, streptogramin B methylase [MLS_B]) mediated by *erm* genes
	Clindamycin	
	Streptogramins	
	Fluoroquinolones	Structural change (mutation) of DNA gyrase or topoisomerase IV
	Glycopeptides	Modification of the D-alanine terminus of cell-wall pentapeptide
	Rifamycins	Mutation on the RNA polymerase β subunit (rpoB)
	Sulfonamides	Structural change in DHPS
	Trimethoprim	Structural change in dihydrofolate reductase
	Tetracycline	Alteration of ribosomal target
	Oxazolidinones	Alterations in 23S rRNA
	Polymyxin	Alterations in binding to outer membrane target
	Daptomycin	Alterations in cell membrane binding sites because of mutations in *mprF* gene

Continued

TABLE 5-1

COMMON MECHANISMS OF MICROBIAL RESISTANCE (Continued)

Resistance Category	Antibiotics	Specific Mechanism
Decreased permeability	β-Lactams	Loss of specific porins caused by mutations
	Aminoglycosides	Lack of production of outer membrane proteins caused by mutations; inner membrane transport changes
	Chloramphenicol	Plasmid-mediated alterations in outer membrane proteins
	Macrolide	Decreased permeability of outer cell membrane of gram-negative rods
	Lincosamide/Streptogramin	Decreased permeability of outer cell membrane of gram-negative rods
	Tetracycline	Alteration of porin channels, e.g., OmpF
	Fluoroquinolone	Modification of porin channels (e.g., decreased expression of OmpF porin in *E. coli*)
	Glycopeptides	Alterations in outer membrane porins
Efflux	Tetracycline	Efflux pumps
	Glycylcyclines (tigecycline)	Efflux pumps
	Macrolides (14- to 15-membered ring)	Efflux pumps (*mef* genes)
	Fluoroquinolones	Efflux pumps
	Carbapenems	Loss of outer membrane porins
	Aminoglycosides	Decreased uptake/accumulation
	Oxazolidinone (linezolid)	Efflux pumps
Protection of target site	Fluoroquinolone	Protection of DNA gyrase from quinolone binding
	Tetracycline	*tetM*-mediated protection of ribosome from tetracycline binding
	Daptomycin	Increased thickness of bacterial cell wall
Overproduction of target	Sulfonamide	Overproduction of the enzyme DHPS
	Trimethoprim	Overproduction of the enzyme dihydrofolate reductase
	Glycopeptide	Overproduction of peptidoglycan
Bypass of inhibited process	Sulfonamide	Development of auxotrophs that have unique growth requirements
	Trimethoprim	
	Metronidazole	Loss of activity of reduced NADPH nitroreductase
Bind-up antibiotic	Glycopeptide	Production of an increased number of false binding sites
	Polymyxin	Binding by polysaccharide capsule

Modified from Opal SM, Pop-Vicas A. Molecular mechanisms of antibiotic resistance in bacteria. In: *Mandell, Douglas and Bennett's Principles and Practice of Infectious Diseases.* 7th ed. Philadelphia: Churchill Livingstone-Elsevier; 2010.

II. DISCORDANCE BETWEEN IN VITRO SUSCEPTIBILITY AND IN VIVO EFFICACY

TABLE 5-2

DISCORDANCE BETWEEN IN VITRO SUSCEPTIBILITY AND IN VIVO EFFICACY

Organisms	May Be Susceptible In Vitro	In Vivo
Salmonella	First and second generation cephalosporins	Poor in vivo efficacy.
Shigella	Aminoglycosides	
Extended-spectrum β-lactamase producing *Klebsiella* spp. *Escherichia coli* *Proteus mirabilis*	Cephalosporins Aztreonam ± β-lactam/β-lactamase inhibitors	Poor in vivo efficacy.
Methicillin-resistant staphylococci	All β-lactam agents, including penicillin, cephalosporins, and carbapenems	Poor in vivo efficacy.
Enterococcus spp.	All cephalosporin, clindamycin, macrolides, trimethoprim/sulfamethoxazole, and aminoglycosides (except high-level gentamicin <500 mcg/mL and streptomycin <2000 mcg/mL)	Poor in vivo efficacy.
Listeria spp.	All cephalosporins	Poor in vivo efficacy.
Clostridium difficile	All antibiotics except metronidazole and vancomycin	Poor in vivo efficacy.
Enterobacter spp. *Citrobacter* spp. *Serratia* spp. *Morganella* spp. *Providencia* spp.	Third generation cephalosporins	Initial susceptibility but rapid emergence of resistance during therapy. Combination therapy usually required.
Pseudomonas aeruginosa	All antimicrobial agents	Emergence of resistance during therapy. Combination therapy usually required.
Staphylococcus spp.	Quinolones, vancomycin (VISA)	Emergence of resistance during prolonged therapy.
Staphylococci, Streptococci	Erythromycin resistant, clindamycin susceptible	Macrolide resistance can be caused by inducible MLS resistance, which can result in clinical failure with clindamycin. Clindamycin susceptibility should be evaluated using the "D" test or similar assay if erythromycin resistant.
Yersinia pestis	All β-lactam agents	Poor in vivo efficacy.

Continued

TABLE 5-2

DISCORDANCE BETWEEN IN VITRO SUSCEPTIBILITY AND IN VIVO EFFICACY (Continued)

Organisms	May Be Susceptible In Vitro	In Vivo
All CSF isolates	All oral antibiotics Clindamycin Tetracyclines Fluoroquinolones First and second generation cephalosporins/cephamycins	Poor penetration/ concentration in CSF. Poor in vivo efficacy.

Chapter 6

Therapeutic Drug Monitoring

Kristine A. Parbuoni, PharmD, BCPS, and Carlton K. K. Lee, PharmD, MPH

I. GENERAL PRINCIPLES

A. Therapeutic Drug Monitoring

Therapeutic drug monitoring uses serum drug concentrations, pharmacokinetics (PK), and pharmacodynamics (PD) to individualize and optimize drug therapy response in patients (Fig. 6-1).

Dosing and frequency of medication administration are governed largely by two principles:

1. **PK:** the effect of the body on the drug disposition (absorption, distribution, metabolism, and excretion). Factors that affect PK are:
   a. Drug's physiochemical characteristics
   b. Maturational physiologic changes
   c. Concomitant disease states/medical conditions
   d. Drug interactions
   e. Pharmacogenomics
2. **PD:** the effect of the drug on the body (clinical effects). Factors that affect PD are:
   a. Concomitant disease states/medical conditions
   b. Drug interactions
   c. Pharmacogenomics

B. Therapeutic Serum Concentrations or Ranges

1. Main goal is to enhance efficacy, prevent toxicity, or both.
2. Therapeutic ranges are based on a strong correlation and probabilities between serum concentration with desired (efficacy) and undesired (toxicity) drug effects. Some patients may still experience toxic reactions within therapeutic ranges, and others may require "supratherapeutic" levels to obtain desired response.
3. Serum drug concentrations serve as a surrogate site for drug measurement because measurement at the site of action is typically not possible.

C. Benefits of Therapeutic Drug Monitoring

1. Promotes optimal pharmacologic outcomes for drugs with unpredictable drug dose–exposure relationship and with known "therapeutic concentrations" (Fig. 6-2).
2. Promotes the safe and efficacious use of drugs with a narrow "therapeutic index" (Fig. 6-3).

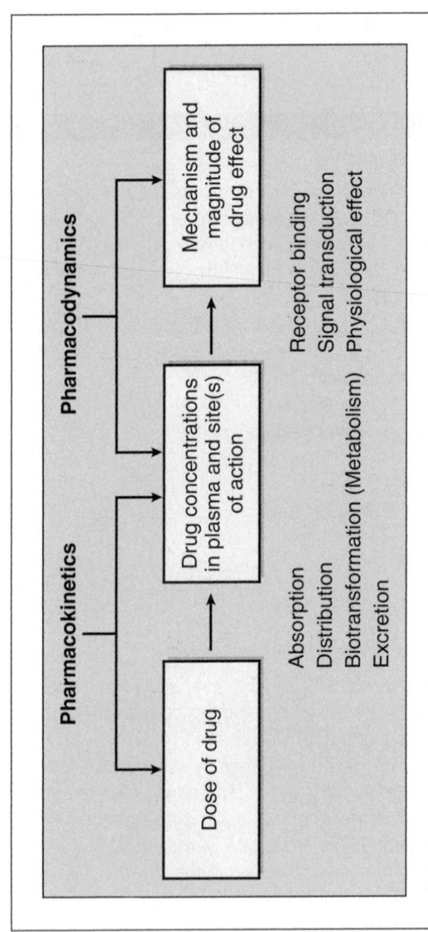

FIGURE 6-1 Relationship between pharmacokinetics and pharmacodynamics. *(From Brenner GM, Stevens C.* Pharmacology *3rd ed. Copyright © 2009 by Saunders, an imprint of Elsevier, Inc. All rights reserved.)*

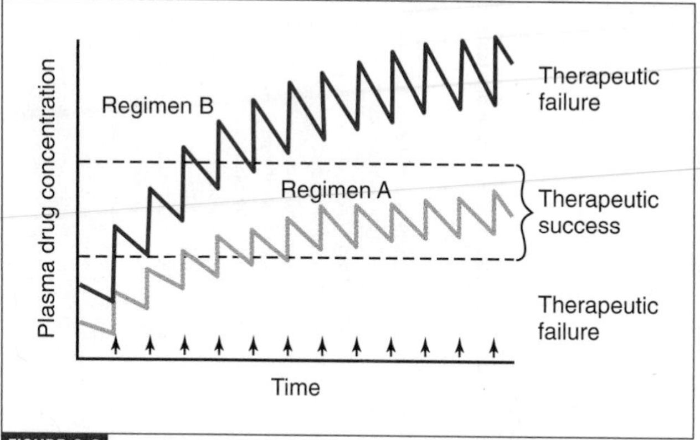

FIGURE 6-2
Therapeutic range. Illustrates the concentration time profile after the administration of two different drug regimens, A and B. The dosing intervals are the same for both regimens; however, the dose for regimen B is twice that given in A.

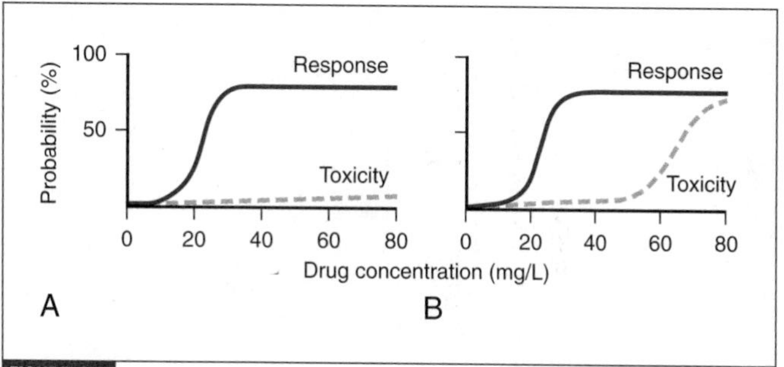

FIGURE 6-3
Therapeutic index. Probability of effect (response and toxicity) with drug concentration for two different drugs. **A,** A hypothetical drug with very little toxicity at concentrations yielding maximum probability of response (wide therapeutic index). **B,** Increasing probability of toxicity as drug concentration increases (narrow therapeutic index). *(From McLeod HL, Evans WE. Pediatric pharmacokinetics and therapeutic drug monitoring. Pediatr Rev. 1992;13(11):413–421.)*

3. Assists in determining patient status trends and/or changes (physiologic organ system changes, dietary changes, patient compliance issues, and drug interactions).
4. Potential economic impact by decreasing length of hospitalization, fewer hospital admissions, and rational use of serum concentration measurements.

Text continued on page 264.

II. ANTIMICROBIALS THAT REQUIRE THERAPEUTIC DRUG MONITORING[1–10]

A. Therapeutic Drug Monitoring Goals and Appropriate Times to Sample Serum Concentrations (Table 6-1)

TABLE 6-1

THERAPEUTIC DRUG MONITORING GOALS AND APPROPRIATE TIMES TO SAMPLE SERUM CONCENTRATIONS (For notes and abbreviations used in this table, see p. xvii.)

Drug	When to Draw Peak Levels	When to Draw Trough Levels	Suggested Peak Levels (mg/L)	Suggested Trough Levels (mg/L)	Half life (hr)*,†	Time to Reach Steady State (hr)‡	Toxicity and Relationship to Serum Concentration
Amikacin	30 min after end of infusion	Within 30 min of next scheduled dose	20–30; 25–30 for CNS, pulmonary, bone, and serious infections, and patients with febrile neutropenia	<10	Neonate: 6 ± 2 Infant: 4 ± 1 Child: 2 ± 1 Adolescent: 1.5 ± 1 Adult: 2 ± 1	Neonate: 20–40 Infant: 15–25 Child: 5–12 Adolescent: 5–8 Adult: 8–10	Toxicity risk factors: >5 days of use; dehydration; existing nephrotoxicities or ototoxicities; and use of other drugs with similar toxicities **Nephrotoxicity:** can be associated with high troughs **Ototoxicity (avoid loop diuretics):** —Cochlear: loss of high-frequency tones and related to high peaks; amikacin is most toxic —Vestibular: include nystagmus and ataxia; gentamicin is most toxic

Chloramphenicol	Capsule: 60 min after dose Suspension: 1.5–3 hr after dose IV: 0.5–1.5 hr after end of infusion	Immediately before next dose	Meningitis: 15–25 Other infections: 10–20	Meningitis: 5–15 Other infections: 5–10	Neonate (1–2 days of age): 24 Neonate (10–16 days of age): 10 Adult: 1.6–3.3	Neonate: 2–3 days All others: 12–24	Reversible bone marrow toxicity and anemia: levels >25 mg/L (*Note:* rare idiosyncratic, irreversible aplastic anemia has been reported) "Gray baby syndrome" due to immature drug metabolism in neonates (cardiovascular-respiratory collapse): levels >50 mg/L
Flucytosine	60–120 min after an oral dose	Immediately before next dose	Invasive candidiasis: 40–60	≥25	Neonate: 4–34 Infant: 7.4 Adult: 2.5–6	Neonate: 16–136 Infant: 44.4 Adult: 6.4–24	Bone marrow toxicity (anemia, leukopenia, thrombocytopenia): levels >100 mg/L for prolonged periods
Gentamicin	30 min after end of infusion	Within 30 min of next scheduled dose	4–10; 8–10 for CNS, pulmonary, bone, and serious infections; and patients with febrile neutropenia	<2	Neonate: 6 ± 2 Infant: 4 ± 1 Child: 2 ± 1 Adolescent: 1.5 ± 1 Adult: 2 ± 1	Neonate: 20–40 Infant: 15–25 Child: 5–12 Adolescent: 5–8 Adult: 8–10	Toxicity risk factors: >5 days of use; dehydration; existing nephrotoxicities or ototoxicities; and use of other drugs with similar toxicities **Nephrotoxicity:** can be associated with high troughs **Ototoxicity (avoid loop diuretics):** —Cochlear: loss of high-frequency tones and related to high peaks; amikacin is most toxic —Vestibular: include nystagmus and ataxia; gentamicin is most toxic

Continued

6

TABLE 6-1

THERAPEUTIC DRUG MONITORING GOALS AND APPROPRIATE TIMES TO SAMPLE SERUM CONCENTRATIONS (Continued)

Drug	When to Draw Peak Levels	When to Draw Trough Levels	Suggested Peak Levels (mg/L)	Suggested Trough Levels (mg/L)	Half life (hr)[*,†]	Time to Reach Steady State (hr)[‡]	Toxicity and Relationship to Serum Concentration
Quinidine	N/A	Within 30 min of next scheduled dose	N/A	<8	Child: 2.5–6.7 Adult: 6–8	Child: 10–34 Adult: 24–40	Cardiac arrhythmias (extrasystoles, atrial flutter, ventricular flutter, or fibrillation): may occur with levels ≥5 mg/L
Tobramycin	30 min after end of infusion	Within 30 min of next scheduled dose	4–10; 8–10 for CNS, pulmonary, bone, and serious infections; and patients with febrile neutropenia	<2	Neonate: 6 ± 2 Infant: 4 ± 1 Child: 2 ± 1 Adolescent: 1.5 ± 1 Adult: 2 ± 1	Neonate: 20–40 Infant: 15–25 Child: 5–12 Adolescent: 5–8 Adult: 8–10	Toxicity risk factors: >5 days of use; dehydration; existing nephrotoxicities or ototoxicities; and use of other drugs with similar toxicities **Nephrotoxicity:** can be associated with high troughs **Ototoxicity (avoid loop diuretics):** —Cochlear: loss of high-frequency tones and related to high peaks; amikacin is most toxic —Vestibular: include nystagmus and ataxia; gentamicin is most toxic

Vancomycin	Monitoring of peak level is not recommended	Within 30 min of next scheduled dose	N/A	10–20[§]; 15–20 for serious infections due to MRSA including bacteremia, infective endocarditis, osteomyelitis, meningitis, pneumonia, and severe SSTI (e.g., necrotizing fasciitis); and MRSA strains with elevated vancomycin MICs of 2 mg/L	Premature neonate[¶] 30–40 wk and <1.2 kg: 7.8 ± 3 30–42 wk and ≥1.2 kg: 3.8 ± 1.4 >42 wk and >2 kg: 2.1 ± 0.8 Full-term neonate: 6.7 Infant: 4.1 Child: 2.6 ± 0.4 Adult ≥16 yr: 7 ± 1.5	Premature neonate[¶] 30–40 wk and <1.2 kg: 23–39 30–42 wk and >1.2 kg: 11–19 >42 wk and >2 kg: 6–11 Full-term neonate: 20–34 Infant: 12–21 Child: 8–13 Adult ≥16 yr: 21–35	Toxicity risk factors: use with aminoglycoside; preexisting ototoxicity or nephrotoxicity; life-threatening *Staphylococcus* infection; intensive care unit stay, and >15–21 days of use Despite the use of current improved purified formulation of the drug (vs. original "Mississippi Mud" formulation), nephrotoxicity risk with use of higher serum trough concentration (≥15 mg/L) and concomitant use of furosemide in the intensive care unit has been reported in children[10]
Voriconazole	N/A	Within 30 min of next scheduled dose	N/A	1–5.5	Variable, dose dependent[6]	Variable, dose dependent	Neurotoxicity may occur with trough levels >5.5 and treatment failures with levels <1

III. SPECIAL TOPICS IN ANTIMICROBIAL THERAPEUTIC DRUG MONITORING

A. High-Dose, Extended-Interval Dosing of Aminoglycosides: Amikacin, Gentamicin, and Tobramycin[11–18]

1. Also known as once-daily or extended-interval dosing.
2. Designed to enhance efficacy by using concentration-dependent bactericidal properties of aminoglycosides and their postantibiotic effects (PAE).
3. May reduce nephrotoxicity by decreasing drug accumulation in renal tubular cells.
4. Goal peak/minimum inhibitory concentration (MIC) ratio of at least 8 to 10 maximizes bacterial killing (equivalent to peak of 16–20 if MIC is 2). Higher milligram per kilogram dosing with high-dose, extended-interval (HDEI) enables the achievement of goal peak/MIC ratios (Fig. 6-4).
5. Adult studies have demonstrated equal efficacy and equal or less nephrotoxicity with HDEI dosing in select patient populations.
6. Rates of ototoxicity have been similar between HDEI dosing and traditional dosing.

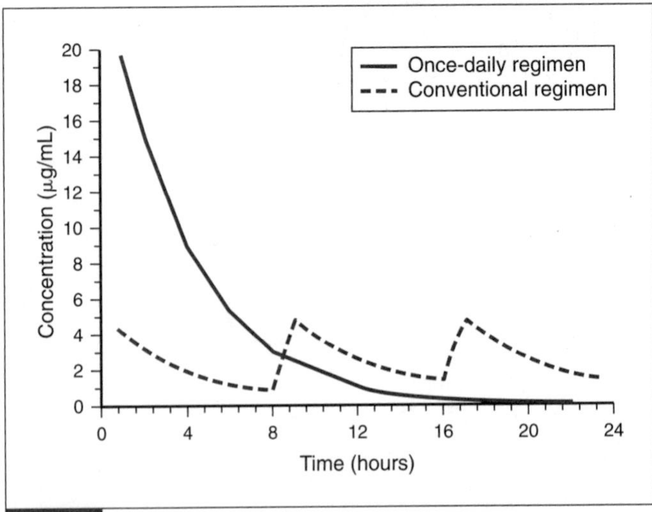

FIGURE 6-4

Simulated gentamicin concentration versus time profile of once-daily dosing and conventional every-8-hour dosing with normal renal function. *(From Nicolau DP, Freeman CD, Belliveau PP, et al. Experience with once daily aminoglycoside program administered to 2,184 adult patients. Antimicrob Agents Chemother. 1995;39(3):650–655.)*

7. Pediatric experience has been limited to patients with cystic fibrosis, pyelonephritis, surgical prophylaxis and treatment, and urinary tract infections, and in the oncology (fever and neutropenia), neonatal intensive care unit, and pediatric intensive care unit populations. A meta-analysis from Contopoulos-Ioannidis et al.[11] comparing HDEI versus traditional multiple daily dosing revealed no differences in clinical and microbiologic failure rates, a statistically significant efficacy benefit for using HDEI with amikacin, no difference in primary nephrotoxicity and ototoxicity, and less secondary nephrotoxicity with HDEI. However, gaps remain in knowledge regarding: (1) the incidence of ototoxicity, (2) the appropriate dose to use with specific clinical conditions, (3) dosage adjustments in renal insufficiency, and (4) the appropriate method of therapeutic drug monitoring with HDEI.
8. HDEI is not recommended in renal insufficiency (glomerular filtration rate <60 mL/min); unstable renal function; pregnancy; extensive burns (>20% body surface area) or trauma; conditions affecting body water such as ascites, extensive edema, and shock; and meningitis.
9. Concerns for using HDEI in children include rapid aminoglycoside clearance, unknown duration of the PAE, safety concerns, and limited clinical and efficacy data.
10. The appropriate HDEI regimen in pediatric patients is unknown and likely varies with age and the patient population. Dosing regimens for gentamicin/tobramycin have ranged from 7.5 to 10.5 mg/kg Q24 hr in febrile neutropenic patients; 7.5 to 9.5 mg/kg Q24 hr in non–cystic fibrosis critically ill patients; and 10 to 15 mg/kg Q24 hr for patients with cystic fibrosis.

B. Vancomycin Serum Monitoring Controversy[3,4]

1. Toxicity relationship with serum levels has not been clearly established. Earlier reports of toxicity may be related to the less purified version of vancomycin ("Mississippi Mud").[19–21]

a. Nephrotoxicity
   (1) A 14% rate of nephrotoxicity has been reported in children from a tertiary care, teaching hospital.[10]
   (2) Higher doses with resultant higher troughs are associated with nephrotoxicity in adults.[22,23] Trough concentrations ≥15 mg/L and receiving concomitant furosemide therapy in the intensive care unit have been associated with nephrotoxicity in children.[10]
   (3) Concomitant use of aminoglycosides or other nephrotoxic drugs, advanced age, or preexisting renal failure can increase risk.
   (4) Usually reversible upon discontinuation.

b. Ototoxicity
   (1) High trough or peak levels have *not* caused ototoxicity.
   (2) Concomitant use of aminoglycosides or other ototoxic drugs, preexisting hearing loss, or kidney dysfunction can increase risk.
   (3) May be reversible upon drug discontinuation.

6

2. **Monitoring controversy**
a. Trough concentrations are the most practical method to guide vancomycin dosing in clinical practice. Monitoring of peak concentrations is not recommended.
   (1) For a pathogen MIC of 1 mg/L, a minimum trough serum vancomycin of 15 mg/L would achieve the targeted area under the serum concentration versus time curve AUC/MIC or ≥400.[24]
b. Wide interpatient variability in PK (especially with neonates and infants) and sites of infection with difficult tissue penetration support the need for serum concentration monitoring. Patients who should be monitored include:
   (1) Patients in intensive care units
   (2) Patients with renal impairment, fluctuating renal function, and advanced renal failure (including patients on dialysis)
   (3) Neonates, infants, or children
   (4) Patients with serious infections (meningitis, pneumonia, osteomyelitis, or endocarditis)
   (5) Patients with poor therapeutic response
   (6) Patients receiving concurrent nephrotoxic medications
   (7) Patients with fluctuating volumes of distribution
   (8) Obese patients

IV. PHARMACOKINETIC MONITORING IN THERAPEUTIC DRUG MONITORING

A. One-Compartment First-Order Elimination Pharmacokinetic Model

The one-compartment first-order elimination pharmacokinetic model assumes the following characteristics:

1. Instantaneous distribution and equilibration to all tissues and fluids
2. Drug removal is constant, independent of the dose, and logarithmic over time

B. Basic Pharmacokinetic Terms

1. **Bioavailability:** percentage or fraction of the administered extravascular dose that reaches the patient's bloodstream. Factors that influence bioavailability include the route of administration, drug's dissolution and absorptive characteristics, and precirculation metabolism of drug. General equation:

$$\text{Amount of drug absorbed or reaching systemic circulation (mg)} = S \times F \times \text{dose (mg)}$$

   where S = salt or ester factor and F = bioavailability factor. Both factors are expressed as fractions.
2. **Volume of distribution (Vd):** a theoretical size of a compartment necessary to account for the total amount of drug in the body if it were present throughout the body at the same concentration found in plasma. General equation:

$$\text{Vd(L)} = \frac{\text{Total amount of drug in body (mg)}}{\text{Serum concentration (mg/L)}}$$

a. Usually expressed in liters (L) or liters/kilogram of body weight (L/kg).
b. Significant changes to just Vd will require a drug dose amount modification with no change in dosage interval. For example, an increase in aminoglycoside Vd caused by edema will result in a dose increase to maintain the desired serum concentration.
c. Loading doses can be determined when a drug's given Vd and desired serum concentration are known. Loading doses are used to shorten the time to achieve a desired serum concentration. Bioavailability (S and F factors, see earlier) of the medication must be included. General equation:

$$\text{Loading dose (mg/kg)} = \frac{\text{Vd (L/kg)} \times [\text{desired serum conc.} - \text{current serum conc.}]\ \text{(mg/L)}}{\text{S} \times \text{F}}$$

3. **Elimination rate constant (Kel):** fraction or percentage of the total amount of drug in the serum removed per unit of time; independent of concentration. General equation:

$$\text{Kel}(\text{hr}^{-1}) = \frac{\text{Ln}[\text{Cp}_1 \div \text{Cp}_2]}{\Delta t_{1-2}}$$

where

Ln = natural log
Cp_1 = serum concentration at time 1 (mg/L)
Cp_2 = serum concentration at time 2 (mg/L)
Cp_1 always > Cp_2
Δt_{1-2} = time interval between Cp_1 and Cp_2 (hours)

4. **Elimination half-life ($T_{1/2}$):** time required for a 50% reduction in serum concentration. General equation:

$$T_{1/2}(\text{hr}) = \frac{0.693}{\text{Kel}(\text{hr}^{-1})}$$

Significant changes to just the elimination $T_{1/2}$ will require a dosage interval modification without a change in dosage amount. For example, an increase in aminoglycoside elimination $T_{1/2}$ because of renal insufficiency will result in an increase in dosage interval to maintain a desired serum trough concentration.

5. **Steady state:** concept is achieved when the rate of drug administration is equal to the rate of drug removal, and the serum concentration of drug (measured at similar times around any given dose) remains constant. This is also the time when drug accumulation is complete.

a. Relationship between elimination $T_{1/2}$ and steady state:

No. of Half-lives ($T_{1/2}$)	% Steady State Achieved
1	50
2	75
3	87.5
4	93.75
5	96.88

b. In clinical practice, steady state is achieved after four to five half-lives.
c. Any changes in drug dose (amount or interval) will require the same four to five half-lives to reach the new steady-state serum concentration.
d. Loading doses do not shorten the time to reach steady state.

6. **Clearance (Cl):** intrinsic ability of the body or its organs of elimination (primarily in liver and kidneys) to remove drug from the blood. Clearance does not represent the amount (mg) of drug removal but describes a theoretical volume of blood being removed (of the drug) per unit time. General equation:

$$Cl\,(L/hr) = Vd(L) \times Kel\,(hr^{-1})$$

a. Usually expressed as a volume per unit time (L/hr)
b. Significant changes to just clearance will require a dosage interval modification, change in dosage amount, or both. For example, increased piperacillin clearance as seen in cystic fibrosis results in higher mg/kg daily dosages, and increased vancomycin clearance as seen in infants results in shorter dosing intervals (e.g., every 6 hours) to prevent subtherapeutic serum levels.

C. Serum Measurement Methods

1. **During steady state** (Fig 6-5):
a. Maintenance dose → "Peak" → Trough: easiest method for calculating elimination rate constant but is not the most efficient method because of the lengthy time interval between the two serum samples.
b. Trough → Maintenance dose → "Peak": commonly used method of serum level determination. Extrapolating (superpositioning) the measured trough as the trough level following the measured peak level is done to facilitate the drug elimination rate constant calculation. Time between serum level measurements is shorter than the preceding method.

2. **Non–steady state**
a. Useful for preventing toxicity, especially in situations of organ dysfunction
b. Assessment methods are different from steady-state methods
c. Non–steady-state levels can be used to predict steady-state levels

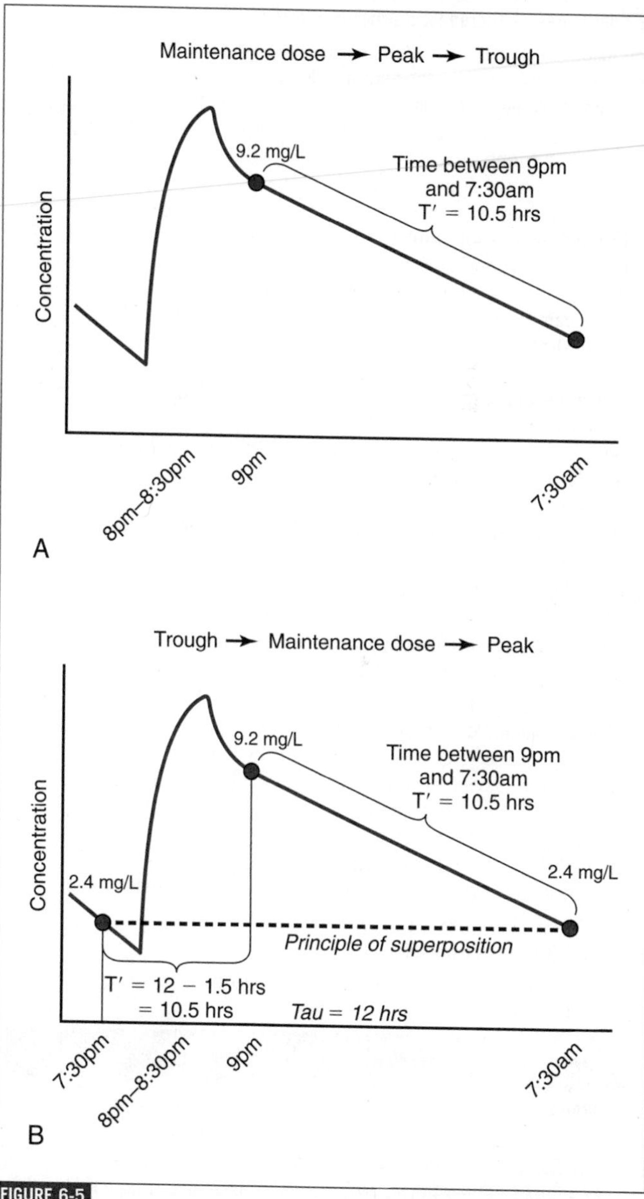

FIGURE 6-5

Serum concentration measurement methods at steady state. **A,** Maintenance dose → Peak → Trough. **B,** Trough → Maintenance dose → Peak.

D. Challenges to Therapeutic Drug Monitoring

The following issues associated with therapeutic drug monitoring may result in an improper assessment and incorrect dosing recommendations.

1. **Improper serum sampling**
   a. Measuring pre–steady-state levels but interpreting as steady state
   b. Sampling during drug infusion
   c. Sampling before drug distribution
   d. Inappropriately flushing/discarding volume from intravenous line
2. **Improper drug administration**
   a. Incorrect dose and time of dose
   b. Improper site of intravenous line administration
3. **Inaccurate time documentation of serum sampling and/or dose administration**
   a. Improper serum level assessment
   b. Will result in incorrect calculation of key individualized pharmacokinetic parameters (Kel, $T_{1/2}$, and Vd)
4. **Drug–drug interactions:** inadequate spacing of aminoglycosides and β-lactam antibiotics can result in falsely lower aminoglycoside serum levels
5. **Food and certain electrolytes can reduce absorption of antibiotics.**
6. **Abnormal PK parameter calculations should be explained by a physiologic process (i.e., edema) or improper serum sampling should be considered.**

E. Additional Considerations in Pharmacokinetic Monitoring

1. **Patient age:** for neonates, reduced renal elimination and protein binding, and increased total body water
2. **Disease-specific pharmacokinetic parameters and empiric dosages**
   a. Burns: dynamic renal elimination and body fluid status
   b. Cystic fibrosis: pancreatic insufficiency, leaner body mass, hypoalbuminemia, and enhanced drug clearance
   c. Oncology: hypoalbuminemia and enhanced drug clearance
   d. Renal failure: reduced drug clearance
3. **Volume status:** fluid overload versus dehydration: increased and decreased Vd of water-soluble drugs, respectively

F. For Additional Assistance

Consult a clinical pharmacist who is knowledgeable in pharmacokinetic therapeutic drug monitoring for assistance.

V. PHARMACOKINETICS/PHARMACODYNAMICS (PK/PD) ANTIMICROBIAL RELATIONSHIPS

A. Pharmacokinetics/Pharmacodynamics Relationship Concept

Specific antimicrobial and pathogen PK/PD targets have been developed from in vitro models to enhance efficacy and reduce development of resistance. Most PK/PD indices use drug blood concentrations that may differ greatly at the targeted site of action depending on drug protein binding and tissue penetration characteristics. Mechanical factors of the organism, such as biofilm, inoculum effects, and stationary growth phase, may also affect the PD target achievement. Synergistic effects of combination antimicrobial therapy should also be considered.

B. Common Pharmacokinetics/Pharmacodynamics Indices (Fig. 6-6)**:**

1. **AUC/MIC:** Area under the serum concentration versus time curve (AUC) to minimum inhibitory concentration (MIC) ratio; also described as concentration-dependent with time-dependence PD
2. **C_{max}/MIC:** maximum serum concentration (C_{max}) to MIC ratio; also described as concentration-dependent PD
3. **T > MIC:** duration of the dosing interval when serum concentrations exceed the MIC; also described as time-dependent PD. As doses are increased to enhance the T > MIC, a colinear effect on increasing the AUC/MIC and C_{max}/MIC may occur.

NOTE: MIC is used as a surrogate marker for predicting microbiologic activity at the infection site. Always consider the antibiotics distributive properties to the desired site of action.

6

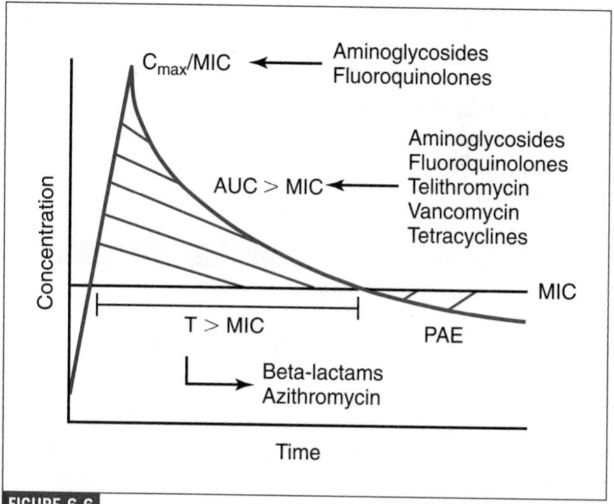

FIGURE 6-6

Concentration versus time curve with minimum inhibitory concentration superimposed and pharmacokinetic and pharmacodynamic markers. *(Adapted from McKinnon PS, Yu VL. Pharmacologic considerations in antimicrobial therapy, with emphasis on pharmacokinetics and pharmacodynamics: Review for the practicing clinician. Eur J Clin Microbiol Infect Dis. 2004;23:271–288.)*

C. Concentration-Independent (Time-Dependent) Antimicrobial Activity

Increasing the dosage of these agents above the MIC of the bacteria will not enhance the bacterial killing rate because the characteristic of killing is not concentration dependent. Time-dependent agents may also have a post-antibiotic effect (PAE).

Antimicrobial	Key Predictor of Outcome*
β-Lactams	T > MIC
Macrolides (Azithromycin†)	T > MIC

*Specific outcome predictor numeric value is dependent on specific drug, microbial organism, and in vitro/in vivo clinical condition.

†Also has a PAE, and its AUC/MIC ratio predicts efficacy against *Streptococcus pneumoniae.*

D. Concentration-Dependent Antimicrobial Activity

Demonstrates increasing bacterial killing with increasing drug concentrations.

Antimicrobial	Key Predictor of Outcome*
Aminoglycosides†	AUC/MIC or C_{max}/MIC
Fluoroquinolones	AUC/MIC or C_{max}/MIC
Glycopeptides (vancomycin‡)	AUC/MIC
Ketolides (telithromycin)	AUC/MIC or C_{max}/MIC
Tetracyclines/Glycylcyclines	AUC/MIC

*Specific outcome predictor numeric value is dependent on specific drug, microbial organism, and in vitro/in vivo clinical condition.

†Also has a PAE.

‡Time-dependent activity (T > MIC) had been previously suggested.

E. Selected Pharmacokinetic and Pharmacodynamic Relationships of Various Antimicrobials

1. **Antibacterials** (Tables 6-2 and 6-3)
2. **Antimycobacterials** (Table 6-4)
3. **Antifungals** (Table 6-5)

VI. DRUG INTERACTIONS

Drug interactions may result in increased drug effects/toxicity or decreased effects because of a variety of mechanisms. They may include alterations in drug absorption, protein binding, metabolism, and clearance; additive/synergistic drug toxicity; and antagonistic effects on efficacy. Major drug–drug interactions are described in specific antimicrobial drug monographs of the formulary section. Table 6-6 is a summary of those drug interactions that are considered contraindicated, where the risks associated with concomitant use usually outweigh the benefits. Data demonstrate the specified agents that may interact with each other in a clinically significant manner.

TABLE 6-2

EFFICACY RELATIONSHIPS IN HUMANS

Antibacterial Agent	PK/PD Parameter Associated with Improved Efficacy	Clinical Condition
Aminoglycosides	C_{max}/MIC >8:1	Gram-negative bacteremia
	C_{max}/MIC ≥10:1	Gram-negative pneumonia
β-Lactams		
Cefepime	T >4 × MIC	Various gram-negative pneumonia
Fluoroquinolones		
Ciprofloxacin	AUC/MIC ≥250	Various gram-negative infections
Levofloxacin/gatifloxacin	AUC/MIC 30–40*	*Streptococcus pneumoniae* in community-acquired pneumonia and chronic bronchitis
Levofloxacin	C_{max}/MIC ≥12:1	*Streptococcus pneumoniae, Staphylococcus aureus, Pseudomonas aeruginosa,* and other gram-negative infections
Glycopeptides		
Vancomycin	AUC/MIC >125	Various *Staphylococcus aureus* infections
	AUC/MIC >400	Methicillin-resistant *Staphylococcus aureus* pneumonia

Adapted from Scheetz MH, Hurt KM, Noskin GA, et al. Applying antimicrobial pharmacodynamics to resistant gram-negative pathogens. *Am J Health Syst Pharm.* 2006;63:1346–1360; and McKinnon PS, Davis SL. Pharmacokinetic and pharmacodynamic issues in the treatment of bacterial infectious diseases. *Eur J Clin Microbiol Infect Dis.* 2004;23:271–288.

*Reflects free-drug concentration measurements.

AUC/MIC, Area under the serum concentration versus time curve to minimum inhibitory concentration ratio; *C_{max}/MIC,* maximum serum concentration to MIC ratio; *T> MIC,* duration of the dosing interval with serum concentrations exceeds the MIC; *PD,* pharmacodynamics; *PK,* pharmacokinetics.

TABLE 6-3

IN VITRO RESISTANCE RELATIONSHIPS

Antibacterial Agent	PK/PD Parameter Associated with Reduced Resistance	Condition
Fluoroquinolones		
Levofloxacin	AUC/MIC ≥157	Mouse model evaluating drug exposure and resistant development in *Pseudomonas aeruginosa*
Glycopeptides		
Vancomycin	AUC/MIC ≥382	Simulated in vitro PK model using an *agr*-null group II *Staphylococcus aureus* strain

Adapted from Rybak MJ. Pharmacodynamics: Relation to antimicrobial resistance. *Am J Med.* 2006;119(6A):S37–S44.

AUC/MIC, Area under the serum concentration versus time curve to minimum inhibitory concentration ratio; *PD,* pharmacodynamics; *PK,* pharmacokinetics.

TABLE 6-4

EFFICACY RELATIONSHIPS OF ANTIMYCOBACTERIAL AGENTS

Antimycobacterial Agent	PK/PD Parameter Associated with Improved Efficacy	Condition
Isoniazid	C_{max}/MIC >15	Mouse model
Rifampin	AUC/MIC ≥500 or AUC_{free}/MIC ≥75–100	Mouse model and human pharmacokinetic simulations

Adapted from Nuermberger E, Grosset J. Pharmacokinetic and pharmacodynamic issues in the treatment of mycobacterial infections. *Eur J Clin Microbiol Infect Dis.* 2004;23:243–255.

AUC/MIC, Area under the serum concentration versus time curve to minimum inhibitory concentration ratio; *C_{max}/MIC,* maximum serum concentration to MIC ratio; *PD,* pharmacodynamics; *PK,* pharmacokinetics.

TABLE 6-5

PHARMACOKINETIC/PHARMACODYNAMIC INDICES OF ANTIFUNGAL DRUG CLASSES FOR *CANDIDA*

Antifungal Class	PK/PD Index	Data Supporting Index
Polyenes (amphotericins)	C_{max}/MIC* >4–10 (neutropenic mouse model)	In vitro and in vivo; neutropenic mouse model and limited clinical data
Flucytosine	T > MIC; >20%–40% of time above MIC	Neutropenic mouse model
Triazoles	AUC/MIC* >25 (free fluconazole concentration)	Animal and clinical data with fluconazole for mucosal and invasive disease
	For aspergillosis: AUC/MIC >167 (posaconazole)	Mouse model and in vitro human alveolus model
Echinocandins	C_{max}/MIC* >10 (aminocandin)	Mouse model
	AUC/MIC* >20 for *C. albicans* and >7 for *C. glabrata* and *C. parapsilosis* (free drug)	Mouse model

Adapted from Sinnollareddy M, Peake SL, Roberts MS, et al. Using pharmacokinetics and pharmacodynamics to optimize dosing of antifungal agents in critically ill patients: A systematic review. *Int J Antimicrob Agents.* 2012:39:1–10; and Lewis RE. Current concepts in antifungal pharmacology. *Mayo Clin Proc.* 2011;86(8):805–817.

*Postantifungal effects have been identified for certain drugs within the indicated antifungal drug class and specific *Candida* strain.

AUC/MIC, Area under the serum concentration versus time curve to minimum inhibitory concentration ratio; *C_{max}/MIC,* maximum serum concentration to MIC ratio; *T > MIC,* duration of the dosing interval with serum concentrations exceeds the MIC; *PD,* pharmacodynamics; *PK,* pharmacokinetics.

TABLE 6-6

CONTRAINDICATED DRUG INTERACTIONS FOR ANTIMICROBIAL AGENTS[25,26]

Antimicrobial	Interacting Drug(s)	Toxic Effect
Acyclovir	Zoster vaccine	Acyclovir may diminish the therapeutic effect of zoster vaccine
Adefovir	Tenofovir	Adefovir may diminish the therapeutic effect of tenofovir; specifically, adefovir-associated mutations in hepatitis B viral reverse transcriptase may decrease viral susceptibility to tenofovir; tenofovir may increase the serum concentration of adefovir; adefovir may increase the serum concentration of tenofovir
Amprenavir	Alcohol (ethyl), disulfiram, or metronidazole	Propylene glycol toxicity (from amprenavir suspension)
	Amiodarone	Bradycardia, hypotension, cardiogenic shock, heart block, QT prolongation, hepatotoxicity (amiodarone toxicity)
	Cisapride	QT prolongation, cardiac arrhythmias
	Ergot derivatives	Vasospasm resulting in peripheral, cardiac, and/or cerebral ischemia; ↑ or ↓ in blood pressure or heart rate; seizures; headache
	Pimozide	QT prolongation, ventricular arrhythmias; hypotension; seizures; anticholinergic and extrapyramidal effects
	Quinidine	Tachycardia, hypotension, heart block, ventricular fibrillation, syncope, vascular collapse (quinidine toxicity)
	St. John's wort	Decreased amprenavir efficacy
Artemether + lumefantrine	Antimalarial agents	Artemether may enhance the adverse/toxic effect of antimalarial agents; may enhance the adverse/toxic effect of lumefantrine
	Halofantrine	Lumefantrine may enhance the QTc-prolonging effect of halofantrine
	Mifepristone	May enhance the QTc-prolonging effect of highest risk QTc-prolonging agents
Atazanavir	Amiodarone	Bradycardia, hypotension, cardiogenic shock, heart block, QT prolongation, hepatotoxicity (amiodarone toxicity)
	Cisapride	QT prolongation, cardiac arrhythmias
	Ergot derivatives	Vasospasm resulting in peripheral, cardiac, and/or cerebral ischemia; ↑ or ↓ in blood pressure or heart rate; seizures; headache
	Etravirine	Atazanavir may increase the serum concentration of etravirine; etravirine may decrease the serum concentration of atazanavir

Continued

TABLE 6-6

CONTRAINDICATED DRUG INTERACTIONS FOR ANTIMICROBIAL AGENTS (Continued)

Antimicrobial	Interacting Drug(s)	Toxic Effect
	Everolimus	CYP3A4 inhibitors (strong) may increase the serum concentration of everolimus
	Fluticasone (inhalation)	CYP3A4 inhibitors (strong) may increase the serum concentration of fluticasone (oral inhalation)
	Halofantrine	CYP3A4 inhibitors (strong) may increase the serum concentration of halofantrine
	Indinavir	Atazanavir may enhance the adverse/toxic effect of indinavir; indinavir may enhance the adverse/toxic effect of atazanavir
	Irinotecan	Atazanavir may increase the serum concentration of irinotecan; the metabolism (via glucuronidation) of the active SN-38 metabolite may be primarily impacted by this interaction
	Lovastatin	Protease inhibitors may increase the serum concentration of lovastatin
	Midazolam	Protease inhibitors may increase the serum concentration of midazolam. Management: oral midazolam contraindicated with all protease inhibitors; IV midazolam contraindicated with fosamprenavir and nelfinavir; other protease inhibitors recommend caution, close monitoring, and consideration of lower IV midazolam doses with concurrent use
	Nevirapine	May decrease the serum concentration of atazanavir; atazanavir may increase the serum concentration of nevirapine
	Pimozide	QT prolongation, ventricular arrhythmias; hypotension; seizures; anticholinergic and extrapyramidal effects
	Quinidine	Tachycardia, hypotension, heart block, ventricular fibrillation, syncope, vascular collapse (quinidine toxicity)
	Rifampin	May decrease the serum concentration of atazanavir
	Salmeterol	CYP3A4 inhibitors (strong) may increase the serum concentration of salmeterol
	Sildenafil	Contraindicated if sildenafil being used for pulmonary arterial hypertension; CYP3A4 inhibitors (strong) may increase the serum concentration of sildenafil
	Simvastatin	Protease inhibitors may increase the serum concentration of simvastatin
	St. John's wort	Decreased atazanavir efficacy

TABLE 6-6

CONTRAINDICATED DRUG INTERACTIONS FOR ANTIMICROBIAL AGENTS (Continued)

Antimicrobial	Interacting Drug(s)	Toxic Effect
Atovaquone and proguanil	Artemether	May enhance the adverse/toxic effect of antimalarial agents
	Lumefantrine	May enhance the adverse/toxic effect of antimalarial agents
Azithromycin	Quinine	Macrolide antibiotics may increase the serum concentration of quinine
Boceprevir	Carbamazepine	May decrease the serum concentration of boceprevir
	Cisapride	Boceprevir may increase the serum concentration of cisapride
	Efavirenz	May decrease the serum concentration of boceprevir; boceprevir may increase the serum concentration of efavirenz
	Ergot derivatives	Vasospasm resulting in peripheral, cardiac, and/or cerebral ischemia; ↑ or ↓ in blood pressure or heart rate; seizures; headache
	Everolimus	CYP3A4 inhibitors (strong) may increase the serum concentration of everolimus
	Fluticasone (inhalation)	CYP3A4 inhibitors (strong) may increase the serum concentration of fluticasone
	Fosphenytoin, phenytoin, phenobarbital, primidone	May decrease the serum concentration of boceprevir
	Halofantrine	CYP3A4 inhibitors (strong) may increase the serum concentration of halofantrine
	Lovastatin	Boceprevir may increase the serum concentration of lovastatin
	Midazolam	Boceprevir may increase the serum concentration of midazolam
	Pimozide	Boceprevir may increase the serum concentration of pimozide
	Rifabutin	May decrease the serum concentration of boceprevir
	Rifampin	May decrease the serum concentration of boceprevir
	Salmeterol	CYP3A4 inhibitors (strong) may increase the serum concentration of salmeterol
	Sildenafil	Contraindicated if sildenafil being used for pulmonary arterial hypertension; CYP3A4 inhibitors (strong) may increase the serum concentration of sildenafil
	Simvastatin	Boceprevir may increase the serum concentration of simvastatin
	St. John's wort	Decreased boceprevir efficacy
	Triazolam	Protease inhibitors may increase the serum concentration of triazolam

Continued

TABLE 6-6

CONTRAINDICATED DRUG INTERACTIONS FOR ANTIMICROBIAL AGENTS (Continued)

Antimicrobial	Interacting Drug(s)	Toxic Effect
Chloramphenicol	Clopidogrel	CYP2C19 inhibitors (strong) may decrease serum concentrations of the active metabolite(s) of clopidogrel
	Clozapine	Myelosuppressive agents may enhance the adverse/toxic effect of clozapine; specifically, the risk for agranulocytosis may be increased
	Everolimus	CYP3A4 inhibitors (strong) may increase the serum concentration of everolimus
	Fluticasone (inhalation)	CYP3A4 inhibitors (strong) may increase the serum concentration of fluticasone
	Halofantrine	CYP3A4 inhibitors (strong) may increase the serum concentration of halofantrine
	Lovastatin	CYP3A4 inhibitors (strong) may increase the serum concentration of lovastatin
	Pimozide	CYP3A4 inhibitors (strong) may increase the serum concentration of pimozide
	Salmeterol	CYP3A4 inhibitors (strong) may increase the serum concentration of salmeterol
	Sildenafil	Contraindicated if sildenafil being used for pulmonary arterial hypertension; CYP3A4 inhibitors (strong) may increase the serum concentration of sildenafil
	Simvastatin	CYP3A4 inhibitors (strong) may increase the serum concentration of simvastatin
Chloroquine HCl/ phosphate	Agalsidase alfa/beta	Chloroquine may diminish the therapeutic effect of agalsidase alfa/beta
	Artemether	May enhance the adverse/toxic effect of antimalarial agents
	Lumefantrine	May enhance the adverse/toxic effect of antimalarial agents
	Mefloquine	Aminoquinolines (antimalarial) may enhance the adverse/toxic effect of mefloquine; specifically, the risk for QTc-prolongation and the risk for convulsions may be increased; mefloquine may increase the serum concentration of aminoquinolines (antimalarial)
	Mifepristone	May enhance the QTc-prolonging effect of moderate-risk QTc-prolonging agents
Clarithromycin	Amiodarone, disopyramide, procainamide, sotalol	QT prolongation, cardiac arrhythmias
	Artemether, halofantrine, lumefantrine	QT prolongation, cardiac arrhythmias
	Cisapride	QT prolongation, cardiac arrhythmias
	Citalopram, escitalopram	QT prolongation, cardiac arrhythmias

TABLE 6-6

CONTRAINDICATED DRUG INTERACTIONS FOR ANTIMICROBIAL AGENTS (Continued)

Antimicrobial	Interacting Drug(s)	Toxic Effect
	Dihydroergotamine, ergotamine	Clarithromycin may increase the serum concentration of Dihydroergotamine
	Everolimus	CYP3A4 inhibitors (strong) may increase the serum concentration of everolimus
	Fluticasone (inhalation)	CYP3A4 inhibitors (strong) may increase the serum concentration of fluticasone
	Lovastatin	CYP3A4 inhibitors (strong) may increase the serum concentration of lovastatin
	Mifepristone	QT prolongation, cardiac arrhythmias
	Paliperidone, pimozide, quetiapine, thioridazine, ziprasidone	QT prolongation, cardiac arrhythmias
	Quinidine, quinine, saquinavir, telithromycin	QT prolongation, cardiac arrhythmias
	Salmeterol	CYP3A4 inhibitors (strong) may increase the serum concentration of salmeterol
	Sildenafil	Contraindicated if sildenafil being used for pulmonary arterial hypertension; CYP3A4 inhibitors (strong) may increase the serum concentration of sildenafil
	Simvastatin	CYP3A4 inhibitors (strong) may increase the serum concentration of simvastatin
Clindamycin	Erythromycin	Clindamycin diminishes erythromycin efficacy
Clotrimazole	Pimozide	CYP3A4 inhibitors (moderate) may increase the serum concentration of pimozide
Cycloserine	Alcohol (ethyl)	May enhance the neurotoxic effect of cycloserine
Darunavir	Amiodarone	Protease inhibitors may decrease the metabolism of amiodarone
	Cisapride	QT prolongation, cardiac arrhythmias
	Ergot derivatives	Protease inhibitors may increase the serum concentration of ergot derivatives
	Everolimus	CYP3A4 inhibitors (strong) may increase the serum concentration of everolimus
	Fluticasone (inhalation)	CYP3A4 inhibitors (strong) may increase the serum concentration of fluticasone
	Fosphenytoin, phenytoin, phenobarbital	May decrease the serum concentration of darunavir
	Halofantrine	CYP3A4 inhibitors (strong) may increase the serum concentration of halofantrine
	Lopinavir	May decrease the serum concentration of darunavir; darunavir may increase the serum concentration of lopinavir

Continued

6

TABLE 6-6

CONTRAINDICATED DRUG INTERACTIONS FOR ANTIMICROBIAL AGENTS (Continued)

Antimicrobial	Interacting Drug(s)	Toxic Effect
	Lovastatin	CYP3A4 inhibitors (strong) may increase the serum concentration of lovastatin
	Midazolam	Protease inhibitors may increase the serum concentration of midazolam
	Pimozide	CYP3A4 inhibitors (strong) may increase the serum concentration of pimozide
	Quinidine	Protease inhibitors may decrease the metabolism of quinidine
	Rifampin	May decrease the serum concentration of darunavir
	Salmeterol	CYP3A4 inhibitors (strong) may increase the serum concentration of salmeterol
	Sildenafil	Contraindicated if sildenafil being used for pulmonary arterial hypertension; CYP3A4 inhibitors (strong) may increase the serum concentration of sildenafil
	Simvastatin	Darunavir may increase the serum concentration of simvastatin
	St. John's wort	Decreased darunavir efficacy
	Triazolam	Protease inhibitors may increase the serum concentration of triazolam
	Voriconazole	Darunavir may decrease the serum concentration of voriconazole
Delavirdine	Clopidogrel	CYP2C19 inhibitors (strong) may decrease serum concentrations of the active metabolite(s) of clopidogrel
	Etravirine	Delavirdine may increase the serum concentration of etravirine
	Everolimus	CYP3A4 inhibitors (strong) may increase the serum concentration of everolimus
	Fluticasone (inhalation)	CYP3A4 inhibitors (strong) may increase the serum concentration of fluticasone
	Fosamprenavir	May decrease the serum concentration of delavirdine; the active metabolite amprenavir is likely responsible for this effect; delavirdine may increase the serum concentration of fosamprenavir; specifically, delavirdine may increase concentrations of the active metabolite amprenavir
	Fosphenytoin, phenytoin	May decrease the serum concentration of delavirdine
	H2 antagonists	May decrease the serum concentration of delavirdine
	Halofantrine	CYP3A4 inhibitors (strong) may increase the serum concentration of halofantrine

TABLE 6-6

CONTRAINDICATED DRUG INTERACTIONS FOR ANTIMICROBIAL AGENTS (Continued)

Antimicrobial	Interacting Drug(s)	Toxic Effect
	Lovastatin	CYP3A4 inhibitors (strong) may increase the serum concentration of lovastatin
	Pimozide	CYP3A4 inhibitors (strong) may increase the serum concentration of pimozide
	Proton pump inhibitors	May decrease the serum concentration of delavirdine
	Rilpivirine	Delavirdine may increase the serum concentration of rilpivirine
	Salmeterol	CYP3A4 inhibitors (strong) may increase the serum concentration of salmeterol
	Sildenafil	Contraindicated if sildenafil being used for pulmonary arterial hypertension; CYP3A4 inhibitors (strong) may increase the serum concentration of sildenafil
	Simvastatin	Boceprevir may increase the serum concentration of simvastatin
	St. John's wort	Decreased delavirdine efficacy
	Tamoxifen	CYP2D6 inhibitors (strong) may decrease serum concentrations of the active metabolite(s) of tamoxifen; specifically, strong CYP2D6 inhibitors may decrease the metabolic formation of highly potent active metabolites
	Thioridazine	QT prolongation, cardiac arrhythmias, hypotension, anticholinergic and extrapyramidal effects, agitation
Demeclocycline	Retinoic acid derivatives	Tetracycline derivatives may enhance the adverse/toxic effect of retinoic acid derivatives; the development of pseudotumor cerebri is of particular concern
Didanosine	Alcohol (ethyl)	May enhance the adverse/toxic effect of didanosine; specifically, the risk for pancreatitis may be increased
	Allopurinol	May increase the serum concentration of didanosine
	Hydroxyurea	An increased risk for pancreatitis, hepatotoxicity, and/or neuropathy may exist
	Ribavirin	May enhance the adverse/toxic effect of didanosine; ribavirin may increase serum concentrations of the active metabolite(s) of didanosine
	Tenofovir	May diminish the therapeutic effect of didanosine; tenofovir may increase the serum concentration of didanosine

Continued

TABLE 6-6

CONTRAINDICATED DRUG INTERACTIONS FOR ANTIMICROBIAL AGENTS (Continued)

Antimicrobial	Interacting Drug(s)	Toxic Effect
Demeclocycline	Pimozide	CYP3A4 inhibitors (weak) may increase the serum concentration of pimozide
	Retinoic acid derivatives	Tetracycline derivatives may enhance the adverse/toxic effect of retinoic acid derivatives; the development of pseudotumor cerebri is of particular concern
Efavirenz	Azelastine	Efavirenz may enhance the CNS depressant effect of azelastine (nasal)
	Boceprevir	Efavirenz may decrease the serum concentration of boceprevir; boceprevir may increase the serum concentration of efavirenz
	Cisapride	QT prolongation, cardiac arrhythmias
	Clopidogrel	CYP2C19 inhibitors (moderate) may decrease serum concentrations of the active metabolite(s) of clopidogrel
	Ergot derivatives	Protease inhibitors may increase the serum concentration of ergot derivatives
	Etravirine	Reverse transcriptase inhibitors (non-nucleoside) may decrease the serum concentration of etravirine
	Ivacaftor	CYP3A4 inducers (strong) may decrease the serum concentration of ivacaftor
	Midazolam	Protease inhibitors may increase the serum concentration of midazolam
	Nevirapine	Efavirenz may enhance the adverse/toxic effect of nevirapine; nevirapine may enhance the adverse/toxic effect of efavirenz; nevirapine may decrease the serum concentration of efavirenz
	Pimozide	CYP3A4 inhibitors (strong) may increase the serum concentration of pimozide
	Posaconazole	Efavirenz may decrease the serum concentration of posaconazole
	Praziquantel	CYP3A4 inducers (strong) may decrease the serum concentration of praziquantel
	Rilpivirine	Reverse transcriptase inhibitors (non-nucleoside) may decrease the serum concentration of rilpivirine; this mechanism applies to coadministration of efavirenz, etravirine, and nevirapine
	St. John's wort	Decreased efavirenz efficacy
	Triazolam	Protease inhibitors may increase the serum concentration of triazolam
Emtricitabine	Lamivudine	May enhance the adverse/toxic effect of emtricitabine

TABLE 6-6

CONTRAINDICATED DRUG INTERACTIONS FOR ANTIMICROBIAL AGENTS (Continued)

Antimicrobial	Interacting Drug(s)	Toxic Effect
Erythromycin ethylsuccinate and acetylsulfisoxazole	Amiodarone, disopyramide, procainamide, sotalol	QT prolongation, cardiac arrhythmias
	Artemether, halofantrine, lumefantrine	QT prolongation, cardiac arrhythmias
	Cisapride	QT prolongation, cardiac arrhythmias
	Lincosamide antibiotics (clindamycin, lincomycin)	Decreased erythromycin efficacy
	Citalopram, escitalopram	QT prolongation, cardiac arrhythmias
	Lovastatin	Erythromycin may increase the serum concentration of lovastatin
	Methenamine	May enhance the adverse/toxic effect of sulfonamide derivatives; specifically, the combination may result in the formation of an insoluble precipitate in the urine
	Mifepristone	QT prolongation, cardiac arrhythmias
	Paliperidone, pimozide, quetiapine, thioridazine, ziprasidone	QT prolongation, cardiac arrhythmias
	Quinidine, quinine, saquinavir, telithromycin	QT prolongation, cardiac arrhythmias
	Simvastatin	Erythromycin may increase the serum concentration of simvastatin
Erythromycin preparations	Amiodarone, disopyramide, procainamide, sotalol	QT prolongation, cardiac arrhythmias
	Artemether, halofantrine, lumefantrine	QT prolongation, cardiac arrhythmias
	Cisapride	QT prolongation, cardiac arrhythmias
	Lincosamide antibiotics (clindamycin, lincomycin)	Decreased erythromycin efficacy
	Citalopram, escitalopram	QT prolongation, cardiac arrhythmias
	Lovastatin	Erythromycin may increase the serum concentration of Lovastatin
	Mifepristone	QT prolongation, cardiac arrhythmias
	Paliperidone, pimozide, quetiapine, thioridazine, ziprasidone	QT prolongation, cardiac arrhythmias
	Quinidine, quinine, saquinavir, telithromycin	QT prolongation, cardiac arrhythmias
	Simvastatin	Erythromycin may increase the serum concentration of simvastatin

Continued

TABLE 6-6

CONTRAINDICATED DRUG INTERACTIONS FOR ANTIMICROBIAL AGENTS (Continued)

Antimicrobial	Interacting Drug(s)	Toxic Effect
Etravirine	Atazanavir	Etravirine may decrease the serum concentration of atazanavir; atazanavir may increase the serum concentration of etravirine
	Carbamazepine	May decrease the serum concentration of etravirine
	Clopidogrel	CYP2C19 inhibitors (moderate) may decrease serum concentrations of the active metabolite(s) of clopidogrel
	Everolimus	CYP3A4 inducers (strong) may decrease the serum concentration of everolimus
	Fosamprenavir	Etravirine may increase the serum concentration of fosamprenavir
	Fosphenytoin, phenytoin, phenobarbital	May decrease the serum concentration of etravirine
	Ivacaftor	CYP3A4 inducers (strong) may decrease the serum concentration of ivacaftor
	Mifepristone	CYP3A4 inducers (strong) may decrease the serum concentration of mifepristone
	Praziquantel	CYP3A4 inducers (strong) may decrease the serum concentration of praziquantel
	Rifampin	May decrease the serum concentration of etravirine
	Rilpivirine	Etravirine may decrease the serum concentration of rilpivirine
	Ritonavir	May decrease the serum concentration of etravirine
	St. John's wort	May decrease the serum concentration of reverse transcriptase inhibitors (non-nucleoside)
	Tipranavir	May decrease the serum concentration of etravirine
Fluconazole	Cisapride	QT prolongation, cardiac arrhythmias
	Clopidogrel	CYP2C19 inhibitors (moderate) may decrease serum concentrations of the active metabolite(s) of clopidogrel
	Pimozide	Fluconazole may decrease the metabolism of pimozide
	Voriconazole	Fluconazole may increase the serum concentration of voriconazole
Flucytosine	Clozapine	Myelosuppressive agents may enhance the adverse/toxic effect of clozapine; specifically, the risk for agranulocytosis may be increased

TABLE 6-6

CONTRAINDICATED DRUG INTERACTIONS FOR ANTIMICROBIAL AGENTS (Continued)

Antimicrobial	Interacting Drug(s)	Toxic Effect
Fosamprenavir	Amiodarone	Bradycardia, hypotension, cardiogenic shock, heart block, QT prolongation, hepatotoxicity (amiodarone toxicity)
	Cisapride	QT prolongation, cardiac arrhythmias
	Delavirdine	Fosamprenavir may decrease the serum concentration of delavirdine; the active metabolite amprenavir is likely responsible for this effect; delavirdine may increase the serum concentration of fosamprenavir; specifically, delavirdine may increase concentrations of the active metabolite amprenavir
	Ergot derivatives	Vasospasm resulting in peripheral, cardiac, and/or cerebral ischemia; ↑ or ↓ in blood pressure or heart rate; seizures; headache
	Etravirine	May increase the serum concentration of fosamprenavir
	Everolimus	CYP3A4 inhibitors (strong) may increase the serum concentration of everolimus
	Flecainide	Fosamprenavir may increase the serum concentration of flecainide
	Fluticasone (inhalation)	CYP3A4 inhibitors (strong) may increase the serum concentration of fluticasone (oral inhalation)
	Halofantrine	CYP3A4 inhibitors (strong) may increase the serum concentration of halofantrine
	Lovastatin	Protease inhibitors may increase the serum concentration of lovastatin.
	Midazolam	Protease inhibitors may increase the serum concentration of midazolam; both IV and oral midazolam are contraindicated with fosamprenavir
	Pimozide	QT prolongation, ventricular arrhythmias; hypotension; seizures; anticholinergic and extrapyramidal effects
	Quinidine	Tachycardia, hypotension, heart block, ventricular fibrillation, syncope, vascular collapse (quinidine toxicity)
	Rifampin	May decrease the serum concentration of fosamprenavir
	Salmeterol	CYP3A4 inhibitors (strong) may increase the serum concentration of salmeterol
	Sildenafil	Contraindicated if sildenafil being used for pulmonary arterial hypertension; CYP3A4 inhibitors (strong) may increase the serum concentration of sildenafil

Continued

TABLE 6-6

CONTRAINDICATED DRUG INTERACTIONS FOR ANTIMICROBIAL AGENTS (Continued)

Antimicrobial	Interacting Drug(s)	Toxic Effect
	Simvastatin	Protease inhibitors may increase the serum concentration of simvastatin
	St. John's wort	May increase the metabolism of protease inhibitors
	Telaprevir	May decrease the serum concentration of fosamprenavir; fosamprenavir may decrease the serum concentration of telaprevir
	Thioridazine	QT prolongation, cardiac arrhythmias, hypotension, anticholinergic and extrapyramidal effects, agitation
	Triazolam	Protease inhibitors may increase the serum concentration of triazolam
Foscarnet	Thioridazine	QT prolongation, cardiac arrhythmias, hypotension, anticholinergic and extrapyramidal effects, agitation
Ganciclovir	Imipenem	Seizures
Gemifloxacin	Amiodarone, disopyramide, procainamide, sotalol	QT prolongation, cardiac arrhythmias
	Artemether, halofantrine, lumefantrine	QT prolongation, cardiac arrhythmias
	Cisapride	QT prolongation, cardiac arrhythmias
	Citalopram, escitalopram	QT prolongation, cardiac arrhythmias
	Mifepristone	QT prolongation, cardiac arrhythmias
	Paliperidone, pimozide, quetiapine, thioridazine, ziprasidone	QT prolongation, cardiac arrhythmias
	Quinidine, quinine, saquinavir, telithromycin	QT prolongation, cardiac arrhythmias
Griseofulvin	Contraceptives (progestins)	Contraceptive failure, breakthrough bleeding
Hydroxychloroquine	Artemether/lumefantrine	Artemether may enhance the adverse/toxic effect of antimalarial agents
	Mefloquine	Aminoquinolines (antimalarial) may enhance the adverse/toxic effect of mefloquine; specifically, the risk for QTc-prolongation and the risk for convulsions may be increased; mefloquine may increase the serum concentration of aminoquinolines (antimalarial)
	Pimecrolimus	Avoid use of pimecrolimus cream in patients receiving immunosuppressants
	Tacrolimus (topical)	Avoid use of tacrolimus ointment in patients receiving immunosuppressants
Imipenem-Cilastatin	Ganciclovir	Seizures

TABLE 6-6

CONTRAINDICATED DRUG INTERACTIONS FOR ANTIMICROBIAL AGENTS (Continued)

Antimicrobial	Interacting Drug(s)	Toxic Effect
Imiquimod	Pimecrolimus	Avoid use of pimecrolimus cream in patients receiving immunosuppressants
	Tacrolimus (topical)	Avoid use of tacrolimus ointment in patients receiving immunosuppressants
Indinavir	Alprazolam	Indinavir may increase the serum concentration of alprazolam
	Amiodarone	Bradycardia, hypotension, cardiogenic shock, heart block, QT prolongation, hepatotoxicity (amiodarone toxicity)
	Atazanavir	Atazanavir may enhance the adverse/toxic effect of indinavir; indinavir may enhance the adverse/toxic effect of atazanavir
	Cisapride	QT prolongation, cardiac arrhythmias
	Ergot derivatives	Vasospasm resulting in peripheral, cardiac, and/or cerebral ischemia; ↑ or ↓ in blood pressure or heart rate; seizures; headache
	Everolimus	CYP3A4 inhibitors (strong) may increase the serum concentration of everolimus
	Fluticasone (inhalation)	CYP3A4 inhibitors (strong) may increase the serum concentration of fluticasone (oral inhalation)
	Halofantrine	CYP3A4 inhibitors (strong) may increase the serum concentration of halofantrine
	Lovastatin	Protease inhibitors may increase the serum concentration of lovastatin
	Midazolam	Protease inhibitors may increase the serum concentration of midazolam; both IV and oral midazolam are contraindicated with fosamprenavir
	Pimozide	QT prolongation, ventricular arrhythmias; hypotension; seizures; anticholinergic and extrapyramidal effects
	Quinidine	Tachycardia, hypotension, heart block, ventricular fibrillation, syncope, vascular collapse (quinidine toxicity)
	Rifampin	May decrease the serum concentration of fosamprenavir
	Salmeterol	CYP3A4 inhibitors (strong) may increase the serum concentration of salmeterol
	Sildenafil	Contraindicated if sildenafil being used for pulmonary arterial hypertension; CYP3A4 inhibitors (strong) may increase the serum concentration of sildenafil

Continued

TABLE 6-6

CONTRAINDICATED DRUG INTERACTIONS FOR ANTIMICROBIAL AGENTS (Continued)

Antimicrobial	Interacting Drug(s)	Toxic Effect
Isoniazid	Clopidogrel	CYP2C19 inhibitors (strong) may decrease serum concentrations of the active metabolite(s) of clopidogrel
	Pimozide	CYP3A4 inhibitors (weak) may increase the serum concentration of pimozide
	Thioridazine	CYP2D6 inhibitors may decrease the metabolism of thioridazine; QT prolongation, cardiac arrhythmias
Itraconazole	Cisapride	QT prolongation, cardiac arrhythmias
	Ergot derivatives	Vasospasm resulting in peripheral, cardiac, and/or cerebral ischemia; ↑ or ↓ in blood pressure or heart rate; seizures; headache
	Everolimus	CYP3A4 inhibitors (strong) may increase the serum concentration of everolimus
	Fluticasone (inhalation)	CYP3A4 inhibitors (strong) may increase the serum concentration of fluticasone (oral inhalation)
	Halofantrine	CYP3A4 inhibitors (strong) may increase the serum concentration of halofantrine
	Lovastatin	CYP3A4 inhibitors (strong) may increase the serum concentration of lovastatin
	Methadone	Itraconazole may increase the serum concentration of methadone
	Nafcillin	CYP3A4 inducers (strong) may decrease the serum concentration of itraconazole
	Nevirapine	Nevirapine may decrease the serum concentration of itraconazole
	Carbamazepine, fosphenytoin, oxcarbazepine, pentobarbital, phenobarbital, phenytoin, primidone	CYP3A4 inducers (strong) may decrease the serum concentration of itraconazole
	Pimozide	QT prolongation, ventricular arrhythmias; hypotension; seizures; anticholinergic and extrapyramidal effects
	Quinidine	Tachycardia, hypotension, heart block, ventricular fibrillation, syncope, vascular collapse (quinidine toxicity)
	Salmeterol	CYP3A4 inhibitors (strong) may increase the serum concentration of salmeterol
	Sildenafil	Contraindicated if sildenafil being used for pulmonary arterial hypertension; CYP3A4 inhibitors (strong) may increase the serum concentration of sildenafil
	Simvastatin	CYP3A4 inhibitors (strong) may increase the serum concentration of simvastatin

TABLE 6-6

CONTRAINDICATED DRUG INTERACTIONS FOR ANTIMICROBIAL AGENTS (Continued)

Antimicrobial	Interacting Drug(s)	Toxic Effect
Ketoconazole	Cisapride	QT prolongation, cardiac arrhythmias
	Clopidogrel	CYP2C19 inhibitors (moderate) may decrease serum concentrations of the active metabolite(s) of clopidogrel
	Ergot derivatives	Vasospasm resulting in peripheral, cardiac, and/or cerebral ischemia; ↑ or ↓ in blood pressure or heart rate; seizures; headache
	Everolimus	CYP3A4 inhibitors (strong) may increase the serum concentration of everolimus
	Fluticasone (inhalation)	CYP3A4 inhibitors (strong) may increase the serum concentration of fluticasone (oral inhalation).
	Halofantrine	CYP3A4 inhibitors (strong) may increase the serum concentration of halofantrine
	Lovastatin	CYP3A4 inhibitors (strong) may increase the serum concentration of lovastatin
	Nevirapine	Nevirapine may decrease the serum concentration of ketoconazole
	Pimozide	QT prolongation, ventricular arrhythmias; hypotension; seizures; anticholinergic and extrapyramidal effects
	Quinidine	Tachycardia, hypotension, heart block, ventricular fibrillation, syncope, vascular collapse (quinidine toxicity)
	Salmeterol	CYP3A4 inhibitors (strong) may increase the serum concentration of salmeterol
	Sildenafil	Contraindicated if sildenafil being used for pulmonary arterial hypertension; CYP3A4 inhibitors (strong) may increase the serum concentration of sildenafil
	Simvastatin	CYP3A4 inhibitors (strong) may increase the serum concentration of simvastatin
Lamivudine	Emtricitabine	Lamivudine may enhance the adverse/toxic effect of emtricitabine
Levofloxacin	Amiodarone, disopyramide, procainamide, sotalol	QT prolongation, cardiac arrhythmias
	Artemether, halofantrine, lumefantrine	QT prolongation, cardiac arrhythmias
	Cisapride	QT prolongation, cardiac arrhythmias
	Citalopram, escitalopram	QT prolongation, cardiac arrhythmias
	Mifepristone	QT prolongation, cardiac arrhythmias
	Pimozide, quetiapine, thioridazine, ziprasidone	QT prolongation, cardiac arrhythmias
	Quinidine, quinine, saquinavir, telithromycin	QT prolongation, cardiac arrhythmias

Continued

TABLE 6-6

CONTRAINDICATED DRUG INTERACTIONS FOR ANTIMICROBIAL AGENTS (Continued)

Antimicrobial	Interacting Drug(s)	Toxic Effect
Linezolid	Anilidopiperidine opioids (alfentanil, fentanyl, remifentanil, sufentanil), buprenorphine, cyclobenzaprine, dextromethorphan, meperidine	Serotonin syndrome (mental status changes, agitation, myoclonus, hyperreflexia, diaphoresis, dilated pupils, shivering, tremor, diarrhea, fever)
	Almotriptan, rizatriptan, sumatriptan, zolmitriptan	MAO inhibitors may decrease the metabolism of serotonin 5-HT1D receptor agonists
	Amphetamine, benzphetamine, dextroamphetamine, lisdexamphetamine, methamphetamine, buspirone, dexmethylphenidate, methylphenidate	Hypertension
	Antidepressants involving serotonin: citalopram, escitalopram, fluoxetine, fluvoxamine, nefazodone, paroxetine, sertraline, trazodone, venlafaxine	Serotonin syndrome (mental status changes, agitation, myoclonus, hyperreflexia, diaphoresis, dilated pupils, shivering, tremor, diarrhea, fever)
	Atomoxetine, bupropion	Nausea, vomiting, flushing, dizziness, tremor, myoclonus, rigidity, diaphoresis, hyperthermia, autonomic instability
	Brimonidine	Hypertension
	Carbamazepine	Carbamazepine may enhance the adverse/toxic effect of MAO inhibitors
	Clozapine	Myelosuppressive agents may enhance the adverse/toxic effect of clozapine; specifically, the risk for agranulocytosis may be increased
	Ephedrine, pseudoephedrine	Hypertension
	Hydromorphone	MAO inhibitors may enhance the adverse/toxic effect of hydromorphone
	Methyldopa	MAO inhibitors may enhance the adverse/toxic effect of methyldopa
	Methylene blue	Serotonin syndrome (mental status changes, agitation, myoclonus, hyperreflexia, diaphoresis, dilated pupils, shivering, tremor, diarrhea, fever)
	Phenylephrine	Hypertension, headache

TABLE 6-6

CONTRAINDICATED DRUG INTERACTIONS FOR ANTIMICROBIAL AGENTS (Continued)

Antimicrobial	Interacting Drug(s)	Toxic Effect
	Tricyclic antidepressants (amitriptyline, clomipramine, desipramine, doxepin, imipramine, nortriptyline, protriptyline, trimipramine)	Hypertensive crisis, serotonin syndrome (mental status changes, agitation, myoclonus, hyperreflexia, diaphoresis, dilated pupils, shivering, tremor, diarrhea, fever)
Lopinavir with ritonavir	Amiodarone	Bradycardia, hypotension, cardiogenic shock, heart block, QT prolongation, hepatotoxicity (amiodarone toxicity)
	Cisapride	QT prolongation, cardiac arrhythmias
	Darunavir	Lopinavir may decrease the serum concentration of darunavir; darunavir may increase the serum concentration of lopinavir
	Disulfiram	Decreased metabolism of ritonavir; decreased metabolism of alcohol contained in Kaletra brand of oral solution with accumulation of acetaldehyde
	Ergot derivatives (bromocriptine, dihydroergotamine; ergoloid mesylates; ergonovine; ergotamine; methylergonovine)	Vasospasm resulting in peripheral, cardiac, and/or cerebral ischemia; ↑ or ↓ in blood pressure or heart rate; seizures; headache
	Everolimus	CYP3A4 inhibitors (strong) may increase the serum concentration of everolimus
	Flecainide	Cardiac arrhythmias (ventricular tachydysrhythmias, severe bradycardia, AV block)
	Fluticasone (inhalation)	CYP3A4 inhibitors (strong) may increase the serum concentration of fluticasone (oral inhalation)
	Halofantrine	CYP3A4 inhibitors (strong) may increase the serum concentration of halofantrine
	Lovastatin	Protease inhibitors may increase the serum concentration of lovastatin
	Midazolam	Protease inhibitors may increase the serum concentration of midazolam
	Pimozide	QT prolongation, ventricular arrhythmias; hypotension; seizures; anticholinergic and extrapyramidal effects
	Quinidine	Tachycardia, hypotension, heart block, ventricular fibrillation, syncope, vascular collapse (quinidine toxicity)

Continued

TABLE 6-6

CONTRAINDICATED DRUG INTERACTIONS FOR ANTIMICROBIAL AGENTS (Continued)

Antimicrobial	Interacting Drug(s)	Toxic Effect
	Quinine	Ritonavir may increase or decrease the serum concentration of quinine; quinine may increase the serum concentration of ritonavir
	Rifampin	Rifampin may enhance the adverse/toxic effect of lopinavir; specifically, the risk for hepatocellular toxicity may be increased; rifampin may decrease the serum concentration of lopinavir
	Salmeterol	CYP3A4 inhibitors (strong) may increase the serum concentration of salmeterol
	Sildenafil	Contraindicated if sildenafil being used for pulmonary arterial hypertension
	Simvastatin	Protease inhibitors may increase the serum concentration of simvastatin
	St. John's wort	Decreased lopinavir/ritonavir efficacy
	Telaprevir	Lopinavir may decrease the serum concentration of telaprevir
	Thioridazine	QT prolongation, cardiac arrhythmias, hypotension, anticholinergic and extrapyramidal effects, agitation
	Voriconazole	Ritonavir may decrease the serum concentration of voriconazole
Maraviroc	St. John's wort	St. John's wort may decrease the serum concentration of maraviroc
Mefloquine HCl	Artemether, halofantrine, lumefantrine	QT prolongation, cardiac arrhythmias
	Chloroquine, hydroxychloroquine, primaquine	Aminoquinolines (antimalarial) may enhance the adverse/toxic effect of mefloquine; specifically, the risk for QTc-prolongation and the risk for convulsions may be increased; mefloquine may increase the serum concentration of aminoquinolines (antimalarial)
	Quinidine, quinine	Quinidine and quinine may enhance the adverse/toxic effect of mefloquine; specifically, the risk for QTc prolongation and the risk for convulsions may be increased
Metronidazole	Amprenavir	Propylene glycol toxicity (from amprenavir suspension)
Methenamine mandelate	Sulfonamide derivatives (sulfacetamide, sulfadiazine, sulfamethoxazole, sulfisoxazole)	Methenamine may enhance the adverse/toxic effect of sulfonamide derivatives; specifically, the combination may result in the formation of an insoluble precipitate in the urine

TABLE 6-6

CONTRAINDICATED DRUG INTERACTIONS FOR ANTIMICROBIAL AGENTS (Continued)

Antimicrobial	Interacting Drug(s)	Toxic Effect
Metronidazole	Disulfiram	Metronidazole may enhance the adverse/toxic effect of disulfiram
	Pimozide	CYP3A4 inhibitors (moderate) may increase the serum concentration of pimozide
Miconazole	Clopidogrel	CYP2C19 inhibitors (moderate) may decrease serum concentrations of the active metabolite(s) of clopidogrel
	Pimozide	QT prolongation, ventricular arrhythmias; hypotension; seizures; anticholinergic and extrapyramidal effects
	Thioridazine	QT prolongation, cardiac arrhythmias, hypotension, anticholinergic and extrapyramidal effects, agitation
Minocycline	Isotretinoin, tretinoin	Tetracycline derivatives may enhance the adverse/toxic effect of retinoic acid derivatives; the development of pseudotumor cerebri is of particular concern
Moxifloxacin	Amiodarone, disopyramide, procainamide, sotalol	QT prolongation, cardiac arrhythmias
	Artemether, halofantrine, lumefantrine	QT prolongation, cardiac arrhythmias
	Cisapride	QT prolongation, cardiac arrhythmias
	Citalopram, escitalopram	QT prolongation, cardiac arrhythmias
	Mifepristone	QT prolongation, cardiac arrhythmias
	Pimozide, quetiapine, thioridazine, ziprasidone	QT prolongation, cardiac arrhythmias
	Quinidine, quinine, saquinavir, telithromycin	QT prolongation, cardiac arrhythmias
Nafcillin	Everolimus	CYP3A4 inhibitors (strong) may increase the serum concentration of everolimus
	Itraconazole	CYP3A4 inducers (strong) may decrease the serum concentration of itraconazole
	Ivacaftor	CYP3A4 inducers (strong) may decrease the serum concentration of ivacaftor
	Lurasidone	CYP3A4 inducers (strong) may decrease the serum concentration of lurasidone
	Mifepristone	CYP3A4 inducers (strong) may decrease the serum concentration of mifepristone
	Praziquantel	CYP3A4 inducers (strong) may decrease the serum concentration of praziquantel
Nelfinavir	Amiodarone	Bradycardia, hypotension, cardiogenic shock, heart block, QT prolongation, hepatotoxicity, (amiodarone toxicity)
	Cisapride	QT prolongation, cardiac arrhythmias

Continued

TABLE 6-6

CONTRAINDICATED DRUG INTERACTIONS FOR ANTIMICROBIAL AGENTS (Continued)

Antimicrobial	Interacting Drug(s)	Toxic Effect
	Ergot derivatives	Vasospasm resulting in peripheral, cardiac, and/or cerebral ischemia; ↑ or ↓ in blood pressure or heart rate; seizures; headache
	Everolimus	CYP3A4 inhibitors (strong) may increase the serum concentration of everolimus
	Fluticasone (inhalation)	CYP3A4 inhibitors (strong) may increase the serum concentration of fluticasone (oral inhalation)
	Halofantrine	CYP3A4 inhibitors (strong) may increase the serum concentration of halofantrine
	Lovastatin	Protease inhibitors may increase the serum concentration of lovastatin
	Lurasidone	CYP3A4 inhibitors (strong) may increase the serum concentration of lurasidone
	Midazolam	Protease inhibitors may increase the serum concentration of midazolam
	Pimozide	QT prolongation, ventricular arrhythmias; hypotension; seizures; anticholinergic and extrapyramidal effects
	Proton pump inhibitors (dexlansoprazole, esomeprazole, lansoprazole, omeprazole, pantoprazole, rabeprazole)	Proton pump inhibitors may decrease serum concentrations of the active metabolite(s) of nelfinavir; proton pump inhibitors may decrease the serum concentration of nelfinavir
	Quinidine	Tachycardia, hypotension, heart block, ventricular fibrillation, syncope, vascular collapse (quinidine toxicity)
	Rifampin	Rifampin may decrease the serum concentration of nelfinavir
	Salmeterol	CYP3A4 inhibitors (strong) may increase the serum concentration of salmeterol
	Sildenafil	Contraindicated if sildenafil being used for pulmonary arterial hypertension; CYP3A4 inhibitors (strong) may increase the serum concentration of sildenafil
	Simvastatin	Protease inhibitors may increase the serum concentration of simvastatin
	St. John's wort	Decreased nelfinavir efficacy
	Triazolam	Protease inhibitors may increase the serum concentration of triazolam

TABLE 6-6

CONTRAINDICATED DRUG INTERACTIONS FOR ANTIMICROBIAL AGENTS (Continued)

Antimicrobial	Interacting Drug(s)	Toxic Effect
Nevirapine	Atazanavir	Nevirapine may decrease the serum concentration of atazanavir; atazanavir may increase the serum concentration of nevirapine
	Efavirenz	Efavirenz may enhance the adverse/toxic effect of nevirapine; nevirapine may enhance the adverse/toxic effect of efavirenz; nevirapine may decrease the serum concentration of efavirenz
	Etravirine	Reverse transcriptase inhibitors (non-nucleoside) may decrease the serum concentration of etravirine
	Everolimus	CYP3A4 inhibitors (strong) may increase the serum concentration of everolimus
	Itraconazole	CYP3A4 inducers (strong) may decrease the serum concentration of itraconazole
	Ivacaftor	CYP3A4 inducers (strong) may decrease the serum concentration of ivacaftor
	Ketoconazole	Nevirapine may decrease the serum concentration of ketoconazole (systemic)
	Lurasidone	CYP3A4 inducers (strong) may decrease the serum concentration of lurasidone
	Mifepristone	CYP3A4 inducers (strong) may decrease the serum concentration of mifepristone
	Pimozide	CYP3A4 inhibitors (weak) may increase the serum concentration of pimozide
	Praziquantel	CYP3A4 inducers (strong) may decrease the serum concentration of praziquantel
	Rilpivirine	Reverse transcriptase inhibitors (non-nucleoside) may decrease the serum concentration of rilpivirine
	St. John's wort	St. John's wort may decrease the serum concentration of reverse transcriptase inhibitors (non-nucleoside)
Nitrofurantoin	Norfloxacin	Nitrofurantoin may diminish the therapeutic effect of norfloxacin
Norfloxacin	Thioridazine	QT prolongation, cardiac arrhythmias, hypotension, anticholinergic and extrapyramidal effects, agitation
Ofloxacin	Amiodarone, disopyramide, procainamide, sotalol	QT prolongation, cardiac arrhythmias
	Artemether, halofantrine, lumefantrine	QT prolongation, cardiac arrhythmias
	Cisapride	QT prolongation, cardiac arrhythmias
	Citalopram, escitalopram	QT prolongation, cardiac arrhythmias
	Mifepristone	QT prolongation, cardiac arrhythmias

Continued

6

TABLE 6-6

CONTRAINDICATED DRUG INTERACTIONS FOR ANTIMICROBIAL AGENTS (Continued)

Antimicrobial	Interacting Drug(s)	Toxic Effect
	Pimozide, quetiapine, thioridazine, ziprasidone	QT prolongation, cardiac arrhythmias
	Quinidine, quinine, saquinavir, telithromycin	QT prolongation, cardiac arrhythmias
Pentamidine	Amiodarone, disopyramide, procainamide, sotalol	QT prolongation, cardiac arrhythmias
	Artemether, halofantrine, lumefantrine	QT prolongation, cardiac arrhythmias
	Cisapride	QT prolongation, cardiac arrhythmias
	Citalopram, escitalopram	QT prolongation, cardiac arrhythmias
	Mifepristone	QT prolongation, cardiac arrhythmias
	Pimozide, quetiapine, thioridazine, ziprasidone	QT prolongation, cardiac arrhythmias
	Quinidine, quinine, saquinavir, telithromycin	QT prolongation, cardiac arrhythmias
Polymyxin B sulfate, neomycin sulfate, hydrocortisone	Vaccines (live organisms)	Vaccinial infections
Posaconazole	Cisapride	QT prolongation, cardiac arrhythmias
	Efavirenz	Efavirenz may decrease the serum concentration of posaconazole
	Ergot derivatives	Vasospasm resulting in peripheral, cardiac, and/or cerebral ischemia; ↑ or ↓ in blood pressure or heart rate; seizures; headache
	Everolimus	CYP3A4 inhibitors (strong) may increase the serum concentration of everolimus
	Fluticasone (inhalation)	CYP3A4 inhibitors (strong) may increase the serum concentration of fluticasone (oral inhalation)
	Halofantrine	CYP3A4 inhibitors (strong) may increase the serum concentration of halofantrine
	Lovastatin	Protease inhibitors may increase the serum concentration of lovastatin
	Lurasidone	CYP3A4 inhibitors (strong) may increase the serum concentration of lurasidone
	Methadone	Posaconazole may enhance the QTc-prolonging effect of methadone; posaconazole may increase the serum concentration of methadone
	Pimozide	QT prolongation, ventricular arrhythmias; hypotension; seizures; anticholinergic and extrapyramidal effects
	Proton pump inhibitors (dexlansoprazole, esomeprazole, lansoprazole, omeprazole, pantoprazole, rabeprazole)	Proton pump inhibitors may decrease the serum concentration of posaconazole

TABLE 6-6

CONTRAINDICATED DRUG INTERACTIONS FOR ANTIMICROBIAL AGENTS (Continued)

Antimicrobial	Interacting Drug(s)	Toxic Effect
	Quinidine	Tachycardia, hypotension, heart block, ventricular fibrillation, syncope, vascular collapse (quinidine toxicity)
	Salmeterol	CYP3A4 inhibitors (strong) may increase the serum concentration of salmeterol
	Sildenafil	Contraindicated if sildenafil being used for pulmonary arterial hypertension; CYP3A4 inhibitors (strong) may increase the serum concentration of sildenafil
	Simvastatin	Protease inhibitors may increase the serum concentration of simvastatin
	Sirolimus	Posaconazole may increase the serum concentration of sirolimus
Praziquantel	Bosentan	CYP3A4 inducers (strong) may decrease the serum concentration of praziquantel
	Carbamazepine, oxcarbazepine	CYP3A4 inducers (strong) may decrease the serum concentration of praziquantel
	Dexamethasone	CYP3A4 inducers (strong) may decrease the serum concentration of praziquantel
	Efavirenz, etravirine, nevirapine	CYP3A4 inducers (strong) may decrease the serum concentration of praziquantel
	Fosphenytoin, phenytoin, pentobarbital, phenobarbital	CYP3A4 inducers (strong) may decrease the serum concentration of praziquantel
	Nafcillin	CYP3A4 inducers (strong) may decrease the serum concentration of praziquantel
	Primidone	CYP3A4 inducers (strong) may decrease the serum concentration of praziquantel
	Rifabutin, rifampin, rifapentine	CYP3A4 inducers (strong) may decrease the serum concentration of praziquantel
Primaquine	Artemether, lumefantrine	QT prolongation, cardiac arrhythmias
	Mefloquine	QTc prolongation and the risk for convulsions may be increased
	Pimozide	CYP3A4 inhibitors (weak) may increase the serum concentration of pimozide
Pyrimethamine +/– sulfadoxine	Artemether, lumefantrine	Artemether/lumefantrine may enhance the adverse/toxic effect of antimalarial agents
	Methenamine	Methenamine may enhance the adverse/toxic effect of sulfonamide derivatives; specifically, the combination may result in the formation of an insoluble precipitate in the urine

Continued

6

TABLE 6-6

CONTRAINDICATED DRUG INTERACTIONS FOR ANTIMICROBIAL AGENTS (Continued)

Antimicrobial	Interacting Drug(s)	Toxic Effect
Quinidine gluconate	Amiodarone, disopyramide, flecainide, procainamide, sotalol	QT prolongation, cardiac arrhythmias
	Artemether, halofantrine, lumefantrine	QT prolongation, cardiac arrhythmias
	Atazanavir, clarithromycin, darunavir, erythromycin, fluconazole, fosamprenavir, gemifloxacin, indinavir, itraconazole, ketoconazole, levofloxacin, lopinavir moxifloxacin, nelfinavir, ofloxacin, pentamidine, posaconazole, quinine, rilpivirine, ritonavir, saquinavir, telithromycin, tipranavir, voriconazole	QT prolongation, cardiac arrhythmias
	Chloroquine, mefloquine	QT prolongation, cardiac arrhythmias
	Cisapride, chlorpromazine, dolasetron, droperidol, granisetron, ondansetron	QT prolongation, cardiac arrhythmias
	Citalopram, escitalopram, trazodone	QT prolongation, cardiac arrhythmias
	Clozapine, haloperidol, Paliperidone, pimozide, quetiapine, risperidone, thioridazine, ziprasidone	QT prolongation, cardiac arrhythmias
	Methadone	QT prolongation, cardiac arrhythmias
	Mifepristone	QT prolongation, cardiac arrhythmias
Quinine sulfate	Amiodarone, disopyramide, flecainide, procainamide, sotalol	QT prolongation, cardiac arrhythmias
	Aluminum hydroxide, magnesium hydroxide,	Antacids may decrease the serum concentration of quinine
	Artemether, halofantrine, lumefantrine	QT prolongation, cardiac arrhythmias
	Atracurium, cisatracurium, pancuronium, rocuronium, succinylcholine, vecuronium	Quinine may enhance the neuromuscular-blocking effect of neuromuscular-blocking agents

TABLE 6-6

CONTRAINDICATED DRUG INTERACTIONS FOR ANTIMICROBIAL AGENTS (Continued)

Antimicrobial	Interacting Drug(s)	Toxic Effect
	Azithromycin, clarithromycin, erythromycin, gemifloxacin, levofloxacin, moxifloxacin, ofloxacin, pentamidine, quinidine, rilpivirine, saquinavir, telithromycin, voriconazole	QT prolongation, cardiac arrhythmias
	Chloroquine, mefloquine	QT prolongation, cardiac arrhythmias
	Cisapride, chlorpromazine, dolasetron, droperidol, granisetron, ondansetron	QT prolongation, cardiac arrhythmias
	Citalopram, escitalopram, trazodone	QT prolongation, cardiac arrhythmias
	Clozapine, haloperidol, paliperidone, pimozide, quetiapine, risperidone, thioridazine, ziprasidone	QT prolongation, cardiac arrhythmias
	Lopinavir, ritonavir	Lopinavir may decrease the serum concentration of quinine; this effect has been seen with lopinavir/ritonavir
	Methadone	QT prolongation, cardiac arrhythmias
	Mifepristone	QT prolongation, cardiac arrhythmias
	Rifampin	Rifampin may decrease the serum concentration of quinine
Quinupristin + dalfopristin	Cisapride	Quinupristin may increase the serum concentration of cisapride
	Pimozide	CYP3A4 inhibitors (weak) may increase the serum concentration of pimozide
Ribavirin	Didanosine	Ribavirin may enhance the adverse/toxic effect of didanosine; ribavirin may increase serum concentrations of the active metabolite(s) of didanosine
Rifabutin	Boceprevir	Rifabutin may decrease the serum concentration of boceprevir; boceprevir may increase the serum concentration of rifabutin
	Everolimus	CYP3A4 inducers (strong) may decrease the serum concentration of everolimus
	Ivacaftor	CYP3A4 inducers (strong) may decrease the serum concentration of ivacaftor
	Lurasidone	CYP3A4 inducers (strong) may decrease the serum concentration of lurasidone
	Mifepristone	CYP3A4 inducers (strong) may decrease the serum concentration of mifepristone

Continued

TABLE 6-6

CONTRAINDICATED DRUG INTERACTIONS FOR ANTIMICROBIAL AGENTS (Continued)

Antimicrobial	Interacting Drug(s)	Toxic Effect
	Mycophenolate	Rifamycin derivatives may decrease the serum concentration of mycophenolate; specifically, rifamycin derivatives may decrease the concentration of the active metabolite mycophenolic acid
	Praziquantel	CYP3A4 inducers (strong) may decrease the serum concentration of praziquantel
	Rilpivirine	Rifamycin derivatives may decrease the serum concentration of rilpivirine
	Telaprevir	Telaprevir may increase the serum concentration of rifabutin; rifabutin may decrease the serum concentration of telaprevir
	Voriconazole	Rifamycin derivatives may decrease the serum concentration of voriconazole; voriconazole may increase the serum concentration of rifamycin derivatives
Rifampin	Atazanavir	Rifampin may decrease the serum concentration of atazanavir
	Boceprevir	Rifampin may decrease the serum concentration of boceprevir
	Darunavir	Rifampin may decrease the serum concentration of darunavir
	Esomeprazole	Rifampin may decrease the serum concentration of esomeprazole
	Etravirine	Rifampin may decrease the serum concentration of etravirine
	Everolimus	CYP3A4 inducers (strong) may decrease the serum concentration of everolimus
	Fosamprenavir	Rifampin may decrease the serum concentration of fosamprenavir; specifically, concentrations of amprenavir (active metabolite) may be decreased
	Indinavir	Rifampin may decrease the serum concentration of indinavir
	Ivacaftor	CYP3A4 inducers (strong) may decrease the serum concentration of ivacaftor
	Lopinavir	Rifampin may enhance the adverse/toxic effect of lopinavir; specifically, the risk for hepatocellular toxicity may be increased; rifampin may decrease the serum concentration of lopinavir
	Lurasidone	CYP3A4 inducers (strong) may decrease the serum concentration of lurasidone
	Mifepristone	CYP3A4 inducers (strong) may decrease the serum concentration of mifepristone

TABLE 6-6

CONTRAINDICATED DRUG INTERACTIONS FOR ANTIMICROBIAL AGENTS (Continued)

Antimicrobial	Interacting Drug(s)	Toxic Effect
	Mycophenolate	Rifamycin derivatives may decrease the serum concentration of mycophenolate; specifically, rifamycin derivatives may decrease the concentration of the active metabolite mycophenolic acid
	Nelfinavir	Rifampin may decrease the serum concentration of nelfinavir
	Omeprazole	Rifampin may decrease the serum concentration of omeprazole
	Praziquantel	CYP3A4 inducers (strong) may decrease the serum concentration of praziquantel
	Quinine	Rifampin may decrease the serum concentration of quinine
	Rilpivirine	Rifamycin derivatives may decrease the serum concentration of rilpivirine
	Ritonavir	Rifampin may decrease the serum concentration of ritonavir
	Saquinavir	Rifampin may enhance the adverse/toxic effect of saquinavir; specifically, the risk for hepatocellular toxicity may be increased; rifampin may decrease the serum concentration of saquinavir
	Telaprevir	Rifampin may decrease the serum concentration of telaprevir
	Voriconazole	Rifamycin derivatives may decrease the serum concentration of voriconazole; voriconazole may increase the serum concentration of rifamycin derivatives
Rifapentine	Etravirine	Rifapentine may decrease the serum concentration of etravirine
	Everolimus	CYP3A4 inducers (strong) may decrease the serum concentration of everolimus
	Ivacaftor	CYP3A4 inducers (strong) may decrease the serum concentration of ivacaftor
	Lurasidone	CYP3A4 inducers (strong) may decrease the serum concentration of lurasidone
	Mifepristone	CYP3A4 inducers (strong) may decrease the serum concentration of mifepristone
	Mycophenolate	Rifamycin derivatives may decrease the serum concentration of mycophenolate; specifically, rifamycin derivatives may decrease the concentration of the active metabolite mycophenolic acid
	Praziquantel	CYP3A4 inducers (strong) may decrease the serum concentration of praziquantel

Continued

TABLE 6-6

CONTRAINDICATED DRUG INTERACTIONS FOR ANTIMICROBIAL AGENTS (Continued)

Antimicrobial	Interacting Drug(s)	Toxic Effect
	Rilpivirine	Rifamycin derivatives may decrease the serum concentration of rilpivirine
	Voriconazole	Rifamycin derivatives may decrease the serum concentration of voriconazole; voriconazole may increase the serum concentration of rifamycin derivatives
Rilpivirine	Amiodarone, disopyramide, procainamide, sotalol	QT prolongation, cardiac arrhythmias
	Artemether, halofantrine, lumefantrine	QT prolongation, cardiac arrhythmias
	Carbamazepine, oxcarbazepine	Carbamazepine/oxcarbazepine may decrease the serum concentration of rilpivirine
	Cisapride	QT prolongation, cardiac arrhythmias
	Citalopram, escitalopram	QT prolongation, cardiac arrhythmias
	Delavirdine	Delavirdine may increase the serum concentration of rilpivirine
	Dexamethasone	Dexamethasone may decrease the serum concentration of rilpivirine
	Efavirenz	Efavirenz may decrease the serum concentration of rilpivirine
	Etravirine	Etravirine may decrease the serum concentration of rilpivirine
	Fosphenytoin, phenytoin, phenobarbital	May decrease the serum concentration of rilpivirine
	Mifepristone	QT prolongation, cardiac arrhythmias
	Nevirapine	Nevirapine may decrease the serum concentration of rilpivirine.
	Proton pump inhibitors (dexlansoprazole, esomeprazole, lansoprazole, omeprazole, pantoprazole, rabeprazole)	Proton pump inhibitors may decrease the serum concentration of rilpivirine
	Pimozide, quetiapine, thioridazine, ziprasidone	QT prolongation, cardiac arrhythmias
	Quinidine, quinine, saquinavir, telithromycin	QT prolongation, cardiac arrhythmias
	Rifabutin, rifampin, rifapentine	Rifamycin derivatives may decrease the serum concentration of rilpivirine
	St. John's wort	St. John's wort may decrease the serum concentration of reverse transcriptase inhibitors (non-nucleoside).
Ritonavir	Amiodarone	Bradycardia, hypotension, cardiogenic shock, heart block, QT prolongation, hepatotoxicity, (amiodarone toxicity)
	Cisapride	QT prolongation, cardiac arrhythmias

TABLE 6-6

CONTRAINDICATED DRUG INTERACTIONS FOR ANTIMICROBIAL AGENTS (Continued)

Antimicrobial	Interacting Drug(s)	Toxic Effect
	Ergot derivatives (bromocriptine, dihydroergotamine; ergoloid mesylates; ergonovine; ergotamine; methylergonovine)	Vasospasm resulting in peripheral, cardiac, and/or cerebral ischemia; ↑ or ↓ in blood pressure or heart rate; seizures; headache
	Etravirine	Ritonavir may decrease the serum concentration of etravirine
	Everolimus	CYP3A4 inhibitors (strong) may increase the serum concentration of everolimus
	Flecainide	Cardiac arrhythmias (ventricular tachydysrhythmias, severe bradycardia, AV block)
	Fluticasone (nasal and inhalation)	CYP3A4 inhibitors (strong) may increase the serum concentration of fluticasone (nasal and oral inhalation)
	Halofantrine	CYP3A4 inhibitors (strong) may increase the serum concentration of halofantrine
	Lovastatin	Protease inhibitors may increase the serum concentration of lovastatin
	Midazolam	Protease inhibitors may increase the serum concentration of midazolam
	Pimozide	QT prolongation, ventricular arrhythmias; hypotension; seizures; anticholinergic and extrapyramidal effects
	Quinidine	Tachycardia, hypotension, heart block, ventricular fibrillation, syncope, vascular collapse (quinidine toxicity)
	Quinine	Ritonavir may increase or decrease the serum concentration of quinine; quinine may increase the serum concentration of ritonavir
	Rifampin	Rifampin may decrease the serum concentration of ritonavir
	Salmeterol	CYP3A4 inhibitors (strong) may increase the serum concentration of salmeterol
	Sildenafil	Contraindicated if sildenafil being used for pulmonary arterial hypertension; CYP3A4 inhibitors (strong) may increase the serum concentration of sildenafil
	Simvastatin	Protease inhibitors may increase the serum concentration of simvastatin
	St. John's wort	Decreased ritonavir efficacy
	Triazolam	Protease inhibitors may increase the serum concentration of triazolam
	Voriconazole	Ritonavir may decrease the serum concentration of voriconazole

Continued

TABLE 6-6

CONTRAINDICATED DRUG INTERACTIONS FOR ANTIMICROBIAL AGENTS (Continued)

Antimicrobial	Interacting Drug(s)	Toxic Effect
Saquinavir mesylate	Amiodarone, disopyramide, flecainide, procainamide, sotalol	Bradycardia, hypotension, cardiogenic shock, heart block, QT prolongation, hepatotoxicity (amiodarone toxicity)
	Artemether, halofantrine, lumefantrine	QT prolongation, cardiac arrhythmias
	Clarithromycin, erythromycin, gemifloxacin, levofloxacin, moxifloxacin, ofloxacin, pentamidine, quinidine, quinine, rilpivirine, telithromycin, voriconazole	QT prolongation, cardiac arrhythmias
	Chloroquine	QT prolongation, cardiac arrhythmias
	Cisapride, chlorpromazine, dolasetron, droperidol, granisetron, ondansetron	QT prolongation, cardiac arrhythmias
	Citalopram, escitalopram, trazodone	QT prolongation, cardiac arrhythmias
	Clozapine, haloperidol, paliperidone, pimozide, quetiapine, risperidone, thioridazine, ziprasidone	QT prolongation, cardiac arrhythmias
	Darunavir	Saquinavir may decrease the serum concentration of darunavir
	Ergot derivatives (bromocriptine, dihydroergotamine; ergoloid mesylates; ergonovine; ergotamine; methylergonovine)	Vasospasm resulting in peripheral, cardiac, and/or cerebral ischemia; ↑ or ↓ in blood pressure or heart rate; seizures; headache
	Everolimus	CYP3A4 inhibitors (strong) may increase the serum concentration of everolimus
	Fluticasone (inhalation)	CYP3A4 inhibitors (strong) may increase the serum concentration of fluticasone (oral inhalation)
	Lovastatin	Protease inhibitors may increase the serum concentration of lovastatin
	Methadone	QT prolongation, cardiac arrhythmias
	Midazolam	Protease inhibitors may increase the serum concentration of midazolam
	Mifepristone	QT prolongation, cardiac arrhythmias
	Rifampin	Rifampin may enhance the adverse/toxic effect of saquinavir; specifically, the risk for hepatocellular toxicity may be increased; rifampin may decrease the serum concentration of saquinavir

TABLE 6-6

CONTRAINDICATED DRUG INTERACTIONS FOR ANTIMICROBIAL AGENTS (Continued)

Antimicrobial	Interacting Drug(s)	Toxic Effect
	Salmeterol	CYP3A4 inhibitors (strong) may increase the serum concentration of salmeterol
	Sildenafil	Contraindicated if sildenafil being used for pulmonary arterial hypertension; CYP3A4 inhibitors (strong) may increase the serum concentration of sildenafil
	Simvastatin	Protease inhibitors may increase the serum concentration of simvastatin
	St. John's wort	Decreased saquinavir efficacy
	Triazolam	Protease inhibitors may increase the serum concentration of triazolam
Stavudine	Hydroxyurea	Pancreatitis, hepatotoxicity, and/or neuropathy
	Zidovudine	Zidovudine may diminish the therapeutic effect of stavudine
Sulconazole	Pimozide	CYP3A4 inhibitors (weak) may increase the serum concentration of pimozide
Sulfadiazine	Methenamine	Methenamine may enhance the adverse/toxic effect of sulfonamide derivatives; specifically, the combination may result in the formation of an insoluble precipitate in the urine
Sulfamethoxazole and trimethoprim	Methenamine	Methenamine may enhance the adverse/toxic effect of sulfonamide derivatives; specifically, the combination may result in the formation of an insoluble precipitate in the urine
Sulfisoxazole	Methenamine	Methenamine may enhance the adverse/toxic effect of sulfonamide derivatives; specifically, the combination may result in the formation of an insoluble precipitate in the urine
Telaprevir	Atorvastatin	Telaprevir may increase the serum concentration of atorvastatin
	Carbamazepine	Telaprevir may increase the serum concentration of carbamazepine; carbamazepine may decrease the serum concentration of telaprevir
	Cisapride	QT prolongation, cardiac arrhythmias
	Darunavir (when with ritonavir), fosamprenavir (when with ritonavir)	Telaprevir may decrease the serum concentration of darunavir/fosamprenavir; darunavir/fosamprenavir may decrease the serum concentration of telaprevir

Continued

TABLE 6-6

CONTRAINDICATED DRUG INTERACTIONS FOR ANTIMICROBIAL AGENTS (Continued)

Antimicrobial	Interacting Drug(s)	Toxic Effect
	Ergot derivatives (bromocriptine, dihydroergotamine; ergoloid mesylates; ergonovine; ergotamine; methylergonovine)	Vasospasm resulting in peripheral, cardiac, and/or cerebral ischemia; ↑ or ↓ in blood pressure or heart rate; seizures; headache
	Etravirine	Telaprevir may decrease the serum concentration of etravirine
	Everolimus	CYP3A4 inhibitors (strong) may increase the serum concentration of everolimus
	Fluticasone (nasal and inhalation)	CYP3A4 inhibitors (strong) may increase the serum concentration of fluticasone (nasal and oral inhalation)
	Fosphenytoin, phenytoin, phenobarbital	Telaprevir may increase or decrease the serum concentration of fosphenytoin/phenytoin/phenobarbital; fosphenytoin/phenytoin/phenobarbital may decrease the serum concentration of telaprevir
	Halofantrine	CYP3A4 inhibitors (strong) may increase the serum concentration of halofantrine
	Lopinavir with ritonavir	Lopinavir may decrease the serum concentration of telaprevir
	Lovastatin	Protease inhibitors may increase the serum concentration of lovastatin
	Midazolam	Protease inhibitors may increase the serum concentration of midazolam
	Pimozide	QT prolongation, ventricular arrhythmias; hypotension; seizures; anticholinergic and extrapyramidal effects
	Rifabutin	Telaprevir may increase the serum concentration of rifabutin; rifabutin may decrease the serum concentration of telaprevir
	Rifampin	Rifampin may decrease the serum concentration of telaprevir
	Salmeterol	CYP3A4 inhibitors (strong) may increase the serum concentration of salmeterol
	Sildenafil	Contraindicated if sildenafil being used for pulmonary arterial hypertension; CYP3A4 inhibitors (strong) may increase the serum concentration of sildenafil
	Simvastatin	Protease inhibitors may increase the serum concentration of simvastatin
	St. John's wort	Decreased telaprevir efficacy
	Triazolam	Protease inhibitors may increase the serum concentration of triazolam

TABLE 6-6

CONTRAINDICATED DRUG INTERACTIONS FOR ANTIMICROBIAL AGENTS (Continued)

Antimicrobial	Interacting Drug(s)	Toxic Effect
Telbivudine	Interferon alfa-2b, peginterferon alfa-2a, peginterferon alfa-2b	Increased risk for peripheral neuropathy
Telithromycin	Amiodarone, disopyramide, flecainide, procainamide, sotalol	Bradycardia, hypotension, cardiogenic shock, heart block, QT prolongation, hepatotoxicity (amiodarone toxicity)
	Artemether, halofantrine, lumefantrine	QT prolongation, cardiac arrhythmias
	Chloroquine	QT prolongation, cardiac arrhythmias
	Cisapride, chlorpromazine, dolasetron, droperidol, granisetron, ondansetron	QT prolongation, cardiac arrhythmias
	Citalopram, escitalopram, trazodone	QT prolongation, cardiac arrhythmias
	Clarithromycin, erythromycin, gemifloxacin, levofloxacin, moxifloxacin, ofloxacin, pentamidine, quinidine, quinine, rilpivirine, saquinavir, voriconazole	QT prolongation, cardiac arrhythmias
	Clozapine, haloperidol, paliperidone, pimozide, quetiapine, risperidone, thioridazine, ziprasidone	QT prolongation, cardiac arrhythmias
	Everolimus	CYP3A4 inhibitors (strong) may increase the serum concentration of everolimus
	Fluticasone (inhalation)	CYP3A4 inhibitors (strong) may increase the serum concentration of fluticasone (oral inhalation)
	Lovastatin	CYP3A4 inhibitors (strong) may increase the serum concentration of lovastatin
	Methadone	QT prolongation, cardiac arrhythmias
	Mifepristone	QT prolongation, cardiac arrhythmias
	Salmeterol	CYP3A4 inhibitors (strong) may increase the serum concentration of salmeterol
	Sildenafil	Contraindicated if sildenafil being used for pulmonary arterial hypertension; CYP3A4 inhibitors (strong) may increase the serum concentration of sildenafil
	Simvastatin	CYP3A4 inhibitors (strong) may increase the serum concentration of simvastatin

Continued

TABLE 6-6

CONTRAINDICATED DRUG INTERACTIONS FOR ANTIMICROBIAL AGENTS (Continued)

Antimicrobial	Interacting Drug(s)	Toxic Effect
Tenofovir	Adefovir	Adefovir may diminish the therapeutic effect of tenofovir; specifically, adefovir-associated mutations in hepatitis B viral reverse transcriptase may decrease viral susceptibility to tenofovir; tenofovir may increase the serum concentration of adefovir; adefovir may increase the serum concentration of tenofovir
	Didanosine	Tenofovir may diminish the therapeutic effect of didanosine; tenofovir may increase the serum concentration of didanosine
Terbinafine	Pimozide	CYP2D6 inhibitors (strong) may increase the serum concentration of pimozide
	Thioridazine	QT prolongation, cardiac arrhythmias, hypotension, anticholinergic and extrapyramidal effects, agitation
Tetracycline	Pimozide	CYP3A4 inhibitors (moderate) may increase the serum concentration of pimozide
	Isotretinoin and tretinoin	Tetracycline derivatives may enhance the adverse/toxic effect of retinoic acid derivatives; the development of pseudotumor cerebri is of particular concern
Thalidomide	Vaccines (live organisms)	Vaccinial infections
	Abatacept, anakinra, canakinumab, rilonacept	An increased risk for serious infection during concomitant use has been reported
	Azelastine (nasal)	CNS depression
	Clozapine	Agranulocytosis
	Methadone	CNS depression
	Pimecrolimus, tacrolimus	Pimecrolimus/tacrolimus may enhance the adverse/toxic effect of immunosuppressants
Tigecycline	Isotretinoin and tretinoin	Tetracycline derivatives may enhance the adverse/toxic effect of retinoic acid derivatives; the development of pseudotumor cerebri is of particular concern
Tinidazole	Alcohol (ethyl), disulfiram	Abdominal pain, cramps, nausea, vomiting, headache, flushing

TABLE 6-6

CONTRAINDICATED DRUG INTERACTIONS FOR ANTIMICROBIAL AGENTS (Continued)

Antimicrobial	Interacting Drug(s)	Toxic Effect
Tipranavir	Amiodarone	Bradycardia, hypotension, cardiogenic shock, heart block, QT prolongation, hepatotoxicity (amiodarone toxicity)
	Cisapride	QT prolongation, cardiac arrhythmias
	Ergot derivatives (bromocriptine; dihydroergotamine; ergoloid mesylates; ergonovine; ergotamine; methylergonovine)	Vasospasm resulting in peripheral, cardiac, and/or cerebral ischemia; ↑ or ↓ in blood pressure or heart rate; seizures; headache
	Etravirine	Tipranavir may decrease the serum concentration of etravirine
	Flecainide	Cardiac arrhythmias (ventricular tachydysrhythmias, severe bradycardia, AV block)
	Lovastatin	Protease inhibitors may increase the serum concentration of lovastatin
	Midazolam	Protease inhibitors may increase the serum concentration of midazolam
	Pimozide	QT prolongation, ventricular arrhythmias; hypotension; seizures; anticholinergic and extrapyramidal effects
	Quinidine	Tachycardia, hypotension, heart block, ventricular fibrillation, syncope, vascular collapse (quinidine toxicity)
	Rifampin	Rifampin may decrease the serum concentration of tipranavir
	Sildenafil	Contraindicated if sildenafil being used for pulmonary arterial hypertension; CYP3A4 inhibitors (strong) may increase the serum concentration of sildenafil
	Simvastatin	Protease inhibitors may increase the serum concentration of simvastatin
	St. John's wort	Decreased tipranavir efficacy
	Thioridazine	CYP2D6 inhibitors may decrease the metabolism of thioridazine
	Triazolam	Protease inhibitors may increase the serum concentration of triazolam
Valganciclovir	Imipenem	Seizures
Voriconazole	Amiodarone, disopyramide, procainamide, sotalol	Bradycardia, hypotension, cardiogenic shock, heart block, QT prolongation, hepatotoxicity (amiodarone toxicity)
	Artemether, halofantrine, lumefantrine	QT prolongation, cardiac arrhythmias
	Barbiturates (amobarbital, butabarbital, phenobarbital)	Barbiturates may decrease the serum concentration of voriconazole

Continued

TABLE 6-6

CONTRAINDICATED DRUG INTERACTIONS FOR ANTIMICROBIAL AGENTS (Continued)

Antimicrobial	Interacting Drug(s)	Toxic Effect
	Carbamazepine	Carbamazepine may decrease the serum concentration of voriconazole
	Cisapride	QT prolongation, cardiac arrhythmias
	Citalopram, Escitalopram	QT prolongation, cardiac arrhythmias
	Clopidogrel	CYP2C19 inhibitors (moderate) may decrease serum concentrations of the active metabolite(s) of clopidogrel
	Darunavir, lopinavir, ritonavir	May decrease the serum concentration of voriconazole
	Ergot derivatives (bromocriptine, dihydroergotamine; ergoloid mesylates; ergonovine; ergotamine; methylergonovine)	Vasospasm resulting in peripheral, cardiac, and/or cerebral ischemia; ↑ or ↓ in blood pressure or heart rate; seizures; headache
	Everolimus	CYP3A4 inhibitors (strong) may increase the serum concentration of everolimus
	Fluconazole	Fluconazole may increase the serum concentration of voriconazole
	Fluticasone (inhalation)	CYP3A4 inhibitors (strong) may increase the serum concentration of fluticasone (oral inhalation)
	Lovastatin	CYP3A4 inhibitors (strong) may increase the serum concentration of lovastatin
	Mifepristone	QT prolongation, cardiac arrhythmias
	Paliperidone, pimozide, quetiapine, thioridazine, ziprasidone	QT prolongation, cardiac arrhythmias
	Quinidine, quinine, saquinavir, telithromycin	QT prolongation, cardiac arrhythmias
	Rifabutin, rifampin, rifapentine	Rifamycin derivatives may decrease the serum concentration of voriconazole; voriconazole may increase the serum concentration of rifamycin derivatives
	Salmeterol	CYP3A4 inhibitors (strong) may increase the serum concentration of salmeterol
	Sildenafil	Contraindicated if sildenafil being used for pulmonary arterial hypertension; CYP3A4 inhibitors (strong) may increase the serum concentration of sildenafil
	Sirolimus	Decreased metabolism of sirolimus, increases sirolimus drug levels
	Simvastatin	CYP3A4 inhibitors (strong) may increase the serum concentration of simvastatin
	St. John's wort	Decreased voriconazole efficacy
Zidovudine	Clozapine	Agranulocytosis
	Stavudine	Zidovudine may diminish the therapeutic effect of stavudine

REFERENCES

1. Hammett-Stabler CA, Johns T. Laboratory guidelines for monitoring of antimicrobial drugs. *Clin Chem.* 1998;44(5):1129–1140.
2. 2012–2013 Antibiotic Guidelines. Treatment Recommendations for Adult Inpatients. The Johns Hopkins Hospital Antibiotic Management Program. Johns Hopkins Medicine. Published June 2012.
3. Liu C, Bayer A, Cosgrove SE, et al. Clinical practice guidelines by the infectious diseases society of America for the treatment of methicillin-resistant Staphylococcus aureus infections in adults and children. *Clin Infect Dis.* 2011;52(3):e18–e55.
4. Rybak M, Lomaestro B, Rotschafer JC, et al. Therapeutic monitoring of vancomycin in adult patients: A consensus review of the American Society of Health-System Pharmacists, the Infectious Diseases Society of America, and the Society of Infectious Diseases Pharmacists. *Am J Health Syst Pharm.* 2009;66(1):82–98.
5. Pascual A, Calandra T, Bolay S, et al. Voriconazole therapeutic drug monitoring in patients with invasive mycoses improves efficacy and safety outcomes. *Clin Infect Dis.* 2008;46(2):201–211.
6. Pascual A, Csajka C, Buclin T, et al. Challenging recommended oral and intravenous voriconazole doses for improved efficacy and safety: Population pharmacokinetics-based analysis of adult patients with invasive fungal infections. *Clin Infect Dis.* 2012;55(3):381–390.
7. Andes D, Lepak A. Antifungal therapeutic drug monitoring progress: Getting it right the first time. *Clin Infect Dis.* 2012;55(3):391–393.
8. Michael C, Bierbach U, Frenzel K, et al. Voriconazole pharmacokinetics and safety in immunocompromised children compared to adult patients. *Antimicrob Agents Chemother.* 2010;54(8):3225–3232.
9. Neely M, Rushing T, Kovacs A, et al. Voriconazole pharmacokinetics and pharmacodynamics in children. *Clin Infect Dis.* 2010;50(1):27–36.
10. McKamy S, Hernandez E, Jahng M, et al. Incidence and risk factors influencing the development of vancomycin nephrotoxicity in children. *J Pediatr.* 2011;158:422–426.
11. Contopoulos-Ioannidis DG, Giotis ND, Baiatsa DV, et al. Extended-interval aminoglycoside administration for children: A meta-analysis. *Pediatrics.* 2004;114(1):e111–e118.
12. Best EJ, Palasanthiran P, Gazaria M. Extended-interval aminoglycoside in children: More guidance is needed. *Pediatrics.* 2005;115(3):827–828.
13. Jenh AM, Tamma PD, Milstone AM. Extended-interval aminoglycoside dosing in pediatrics. *Pediatr Infect Dis J.* 2011;30(4):338–339.
14. Knoderer CA, Everett JA, Buss WF. Clinical issues surrounding once-daily aminoglycoside dosing in children. *Pharmacotherapy.* 2003;23(1):44–56.
15. Lopez SA, Mulla H, Durward A, et al. Extended-interval gentamicin: Population pharmacokinetics in pediatric critical illness. *Pediatr Crit Care Med.* 2010;11(2):267–274.
16. Prescott Jr WA, Nagel JL. Extended-interval once-daily dosing of aminoglycosides in adult and pediatric patients with cystic fibrosis. *Pharmacotherapy.* 2010;30(1):95–108.
17. McDade EJ, Wagner JL, Moffett BS, et al. Once-daily gentamicin dosing in pediatric patients without cystic fibrosis. *Pharmacotherapy.* 2010; 30(3):248–253.

18. Inparajah M, Wong C, Sibbald C, et al. Once-daily gentamicin dosing in children with febrile neutropenia resulting from antineoplastic therapy. *Pharmacotherapy.* 2010;30(1):43–51.
19. Darko W, Medicis JJ, Smith A, et al. Mississippi mud no more: Cost-effectiveness of pharmacokinetic dosage adjustment of vancomycin to prevent nephrotoxicity. *Pharmacotherapy.* 2003;23(5):643–650.
20. Rodvold KA, Zokufa H, Rotschafer JC. Routine monitoring of serum vancomycin concentrations: Can waiting be justified? *Clin Pharm.* 1987;6:655–658.
21. Edwards DJ. Therapeutic drug monitoring of aminoglycosides and vancomycin: Guidelines and controversies. *J Pharm Pract.* 1991;4:211–214.
22. Lodise TP, Lomaestro B, Graves J, Drusano GL. Larger vancomycin doses (at least 4 grams per day) are associated with an increased incidence of nephrotoxicity. *Antimicrob Agents Chemother.* 2008;52:1330–1336.
23. Hermsen ED, Hanson M, Sankaranarayanan J, et al. Clinical outcomes and nephrotoxicity associated with vancomycin trough concentrations during treatment of deep-seated infections. *Expert Opin Drug Saf.* 2010;9:9–14.
24. Rybak M, Lomaestro B, Rotschafer JC, et al. Therapeutic monitoring of vancomycin in adult patients: A consensus review of the American Society of Health-System Pharmacists, the Infectious Diseases Society of America, and the Society of Infectious Diseases Pharmacists. *Am J Health Syst Pharm.* 2009;66:82–98.
25. Lexi-Comp's Comprehensive Interaction Analysis Program [Intranet database]. Accessed August 20, 2012.
26. Micromedex Healthcare Series [Intranet database]. Version 133. Greenwood Village, CO: Thomson Micromedex; Accessed August 20, 2012.

Chapter 7

Adverse Drug Reactions

Melissa D. Makii, PharmD, BCPS,
and Carlton K. K. Lee, PharmD, MPH

Tables 7-1 through 7-13 list common antimicrobial adverse drug reactions with a 1% or greater incidence rate. These tables are limited to those adverse reactions for which such incidence has been published. Adverse drug reactions specific to a route of administration have been noted (i.e., inhaled, intravenous, oral). The specific incidences of adverse drug reactions in children have been provided in parentheses when available. Drugs are categorized by organ system. For additional information, see the specific drug monograph in Chapter 10 or the package insert.

I. BLOOD

TABLE 7-1

ADVERSE DRUG EFFECTS ON BLOOD

Adverse Effect	Medication
Anemia	Amphotericin B, amphotericin B (liposomal), artemether + lumefantrine, atazanavir, atovaquone, boceprevir, botulinum immunoglobulin IV, caspofungin, cefuroxime, cidofovir, dapsone, daptomycin, delavirdine, doripenem, emtricitabine (children 7%), ertapenem, fidaxomicin, flucytosine, foscarnet, ganciclovir, linezolid, meropenem, micafungin, miconazole, moxifloxacin, pentamidine isethionate, posaconazole, quinupristin + dalfopristin, ribavirin (Inh, PO), rifapentine, rifaximin, telaprevir, thalidomide, tigecycline, tipranavir, trimethoprim, valganciclovir, zalcitabine, zidovudine (neonates 22%, children 4%, adults 1%)
Eosinophilia	Aztreonam (IV) (children 6%, adults <1%), capreomycin, cefaclor, cefdinir, cefepime, ceftibuten, ceftriaxone, cefuroxime, daptomycin, ertapenem, enfuvirtide, ivermectin, norfloxacin, ticarcillin, vancomycin
Increased prothrombin time	Cefepime, clarithromycin, delavirdine, ertapenem, piperacillin + tazobactam
Leukopenia	Amphotericin B (liposomal), caspofungin, ceftriaxone, dapsone, ertapenem, famciclovir, flucytosine, foscarnet, ganciclovir, ivermectin, linezolid, pentamidine isethionate (IV), pyrimethamine, ribavirin (PO), rifabutin, rifapentine, ritonavir, silver sulfadiazine, sulfadiazine, sulfisoxazole, thalidomide, zidovudine
Neutropenia	Atazanavir (children 9%, adults 3%–7%), aztreonam (IV) (children 3%–11%, adults <1%), atovaquone, boceprevir, caspofungin, cephapirin, cidofovir, efavirenz, emtricitabine (children 2%, adults 5%), ertapenem, famciclovir, fidaxomicin, fosamprenavir (children up to 16%, adults 3%), ganciclovir, gemifloxacin, indinavir, lamivudine, linezolid, lopinavir + ritonavir (children 9%), maraviroc, micafungin, miconazole, moxifloxacin, nelfinavir, nevirapine, posaconazole, raltegravir, ribavirin (PO), rifabutin, rifapentine, ritonavir, telbivudine, tenofovir disoproxil fumarate, thalidomide, tipranavir, valganciclovir, vancomycin, zidovudine (children 8%)
Positive Coombs test	Cefepime, ceftaroline, ceftazidime
Thrombocytopenia	Abacavir sulfate, amphotericin B (cholesteryl sulfate), amphotericin B (liposomal), atazanavir, boceprevir, caspofungin, ertapenem, flucytosine, foscarnet, ganciclovir, lamivudine, linezolid, lopinavir + ritonavir (children 4%), micafungin, pentamidine isethionate (IV), posaconazole, pyrimethamine, raltegravir, ribavirin (PO), rifabutin, rifapentine, sulfadiazine, sulfisoxazole, suramin, telaprevir, telavancin, trimetrexate, valacyclovir, valganciclovir, voriconazole, zidovudine
Thrombocytosis	Aztreonam (IV) (children 4%, adults <1%), cefdinir, ceftriaxone, ertapenem, gemifloxacin

Data from Lexi-Comp Online (http://online.lexi.com/crlonline), accessed 27 August 2012; and Micromedex Healthcare Series (http://www.thomsonhc.com), accessed 27 August 2012.

Inh, Inhaled; *IV*, intravenous; *PO*, oral.

II. CARDIOVASCULAR

TABLE 7-2

ADVERSE DRUG EFFECTS ON CARDIOVASCULAR SYSTEM

Adverse Effect	Medication
Arrhythmia	Amphotericin B (liposomal), melarsoprol, micafungin, quinidine
Bradycardia	Micafungin
Chest pain	Amphotericin B (liposomal), daptomycin, ertapenem, foscarnet, imiquimod, immune globulin IV (human), itraconazole, levofloxacin, ofloxacin, pentamidine isethionate (Inh), quinidine, ribavirin (PO), rifaximin, saquinavir, tenofovir disoproxil fumarate, zidovudine
Edema	Amantadine, amphotericin B (liposomal), atazanavir (children 7%), botulinum immune globulin IV, caspofungin, daptomycin, entecavir, ertapenem, foscarnet, gatifloxacin, itraconazole, ivermectin, levofloxacin, micafungin, posaconazole, rifaximin, thalidomide, zidovudine (children <6%)
Flushing	Amphotericin B, amphotericin B (liposomal), cytomegalovirus immune globulin IV, foscarnet, immune globulin IV (human), micafungin, ribavirin (PO)
Hypertension	Amphotericin B, amphotericin B (liposomal), botulinum immune globulin IV, caspofungin (children 9%–10%, adults 5%–6%), daptomycin, ertapenem, foscarnet, itraconazole, lopinavir + ritonavir, maraviroc, melarsoprol, micafungin, piperacillin + tazobactam, posaconazole, Rho(D) immune globulin IV (human), rifapentine, valganciclovir, voriconazole
Hypotension	Amantadine, amphotericin B, amphotericin B (cholesteryl sulfate), amphotericin B (lipid), amphotericin B (liposomal), botulinum immune globulin IV, caspofungin, clindamycin, daptomycin, ertapenem, ethionamide, foscarnet, immune globulin IV (human), ivermectin, micafungin, pentamidine isethionate (IV), posaconazole, quinidine, Rho(D) immune globulin IV (human), rifaximin, thalidomide, vancomycin, voriconazole
QTc prolongation	Posaconazole, quinidine
Tachycardia	Amphotericin B, amphotericin B (cholesteryl sulfate), amphotericin B (liposomal), botulinum immune globulin IV, caspofungin, ertapenem, imipenem + cilastatin (infants 2%, adults <1%), immune globulin IV (human), micafungin, ivermectin, posaconazole, Rho(D) immune globulin IV (human), voriconazole

Data from Lexi-Comp Online (http://online.lexi.com/crlonline), accessed 27 August 2012; and Micromedex Healthcare Series (http://www.thomsonhc.com), accessed 27 August 2012.

Inh, Inhaled; *IV*, intravenous; *PO*, oral.

III. CENTRAL NERVOUS SYSTEM

TABLE 7-3

ADVERSE DRUG EFFECTS ON THE CENTRAL NERVOUS SYSTEM

Adverse Effect	Medication
Agitation/Irritability	Amantadine, boceprevir, botulinum immune globulin IV, ribavirin (PO)
Anxiety	Abacavir sulfate, amantadine, amphotericin B (liposomal), atovaquone, ciprofloxacin, daptomycin, delavirdine, efavirenz, ertapenem, foscarnet, imiquimod, itraconazole, maraviroc, micafungin, ofloxacin, posaconazole, quinidine, ribavirin (PO), rimantadine, ritonavir, saquinavir, tenofovir disoproxil fumarate, thalidomide, zidovudine
Ataxia	Amantadine, foscarnet
Chills/Rigors	Abacavir (children 9%, adults 6%), amphotericin B (conventional), amphotericin B (cholesteryl sulfate), amphotericin B (lipid), amphotericin B (liposomal), artemether + lumefantrine (children 5%, adults 23%), boceprevir, caspofungin, cidofovir, cytomegalovirus immune globulin IV (human), foscarnet, ganciclovir, hepatitis B immune globulin IV (human), iodoquinol, immune globulin IV (human), lamivudine, lopinavir + ritonavir, mefloquine HCl, Rho(D) immune globulin IV (human), ribavirin (PO), terconazole, vancomycin, voriconazole, zanamivir, zidovudine
Confusion	Amantadine, amphotericin B, amphotericin B (liposomal), ertapenem, ethambutol HCL, foscarnet, ganciclovir, griseofulvin, pentamidine isethionate (IV), thalidomide, valganciclovir, zidovudine
Depression	Abacavir sulfate, amantadine, amphotericin B (liposomal), atazanavir, atovaquone, delavirdine, efavirenz, emtricitabine, foscarnet, itraconazole, lamivudine, lopinavir + ritonavir, maraviroc, ribavirin (PO), rifaximin, rilpivirine, saquinavir, tenofovir disoproxil fumarate, valacyclovir, zidovudine
Dizziness	Artemether + lumefantrine (children 4%, adults 39%), abacavir sulfate, albendazole, amantadine, amphotericin B (liposomal), atazanavir, atovaquone, atovaquone + proguanil, boceprevir, caspofungin, cefprozil, ceftibuten, ciprofloxacin, colistimethate sodium, daptomycin, efavirenz (children 16%, adults 2%–28%), emtricitabine, entecavir, ertapenem, foscarnet, fosfomycin, gemifloxacin, griseofulvin, halofantrine, hepatitis B immune globulin IV (human), hydroxychloroquine, imiquimod, indinavir, itraconazole, ivermectin, lamivudine, levofloxacin, lindane, linezolid, maraviroc, mefloquine, metronidazole, micafungin, minocycline, moxifloxacin, nifurtimox, norfloxacin, ofloxacin, pentamidine isethionate, phenazopyridine HCl, posaconazole, praziquantel, Rho(D) immune globulin IV (human), ribavirin (PO), rifapentine, rifaximin, rimantadine, ritonavir, telavancin, telbivudine, telithromycin, tenofovir disoproxil fumarate, thalidomide, thiabendazole, tigecycline, tinidazole, valacyclovir, zanamivir, zidovudine

TABLE 7-3

ADVERSE DRUG EFFECTS ON THE CENTRAL NERVOUS SYSTEM (Continued)

Adverse Effect	Medication
Fatigue	Abacavir, amantadine, artemether + lumefantrine (children 3%, adults 17%), boceprevir, darunavir (children 3%, adults ≤2%), delavirdine, efavirenz, enfuvirtide, entecavir, ertapenem, famciclovir, foscarnet, imiquimod, immune globulin IV (human), indinavir, itraconazole, lamivudine, levofloxacin, mefloquine, micafungin, miconazole, nelfinavir, nevirapine, ofloxacin, pentamidine isethionate (Inh), posaconazole, quinidine, raltegravir, ribavirin (Inh, PO; children 25%), rifaximin, saquinavir, telaprevir, telbivudine, tenofovir disoproxil fumarate, thalidomide, tipranavir, valacyclovir, zanamivir
Fever	Artemether + lumefantrine (children 29%, adults 25%), abacavir sulfate (children 9%, adults 6%), albendazole, amphotericin B, amphotericin B (cholesteryl sulfate), amphotericin B (lipid), atazanavir (children 19%, adults 2%), atovaquone, aztreonam (Inh), caspofungin, cefepime, cidofovir, ciprofloxacin (children 2%), cytomegalovirus immune globulin IV (human), daptomycin, delavirdine, diphtheria antitoxin, efavirenz (children 21%), emtricitabine (children 18%), entecavir, ertapenem, foscarnet, ganciclovir, hepatitis B immune globulin IV (human), imiquimod, immune globulin IV (human), indinavir, iodoquinol, itraconazole, ivermectin, lamivudine (children 25%, adults 10%), linezolid (children ≤14.1%, adults 1.6%), lopinavir + ritonavir, maraviroc, mefloquine HCl, melarsoprol, micafungin, palivizumab, pentamidine isethionate (Inh), piperacillin + tazobactam, posaconazole, praziquantel, rabies immune globulin IV (human), Rho(D) immune globulin IV (human), ribavirin (PO), rifabutin, rifaximin, ritonavir, saquinavir, sulfadiazine, sulfisoxazole, suramin, telbivudine, tenofovir disoproxil fumarate, terbinafine, terconazole, tetanus immune globulin IV (human), thalidomide, tipranavir, trimetrexate, valacyclovir, valganciclovir, vancomycin, voriconazole, zanamivir, zidovudine (children 25%)
Hallucinations	Amantadine, efavirenz, foscarnet, pentamidine isethionate (IV), voriconazole

Continued

TABLE 7-3

ADVERSE DRUG EFFECTS ON THE CENTRAL NERVOUS SYSTEM (Continued)

Adverse Effect	Medication
Headache	Abacavir sulfate, acyclovir, adefovir, albendazole, amantadine, amphotericin B, amphotericin B (cholesteryl sulfate), amphotericin B (lipid), amphotericin B (liposomal), amprenavir, artemether + lumefantrine (children 13%, adults 56%), atazanavir (children 8%, adults 25%), atovaquone, atovaquone + proguanil, azithromycin, boceprevir, caspofungin, cefdinir, cefditoren, cefepime, ceftaroline, ceftibuten, cidofovir, ciprofloxacin, clarithromycin, daptomycin, darunavir (children 9%, adults 3%–6%), delavirdine, didanosine, doripenem, efavirenz (children 11%, adults 2%–8%), emtricitabine, entecavir, ertapenem, ethambutol HCl, famciclovir, fluconazole, fosamprenavir, foscarnet, fosfomycin, furazolidone, gemifloxacin, griseofulvin, halofantrine, hepatitis B immune globulin IV (human), hydroxychloroquine, imiquimod, immune globulin IV (human), indinavir, iodoquinol, itraconazole, lamivudine, levofloxacin, linezolid, lopinavir + ritonavir, mefloquine HCl, melarsoprol, meropenem, metronidazole, micafungin, miconazole, mupirocin, nevirapine, nifurtimox, nitazoxanide, nitrofurantoin, norfloxacin, ofloxacin, penciclovir, pentamidine isethionate (Inh), phenazopyridine, piperacillin + tazobactam, posaconazole, praziquantel, quinidine, quinine, quinupristin + dalfopristin, rabies immune globulin IV (human), raltegravir, retapamulin, Rho(D) immune globulin IV (human), ribavirin (Inh, PO), rifabutin, rifapentine, rifaximin, rilpivirine, rimantadine, ritonavir, saquinavir, stavudine, sulfadiazine, sulfisoxazole, suramin, telavancin, telbivudine, telithromycin, tenofovir disoproxil fumarate, terbinafine, terconazole, thalidomide, thiabendazole, tigecycline, tinidazole, tipranavir, valacyclovir, valganciclovir, varicella zoster immune globulin IV (human), voriconazole, zalcitabine, zanamivir, zidovudine
Increased intracranial pressure	Albendazole
Insomnia	Amantadine, amphotericin B (liposomal), artemether + lumefantrine, atazanavir, atovaquone, boceprevir, caspofungin, ceftaroline, ciprofloxacin, daptomycin, efavirenz, emtricitabine, enfuvirtide, ertapenem, foscarnet, griseofulvin, lamivudine, levofloxacin, linezolid, lopinavir + ritonavir, maraviroc, micafungin, ofloxacin, piperacillin + tazobactam, posaconazole, raltegravir, ribavirin (Inh, PO), rilpivirine, rimantadine, ritonavir, saquinavir, telavancin, telbivudine, tenofovir disoproxil fumarate, thalidomide, valganciclovir, zidovudine
Malaise	Acyclovir, amantadine, amphotericin B, amphotericin B (liposomal), artemether + lumefantrine, foscarnet, hepatitis B immune globulin IV (human), imiquimod, indinavir, itraconazole, lamivudine, praziquantel, pyrazinamide, Rho(D) immune globulin IV (human), ribavirin (PO), thalidomide, tinidazole, zanamivir, zidovudine

TABLE 7-3

ADVERSE DRUG EFFECTS ON THE CENTRAL NERVOUS SYSTEM (Continued)

Adverse Effect	Medication
Neuropathy	Amphotericin B, atazanavir, didanosine, emtricitabine, etravirine, famciclovir, foscarnet, ganciclovir, isoniazid, iodoquinol, lamivudine, maraviroc, melarsoprol, ritonavir, saquinavir, stavudine, suramin, telavancin, tenofovir disoproxil fumarate, thalidomide, valganciclovir, zalcitabine
Neurotoxicity	Amikacin, gentamicin, kanamycin, melarsoprol (encephalopathy), streptomycin sulfate, tobramycin
Pain, unspecified	Amphotericin B, amphotericin B (lipid), amphotericin B (liposomal), atovaquone, ciclopirox, cidofovir, efavirenz (children 14%, adults 1%–13%), foscarnet, fosfomycin, imiquimod, itraconazole, kunecatechins, levofloxacin, maraviroc, meropenem, miconazole, piperacillin, piperacillin + tazobactam, podofilox, polymyxin B sulfate + neomycin sulfate + hydrocortisone, posaconazole, quinupristin + dalfopristin, ribavirin (PO), rifapentine, saquinavir, tenofovir disoproxil fumarate, terconazole, tetanus immune globulin IV (human), thalidomide, ticarcillin, varicella zoster immune globulin IV (human)
Seizure	Foscarnet, imipenem + cilastatin (infants 6%, adults <1%), lindane, linezolid, melarsoprol, valganciclovir, zalcitabine, zidovudine
Somnolence	Amantadine, amphotericin B (liposomal), ciprofloxacin, efavirenz, foscarnet, indinavir, ofloxacin, posaconazole, Rho(D) immune globulin IV (human), ritonavir, thalidomide
Weakness	Adefovir, amphotericin B (liposomal), artemether + lumefantrine (children 5%, adults 38%), atovaquone, atovaquone + proguanil, boceprevir, cidofovir, daptomycin, darunavir, emtricitabine, ertapenem, foscarnet, fosfomycin, indinavir, iodoquinol, isoniazid, itraconazole, lopinavir + ritonavir, posaconazole, quinidine, ribavirin (PO), rimantadine, ritonavir, saquinavir, tenofovir disoproxil fumarate, thalidomide, tigecycline, tinidazole, zidovudine

Data from Lexi-Comp Online (http://online.lexi.com/crlonline), accessed 27 August 2012; and Micromedex Healthcare Series (http://www.thomsonhc.com), accessed 27 August 2012.

Inh, Inhaled; *IV,* intravenous; *PO,* oral.

7

IV. SKIN

TABLE 7-4

SKIN ADVERSE DRUG EFFECTS

Adverse Effect	Medication
Alopecia	Albendazole, amphotericin B (liposomal), boceprevir, cidofovir, hydroxychloroquine, imiquimod, ribavirin (PO), selenium sulfide
Angioedema	Hepatitis B immune globulin IV (human), zidovudine
Dermatitis	Amoxicillin, ampicillin, botulinum immune globulin IV, butenafine, gatifloxacin, ketoconazole, lindane, maraviroc, neomycin sulfate + polymyxin B sulfate ± bacitracin, nystatin, penciclovir, polymyxin B sulfate + neomycin sulfate + hydrocortisone, pyrethrins, retapamulin, ribavirin (PO), sertaconazole, thalidomide, undecylenic acid
Erythema multiforme	Efavirenz, kunecatechins, silver sulfadiazine
Hives/Rash	Abacavir sulfate (children 7%, adults 5%–6%), acyclovir, adefovir, amoxicillin, amoxicillin + clavulanic acid, amphotericin B (cholesteryl sulfate), amphotericin B (lipid), amphotericin B (liposomal), ampicillin, ampicillin + sulbactam, amprenavir, artemether + lumefantrine, atazanavir (children 14%, adults 20%–21%), atovaquone, azithromycin, aztreonam, bacitracin ± polymyxin B sulfate, benzyl alcohol, boceprevir, botulinum immune globulin IV, caspofungin, cefaclor, cefdinir, cefepime, cefotaxime, cefpodoxime proxetil, cefprozil, ceftaroline, ceftriaxone, cefuroxime, cidofovir, ciprofloxacin (children 2%, adults 1%), clarithromycin (children 3%), clindamycin, clofazimine, daptomycin, darunavir (children 5%–10%, adults 6%–7%), delavirdine, didanosine, doripenem, etravirine, efavirenz (children ≤46%, adults 5%–26%), emtricitabine, ertapenem, etravirine (children 15%, adults 10%), famciclovir, fluconazole, fosamprenavir, foscarnet, fosfomycin, ganciclovir, gemifloxacin, griseofulvin, hepatitis B immune globulin IV (human), hydroxychloroquine, immune globulin IV (human), imipenem + cilastatin (children 2%, adults ≤1%), imiquimod, indinavir, iodoquinol, itraconazole, kunecatechins, lamivudine, levofloxacin, linezolid, lopinavir + ritonavir (children 12%, adults ≤5%), maraviroc, mefloquine HCl, melarsoprol, meropenem, methenamine mandelate, micafungin, miconazole, mupirocin, nafcillin, nelfinavir, neomycin sulfate + polymyxin B sulfate ± bacitracin, nevirapine, nifurtimox, ofloxacin, palivizumab, pentamidine, permethrin, piperacillin, piperacillin + tazobactam, polymyxin B sulfate + neomycin sulfate + hydrocortisone, posaconazole, quinidine, quinupristin + dalfopristin, Rho(D) immune globulin IV (human), ribavirin (PO), rifabutin, rifampin, rifapentine, rifaximin, rilpivirine, ritonavir, saquinavir, silver sulfadiazine, spinosad, stavudine, sulfadiazine, sulfamethoxazole + trimethoprim, sulfisoxazole, suramin, telaprevir, telavancin, telbivudine, tenofovir disoproxil fumarate, terbinafine, thalidomide, thiabendazole, tigecycline, trimethoprim, trimetrexate, undecylenic acid, valacyclovir, vancomycin, varicella zoster immune globulin IV (human), voriconazole, zidovudine (children 12%)

TABLE 7-4

SKIN ADVERSE DRUG EFFECTS (Continued)

Adverse Effect	Medication
Itching/Pruritus	Acyclovir, adefovir, amoxicillin + clavulanate, amphotericin B (liposomal), artemether + lumefantrine, atovaquone, atovaquone + proguanil (children 6%), azithromycin, bacitracin ± polymyxin B sulfate, benzyl alcohol, butenafine, caspofungin, cefepime, cefotaxime, ceftaroline, ciclopirox, clofazimine, daptomycin, didanosine, doripenem, econazole, efavirenz, ertapenem, famciclovir, fosamprenavir, foscarnet, ganciclovir, halofantrine, hydroxychloroquine, imiquimod, indinavir, itraconazole, ivermectin, ketoconazole, kunecatechins, levofloxacin, maraviroc, meropenem, micafungin, miconazole, mupirocin, naftifine, ofloxacin, oxiconazole, permethrin, piperacillin + tazobactam, podofilox, polymyxin B sulfate + neomycin sulfate + hydrocortisone, posaconazole, pyrethrins + piperonyl butoxide, quinupristin + dalfopristin, retapamulin, ribavirin (PO), rifapentine, rifaximin, saquinavir, silver sulfadiazine, sulconazole, sulfacetamide sodium, sulfadiazine, sulfisoxazole, telaprevir, telbivudine, telavancin, tenofovir disoproxil fumarate, terbinafine, thalidomide, tioconazole, tolnaftate, trimetrexate, varicella zoster immune globulin IV (human)
Stevens–Johnson syndrome	Amprenavir, clindamycin, nystatin, sulfacetamide, sulfadiazine, sulfisoxazole, sulfamethoxazole + trimethoprim, zidovudine
Toxic epidermal necrolysis syndrome	Zidovudine
Phlebitis/ Thrombophlebitis and/or injection site reactions	Acyclovir, amphotericin B, amphotericin B (liposomal), ampicillin + sulbactam, azithromycin, aztreonam (IV) (children 12%, adults 2%), botulinum immune globulin IV, caspofungin, cefepime, cefotaxime, ceftaroline, ceftazidime, cefuroxime, cephapirin, ciprofloxacin, clindamycin, daptomycin, doripenem, enfuvirtide, ertapenem, erythromycin, imipenem + cilastatin, meropenem, micafungin, piperacillin, piperacillin + tazobactam, quinupristin + dalfopristin, ribavirin (IV; children 44%), ticarcillin, tigecycline, vancomycin

Data from Lexi-Comp Online (http://online.lexi.com/crlonline), accessed 27 August 2012; and Micromedex Healthcare Series (http://www.thomsonhc.com), accessed 27 August 2012.

IV, Intravenous; *PO,* oral.

V. GASTROINTESTINAL

TABLE 7-5

ADVERSE DRUG EFFECTS ON THE GASTROINTESTINAL SYSTEM

Adverse Effect	Medication
Abdominal pain	Adefovir, albendazole, amoxicillin + clavulanic acid, amphotericin B, amphotericin B (cholesteryl sulfate), amphotericin B (lipid), amphotericin B (liposomal), ampicillin, artemether + lumefantrine (children 8%, adults 17%), atazanavir, atovaquone, atovaquone + proguanil, azithromycin (children 2%–4%, adults 1.9%–14%), caspofungin, cefdinir, cefditoren, cefixime, cefpodoxime proxetil, cefprozil, ceftibuten, ciprofloxacin (children 3%, adults <1%), clarithromycin (children 3%, adults 2%), clindamycin, clofazimine, cloxacillin, daptomycin, darunavir (children 10%, adults 5%–6%), delavirdine, dicloxacillin sodium, didanosine, efavirenz, emtricitabine, enfuvirtide, ertapenem, erythromycin, ethambutol HCl, famciclovir, fidaxomicin, fluconazole, flucytosine, fosamprenavir, foscarnet, fosfomycin, furazolidone, gemifloxacin, griseofulvin, halofantrine, hydroxychloroquine, indinavir, iodoquinol, isoniazid, itraconazole, ketoconazole, lamivudine, levofloxacin, lopinavir + ritonavir, mebendazole, mefloquine HCl, micafungin, miconazole, nevirapine, nitazoxanide, norfloxacin, nystatin, ofloxacin, oseltamivir phosphate, para-aminosalicylic acid, paromomycin sulfate, phenazopyridine HCl, piperacillin + tazobactam, posaconazole, praziquantel, primaquine phosphate, pyrantel pamoate, quinidine, Rho(D) immune globulin IV (human), ribavirin (PO), rifabutin, rifampin, rifaximin, rimantadine, ritonavir, saquinavir, telavancin, telbivudine, tenofovir disoproxil fumarate, terbinafine, terconazole, tigecycline, tinidazole, tipranavir, valacyclovir, valganciclovir, zalcitabine, zanamivir
Amylase increased	Abacavir, atazanavir, atovaquone, darunavir, delavirdine, didanosine, efavirenz, emtricitabine (children 9%, adults 2%–5%), entecavir, etravirine, indinavir, linezolid, lopinavir + ritonavir, raltegravir, saquinavir, stavudine, tenofovir disoproxil fumarate, tigecycline, tipranavir
Lipase increased	Atazanavir, darunavir, emtricitabine, entecavir, fosamprenavir, linezolid, lopinavir + ritonavir, raltegravir, stavudine, telbivudine
Anorexia/Loss of appetite	Amantadine, amphotericin B, amphotericin B (liposomal), artemether + lumefantrine (children 13%, adults 40%), atovaquone, atovaquone + proguanil, azithromycin, boceprevir, caspofungin, cidofovir, darunavir, efavirenz, enfuvirtide, ethambutol HCl, ethionamide, flucytosine, foscarnet, ganciclovir, hydroxychloroquine, imiquimod, indinavir, isoniazid, lamivudine, lopinavir + ritonavir, mefloquine HCl, metronidazole, micafungin, nifurtimox, pentamidine isethionate, posaconazole, pyrantel pamoate, pyrazinamide, pyrimethamine, quinidine, ribavirin (Inh, PO), rifabutin, rifampin, rifapentine, rimantadine, ritonavir, sulfadiazine, sulfamethoxazole + trimethoprim, sulfisoxazole, tenofovir disoproxil fumarate, terbinafine, thalidomide, thiabendazole, tinidazole, tipranavir, zanamivir, zidovudine

TABLE 7-5

ADVERSE DRUG EFFECTS ON THE GASTROINTESTINAL SYSTEM (Continued)

Adverse Effect	Medication
Colitis/ Pseudomembranous enterocolitis	Cefotaxime, clindamycin, rifampin
Constipation	Amantadine, amphotericin B (liposomal), atovaquone, ceftaroline, daptomycin, ertapenem, foscarnet, itraconazole, levofloxacin, linezolid, maraviroc, meropenem, micafungin, piperacillin + tazobactam, posaconazole, ribavirin (PO), rifaximin, saquinavir, thalidomide, tinidazole, zidovudine
Diarrhea	Abacavir sulfate, acyclovir, adefovir, amantadine, amoxicillin + clavulanic acid, amphotericin B, amphotericin B (cholesteryl sulfate), amphotericin B (lipid), amphotericin B (liposomal), ampicillin, ampicillin + sulbactam, amprenavir, anidulafungin, artemether + lumefantrine (children 8%, adults 7%), atazanavir (children 8%, adults 1%–3%), atovaquone, atovaquone + proguanil (children 6%, adults 8%), azithromycin (children 7%–10%, adults 4.3%–12%), aztreonam, boceprevir, botulinum immune globulin IV, caspofungin, cefaclor, cefadroxil, cefazolin, cefdinir, cefditoren, cefepime, cefixime, cefotaxime, cefotetan, cefoxitin, cefpodoxime proxetil, cefprozil, ceftaroline, ceftazidime, ceftibuten, ceftriaxone, cefuroxime, cephalexin, chloroquine phosphate, cidofovir, ciprofloxacin (children 5%, adults 2%), clarithromycin (children 6%, adults 3%–6%), clindamycin, clofazimine, cloxacillin, daptomycin, darunavir (children 11%–19%, adults 9%–14%), delavirdine, dicloxacillin sodium, didanosine, doripenem, doxycycline, efavirenz (children ≤39%, adults 3%–14%), emtricitabine (children 20%, adults 9%–23%), enfuvirtide, ertapenem, ethionamide, etravirine (children and adolescents ≥2%), famciclovir, fluconazole, flucytosine, fosamprenavir, foscarnet, fosfomycin, furazolidone, ganciclovir, gemifloxacin, griseofulvin, halofantrine, hydroxychloroquine, imipenem + cilastatin (children 3%–4%, adults 1%–2%), imiquimod, immune globulin IV (human), indinavir, iodoquinol, itraconazole, ivermectin, lamivudine (children 8%, adults 18%), levofloxacin, linezolid, lopinavir + ritonavir, mebendazole, mefloquine HCl, meropenem, metronidazole, micafungin, miconazole, minocycline, moxifloxacin, nelfinavir (children 39%–47%, adults 14%–20%), neomycin sulfate, nevirapine, nitazoxanide, nystatin, ofloxacin, oseltamivir, oxacillin, palivizumab, para-aminosalicylic acid, paromomycin sulfate, penicillin V potassium, pentamidine isethionate (Inh), piperacillin, piperacillin + tazobactam, posaconazole, pyrantel pamoate, quinidine, quinine, quinupristin + dalfopristin, retapamulin, ribavirin (PO), rifabutin, rifampin, rifapentine, ritonavir, saquinavir, stavudine, sulfadiazine, sulfisoxazole, telaprevir, telavancin, telbivudine, telithromycin, tenofovir disoproxil fumarate, terbinafine, tetracycline HCl, thalidomide, thiabendazole, tipranavir (children 4%), valacyclovir (children 5%, adults <1%), valganciclovir, zalcitabine, zanamivir, zidovudine (children 8%)

Continued

TABLE 7-5

ADVERSE DRUG EFFECTS ON THE GASTROINTESTINAL SYSTEM (Continued)

Adverse Effect	Medication
Dyspepsia	Adefovir, amphotericin B, amphotericin B (liposomal), atovaquone, cefditoren, cefixime, ceftibuten, ciprofloxacin (children 3%), clarithromycin, daptomycin, darunavir, efavirenz, emtricitabine, ertapenem, foscarnet, fosfomycin, imiquimod, indinavir, itraconazole, lamivudine, levofloxacin, lopinavir + ritonavir, methenamine mandelate, micafungin, piperacillin + tazobactam, posaconazole, ribavirin (PO), rifapentine, ritonavir, saquinavir, telbivudine, tenofovir disoproxil fumarate, terbinafine, tigecycline, tinidazole, zidovudine
Flatulence	Adefovir, azithromycin, cefixime, famciclovir, foscarnet, lopinavir + ritonavir, nelfinavir, ofloxacin
Nausea	Abacavir sulfate (children 9%, adults 7%–19%), acyclovir, adefovir, albendazole, amantadine, amoxicillin + clavulanic acid, amphotericin B, amphotericin B (cholesteryl sulfate), amphotericin B (lipid), amphotericin B (liposomal), amprenavir, artemether + lumefantrine (children 5%, adults 26%), atazanavir, atovaquone, atovaquone + proguanil, azithromycin (children 4%, adults 3%–14%), aztreonam, boceprevir, caspofungin, cefdinir, cefditoren, cefepime, cefixime, cefotaxime, cefpodoxime proxetil, cefprozil, ceftaroline, ceftibuten, cefuroxime, chloroquine phosphate, cidofovir, ciprofloxacin, clarithromycin, clindamycin, clofazimine, clotrimazole, cytomegalovirus immune globulin IV (human), daptomycin, darunavir (children 11%–19%, adults 8%–14%), darunavir, delavirdine, dicloxacillin sodium, didanosine, doripenem, efavirenz (children 12%, adults 2%–12%), emtricitabine, enfuvirtide, entecavir, ertapenem, erythromycin, ethambutol HCl, ethionamide, etravirine, famciclovir, fidaxomicin, fluconazole, flucytosine, fosamprenavir, foscarnet, fosfomycin, furazolidone, gemifloxacin, griseofulvin, halofantrine, hepatitis B immune globulin IV (human), hydroxychloroquine, imipenem + cilastatin, imiquimod, immune globulin IV (human), indinavir, iodoquinol, isoniazid, itraconazole, ivermectin, ketoconazole, lamivudine, levofloxacin, linezolid, lopinavir + ritonavir, mefloquine HCl, meropenem, methenamine mandelate, metronidazole, micafungin, miconazole, minocycline, moxifloxacin, mupirocin, nelfinavir, neomycin sulfate, nevirapine, nifurtimox, nitazoxanide, nitrofurantoin, norfloxacin, nystatin, ofloxacin, oseltamivir phosphate, oxacillin, para-aminosalicylic acid, paromomycin sulfate, penicillin V potassium, pentamidine isethionate, piperacillin + tazobactam, podofilox, posaconazole, praziquantel, primaquine phosphate, pyrantel pamoate, pyrazinamide, quinidine, quinine, quinupristin + dalfopristin, raltegravir, retapamulin, Rho(D) immune globulin IV (human), ribavirin (Inh, PO), rifabutin, rifampin, rifapentine, rifaximin, rimantadine, ritonavir, saquinavir, stavudine, sulfadiazine, sulfamethoxazole + trimethoprim, sulfisoxazole, suramin, telaprevir, telavancin, telbivudine, telithromycin, tenofovir disoproxil fumarate, terbinafine, tetracycline HCl, thalidomide, thiabendazole, tinidazole, tipranavir, trimetrexate, valacyclovir, valganciclovir, vancomycin, varicella zoster immune globulin IV (human), voriconazole, zanamivir, zidovudine (children 8%, adults 51%)

TABLE 7-5

ADVERSE DRUG EFFECTS ON THE GASTROINTESTINAL SYSTEM (Continued)

Adverse Effect	Medication
Pancreatitis	Didanosine, enfuvirtide, foscarnet, lamivudine, linezolid, rifampin, stibogluconate
Taste disturbance	Atovaquone, boceprevir, clarithromycin, foscarnet, gatifloxacin, indinavir, linezolid, lopinavir + ritonavir (children 22%, adults <2%), miconazole, ofloxacin, pentamidine isethionate, ribavirin (PO), rifabutin, ritonavir, saquinavir, telaprevir, telavancin, terbinafine, tinidazole
Vomiting	Abacavir sulfate (children 9%), acyclovir, adefovir, albendazole, amoxicillin + clavulanic acid, amphotericin B, amphotericin B (lipid), amphotericin B (liposomal), ampicillin, amprenavir, artemether + lumefantrine (children 18%, adults 17%), atazanavir (children 8%, adults 3%–4%), atovaquone, atovaquone + proguanil (children 10%–13%, adults 12%), azithromycin (children 11%–14%, adults ≤13%), aztreonam, bacitracin ± polymyxin B sulfate, boceprevir, botulinum immune globulin IV, caspofungin, cefdinir, cefditoren, cefepime, cefotaxime, cefpodoxime proxetil, cefprozil, ceftaroline, ceftibuten (children 2%, adults ≤13%), cefuroxime, cidofovir, ciprofloxacin (children 5%, adults 1%), clarithromycin (children 6%), clindamycin, clofazimine, clotrimazole, cloxacillin, cytomegalovirus immune globulin IV (human), daptomycin, darunavir (children 13%–14%, adults 2%–5%), delavirdine, efavirenz (children 12%, adults 3%–6%), emtricitabine (children 23%, adults 9%), ertapenem, erythromycin, ethambutol HCl, ethionamide, famciclovir, fluconazole, flucytosine, fosamprenavir (children 20%–60%, adults 2%–16%), foscarnet, furazolidone, ganciclovir, griseofulvin, halofantrine, hepatitis B immune globulin IV (human), hydroxychloroquine, imipenem + cilastatin, imiquimod, immune globulin IV (human), indinavir, iodoquinol, isoniazid, itraconazole, ketoconazole, lamivudine, levofloxacin, linezolid, lopinavir + ritonavir (children 21%, adults 2%–6%), mefloquine HCl, meropenem, metronidazole, micafungin, miconazole, neomycin sulfate, nifurtimox, nitazoxanide, nystatin, ofloxacin, oseltamivir phosphate, palivizumab, para-aminosalicylic acid, paromomycin sulfate, penicillin V potassium, pentamidine isethionate, piperacillin + tazobactam, podofilox, posaconazole, praziquantel, primaquine phosphate, pyrantel pamoate, pyrazinamide, pyrimethamine, quinidine, quinine, quinupristin + dalfopristin, ribavirin (PO), rifabutin, rifampin, rifapentine, rimantadine, ritonavir, saquinavir, stavudine, sulfadiazine, sulfamethoxazole + trimethoprim, sulfisoxazole, suramin, telaprevir, telavancin, tenofovir disoproxil fumarate, terbinafine, thiabendazole, tinidazole, tipranavir, trimetrexate, valacyclovir, valganciclovir, vancomycin, voriconazole, zalcitabine, zanamivir, zidovudine (children 8%, adults 17%)
Xerostomia	Amantadine, boceprevir, enfuvirtide, foscarnet, miconazole

Data from Lexi-Comp Online (http://online.lexi.com/crlonline), accessed 27 August 2012; and Micromedex Healthcare Series (http://www.thomsonhc.com), accessed 27 August 2012.

Inh, Inhaled; *IV,* intravenous; *PO,* oral.

VI. ENDOCRINE/METABOLIC

TABLE 7-6

ADVERSE DRUG EFFECTS ON THE ENDOCRINE/METABOLIC SYSTEM

Adverse Effect	Medication
Hyperglycemia	Amphotericin B (liposomal), amprenavir, atazanavir, atovaquone, caspofungin, cefditoren, clofazimine, darunavir, efavirenz, entecavir, ertapenem, etravirine, fosamprenavir, imiquimod, itraconazole, lopinavir + ritonavir, micafungin, posaconazole, quinupristin + dalfopristin, raltegravir, ritonavir, saquinavir, tenofovir disoproxil fumarate, zalcitabine
Hypoglycemia	Atovaquone, meropenem, micafungin, moxifloxacin, pentamidine isethionate (IV), saquinavir, zalcitabine
Hypocalcemia	Amphotericin B (liposomal), foscarnet, posaconazole, thalidomide
Hyperkalemia	Amphotericin B (liposomal), daptomycin, micafungin, rifaximin, saquinavir
Hypokalemia	Amphotericin B, amphotericin B (cholesteryl sulfate), amphotericin B (lipid), amphotericin B (liposomal), anidulafungin, caspofungin, ceftaroline, daptomycin, ertapenem, foscarnet, itraconazole, micafungin, posaconazole, telavancin, voriconazole
Hypomagnesemia	Amphotericin B, amphotericin B (cholesteryl sulfate), amphotericin B (liposomal), caspofungin, foscarnet, micafungin, posaconazole
Hypernatremia	Amphotericin B (liposomal), micafungin
Hyponatremia	Amphotericin B (liposomal), atovaquone, botulinum immune globulin IV, foscarnet, rifaximin, zalcitabine
Hyperphosphatemia	Daptomycin
Hypophosphatemia	Adefovir, cefepime, foscarnet
Hyperuricemia	Didanosine, ethambutol HCl, lopinavir/ritonavir, ribavirin (PO), rifapentine, ritonavir, telaprevir
Increased HDL	Efavirenz
Hypercholesterolemia	Amprenavir, atazanavir, darunavir, efavirenz, etravirine, lopinavir + ritonavir, rilpivirine, ritonavir, tipranavir
Hypertriglyceridemia	Abacavir sulfate, amprenavir, atazanavir, darunavir, efavirenz, emtricitabine, etravirine, fosamprenavir, itraconazole, lopinavir + ritonavir, rilpivirine, ritonavir, tenofovir disoproxil fumarate, tipranavir
Lipodystrophy	Maraviroc, saquinavir

HDL, High-density lipoprotein; *IV*, intravenous; *PO*, oral.

VII. RENAL/GENITOURINARY

TABLE 7-7

ADVERSE DRUG EFFECTS ON THE RENAL/GENITOURINARY SYSTEM

Adverse Effect	Medication
Azotemia	Amphotericin B, pentamidine isethionate (IV)
Hematuria	Adefovir, amphotericin B (liposomal), caspofungin, cefdinir, cefditoren, emtricitabine, entecavir, rifapentine, tenofovir disoproxil fumarate, thalidomide
Interstitial nephritis	Silver sulfadiazine, sulfadiazine
Nephrotoxicity/Renal failure	Acyclovir, adefovir, amikacin, amphotericin B, amphotericin B (cholesteryl sulfate), amphotericin B (lipid), amphotericin B (liposomal), aztreonam (children 6%), capreomycin, caspofungin, cidofovir, colistimethate sodium, daptomycin, doripenem, entecavir, etravirine, foscarnet, ganciclovir, gentamicin, kanamycin, melarsoprol, neomycin sulfate + polymyxin B sulfate ± bacitracin, pentamidine isethionate (IV), Rho(D) immune globulin IV (human), rilpivirine, streptomycin sulfate, sulfadiazine, suramin, telavancin, tenofovir disoproxil fumarate, tobramycin, valganciclovir, voriconazole
Renal tubular acidosis	Amphotericin B
Vaginitis	Amoxicillin + clavulanic acid, azithromycin, cefaclor, cefdinir, cefprozil, cefuroxime, ertapenem, fosfomycin, levofloxacin, metronidazole, ofloxacin, terconazole, tinidazole, tioconazole

Data from Lexi-Comp Online (http://online.lexi.com/crlonline), accessed 27 August 2012.
IV, Intravenous.

7

VIII. RESPIRATORY

TABLE 7-8

ADVERSE DRUG EFFECTS ON THE RESPIRATORY SYSTEM

Adverse Effect	Medication
Bronchospasm	Atovaquone, aztreonam (Inh), foscarnet, maraviroc
Cough	Adefovir, amphotericin B (liposomal), artemether + lumefantrine (children 23%, adults 6%), atazanavir (children 21%), atovaquone + proguanil, aztreonam (Inh), botulinum immune globulin IV, caspofungin, cidofovir, daptomycin, efavirenz, emtricitabine (children 28%, adults 14%), enfuvirtide, ertapenem, foscarnet, imiquimod, immune globulin IV (human), indinavir, itraconazole, lamivudine (children 15%, adults 18%), maraviroc, micafungin, miconazole, pentamidine isethionate (Inh), posaconazole, ribavirin (PO), telbivudine, terbinafine, tipranavir (children 6%), valganciclovir (children >10%), zanamivir, zidovudine (children 15%)
Dyspnea	Amphotericin B (cholesteryl sulfate), amphotericin B (lipid), amphotericin B (liposomal), atovaquone, boceprevir, botulinum immune globulin IV, caspofungin, cidofovir, daptomycin, ertapenem, foscarnet, immune globulin IV (human), itraconazole, levofloxacin, micafungin, pentamidine isethionate (Inh), piperacillin + tazobactam, posaconazole, ribavirin (PO), rifaximin, telavancin, thalidomide, tipranavir
Pharyngitis	Artemether + lumefantrine, doxycycline, emtricitabine, ertapenem (infants, children, adolescents <2%), foscarnet, fosfomycin, imiquimod, itraconazole, levofloxacin, meropenem, ofloxacin, pentamidine isethionate (Inh), piperacillin + tazobactam, posaconazole, ribavirin (PO), rifaximin, tenofovir disoproxil fumarate, terbinafine, thalidomide, valacyclovir
Pulmonary fibrosis	Nitrofurantoin (long-term use)
Rhinitis	Adefovir, artemether + lumefantrine, atazanavir (children 6%), atovaquone, aztreonam (Inh), botulinum immune globulin IV, ciprofloxacin, emtricitabine (children 20%, adults 12%–18%), ertapenem (infants, children, adolescents <2%), fosfomycin, gatifloxacin, imiquimod, immune globulin IV, itraconazole, ribavirin (PO), valacyclovir, zidovudine (children 8%)
Sinusitis	Atovaquone, emtricitabine, enfuvirtide, foscarnet, itraconazole, maraviroc, pentamidine isethionate (Inh), ribavirin (PO), saquinavir, tenofovir disoproxil fumarate, thalidomide, zanamivir
Stridor	Botulinum immune globulin IV, foscarnet
Tachypnea	Amphotericin B, botulinum immune globulin IV
Upper respiratory infection	Abacavir, emtricitabine, entecavir, ertapenem (infants, children, adolescents <2%), imiquimod, itraconazole, maraviroc, miconazole, pentamidine isethionate (Inh), posaconazole, tenofovir disoproxil fumarate, terbinafine, tinidazole, valganciclovir (children >10%)

Data from Lexi-Comp Online (http://online.lexi.com/crlonline), accessed 27 August 2012; and Micromedex Healthcare Series (http://www.thomsonhc.com), accessed 27 August 2012.

Inh, Inhaled; *IV*, intravenous; *PO*, oral.

IX. HEPATIC

TABLE 7-9

ADVERSE DRUG EFFECTS ON THE HEPATIC SYSTEM

Adverse Effect	Medication
Liver enzyme elevation (see medication package insert for specific enzyme affected)	Abacavir sulfate (AST), acyclovir, adefovir (ALT), albendazole, amphotericin B (cholesteryl sulfate), amphotericin B (liposomal), anidulafungin, atazanavir, artemether + lumefantrine (AST), atovaquone + proguanil, azithromycin, aztreonam IV (children 4%–6%), caspofungin, cefaclor, cefdinir (ALT), cefepime, ceftaroline, ceftriaxone, cefotetan, cefprozil, ceftibuten (ALT), cefuroxime, ciprofloxacin, clotrimazole, daptomycin, darunavir, delavirdine, didanosine, doripenem, entecavir (ALT), isoniazid, efavirenz, emtricitabine, enfuvirtide, ertapenem, etravirine, famciclovir, fosamprenavir, foscarnet, gemifloxacin, indinavir, itraconazole, ivermectin, lopinavir + ritonavir, lamivudine, linezolid, maraviroc, micafungin, nevirapine, norfloxacin, palivizumab (AST), pentamidine isethionate (IV), posaconazole, raltegravir, ribavirin (PO), rilpivirine, rifabutin, rifampin, rifapentine, ritonavir (AST), saquinavir, stavudine, telbivudine, tenofovir disoproxil fumarate, terbinafine, thalidomide, tigecycline, tipranavir, trimetrexate, valacyclovir, voriconazole, zidovudine
Alkaline phosphatase elevation	Amphotericin B (cholesteryl sulfate), amphotericin B (liposomal), caspofungin, cefdinir, cefuroxime, daptomycin, darunavir, didanosine, ertapenem, foscarnet, linezolid, micafungin, posaconazole, raltegravir, tigecycline, valacyclovir, voriconazole
GGT elevation	Efavirenz, gemifloxacin, lopinavir + ritonavir, miconazole, quinupristin + dalfopristin, stavudine, tipranavir
Hepatitis	Adefovir, ethionamide, isoniazid, silver sulfadiazine, sulfadiazine, sulfisoxazole, sulfamethoxazole + trimethoprim, zidovudine
Hepatic failure/hepatic toxicity	Abacavir sulfate, melarsoprol, nevirapine, para-aminosalicylic acid, rifampin, stibogluconate
Hyperbilirubinemia/Jaundice	Amphotericin B (cholesteryl sulfate), amphotericin B (lipid), amphotericin B (liposomal), atazanavir [children 13%, adults 5%–9% (jaundice)], [children 58% (hyperbilirubinemia)], caspofungin, ceftibuten, delavirdine, emtricitabine, entecavir, ertapenem, erythromycin, ethionamide, famciclovir, flucytosine, indinavir, linezolid, lopinavir + ritonavir, maraviroc, micafungin, posaconazole, quinupristin + dalfopristin, raltegravir, ribavirin (PO), rilpivirine, saquinavir, stavudine, suramin, thalidomide, tigecycline, trimetrexate, voriconazole, zidovudine

Data from Lexi-Comp Online (http://online.lexi.com/crlonline), accessed 27 August 2012; and Micromedex Healthcare Series (http://www.thomsonhc.com), accessed 27 August 2012.

ALT, Alanine aminotransferase; *AST,* aspartate aminotransferase; *GGT,* gamma-glutamyl transpeptidase; *IV,* intravenous; *PO,* oral.

X. OCULAR

TABLE 7-10

OCULAR ADVERSE DRUG EFFECTS

Adverse Effect	Medication
Blurred vision	Ivermectin, quinidine, quinine, ribavirin (PO), voriconazole
Photophobia	Levofloxacin, ofloxacin, voriconazole
Retinal detachment	Ciprofloxacin, ganciclovir, gatifloxacin, levofloxacin, norfloxacin, valganciclovir
Visual disturbances	Azithromycin, foscarnet, gatifloxacin, hydroxychloroquine, iodoquinol, levofloxacin, ofloxacin, terbinafine, voriconazole

PO, Oral.

XI. MUSCULOSKELETAL

TABLE 7-11

ADVERSE DRUG EFFECTS ON THE MUSCULOSKELETAL SYSTEM

Adverse Effect	Medication
Arthralgia	Abacavir sulfate, amphotericin B, amphotericin B (liposomal), artemether + lumefantrine (children 3%, adults 34%), boceprevir, cytomegalovirus immune globulin IV (human), daptomycin, emtricitabine, ertapenem (infants, children, adolescents <2%) foscarnet, hepatitis B immune globulin IV (human), immune globulin IV (human), ivermectin, lamivudine, posaconazole, pyrazinamide, quinupristin + dalfopristin, Rho(D) immune globulin IV (human), ribavirin (PO), rifapentine, rifaximin, ritonavir, stibogluconate, telbivudine, thalidomide, valacyclovir, zanamivir, zidovudine
Back pain	Adefovir, amphotericin B (liposomal), cytomegalovirus immune globulin IV (human), daptomycin, foscarnet, fosfomycin, imiquimod, immune globulin IV (human), indinavir, micafungin, posaconazole, ribavirin (PO), saquinavir, telbivudine, tenofovir disoproxil fumarate, thalidomide
CPK elevation	Atazanavir, daptomycin, emtricitabine, enfuvirtide, gemifloxacin, lamivudine, saquinavir, telbivudine, tipranavir
Myalgia	Abacavir sulfate, amphotericin B, amphotericin B (liposomal), artemether + lumefantrine (children 3%, adults 32%), atazanavir, atovaquone, emtricitabine, enfuvirtide, foscarnet, halofantrine, hepatitis B immune globulin IV (human), imiquimod, itraconazole, lamivudine, lopinavir + ritonavir, maraviroc, mefloquine HCl, pyrazinamide, quinupristin + dalfopristin, Rho(D) immune globulin IV (human), ribavirin (PO), rifabutin, rifaximin, ritonavir, stibogluconate, suramin, telbivudine, tenofovir disoproxil fumarate, thalidomide, tipranavir, varicella-zoster immune globulin IV (human), zalcitabine, zanamivir, zidovudine
Rhabdomyolysis	Zidovudine

Data from Lexi-Comp Online (http://online.lexi.com/crlonline), accessed 27 August 2012.

CPK, Creatine phosphokinase; *IV,* intravenous; *PO,* oral.

XII. HYPERSENSITIVITY

TABLE 7-12

HYPERSENSITIVITY TO DRUGS

Adverse Effect	Medication
Anaphylaxis	Abacavir, amoxicillin, ampicillin, ampicillin + sulbactam, bacitracin + polymyxin B sulfate, diphtheria antitoxin, erythromycin, hepatitis B immune globulin IV, miconazole, neomycin sulfate + polymyxin B sulfate ± bacitracin, penicillin G (benzathine), Rho(D) immune globulin IV, tetanus immune globulin IV, trimetrexate, varicella zoster immune globulin IV, zidovudine
Serum sickness	Diphtheria antitoxin, immune globulin IV

IV, Intravenous.

XIII. OTHER

TABLE 7-13

OTHER ADVERSE DRUG EFFECTS

Adverse Effect	Medication
Ototoxicity (hearing loss)	Amikacin, capreomycin, gentamicin, streptomycin sulfate, tobramycin
Tinnitus	Mefloquine, minocycline, quinidine
Vestibular toxicity	Amikacin, gentamicin, minocycline, streptomycin sulfate, tobramycin

REFERENCES

1. Lexi-Comp Online (website): http://online.lexi.com/crlonline. Accessed 27 August 2012.
2. Micromedex Healthcare Series (website): http://www.thomsonhc.com. Accessed 27 August 2012.
3. *Drug Facts and Comparisons*, CliniSphere version, St. Louis, MO, Wolters Kluwer Health, Inc. (Available online at http://online.factsandcomparisons.com. Accessed 27 August 2012.)

Chapter 8

Recommended Antimicrobial Prophylaxis for Selected Infectious Agents and Conditions

Julia A. McMillan, MD, and George K. Siberry, MD, MPH

TABLE 8-1

RECOMMENDED ANTIMICROBIAL PROPHYLAXIS FOR SELECTED INFECTIOUS AGENTS AND CONDITIONS

Exposure	Recommended Empiric Preventive Therapy	Alternative Preventive Therapy	Comments
SITUATIONAL			
Bite, animal	Amoxicillin/clavulanate × 3–5 days	[Third generation cephalosporin or TMP/SMX] + clindamycin	Consider need for tetanus and rabies prophylaxis. Longer treatment indicated for immunocompromised patients and wounds that penetrate joints.
Bite, human	Amoxicillin/clavulanate × 3–5 days	[Third generation cephalosporin or TMP/SMX] + clindamycin	Consider need for tetanus prophylaxis. Longer treatment indicated for immunocompromised patients and wounds that penetrate joints.
CSF leak	23-valent pneumococcal polysaccharide vaccine + meningococcal vaccine (conjugate preferred) if ≥2 years old, in addition to conjugated *Haemophilus influenzae* type b and conjugated pneumococcal vaccines routinely recommended for all infants		Some experts recommend penicillin prophylaxis for traumatic CSF leak, but evidence of benefit is lacking.

Endocarditis	For dental, oral, or upper respiratory tract or esophageal procedures: amoxicillin *Penicillin-allergic* Clindamycin *or* Cephalexin *or* Cefadroxil *or* Azithromycin *or* Clarithromycin	Clindamycin *or* Cefazolin IV *or* Ampicillin IV *or* Ceftriaxone	A single antibiotic dose should be administered 30–60 min before the procedure. Cephalosporins should not be used for people with immediate-type hypersensitivity to penicillin. Efficacy of prophylaxis is not proved for all circumstances. See the American Heart Association guidelines[1] for a list of conditions and procedures for which prophylaxis is recommended.
	Cardiac surgery with placement of intracardiac or intravascular material: first-generation cephalosporin	Vancomycin	Administer antibiotic immediately before the procedure; repeat dose every one to two half-lives of the antibiotic during prolonged procedures; continue prophylaxis no more than 48 hr. Vancomycin should be used if the prevalence of methicillin-resistant *Staphylococcus aureus* is high.
Immunocompromised host	Asplenic states Penicillin V <5 yr, 125 mg twice daily ≥5 yr, 250 mg twice daily		Age-appropriate immunization against *Streptococcus pneumoniae*, *H. influenzae*, and *Neisseria meningitidis* is recommended in addition to chemoprophylaxis. ≥2 yr old: pneumococcal polysaccharide vaccine and meningococcal conjugate vaccine.
	Phagocyte function defect TMP/SMX		Interferon-γ has been shown to prolong infection-free periods for children with chronic granulomatous disease.

Continued

8

TABLE 8-1

RECOMMENDED ANTIMICROBIAL PROPHYLAXIS FOR SELECTED INFECTIOUS AGENTS AND CONDITIONS (Continued)

Exposure	Recommended Empiric Preventive Therapy	Alternative Preventive Therapy	Comments
Needlestick (hepatitis B, hepatitis C, HIV)	Immediate cleaning with copious soap and water indicated for all needlesticks **Hepatitis B** No action if exposed person already hepatitis B immune *Source with unknown infection status:* hepatitis B vaccine series for nonimmune contact *Source HBsAg+:* one dose of hepatitis B immune globulin *plus* hepatitis B vaccine series **HIV** Known HIV^+ source: two- to three-drug regimen for 4 wk depending on volume of exposure and HIV class status of source (see Panlilio and colleagues[2] and Havens[3]) Postexposure prophylaxis is generally not recommended after needlestick injury from unknown, nonoccupational source		Exposed person should be tested for HIV and hepatitis C at baseline and 4–6 and 12 wk and at 6 mo after exposure. Risk for HIV infection after percutaneous occupational exposure to HIV-infected blood is 0.3%; 0.09% after mucous membrane exposure. Risk after nonoccupational exposure is lower. Risk for transmission after an episode of receptive penile-anal sexual exposure is estimated to be 50 per 10,000 episodes; the risk after an episode of receptive vaginal exposure is estimated to be 10 per 10,000 exposures. CDC National Clinician's Postexposure hotline: 888-448-4911 (or http://www.nccc.ucsf.edu/about_nccc/).

Ophthalmia neonatorum	Topical: silver nitrate (1%) *or* erythromycin ointment (0.5%) *or* tetracycline ointment or suspension (1%)		Prophylactic topical therapy is used to prevent gonococcal ophthalmia. None of the three agents listed prevents mother-to-infant transmission of *Chlamydia trachomatis* infection. For healthy infants born to mother with untreated gonococcal infection, administer one dose of ceftriaxone IM or IV (25–50 mg/kg) or cefotaxime IV or IM (100 mg/kg). Topical therapy is inadequate and not needed in these patients.
Recurrent otitis media	Amoxicillin *or* sulfisoxazole *or* TMP/SMX	Xylitol	Chemoprophylaxis is of greatest benefit in children 6–24 mo old.
Rheumatic fever	Penicillin G benzathine 1.2 million U Q4 wk *or* Penicillin V, 250 mg twice daily *or* Sulfadiazine *or* sulfisoxazole ≤27 kg: 0.5 g once daily >27 kg: 1 g once daily *Penicillin-allergic:* clarithromycin *or* azithromycin		Prophylaxis should continue for at least 5 years in all patients after the most recent episode of rheumatic fever or until age 21, whichever is longer. Individuals with carditis should continue to receive prophylaxis for at least 10 years; patients with residual or persistent cardiac disease should continue prophylaxis until age 40 yr.

Continued

8

TABLE 8-1

RECOMMENDED ANTIMICROBIAL PROPHYLAXIS FOR SELECTED INFECTIOUS AGENTS AND CONDITIONS (Continued)

Exposure	Recommended Empiric Preventive Therapy	Alternative Preventive Therapy	Comments
Sexual contact or assault	Prepubertal victim: ceftriaxone × 1 dose (prevention of gonorrhea) + [azithromycin (single dose) *or* Erythromycin base *or* ethylsuccinate × 14 days *or* doxycycline × 7 days (if at least 8 yr old) (prevention of *C. trachomatis*)] + Consideration of metronidazole TID × 7 days (trichomoniasis and bacterial vaginosis) Adolescent victim: [ceftriaxone × 1 dose (250 mg) (gonorrhea)] + [azithromycin (1 g × 1 dose) *or* doxycycline 100 mg BID × 7 days *if not pregnant* (*C. trachomatis*)] + metronidazole (2 g × 1 dose) (trichomoniasis and bacterial vaginosis)		Chemoprophylaxis of prepubertal, asymptomatic child may not be indicated if follow-up is ensured. Laboratory tests for sexually transmitted infections should be performed before chemoprophylaxis. Consider HIV chemoprophylaxis, depending on circumstances of exposure. Risk for transmission after an episode of receptive penile-anal sexual exposure is estimated to be 50 per 10,000 episodes; the risk after an episode of receptive vaginal exposure is estimated to be 10 per 10,000 exposures. Consider emergency contraception. Initiate hepatitis B vaccine series if not immune.
Urinary tract infection	Nitrofurantoin *or* TMP/SMX		Amoxicillin for neonates. Benefit of antimicrobial prophylaxis to prevent urinary tract infection in infants with mild-to-moderate vesico-ureteral reflux (Grades I–IV) has not been demonstrated.

PREVENTION OF INFECTION CAUSED BY SPECIFIC BACTERIAL PATHOGENS

NOTE: Many of the following infections must be reported to the Health Department. Contact your local Health Department for the list of reportable diseases in your jurisdiction.

Anthrax	[Ciprofloxacin *or* Doxycycline (for those ≥8 yr)] for 60 days	If susceptibility testing confirms penicillin susceptibility, therapy can be changed to amoxicillin (80 mg/kg/day divided Q8 hr (max 500 mg/dose).
Diphtheria	Erythromycin 50 mg/kg/day (maximum 2 g/day) × 10 days *or* IM benzathine penicillin G (600,000 U for children <30 kg and 1.2 million U for those ≥30 kg) + DTaP, dT, *or* Tdap as appropriate for age	Pharyngeal cultures should be obtained from all contacts before chemoprophylaxis. Follow-up cultures should also be obtained after therapy, and, if positive, a second 10-day course of erythromycin should be given.
H. influenzae type b	Rifampin 20 mg/kg/day (in 1 dose/day) × 4 days (maximum 600 mg/day)	Prophylaxis is recommended *only* for household contacts in which there is at least 1 contact <4 yr old who is incompletely immunized *or* an infant <1 yr old who has not completed the primary series, *or* an immunocompromised child of any age or immunization status; and in nursery schools and child care centers with ≥2 cases of invasive disease within 60 days. Index patient should receive prophylaxis *only if* <2 yr old *and* lives in a household with a susceptible contact *and* was treated with antibiotic other than ceftriaxone or cefotaxime. Index patient <2 years old should be *reimmunized* against Hib.

Continued

TABLE 8-1

RECOMMENDED ANTIMICROBIAL PROPHYLAXIS FOR SELECTED INFECTIOUS AGENTS AND CONDITIONS (Continued)

Exposure	Recommended Empiric Preventive Therapy	Alternative Preventive Therapy	Comments
Mycobacterium avium complex	Azithromycin (20 mg/kg by mouth weekly, maximum 1200 mg) *or* Azithromycin (5 mg/kg by mouth daily, maximum 250 mg) *or* Clarithromycin (7.5 mg/kg by mouth twice daily, maximum 500 mg)	Rifabutin	Rifabutin should be used **only** after tuberculosis disease has been excluded. Prophylaxis is recommended for HIV-infected children if ≥6 yr old with CD4 T lymphocytes <50/μl; 2–5 yr with CD4 T lymphocytes <75/μl; 1–2 yr with CD4 T lymphocytes <500/μl; <12 mo with CD4 T lymphocytes <750/μl.
Mycobacterium tuberculosis	Isoniazid for all exposed contacts with impaired immunity or with age <4 yr Rifampin if contact's isolate is isoniazid resistant		TST should be performed at baseline and 12 wk after contact. If TST is negative at 12 wk and subject is immunocompetent, discontinue isoniazid. If TST is positive or if subject's TST cannot be interpreted because of immune impairment, continue isoniazid for 9 mo (4 mo if rifampin or rifabutin is used because of isoniazid resistance). Tuberculosis specialist should be consulted in cases of exposure to rifampin-resistant organism. For ≥12 yr old: Isoniazid *plus* rifapentine with DOT for 12 wk is an effective alternative to isoniazid for 9 mo.

N. meningitidis	Rifampin <1 mo old: 5 mg/kg Q12 hr × 2 days ≥1 mo old: 10 mg/kg (maximum 600 mg) Q12 hr × 2 days *or* Ceftriaxone <15 yr old: 125 mg IM × 1 dose ≥15 yr old: 250 mg IM × 1 dose *or* Ciprofloxacin ≥18 yr old: 500 mg × 1 dose	Azithromycin <15 yr: 10 mg/kg × 1 dose ≥15 yr: 500 mg × 1 dose	Prophylaxis recommended *only* for household contacts *and* those with the following exposure within 7 days of index patient's illness onset: Child care or nursery school contact Direct exposure to patient secretions Mouth-to-mouth resuscitation Frequently slept in the same dwelling Passenger seated next to index patient on an airline flight of more than 8 hr.
Pertussis	Azithromycin <6 mo old: 10 mg/kg/day in 1 dose × 5 days ≥6 mo old: 10 mg/kg in 1 dose on day 1 (maximum dose 500 mg); then 5 mg/kg/day (maximum 250 mg/day) in 1 dose for 4 days *or* Erythromycin Infants and children: 40–50 mg/kg/day (maximum 2 g/day) in 4 divided doses × 14 days Adolescents and adults: 2 g/day in 4 divided doses × 14 days *or* Clarithromycin: 15 mg/kg/day (maximum 1 g/day) in 2 divided doses × 7 days	TMP/SMX: (must be ≥2 mo old); TMP (8 mg/kg/day, maximum 300 mg/day); SMX (40 mg/kg/day; maximum 1600 mg/day) in 2 divided doses × 14 days	Antibiotic prophylaxis is recommended for all household contacts and other close contacts (including child care) regardless of immunization status. Clarithromycin is not recommended for infants <1 mo old; TMP/SMX is not recommended for infants <2 mo old. Erythromycin may increase risk for pyloric stenosis for infants <6 wk old. Azithromycin is preferred for infants <1 mo.

Continued

TABLE 8-1

RECOMMENDED ANTIMICROBIAL PROPHYLAXIS FOR SELECTED INFECTIOUS AGENTS AND CONDITIONS (Continued)

Exposure	Recommended Empiric Preventive Therapy	Alternative Preventive Therapy	Comments
Tetanus	For clean wound: If <3 prior doses of tetanus toxoid or if history of vaccination is not known, give Td or Tdap. If ≥3 doses of tetanus toxoid is confirmed, Td or Tdap if ≥10 years since last tetanus vaccine. For dirty wound: If <3 prior doses of tetanus toxoid or history (depending on age) of vaccination is not known, give DTaP *or* Td *or* Tdap *plus* tetanus immune globulin (250 U IM); if >3 prior doses, give Td *or* Tdap if ≥5 years since last tetanus vaccine	IV immune globulin can be used if tetanus immune globulin is indicated and not available	If both tetanus toxoid and tetanus immune globulin are indicated, they should be injected in separate syringes and at different sites.
PREVENTION OF INFECTION CAUSED BY SPECIFIC VIRAL PATHOGENS			
Cytomegalovirus (CMV)	Prevention of transmission to transplant recipient: ganciclovir *or* valganciclovir	Foscarnet	CMV immune globulin is moderately effective in preventing CMV in seronegative liver and kidney transplant recipients.
Herpes simplex	Prevention of recurrences: acyclovir *or* famciclovir *or* valacyclovir		Famciclovir is not approved for <18 yr; valacyclovir is not approved for <12 yr.

Hepatitis A	Before exposure: <12 mo: immunoglobulin (IM) 0.02 mL/kg for trips <3 mo; 0.06 mL/kg at departure and every 5 mo if exposure extends ≥3 mo. ≥12 mo: hepatitis A vaccine After exposure in nonimmune person: Hepatitis A vaccine (if ≥1 yr) Immune globulin alone if <1 yr	Postexposure prophylaxis is not recommended if the time since exposure is more than 2 wk; hepatitis A vaccine is recommended as protection against subsequent exposure.
Hepatitis B	After exposure: Source with unknown infection status: hepatitis B vaccine series for nonimmune contact HBsAg$^+$ source: one dose of hepatitis B immune globulin + hepatitis B vaccine series	

Continued

8

TABLE 8-1

RECOMMENDED ANTIMICROBIAL PROPHYLAXIS FOR SELECTED INFECTIOUS AGENTS AND CONDITIONS (Continued)

Exposure	Recommended Empiric Preventive Therapy	Alternative Preventive Therapy	Comments
HIV	Prevention of maternal-to-child transmission: combination antiretroviral regimen that includes zidovudine (see perinatal guidelines at the U.S. Department of Health and Human Services website: http://www.aidsinfo.nih.gov) Sexual, occupational, or nonoccupational exposure: known HIV^+ source: two- to three-drug regimen depending on volume of exposure and HIV class status of source (see Panlilio and colleagues[2] and Havens[3]) Postexposure prophylaxis is generally not recommended after needlestick injury from unknown, nonoccupational source		Exposed person should be tested for HIV at baseline, 4–6 and 12 wk, and at 6 mo after exposure. Risk for HIV infection after percutaneous occupational exposure to HIV-infected blood is 0.3%; 0.09% after mucous membrane exposure. Risk for nonoccupational exposure is lower. CDC National Clinician's Postexposure hotline: 888-448-4911.
Influenza	Zanamivir (≥5 yr) *or* Oseltamivir (≥1 yr)		Rimantadine or amantadine if circulating influenza known to be susceptible; these two agents are not active against influenza B. Recommendations for chemoprophylaxis against influenza vary depending on the susceptibility of the circulating strains. For further information, see CDC website (http://www.cdc.gov/flu/professionals/antivirals/summary-clinicians.htm).

Measles	Measles vaccine (within 72 hr of exposure) *or* immune globulin (within 6 days of exposure)		Immune globulin is recommended for high-risk, susceptible household contacts (<1 yr old, pregnant women, immunocompromised). The usual dose of IVIg used for immunocompromised people who receive it regularly should provide protection against measles as well. IG to prevent measles should be given within 6 days of exposure, usually at 0.25 mL/kg IM, but at 0.5 mL/kg IM for immunocompromised children (maximum dose: 15 mL). If IG is given, delay measles vaccine for 5 mo (if 0.25 mL/kg IM) or 6 mo (if 0.5 mL/kg IM) or 8–11 mo (if IVIg given, depending on dose).
Rubella	IM immune globulin (0.55 mL/kg, max 15 mL)	Rubella vaccine	Immune globulin does not prevent rubella infection and does not reliably prevent in utero transmission from an infected mother to her fetus. It should be offered only as a possible means of reducing the likelihood of fetal infection for susceptible, exposed pregnant women who decline termination of pregnancy. Rubella vaccine (for nonpregnant, exposed people) has not been shown to prevent illness, but if given within 72 hr of exposure, it may be preventative.
Varicella	After exposure: varicella zoster immune globulin (125 U per 10 kg, maximum 625 U) *or* acyclovir (beginning within 10 days of exposure) *or* varicella immunization (within 3–5 days of exposure)	IVIg (400 mg/kg)	Varicella zoster immune globulin (VariZIG) must be administered within 10 days of exposure, and preferably within 96 hr. IVIG can be used (1 dose ≤96 hr after exposure) if varicella zoster immune globulin is not available. If IVIg is used to prevent varicella, measles vaccine should not be administered until at least 5 mo after IVIg administration.

Continued

TABLE 8-1

RECOMMENDED ANTIMICROBIAL PROPHYLAXIS FOR SELECTED INFECTIOUS AGENTS AND CONDITIONS (Continued)

Exposure	Recommended Empiric Preventive Therapy	Alternative Preventive Therapy	Comments
PREVENTION OF INFECTION CAUSED BY SPECIFIC FUNGAL PATHOGENS			
Candida	Fluconazole	Micafungin	Recommended during periods of neutropenia for children undergoing allogeneic stem-cell transplantation.
Pneumocystis	TMP/SMX	Dapsone (≥1 mo) *or* aerosolized Pentamidine (≥5 yr) *or* atovaquone	Recommended for HIV-infected or indeterminant infants aged 1–12 mo and for HIV-infected children with following CD4 T-lymphocyte counts: 1–5 yr: <500/μl; 6–12 yr: <200/μl. Recommended for children with a variety of immunocompromising conditions.
PREVENTION OF INFECTION CAUSED BY SPECIFIC PARASITIC PATHOGENS			
Malaria	Travel to areas without reported chloroquine-resistant malaria: Chloroquine *or* mefloquine (see later) *or* doxycycline (see later) *or* atovaquone-proguanil (see later)		Begin chloroquine prophylaxis 1 wk before travel and continue for 4 wk after exposure has ended.
	Travel to areas with chloroquine-resistant malaria: Atovaquone-proguanil daily		Begin prophylaxis 1 day before exposure and for 1 wk after exposure has ended. Contraindicated in pregnancy.

	or Doxycycline (≥8 yr) daily		Begin prophylaxis 1–2 days before exposure and continue 4 wk after exposure has ended. Contraindicated in pregnancy; caution about diarrhea, photosensitivity, and monilial vaginitis.
	or Mefloquine weekly		Begin prophylaxis 2 wk before travel and continue 4 wk after exposure has ended. Contraindicated for people with anxiety disorders, psychosis, schizophrenia, and other major psychiatric disturbances and in those with a history of seizures.
Toxoplasmosis	Prevention of first episode in HIV-infected people: TMP/SMX: (indicated for infants and children 1–5 yr old if CD4 <15%; for children ≥6 yr old if CD4 count <100/mm^3) Prevention of recurrence in HIV-infected people: [sulfadiazine + pyrimethamine + leucovorin]	[Dapsone (≥1 mo) + pyrimethamine + leucovorin] *or* Atovaquone *or* [Clindamycin + pyrimethamine + leucovorin]	

CDC, Centers for Disease Control and Prevention; *CMV,* cytomegalovirus; *CSF,* cerebrospinal fluid; *DTaP,* diphtheria and tetanus toxoids and acellular pertussis vaccine; *Ig,* immunoglobulin; *IM,* intramuscular; *IV,* intravenous; *IVIg,* intravenous immunoglobulin; *max,* maximum; *Td,* adult-type diphtheria and tetanus toxoids vaccine; *Tdap,* tetanus toxoid, reduced diphtheria toxoid, and acellular pertussis vaccine; *TMP/SMX,* trimethoprim/sulfamethoxazole; *TST,* tuberculin skin test.

REFERENCES

1. Wilson W, Taubert KA, Gewitz M, et al. Prevention of infective endocarditis: Guidelines from the American Heart Association. *Circulation.* 2007;116:1736–1754.
2. Panlilio AL, Cardo DM, Grohskopf LA, et al. Updated U.S. Public Health Service guidelines for the management of occupational exposures to HIV and recommendations for postexposure prophylaxis. *MMWR Recomm Rep.* 2005;54(RR09):1–17. (or http://www.cdc.gov/mmwr/preview/mmwrhtml/rr5409a1.htm).
3. Havens PL; Committee on Pediatric AIDS. Postexposure prophylaxis in children and adolescents for nonoccupational exposure to human immunodeficiency virus. *Pediatrics.* 2003;111:1475–1489.
4. Pickering LK, Baker CJ, Kimberlin DW, Long SS, eds. *Red Book 2012 Report of the Committee on Infectious Diseases.* 29th ed. Elk Grove Village, IL: American Academy of Pediatrics; 2012.

Chapter 9

Antimicrobial Desensitization Protocols

Lisa A. Degnan, PharmD, BCPS, and
Carlton K. K. Lee, PharmD, MPH

Rapid desensitization is intended for patients who have or who are strongly suspected of having antibiotic-specific immunoglobulin E (IgE) antibodies. Desensitization does not prevent non–IgE-mediated allergic reactions. Patients with antibiotic-induced Stevens–Johnson syndrome or toxic epidermal necrolysis **should not** receive the antibiotic under any circumstances because of the risk for inducing a progressive life-threatening reaction.[1] Discontinue all β-blockers before desensitization and do not pretreat (unless indicated) with systemic corticosteroids and antihistamines.

Have patient-specific doses of injectable epinephrine, diphenhydramine, and corticosteroid and appropriate resuscitative equipment available at the bedside. For all injectable infusions, rates should be regulated with a syringe pump.

Most protocols are designed for adults. Please note the cumulative desensitization doses of the following protocols may exceed your patient's dosage. Proportional dose reductions are necessary for pediatric patients, as the final cumulative dose should equal the patient's individualized divided dose. For example, if the antibiotic's usual dose is 30 mg/kg/24 hr divided every 12 hours, the final cumulative dose should be 15 mg/kg. Desensitization may be achieved by intermittent intravenous (IV) infusion, continuous IV infusion, or by the oral route. The oral route is less expensive and safer.

I. PENICILLIN

Mild allergic reactions should be treated; if symptoms do not progress, repeat the same dose or drop back one dose before proceeding. At the completion of desensitization, the therapeutic dose of penicillin may be administered.[2] Continuous penicillin treatment is required to maintain the desensitized state. Unless a long-acting preparation is used, oral penicillin should be taken on a twice-daily basis. If penicillin is discontinued for more than 48 hours, the patient is again at risk for anaphylaxis and desensitization should be repeated.[2]

A. Intermittent Intravenous Infusion[1]

TABLE 9-1

PENICILLIN INTRAVENOUS DESENSITIZATION PROTOCOL WITH DRUG ADDED BY PIGGYBACK INFUSION

Step*	Penicillin (mg/mL)	Amount (mL)	Dose (mg)	Cumulative Dose (mg)
1	0.1	0.1	0.01	0.01
2	0.1	0.2	0.02	0.03
3	0.1	0.4	0.04	0.07
4	0.1	0.8	0.08	0.15
5	0.1	1.6	0.16	0.31
6	1	0.32	0.32	0.63
7	1	0.64	0.64	1.27
8	1	1.2	1.2	2.47
9	10	0.24	2.4	4.87
10	10	0.48	4.8	10
11	10	1	10	20
12	10	2	20	40
13	100	0.4	40	80
14	100	0.8	80	160
15	100	1.6	160	320
16	1000	0.32	320	640
17	1000	0.64	640	1280

Observe patient for 30 min, then give full therapeutic dose by the desired route.
From Solensky R. Drug desensitization. *Immunol Allergy Clin N Am.* 2004;24:425–443.
*Interval between doses is 15 min.

B. Continuous Intravenous Infusion[1,2]

TABLE 9-2

PENICILLIN INTRAVENOUS DESENSITIZATION PROTOCOL USING A CONTINUOUS INFUSION PUMP

Step*	Penicillin (mg/mL)	Flow Rate (mL/hr)	Dose (mg)	Cumulative Dose (mg)
1	0.01	6	0.015	0.015
2	0.01	12	0.03	0.045
3	0.01	24	0.06	0.105
4	0.1	5	0.125	0.23
5	0.1	10	0.25	0.48
6	0.1	20	0.5	1
7	0.1	40	1	2
8	0.1	80	2	4
9	0.1	160	4	8
10	10	3	7.5	15
11	10	6	15	30
12	10	12	30	60
13	10	25	62.5	123
14	10	50	125	250
15	10	100	250	500
16	10	200	500	1000

Observe patient for 30 min, then give full therapeutic dose by the desired route.
From Solensky R. Drug desensitization. *Immunol Allergy Clin N Am.* 2004;24:425–443.
*Interval between doses is 15 min.

C. Oral[1,2]

TABLE 9-3

PENICILLIN ORAL DESENSITIZATION PROTOCOL

Step*	Penicillin (mg/mL)	Amount (mL)	Dose (mg)	Cumulative Dose (mg)
1	0.5	0.1	0.05	0.05
2	0.5	0.2	0.1	0.15
3	0.5	0.4	0.2	0.35
4	0.5	0.8	0.4	0.75
5	0.5	1.6	0.8	1.55
6	0.5	3.2	1.6	3.15
7	0.5	6.4	3.2	6.35
8	5	1.2	6	12.35
9	5	2.4	12	24.35
10	5	5	25	49.35
11	50	1	50	100
12	50	2	100	200
13	50	4	200	400
14	50	8	400	800

Observe patient for 30 min, then give full therapeutic dose by the desired route.

From Solensky R. Drug desensitization. *Immunol Allergy Clin N Am.* 2004;24:425–443.

*Interval between doses is 15 min.

9

II. AMOXICILLIN

A graded challenge method differs from desensitization because the immunological response to the drug is not modified by a graded challenge. Therefore, a graded challenge may be used in patients with a low likelihood of having an allergy to the medication, whereas desensitization is performed on a patient who is assumed to have a type I allergy.[3] Graded challenges may be appropriate in patients with distant type I allergic reactions to penicillin because penicillin-specific IgE antibodies wane over time.[3] Table 9-4 is an example of a graded challenge with oral amoxicillin for a patient with a distant reaction history to penicillin.[3]

TABLE 9-4

GRADED CHALLENGE WITH ORAL AMOXICILLIN FOR PATIENTS WITH DISTANT REACTION HISTORY TO PENICILLIN

Dose*	Amoxicillin (mg/mL)	Amount (mL)	Dose (mg)
1	5	0.5	2.5
2	50	0.5	25
3	50	5	250

From Solensky R. Desensitization with antibiotics. In Pichler WJ, ed. *Drug Hypersensitivity.* Basel, Switzerland: Karger; 2007:404–412.

*Interval between doses is 30 min.

III. CEPHALOSPORINS

Desensitization protocol generally parallels that of penicillin with progressively increasing doses administered in frequent time intervals. Examples of the intermittent IV infusion and continuous IV infusion methods are described in the following sections.

A. Intermittent Intravenous Infusion[4]

TABLE 9-5

RAPID INTRAVENOUS CEPHALOSPORIN DESENSITIZATION PROTOCOL: GOAL DOSE, 1 g AND 2 g INTRAVENOUSLY

	Goal Dose: 1 g IV		Goal Dose: 2 g IV	
Dose	**mg**	**mg, rounded**	**mg, rounded**	**Time**
1	0.1	0.1	0.1	15 min
2	0.2	0.2	0.4	15 min
3	0.7	1	1	15 min
4	2.2	2	4	15 min
5	6.9	10	10	15 min
6	21.8	20	40	15 min
7	69	70	140	15 min
8	218.1	200	400	15 min
9	689.7	700	1400	15 min
Cumulative	1008.6	1003.3	1995.5	2 hr, 15 min

From Win PH, Brown H, Zankar A, et al. Rapid intravenous cephalosporin desensitization. *J Allergy Clin Immunol.* 2005;116(1):225–227.

B. Continuous Intravenous Infusion[1]

TABLE 9-6

INTRAVENOUS CEPHALOSPORIN DESENSITIZATION PROTOCOL USING A CONTINUOUS INFUSION PUMP: GOAL DOSE, 2 g INTRAVENOUSLY

Step*	Cephalosporin mg/mL	Flow Rate (mL/hr)	Dose (mg)	Cumulative Dose (mg)
1	0.01	6	0.015	0.015
2	0.01	12	0.03	0.045
3	0.01	24	0.06	0.105
4	0.1	5	0.125	0.23
5	0.1	10	0.25	0.48
6	0.1	20	0.5	1
7	0.1	40	1	2
8	0.1	80	2	4
9	0.1	160	4	8
10	10	3	7.5	15
11	10	6	15	30
12	10	12	30	60
13	10	25	62.5	123
14	10	50	125	250
15	100	10	250	500
16	100	20	500	1000
17	100	40	1000	2000

From Solensky R. Drug desensitization. *Immunol Allergy Clin N Am.* 2004;24:425–443.
*Interval between doses is 15 min.

IV. TRIMETHOPRIM/SULFAMETHOXAZOLE ORAL

Patients with allergic reactions such as serum sickness, vasculitis, hypersensitivity syndrome, pneumonitis, interstitial nephritis, immune-mediated hematological disorders, drug fever, Stevens–Johnson syndrome, and toxic epidermal necrolysis **are not candidates for desensitization.**

A. Patients with a Previous (Distant) Reaction Consistent with an IgE-Mediated Mechanism[1]

TABLE 9-7

EXAMPLE OF GRADED CHALLENGE WITH ORAL TRIMETHOPRIM/SULFAMETHOXAZOLE IN A PATIENT WITH A DISTANT MILD IMMEDIATE-TYPE ALLERGIC REACTION

Step*	TMP/SMX (SMX mg/mL)	Amount (mL)	SMX Dose (mg)
1	4	0.25	1
2	4	1	4
3	40	0.5	20
4	40	2	80
5	NA	1 tablet	400

From Solensky R. Drug desensitization. *Immunol Allergy Clin N Am.* 2004;24:425–443.

*Interval between doses is 30 min. Dose is expressed as sulfamethoxazole portion of trimethoprim/sulfamethoxazole (TMP/SMX). If an allergic reaction occurs, formal desensitization should be performed.

NA, Not applicable.

9

B. Patients with a History of Typical Delayed Maculopapular Reaction

Cutaneous reactions occur in 40% to 80% of HIV-positive patients compared with 3.3% in non-HIV individuals. Many different TMP/SMX desensitization protocols for HIV are reported in the literature. Tables 9-8 to 9-10 are examples of oral adult regimens.[5]

TABLE 9-8

DILUTION FOR TRIMETHOPRIM/SULFAMETHOXAZOLE DESENSITIZATION

Final Concentration of TMP/SMZ	Bottle Assignment	Procedure
200/40 mg per 5 mL	A	Conventional oral TMP/SMZ suspension 5 mL = 200/40 mg
2/0.4 mg per 1 mL	B	1. Add 5 mL of conventional oral TMP/SMZ suspension (from bottle A) to 95 mL sterile water. 2. Shake well. Recipe will equal 2/0.4 mg per 1 mL.
0.02/0.004 mg per 1 mL	C	1. Add 1 mL of bottle B to 99 mL sterile water. 2. Shake well. Recipe will equal 0.02/0.004 mg per 1 mL.

TABLE 9-9

ADVERSE REACTIONS AND RESPONSE DURING TRIMETHOPRIM/SULFAMETHOXAZOLE DESENSITIZATION

Type of Reaction	Alteration of Protocol
Mild (rash, fever, nausea)	Diphenhydramine (PO) *or* ibuprofen (PO)
Urticaria, dyspnea, severe vomiting, and/or hypotension	**Stop** the desensitization **immediately.** Treat with epinephrine and corticosteroid.

TABLE 9-10

ORAL TRIMETHOPRIM/SULFAMETHOXAZOLE DESENSITIZATION PROTOCOL

Hour	Dose of TMP/SMZ	Form/Bottle No.	Suggested Volume
0	0.02/0.004 mg	C	1 mL
1	0.2/0.04 mg	C	10 mL
2	2/0.4 mg	B	1 mL
3	20/4 mg	B	10 mL
4	200/40 mg	A	5 mL
5	800/160 mg	NA	1 single-strength tablet

Drink 180 mL water after each dose of trimethoprim/sulfamethoxazole (TMP/SMX). Subjects tolerating this protocol were prescribed 800/160 mg TMP/SMZ every Monday, Wednesday, and Friday for low-dose *Pneumocystis carinii* prophylaxis.

From Gluckstein D, Ruskin J. Rapid oral desensitization to trimethoprim-sulfamethoxazole (TMP-SMZ): Use in prophylaxis for *Pneumocystis jiroveci (carinii)* pneumonia in patients with AIDS who were previously intolerant to TMP-SMZ. *Clin Infect Dis.* 1995;20:849–853.

NA, Not applicable.

V. FLUOROQUINOLONE

A. Intravenous Ciprofloxacin Desensitization Protocol

Table 9-11 is an example of a successful IV ciprofloxacin desensitization protocol from a 29-month-old with a gluteal abscess and chronic osteomyelitis experiencing anaphylaxis.[6]

TABLE 9-11

SAMPLE INTRAVENOUS CIPROFLOXACIN DESENSITIZATION PROTOCOL

Dose*	Concentration (mg/mL)	Volume Given (mL)	Absolute Amount (mg)	Cumulative Total Dose (mg)
1	0.000002	5	0.00001	0.00001
2	0.00002	5	0.0001	0.0001
3	0.0002	5	0.001	0.001
4	0.002	5	0.01	0.01
5	0.004	5	0.02	0.03
6	0.008	5	0.04	0.07
7	0.016	5	0.08	0.15
8	0.032	5	0.16	0.31
9	0.064	5	0.32	0.63
10	0.128	5	0.64	1.27
11	0.256	5	1.28	2.55
12	0.512	5	2.56	5.11
13	1.024	5	5.12	10.23
14	2	5	10	20.23
15	2	10	20	40.23
16	2	20	40	80.23
17	2	40	80	160.23

From Erdem G, Staat MA, Connelly BL, et al. Anaphylactic reaction to ciprofloxacin in a toddler: Successful desensitization. *Pediatr Infect Dis J.* 1999;18(6):563–564.

*Administer doses as continuous 15-min infusions, except for the last three doses, which are given as 30-min infusions with no intervals between the doses.

B. Oral Ciprofloxacin Desensitization Protocol

Table 9-12 is an example of a successful oral ciprofloxacin desensitization protocol from a 15-year-old with cystic fibrosis experiencing urticarial reaction.[7]

TABLE 9-12

CIPROFLOXACIN ORAL DESENSITIZATION PROTOCOL

Step*	Ciprofloxacin (mg/mL)	Amount (mL)	Dose (mg)	Cumulative Dose (mg)
1	0.1	0.5	0.05	0.05
2	0.1	1	0.1	0.15
3	0.1	2	0.2	0.35
4	0.1	4	0.4	0.75
5	0.1	8	0.8	1.55
6	1	1.6	1.6	3.15
7	1	3.2	3.2	6.35
8	1	6.4	6.4	12.75
9	1	12.8	12.8	25.55
10	10	2.5	25	50.55
11	10	5	50	100.55
12	10	10	100	200.55
13	NA	1 tablet	250	450.55

From Lantner RR. Ciprofloxacin desensitization in a patient with cystic fibrosis. *J Allergy Clin Immunol.* 1995;96:1001–1002.

*Interval between doses is 15 min.

NA, Not applicable.

VI. VANCOMYCIN

Desensitization should be considered in hypersensitivity reactions, red-man syndrome that does not respond to the usual treatment measures, and vancomycin-induced anaphylaxis.[8] Concomitant use of medications that induce mast-cell degranulation may lead to an unsuccessful desensitization.[8] These medications include ciprofloxacin, barbiturates, narcotic analgesics (fentanyl rarely induces histamine release), atracurium, cisatracurium, succinylcholine, propofol, dextran, and radiocontrast agents.[8] Concurrent use of opioids has produced a synergistic response.[9]

A. Rapid Vancomycin Desensitization[10]

Rapid desensitization is the preferred method that is effective in most patients (Table 9-13). Preparation of vancomycin injections for desensitization:

1. Prepare a standard bag of vancomycin (500 mg in 250 mL normal saline [NS; NaCl 0.9%] or dextrose 5% in water [D5W]); label as infusion no. 5 (vancomycin 2 mg/mL).
2. Draw up 10 mL from infusion no. 5 (vancomycin 2 mg/mL) and place in a 100-mL bag of NS or D5W; label as infusion no. 4 (vancomycin 0.2 mg/mL).

3. Draw up 10 mL from infusion no. 4 (vancomycin 0.2 mg/mL) and place in a 100-mL bag of NS or D5W; label as infusion no. 3 (vancomycin 0.02 mg/mL).
4. Draw up 10 mL from infusion no. 3 (vancomycin 0.02 mg/mL) and place in a 100-mL bag of NS or D5W; label as infusion no. 2 (vancomycin 0.002 mg/mL).
5. Draw up 10 mL from infusion no. 2 (vancomycin 0.002 mg/mL) and place in a 100-mL bag of NS or D5W; label as infusion no. 1 (vancomycin 0.0002 mg/mL).

TABLE 9-13

RAPID VANCOMYCIN DESENSITIZATION PROTOCOL

Infusion No.	Dilution	Vancomycin Dose (mg)	Vancomycin Concentration (mg/mL)
1	1:10,000	0.02	0.0002
2	1:1000	0.2	0.002
3	1:100	2	0.02
4	1:10	10	0.2
5	Standard	500	2

From Lerner A, Dwyer JM. Desensitization to vancomycin [letter]. *Ann Intern Med.* 1984;100:157.

Infusion Directions:

1. Diphenhydramine and hydrocortisone injections are given 15 minutes before initiation of this desensitization protocol and then every 6 hours throughout the protocol.
2. Initiate infusion rate at 0.5 mL/min (30 mL/hr) and increase by 0.5 mL/min (30 mL/hr) as tolerated every 5 minutes to a maximum rate of 5 mL/min (300 mL/hr). If pruritus, hypotension, rash, or difficulty breathing occurs, stop infusion and reinfuse the previously tolerated infusion at the highest tolerated rate. This step may be repeated up to three times for any given concentration.
3. On completion of infusion no. 5, immediately administer the required dose of vancomycin in the usual dilution of NS or D5W over 2 hours. Decrease rate if patient becomes symptomatic or, alternatively, increase rate if patient tolerates dose. Administer diphenhydramine orally 60 minutes before each dose.

B. Slow Desensitization[11]

Use of slow desensitization should be reserved **only** for patients who do not respond positively to the rapid desensitization protocol (Table 9-14).

Infusion Directions:

1. Infuse each dose over 5 hours. If pruritus, hypotension, rash, or difficulty breathing occurs, stop the infusion and reinfuse the previously tolerated infusion.
2. On day 14, administer the required dose of vancomycin in the usual dilution of NS or D5W (e.g., 1000 mg in 250 mL) at a rate of 100 mL/hr. Decrease rate if patient becomes symptomatic or,

TABLE 9-14

SLOW VANCOMYCIN DESENSITIZATION PROTOCOL

Day	Infusion No.	Dose Provided	Vancomycin Dose (mg)	Concentration (mg/mL)
Premedication: Diphenhydramine 1.25 mg/kg (maximum dose 50 mg) IV 15 min before protocol initiation, then Q6 hr throughout protocol.				
1	1	0.5 mg in 500 mL	0.5	0.001
2	2	5 mg in 500 mL	5	0.01
3	3	10 mg in 500 mL	10	0.02
4	4	50 mg in 500 mL	50	0.1
5	4	50 mg in 500 mL	50	0.1
6	5	100 mg in 500 mL	100	0.2
7*	6	100 mg in 250 mL × 2	200	0.4
8	7	150 mg in 250 mL × 2	300	0.6
9	8	250 mg in 250 mL × 2	500	1
10	9	500 mg in 250 mL × 2	1000	2
11	9	500 mg in 250 mL × 2	1000	2
12	9	500 mg in 250 mL × 2	1000	2
13	10	1000 mg in 250 mL	1000	4

From Lin RY. Desensitization in the management of vancomycin hypersensitivity. *Arch Intern Med.* 1990;150:2197–2198.

*Beginning on day 7, doses infused consecutively.

IV, Intravenously.

alternatively, increase rate if patient tolerates dose. Consider oral antihistamine before each dose.

VII. AMINOGLYCOSIDES

A. Intravenous Tobramycin Desensitization Protocol

Following is an example of a successful IV tobramycin desensitization protocol from a 15-year-old with cystic fibrosis experiencing urticarial reactions to tobramycin and gentamicin.[12]

Directions (Table 9-15):

1. Each tobramycin dose should be diluted in 20 mL NS.
2. Each tobramycin dose should be infused over 20 minutes and then flushed with 10 mL NS.
3. Subsequent desensitization dosages should be given 10 minutes after the completion of the prior infusion (time from beginning of infusion to next infusion = 30 minutes).

B. Inhaled Tobramycin Desensitization Protocol

Following is an example of a successful inhaled tobramycin desensitization protocol from a 9-year-old with cystic fibrosis experiencing a rash after a course of IV gentamicin.[13]

Directions (Table 9-16):

1. Each inhaled tobramycin dose should be diluted in 5 mL NS.
2. Each dose is nebulized on an every 2-hour schedule until the full dose of 300 mg is given.

TABLE 9-15

SAMPLE INTRAVENOUS TOBRAMYCIN DESENSITIZATION PROTOCOL

Dose	Elapsed Time (hr)	Tobramycin (mg)	Cumulative Dose (mg)
1	0	0.001	0.001
2	0.5	0.002	0.003
3	1	0.004	0.007
4	1.5	0.008	0.015
5	2	0.016	0.031
6	2.5	0.032	0.063
7	3	0.064	0.127
8	3.5	0.125	0.255
9	4	0.256	0.511
10	4.5	0.512	1.023
11	5	1	2.023
12	5.5	2	4.023
13	6	4	8.023
14	6.5	8	16.023
15	7	16	32.023
16	7.5	32	64.023
17	8	16	80.023

From Earl HS, Sullivan TJ. Acute desensitization of a patient with cystic fibrosis allergic to both beta-lactam and aminoglycoside antibiotics. *J Allergy Clin Immunol.* 1987;79:477–483.

TABLE 9-16

INHALED TOBRAMYCIN DESENSITIZATION PROTOCOL

Treatment No.	Dose (mg)
1	0.3
2	0.6
3	0.9
4	1.2
5	1.5
6	3
7	6
8	12
9	24
10	48
11	96
12	150
13	200
14	250
15	300

From Spigarelli MG, Hurwitz ME, Nasr SZ. Hypersensitivity to inhaled TOBI following reaction to gentamicin. *Pediatr Pulmonol.* 2002;33:311–314.

VIII. CLINDAMYCIN

Clindamycin is not a frequent cause of drug hypersensitivity reactions. Therefore, there is limited data on managing patients who have these reactions to clindamycin.[14] Table 9-17 is an example of a successful oral clindamycin desensitization protocol from a 35-year-old patient with HIV with toxoplasmic encephalitis who experienced a generalized cutaneous eruption with clindamycin.[14]

TABLE 9-17

ORAL CLINDAMYCIN DESENSITIZATION PROTOCOL

Day	Doses* (mg)
1	20, 20, 20
2	40, 40, 40
3	80, 80, 80
4	150, 150, 150
5	300, 300, 300
6	600, 600, 600
7	600, 600, 600, 600

From Marcos C, Sopena B, Luna I, et al. Clindamycin desensitization in an AIDS patient. *AIDS.* 1995;9:1201–1202.
*Interval between doses is 8 hours.

9

IX. LINEZOLID

Patients with multidrug-resistant infections and hypersensitivity to linezolid may benefit from linezolid desensitization. Table 9-18 is an example of a successful oral linezolid desensitization protocol from a 41-year-old with a multidrug-resistant bacteremia who experienced a hypersensitivity reaction consistent with an IgE-mediated response to her first dose of linezolid. In this protocol, the IV formulation of linezolid was given orally because of lack of IV access and unavailability of an oral solution.[15] The first 12 doses were compounded from a premixed IV solution of linezolid 600 mg/300 mL, with sterile water for injection added for a final volume of each dose of at least 2 mL. One milliliter simple syrup was added to doses 10 to 12 to enhance palatability. Doses 13 and 14 were provided by splitting a 600 mg tablet.[15]

X. DARUNAVIR

Drug hypersensitivity reactions can be an issue in managing HIV-positive patients. Table 9-19 is an example of a successful oral darunavir desensitization protocol from a 17-year-old HIV-positive patient who had experienced a pruritic papular erythematous eruption on darunavir.[16] An initial dose of ritonavir 100 mg was given before the first darunavir dose of the desensitization protocol.[16] Doses one to five were provided by dissolving darunavir in saline to a concentration of 20 mcg/mL.[16]

TABLE 9-18

ORAL LINEZOLID DESENSITIZATION PROTOCOL

Dose No.*	Dose (mg)	Final Volume (mL)
1	0.0366	2
2	0.0732	2
3	0.146	2
4	0.293	2
5	0.586	2
6	1.17	2
7	2.34	3
8	4.69	5
9	9.38	10
10	18.8	15
11	37.5	25
12	75	50
13	200	NA (use 1/3 of 600 mg tablet)
14	400	NA (use 2/3 of 600 mg tablet)

From Cawley MJ, Lipka O. Intravenous linezolid administered orally: A novel desensitization strategy. *Pharmacotherapy.* 2006;26(4):563–568.

*Goal interval between doses is 20 minutes.

NA, Not applicable.

TABLE 9-19

ORAL DARUNAVIR DESENSITIZATION PROTOCOL

Dose No.*	Dose Administered
1	25 mcg
2	250 mcg
3	500 mcg
4	1 mg
5	2 mg
6	5 mg
7	10 mg
8	25 mg
9	50 mg
10	100 mg
11	200 mg
12	300 mg

From Marcos Bravo MC, Ocampo Hermida A, Martinez Vilela J, et al. Hypersensitivity reaction to darunavir and desensitization protocol. *J Investig Allergol Clin Immunol.* 2009;19(3):250–251.

*Interval between doses is 30 minutes.

REFERENCES

1. Solensky R. Drug desensitization. *Immunol Allergy Clin N Am.* 2004;24: 425–443.
2. Sullivan TJ. Drug allergy. In: Middleton E, Reed CE, Ellis EF, et al, eds. *Allergy: Principles and Practice.* 4th ed. St. Louis, MO: Mosby; 1993:1726–1746.
3. Solensky R. Desensitization with antibiotics. In: Pichler WJ, ed. *Drug Hypersensitivity.* Basel, Switzerland: Karger; 2007:404–412.
4. Win PH, Brown H, Zankar A, et al. Rapid intravenous cephalosporin desensitization. *J Allergy Clin Immunol.* 2005;116(1):225–227.
5. Gluckstein D, Ruskin J. Rapid oral desensitization to trimethoprim-sulfamethoxazole (TMP-SMZ): Use in prophylaxis for *Pneumocystis carinii* pneumonia in patients with AIDS who were previously intolerant to TMP-SMZ. *Clin Infect Dis.* 1995;20:849–853.
6. Erdem G, Staat MA, Connelly BL, et al. Anaphylactic reaction to ciprofloxacin in a toddler: Successful desensitization. *Pediatr Infect Dis J.* 1999;18(6):563–564.
7. Lantner RR. Ciprofloxacin desensitization in a patient with cystic fibrosis. *J Allergy Clin Immunol.* 1995;96:1001–1002.
8. Wazny LD, Daghigh B. Desensitization protocols for vancomycin hypersenstivity. *Ann Pharmacother.* 2001;35(11):1458–1464.
9. Wong JT, Ripple RE, MacLean JA, et al. Vancomycin hypersensitivity: Synergism with narcotics and desensitization by a rapid continuous intravenous protocol. *J Allergy Clin Immunol.* 1994;94(2):189–194.
10. Lerner A, Dwyer JM. Desensitization to vancomycin [letter]. *Ann Intern Med.* 1984;100:157.
11. Lin RY. Desensitization in the management of vancomycin hypersensitivity. *Arch Intern Med.* 1990;150:2197–2198.
12. Earl HS, Sullivan TJ. Acute desensitization of a patient with cystic fibrosis allergic to both beta-lactam and aminoglycoside antibiotics. *J Allergy Clin Immunol.* 1987;79:477–483.
13. Spigarelli MG, Hurwitz ME, Nasr SZ. Hypersensitivity to inhaled TOBI® following reaction to gentamicin. *Pediatr Pulmonol.* 2002;33:311–314.
14. Marcos C, Sopena B, Luna I, et al. Clindamycin desensitization in an AIDS patient. *AIDS.* 1995;9:1201–1202.
15. Cawley MJ, Lipka O. Intravenous linezolid administered orally: A novel desensitization strategy. *Pharmacotherapy.* 2006;26(4):563–568.
16. Marcos Bravo MC, Ocampo Hermida A, Martinez Vilela J, et al. Hypersensitivity reaction to darunavir and desensitization protocol. *J Investig Allergol Clin Immunol.* 2009;19(3):250–251.

Chapter 10

Formulary

Carlton K. K. Lee, PharmD, MPH

I. NOTE TO READER

The author has made every attempt to check dosages and medical content for accuracy. Because of the incomplete data on pediatric dosing, many drug dosages may be modified after the publication of this text. We recommend that the reader check product information and published literature for changes in dosing, especially for newer medicines. The Food and Drug Administration (FDA) provides the following Pediatric Drug Information data sources:

New Pediatric Labeling Information:
www.accessdata.fda.gov/scripts/sda/sdNavigation.cfm?sd=labelingdatabase

Drug Safety Reporting Updates:
www.fda.gov/ScienceResearch/SpecialTopics/PediatricTherapeuticsResearch/ucm123229.htm

Pediatric Study Characteristics Database:
www.accessdata.fda.gov/scripts/sda/sdNavigation.cfm?sd=fdaaadescriptorssortablewebdatabase

To prevent prescribing errors, the use of abbreviations has been greatly discouraged. Following is a list of abbreviations The Joint Commission considers prohibited for use.

THE JOINT COMMISSION

Official "Do Not Use" List*

Do Not Use	Potential Problem	Use Instead
U (unit)	Mistaken for "0" (zero), the numeral "4" (four), or "cc"	Write "unit"
IU (International Unit)	Mistaken for "IV" (intravenous) or the number 10 (ten)	Write "International Unit"
Q.D., QD, q.d., qd (daily) Q.O.D., QOD, q.o.d., qod (every other day)	Mistaken for each other Period after the Q mistaken for "I" and the "O" mistaken for "I"	Write "daily" Write "every other day"
Trailing zero (X.0 mg)[†] Lack of leading zero (.X mg)	Decimal point is missed	Write "X mg" Write "0.X mg"
MS MSO_4 and $MgSO_4$	Can mean "morphine sulfate" or "magnesium sulfate"	Write "morphine sulfate" Write "magnesium sulfate"

*Applies to all orders and all medication-related documentation that is handwritten (including free-text computer entry) or on preprinted forms.

[†]**Exception:** A "trailing zero" may be used only where required to demonstrate the level of precision of the value being reported, such as for laboratory results, imaging studies that report size of lesions, or catheter/tube sizes. It may not be used in medication orders or other medication-related documentation.

Additional Abbreviations, Acronyms, and Symbols for *Possible* Future Inclusion in the Official "Do Not Use" List

Do Not Use	Potential Problem	Use Instead
> (greater than) < (less than)	Misinterpreted as the number "7" or the letter "L" Confused for one another	Write "greater than" Write "less than"
Abbreviations for drug names	Misinterpreted because of similar abbreviations for multiple drugs	Write drug names in full
Apothecary units	Unfamiliar to many practitioners Confused with metric units	Use metric units
@	Mistaken for the numeral "2" (two)	Write "at"
cc	Mistaken for U (units) when poorly written	Write "mL" or "ml" or "milliliters" ("mL" is preferred)
μg	Mistaken for mg (milligrams) resulting in 1000-fold overdose	Write "mcg" or "micrograms"

II. SAMPLE ENTRY

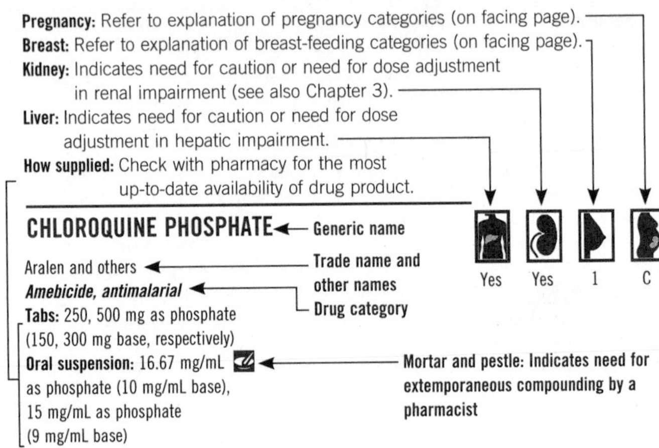

Doses expressed in milligrams of chloroquine base:

Malaria prophylaxis (start 1 week before exposure and continue for 4 weeks after leaving endemic area):

Infant and child: 5 mg/kg/dose PO every wk; **max. dose:** 300 mg/dose

Adult: 300 mg/dose PO every wk

Malaria treatment (chloroquine-sensitive strains):

For treatment for malaria, consult with ID specialist or see the latest edition of the *AAP Red Book*.

Infant and child: 10 mg/kg/dose (**max. dose:** 600 mg/dose) PO × 1; followed by 5 mg/kg/dose (**max. dose:** 300 mg/dose) 6 hr later and then once daily for 2 days

Adult: 600 mg/dose PO × 1; followed by 300 mg/dose 6 hr later and then once daily for 2 days

Drug dosing

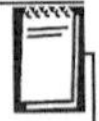

Contraindications: Hypersensitivity to 4-aminoquinoline compounds and retinal/visual changes

Warnings/Precautions: Use with **caution** in liver disease, preexisting auditory damage or seizures, G6PD deficiency, psoriasis, porphyria, or concomitant hepatotoxic drugs. **Adjust dose in renal failure (see Chapter 3).**

Adverse effects: ECG abnormalities, prolonged QT interval, pruritus, GI disturbances, increased liver enzymes, skeletal muscle weakness, amnesia, blurred vision, retinal changes, and corneal changes. Headaches, TEN, Stevens–Johnson syndrome, reversible corneal opacities, confusion, and hair depigmentation have been reported.

Drug interactions: Chloroquine is a substrate for CYP 450 2D6 and 3A4, and inhibitor of CYP 2D6. Antacids, ampicillin, and kaolin may decrease the absorption of chloroquine (allow 4-hour interval between these drugs and chloroquine). May increase serum cyclosporine levels. Cimetidine may increase effects/toxicity of chloroquine. May increase cyclosporine levels. Use with mefloquine may increase risk for convulsions. May reduce the antibody response to intradermal human diploid-cell rabies vaccine.

Drug administration: Administer oral doses with meals to reduce GI complications. Mixing tablets with chocolate syrup or placing tablets in capsules may be used to mask bitter-tasting tablets.

Brief remarks about contraindications, warning/precautions (including therapeutic drug monitoring), adverse effects, drug interactions, and drug administration.

III. EXPLANATION OF BREAST-FEEDING CATEGORIES

See sample entry.

1 Compatible
2 Use with caution
3 Unknown with concerns
X Contraindicated
? Safety not established

IV. EXPLANATION OF PREGNANCY CATEGORIES

A Adequate studies in pregnant women have not demonstrated a risk to the fetus in the first trimester of pregnancy, and there is no evidence of risk in later trimesters.

B Animal studies have not demonstrated a risk to the fetus, but there are no adequate studies in pregnant women; or animal studies have shown an adverse effect, but adequate studies in pregnant women have not demonstrated a risk to the fetus during the first trimester of pregnancy, and there is no evidence of risk in later trimesters.

C Animal studies have shown an adverse effect on the fetus, but there are no adequate studies in humans; or there are no animal reproduction studies and no adequate studies in humans.

D There is evidence of human fetal risk, but the potential benefits from the use of the drug in pregnant women may be acceptable despite its potential risks.

X Studies in animals or humans demonstrate fetal abnormalities or adverse reaction; reports indicate evidence of fetal risk. The risk of use in pregnant women clearly outweighs any possible benefit.

V. DRUG INDEX

Trade Name(s)	Generic Name
1-Day	Tioconazole
3TC*	Lamivudine
5-FC*, 5-Fluorocytosine	Flucytosine
A-200	Pyrethrins with piperonyl butoxide
ABCD*	Amphotericin B cholesteryl sulfate
Abelcet	Amphotericin B lipid complex
ABLC*	Amphotericin B lipid complex
Abreva	Docosanol
Acticin	Permethrin
Aczone	Dapsone
Aftate	Tolnaftate
Agenerase	Amprenavir
AK-Poly-Bac Ophthalmic	Bacitracin + polymyxin B
AK-Spore H.C. Otic	Polymyxin B sulfate, neomycin sulfate, and hydrocortisone
AKTob	Tobramycin
AK-Tracin Ophthalmic	Bacitracin
Albenza	Albendazole
Aldara	Imiquimod
Alinia	Nitazoxanide
Altabax	Retapamulin
AmBisome	Amphotericin B, liposomal
Amikin	Amikacin sulfate
Aminosalicylic acid	Para-aminosalicylic acid
Amoclan	Amoxicillin with clavulanic acid
Amoxil	Amoxicillin
Amphocin	Amphotericin B
Amphotec	Amphotericin B cholesteryl sulfate
Ancef	Cefazolin
Ancobon	Flucytosine
Antiminth	Pyrantel pamoate
Antrypol	Suramin
Aptivus	Tipranavir
APV*	Amprenavir
Aralen	Chloroquine HCL/Phosphate
Arestin	Minocycline
Arsobal	Melarsoprol
Arsobal	Suramin
ATV*	Atazanavir
Augmentin, Augmentin ES-600, Augmentin XR	Amoxicillin with clavulanic acid
Avagard	Chlorhexidine gluconate
AVC Vaginal	Sulfanilamide
Avelox, Avelox IV	Moxifloxacin
Azactam	Aztreonam
Azasite	Azithromycin
AZT*	Zidovudine

*Common abbreviation or other name (not recommended for use when writing a prescription).

Trade Name(s)	Generic Name
Azo-Urinary Pain Relief	Phenazopyridine HCl
BabyBIG	Botulinum immune globulin intravenous, human
Baciguent Topical	Bacitracin
BACiiM	Bacitracin
Bactoshield	Chlorhexidine gluconate
Bactrim	Sulfamethoxazole and trimethoprim
Bactroban, Bactroban Nasal	Mupirocin
Baraclude	Entecavir
Bayer 205	Suramin
Bayer 2502	Nifurtimox
Behenyl alcohol	Docosanol
Belganyl	Suramin
Besivance	Besifloxacin
Betasept	Chlorhexidine gluconate
Biaxin, Biaxin XL	Clarithromycin
Bicillin C-R, Bicillin C-R 900/300	Penicillin G preparations—Penicillin G benzathine and Penicillin G procaine
Bicillin L-A	Penicillin G preparations—Benzathine
BIG-IV	Botulinum immune globulin intravenous, human
Biltricide	Praziquantel
Bleph 10	Sulfacetamide sodium, ophthalmic
Caldesene	Undecylenic acid
Cancidas	Caspofungin
Capastat	Capreomycin
Carbamazine	Diethylcarbamazine
Cayston	Aztreonam
Ceclor, Ceclor CD	Cefaclor
Cedax	Ceftibuten
Cefotan	Cefotetan
Ceftin	Cefuroxime axetil (PO)
Cefzil	Cefprozil
Ceptaz (arginine salt)	Ceftazidime
Cetraxal	Ciprofloxacin
Chloromycetin	Chloramphenicol
Ciclodan	Ciclopirox/ciclopirox olamine
Ciloxan ophthalmic	Ciprofloxacin
Cipro, Cipro XR, Ciprodex, Cipro HC Otic	Ciprofloxacin
Claforan	Cefotaxime
Cleocin, Cleocin-T	Clindamycin
Coartem	Artemether with lumefantrine
Colistin, Colistin Sodium Methanesulfonate	Colistimethate sodium
Coly-Mycin M Parenteral	Colistimethate sodium
Coly-Mycin S Otic with Neomycin and Hydrocortisone	Neomycin/Colistin/Hydrocortisone
Condylox	Podofilox
Copegus	Ribavirin
Cortisporin Otic	Neomycin/Polymyxin B/Hydrocortisone

*Common abbreviation or other name (not recommended for use when writing a prescription).

Trade Name(s)	Generic Name
Cortisporin Otic	Polymyxin B sulfate, neomycin sulfate, and hydrocortisone
Cortisporin TC Otic	Neomycin/Colistin/Hydrocortisone
Cortomycin	Neomycin/Polymyxin B/Hydrocortisone
Cortomycin	Polymyxin B sulfate, neomycin sulfate, and hydrocortisone
Crixivan	Indinavir
Cruex	Clotrimazole
Cruex	Undecylenic acid
Cubicin	Daptomycin
CytoGam	Cytomegalovirus immune globulin
Cytovene	Ganciclovir
d4T*	Stavudine
Daraprim	Pyrimethamine
ddI*	Didanosine
DDS*	Dapsone
DEC*	Diethylcarbamazine
Declomycin	Demeclocycline
Declostatin	Demeclocycline
Denavir	Penciclovir
Diaminodiphenylsulfone	Dapsone
Dideoxyinosine	Didanosine
Diethylcarbamazine citrate	Diethylcarbamazine
Dificid	Fidaxomicin
Diflucan	Fluconazole
Diiodhydroxyquin	Iodoquinol
Diiodohydroxyquinoline	Iodoquinol
Diquinol	Iodoquinol
DLV*	Delavirdine
DMP-266*	Efavirenz
Doribax	Doripenem
DRV*	Darunavir
Duricef	Cefadroxil
Dycill	Dicloxacillin sodium
Dynacin	Minocycline
Dyna-Hex	Chlorhexidine gluconate
Edurant	Rilpivirine
Elimite	Permethrin
Elon Dual Defense Anti-Fungal Formula	Undecylenic acid
Emtriva	Emtricitabine
E-Mycin	Erythromycin preparations
Epivir, Epivir-HBV	Lamivudine
Eraxis	Anidulafungin
Ertaczo	Sertaconazole nitrate
Ery-Ped	Erythromycin preparations
Erythrocin	Erythromycin preparations
Eryzole	Erythromycin ethylsuccinate and acetylsulfisoxazole

*Common abbreviation or other name (not recommended for use when writing a prescription).

Trade Name(s)	Generic Name
Exelderm	Sulconazole
Extina	Ketoconazole
Factive	Gemifloxacin
Famvir	Famciclovir
f-APV*	Fosamprenavir
Flagyl, Flagyl ER	Metronidazole
Floxin, Floxin Otic	Ofloxacin
Flumadine	Rimantadine
Fortaz	Ceftazidime
Foscavir	Foscarnet
Fourneau 309	Suramin
FTC*	Emtricitabine
Fungizone	Amphotericin B
Fungoid AF	Undecylenic acid
Furadantin	Nitrofurantoin
Fuzeon	Enfuvirtide
Gamma benzene hexachloride	Lindane
Garamycin	Gentamicin
Germanin	Suramin
Goordochom	Undecylenic acid
Grifulvin V	Griseofulvin
Grisactin	Griseofulvin
Griseofulvin Microsize	Griseofulvin
Gris-PEG	Griseofulvin
Gyne-Lotrimin 3	Clotrimazole
Gyne-Lotrimin 7	Clotrimazole
HBIG*	Hepatitis B immune globulin
HepaGam	B Hepatitis B immune globulin
Hespera	Adefovir/dipivoxil
Hetrazan	Diethylcarbamazine
Hibiclens	Chlorhexidine gluconate
Hiprex	Methenamine hippurate
Humatin	Paromomycin sulfate
HyperHEP B S/D	Hepatitis B immune globulin
HyperRAB S/D	Rabies immune globulin (human)
HyperTET S/D	Tetanus immune globulin
IDV*	Indinavir
Imogam Rabies-HT	Rabies immune globulin (human)
Incivek	Telaprevir
INH*	Isoniazid
Intelence	Etravirine
Invanz	Ertapenem
Invirase	Saquinavir mesylate
losat	Potassium iodide
Iquix	Levofloxacin
Isentress	Raltegravir
Kaletra	Lopinavir with ritonavir
Kantrex	Kanamycin

*Common abbreviation or other name (not recommended for use when writing a prescription).

Trade Name(s)	Generic Name
Keflex	Cephalexin
Ketek	Telithromycin
Klout	Pyrethrins with piperonyl butoxide
Lamisil, Lamisil AT	Terbinafine
Lampit	Nifurtimox
Lamprene	Clofazimine
Laniazid	Isoniazid
Lariam	Mefloquine HCL
Levaquin	Levofloxacin
Lexiva	Fosamprenavir
Loprox	Ciclopirox/Ciclopirox olamine
Lotrimim Ultra	Butenafine
Lotrimin AF	Miconazole
Lotrimin AF	Clotrimazole
LPV/RTV*	Lopinavir with ritonavir
Macrobid	Nitrofurantoin
Macrodantin	Nitrofurantoin
Malarone Pediatric Tablets, Malarone Tablets	Atovaquone + proguanil
Maxipime	Cefepime
Mefoxin	Cefoxitin
Mel B	Melarsoprol
Mel B	Suramin
Melarsen Oxide-BAL	Melarsoprol
Mentax	Butenafine
Mepron	Atovaquone
Merrem	Meropenem
Methenamine Mandelate	Methenamine preparations
MetroGel, MetroLotion, MetroCream, MetroGel-Vaginal	Metronidazole
Micatin	Miconazole
Minocin	Minocycline
Monistat	Miconazole
Monurol	Fosfomycin tromethamine
Moranyl	Suramin
Moxatag	Amoxicillin
Moxeza	Moxifloxacin
Myambutol	Ethambutol HCL
Mycamine	Micafungin sodium
Mycelex, Mycelex-7	Clotrimazole
Mycifradin	Neomycin sulfate
Mycobutin	Rifabutin
Mycostatin	Nystatin
Nabi-HB	Hepatitis B immune globulin
Naftin Cream, Naftin Gel	Naftifine
Nallpen	Nafcillin
Naphuride	Suramin
Natacyn	Natamycin
Natroba	Spinosad

*Common abbreviation or other name (not recommended for use when writing a prescription).

Trade Name(s)	Generic Name
Nebcin	Tobramycin
NebuPent	Pentamidine isethionate
Neo-Fradin, Neo-Tabs	Neomycin sulfate
Neosporin, Neo To Go, Neo-Polycin, Neosporin Ophthalmic	Neomycin/Polymyxin B/+ Bacitracin
Neosporin GU Irrigant	Neomycin/Polymyxin B/± Bacitracin
NeuTrexin	Trimetrexate glucuronate
NFV*	Nelfinavir
Nilstat	Nystatin
Nix	Permethrin
Nizoral, Nizoral A-D	Ketoconazole
Noritate	Metronidazole
Noroxin	Norfloxacin
Norvir	Ritonavir
Noxafil	Posaconazole
NVP*	Nevirapine
Nydrazid	Isoniazid
Ocuflox	Ofloxacin
Omnicef	Cefdinir
Omnipen	Ampicillin
Ovide	Malathion
Oxistat	Oxiconazole
Pamix	Pyrantel pamoate
PAS*	Para-aminosalicylic acid
Paser Granules	Para-aminosalicylic acid
Pathocil	Dicloxacillin sodium
Pediamycin	Erythromycin preparations
Pediazole	Erythromycin ethylsuccinate and acetylsulfisoxazole
PediOtic	Polymyxin B sulfate, neomycin sulfate, and hydrocortisone
Penlac	Ciclopirox/Ciclopirox olamine
Pentam 300	Pentamidine isethionate
Pentavalent antimony	Stibogluconate
Pentostam	Stibogluconate
Peridex	Chlorhexidine gluconate
PerioGard	Chlorhexidine gluconate
Periostat	Doxycycline
Pfizerpen	Penicillin G preparations—Aqueous potassium and sodium
pHisoHex	Hexachlorophene
Pima	Potassium iodide
Pin-Rid	Pyrantel pamoate
Pin-X	Pyrantel pamoate
Pipracil	Piperacillin
Plaquenil	Hydroxychloroquine
PMPA*	Tenofovir disoproxil fumarate
Podocon-25	Podophyllin/Podophyllum resin

*Common abbreviation or other name (not recommended for use when writing a prescription).

Trade Name(s)	Generic Name
Polymox	Amoxicillin
Polysporin Ophthalmic, Polysporin Topical	Bacitracin + polymyxin B
Polytrim Ophthalmic Solution	Polymyxin B sulfate and bacitracin
Prezista	Darunavir
Priftin	Rifapentine
Primaxin IV	Imipenem-Cilastatin
Primsol	Trimethoprim
Principen	Ampicillin
Proloprim	Trimethoprim
Pronto	Pyrethrins with piperonyl butoxide
Prostat	Metronidazole
Pyrazinoic acid amide	Pyrazinamide
Pyridium	Phenazopyridine HCL
Qualaquin	Quinine sulfate
Quixin	Levofloxacin
Raniclor	Cefaclor
Rebetol	Ribavirin
Reese's Pinworm	Pyrantel pamoate
Relenza	Zanamivir
Rescriptor	Delavirdine
Retrovir	Zidovudine
Reyataz	Atazanavir
Ribasphere	Ribavirin
Ribasphere RibaPak	Ribavirin
RID	Pyrethrins with piperonyl butoxide
Rifadin	Rifampin
Rimactane	Rifampin
Rocephin	Ceftriaxone
Selsun	Selenium sulfide
Selzentry	Maraviroc
Septra	Sulfamethoxazole and trimethoprim
Seromycin	Cycloserine
Silvadene	Silver sulfadiazine
Sinecatechins	Kunecatechins
Solodyn	Minocycline
Spectazole	Econazole nitrate
Spectracef	Cefditoren pivoxil
Sporanox	Itraconazole
SSD Cream, SSD AF Cream	Silver sulfadiazine
SSKI	Potassium iodide
Stromectol	Ivermectin
Sulfamide	Sulfacetamide sodium, ophthalmic
Sulfatrim	Sulfamethoxazole and trimethoprim
Suprax	Cefixime
Sustiva	Efavirenz
Symmetrel	Amantadine hydrochloride
Synagis	Palivizumab
Synercid	Quinupristin with dalfopristin

*Common abbreviation or other name (not recommended for use when writing a prescription).

Trade Name(s)	Generic Name
T-20*	Enfuvirtide
Tamiflu	Oseltamivir phosphate
Tazicef	Ceftazidime
Tazidime	Ceftazidime
TDF*	Tenofovir disoproxil fumarate
Teflaro	Cefteroline fosamil
Terazol 3, Terazol 7	Terconazole
Terbinex	Terbinafine
Thalomid	Thalidomide
Thermazene	Silver sulfadiazine
ThyroSafe	Potassium iodide
ThyroShield	Potassium iodide
Timentin	Ticarcillin with clavulanate
Tinactin	Tolnaftate
Tindamax	Tinidazole
Tisit	Pyrethrins with piperonyl butoxide
TMC 114*	Darunavir
TMC 125	Etravirine
TMP*	Trimethoprim
TMP-SMX*	Sulfamethoxazole and trimethoprim
TOBI	Tobramycin
Tobrex	Tobramycin
Totacillin	Ampicillin
TPV*	Tipranavir
Trecator	Ethionamide
Trifluorothymidine	Trifluridine
Trimethoprim-sulfamethoxazole	Sulfamethoxazole and trimethoprim
Trimox	Amoxicillin
Trobicin	Spectinomycin
Tygacil	Tigecycline
Tyzeka	Telbivudine
Ulesfia	Benzyl alcohol
Unasyn	Ampicillin with sulbactam
Unipen	Nafcillin
Urex	Methenamine hippurate
Uroqid#2	Methenamine mendelate
Vagistat-1	Tioconazole
Vagistat-3	Miconazole
Valcyte	Valganciclovir
Valtrex	Valacyclovir
Vancocin	Vancomycin
Vantin	Cefpodoxime proxetil
VariZig	Varicella-Zoster immune globulin (human)
Veetids	Penicillin V potassium
Veregen	Kunecatechins
Vermox	Mebendazole
Vfend	Voriconazole
Vibativ	Telavancin

*Common abbreviation or other name (not recommended for use when writing a prescription).

Trade Name(s)	Generic Name
Vibramycin	Doxycycline
Victrelis	Boceprevir
Videx, Videx EC	Didanosine
Vigamox	Moxifloxacin
Viracept	Nelfinavir
Viramune, Viramune XR	Nevirapine
Virazole	Ribavirin
Viread	Tenofovir disoproxil fumarate
Viroptic	Trifluridine
Vistide	Cidofovir
Vitrasert	Ganciclovir
VZIG*	Varicella-Zoster immune globulin (human)
Wycillin	Penicillin G preparations—Procaine
Wymox	Amoxicillin
Xifaxan	Rifaximin
Xolegel	Ketoconazole
Yodoxin	Iodoquinol
Zerit	Stavudine
Zinacef	Cefuroxime (IV, IM)
Zirgan	Ganciclovir
Zithromax, Zithromax TRI-PAK	Azithromycin
Zolicef	Cefazolin
Zosyn	Piperacillin/Tazobactam
Zovirax	Acyclovir
Z-PAK, Zmax	Azithromycin
Zymaxid	Gatifloxacin
Zyvox	Linezolid

*Common abbreviation or other name (not recommended for use when writing a prescription).

ABACAVIR SULFATE
Ziagen, 1592
In combination with lamivudine: Epzicom
In combination with zidovudine and lamivudine: Trizivir
Antiviral, nucleoside analogue reverse transcriptase inhibitor

Yes No 3 C

Tabs: 300 mg (scored)
Oral solution: 20 mg/mL (240 mL)
In combination with lamivudine (3TC) as Epzicom:
Tabs: 600 mg abacavir + 300 mg lamivudine
In combination with zidovudine (AZT) and lamivudine (3TC) as Trizivir:
Tabs: 300 mg abacavir + 300 mg zidovudine + 150 mg lamivudine

Use in combination with other HIV antiretroviral agents.
Infant 1–3 mo (investigational dose): 8 mg/kg/dose PO BID
≥3 mo–16 yr (see remarks): 8 mg/kg/dose PO BID; **max dose:** 300 mg BID. Clinically stable patients with undetectable viral load and stable CD4 count may consider using a once daily regimen of 16–20 mg/kg/24 hr PO (**max. dose:** 600 mg).
≥16 yr and adult: 600 mg/24 hr PO ÷ once daily–BID
Mild hepatic impairment (Child-Pugh score 5 to 6): 200 mg PO BID
Alternative dosing using 300 mg tablet dosage form for patients ≥14 kg:
14–21 kg: 150 mg PO BID
>21 to < 30 kg: 150 mg PO every morning and 300 mg PO every evening
≥30 kg: 300 mg PO BID
Epzicom (see remarks):
≥16 yr and adult: 1 tablet PO once daily
Trizivir (see remarks):
Adolescent and adult (≥40 kg): 1 tablet PO BID

Contraindications: Hypersensitivity to abacavir or any other components in the formulation; moderate/severe hepatic impairment.

Warnings/Precautions: Patients with the HLA-B*5701 allele should not be given abacavir due to the risk for hypersensitivity reactions; therapy-naïve patients should be tested for the allele prior to therapy. Fatal hypersensitivity reaction (5%) is characterized by a sign or symptom in 2 or more of the following groups: (1) fever; (2) skin rash; (3) gastrointestinal, including nausea, vomiting, diarrhea, or abdominal pain; (4) constitutional, including malaise, fatigue, or achiness; and (5) respiratory, including cough, dyspnea, and pharyngitis. Discontinue use of drug as soon as hypersensitivity reaction is suspected, and monitor closely. **Do not** restart medication following hypersensitivity reaction, because more severe life-threatening symptoms will recur.

Suboptimal virologic response has been reported with once daily three-drug combination therapy with lamivudine and tenofovir in therapy-naïve adults.

Use of combination products: For Epzicom: **do not** use in patients with creatinine clearance <50 mL/min. For Trizivir, **do not** use in patients with creatinine clearance <50 mL/min or patients with impaired hepatic function. No dosing information is currently available for children with mild hepatic impairment. See http://aidsinfo.nih.gov/guidelines for the latest information

Adverse Effects: In addition to hypersensitivity (see Warnings/Precautions), nausea, vomiting, diarrhea, mild hyperglycemia (more common in children), mild triglyceride elevation, decreased appetite, and insomnia may occur. Lactic acidosis and severe hepatomegaly with steatosis have also been reported.

Drug Interactions: Ethanol decreases the elimination of abacavir. Abacavir may increase the clearance of methadone.

Drug Administration: Doses may be administered with food or on an empty stomach.

For explanation of icons, see p. 364.

ACYCLOVIR
Zovirax and other generics
Antiviral

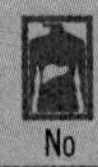
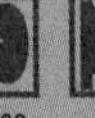
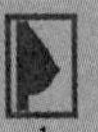
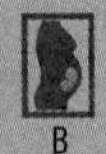
No Yes 1 B

Capsules: 200 mg
Tabs: 400, 800 mg
Oral suspension: 200 mg/5 mL (473 mL); may contain parabens
Ointment: 5% (15, 30 g)
Cream: 5% (2, 5 g)
Injection in powder (with sodium): 500, 1000 mg
Injection in solution (with sodium): 50 mg/mL
Contains 4.2 mEq Na/1 g drug

IMMUNOCOMPETENT:
Neonatal (HSV and HSV encephalitis; birth to 3 mo):
<35 wk postconceptional age: 40 mg/kg/24 hr ÷ Q12 hr IV × 14–21 days
≥35 wk postconceptional age: 60 mg/kg/24 hr ÷ Q8 hr IV × 14–21 days
Oral therapy for HSV suppression and neurodevelopment after treatment with IV acyclovir for 14–21 days: 300 mg/m²/dose Q8 hr PO × 6 mo
HSV encephalitis (duration of therapy: 14–21 days):
Birth to 3 mo: Use above IV dosage.
3 mo–12 yr: 60 mg/kg/24 hr ÷ Q8 hr IV; some experts recommend 45 mg/kg/24 hr ÷ Q8 hr IV
≥12 yr: 30 mg/kg/24 hr ÷ Q8 hr IV
Mucocutaneous HSV (including genital, ≥12 yr):
Initial infection:
IV: 15 mg/kg/24 hr or 750 mg/m²/24 hr ÷ Q8 hr × 5–7 days
PO: 1000–1200 mg/24 hr ÷ 3–5 doses per 24 hr × 7–10 days. For pediatric dosing, use 40–80 mg/kg/24 hr ÷ Q6–8 hr × 5–10 days (**max. pediatric dose:** 1000 mg/24 hr)
Recurrence (≥12 yr):
PO: 1000 mg/24 hr ÷ 5 doses per 24 hr × 5 days, or 1600 mg/24 hr ÷ Q12 hr × 5 days, or 2400 mg/24 hr ÷ Q8 hr × 2 days
Chronic suppressive therapy (≥12 yr):
PO: 800 mg/24 hr ÷ Q12 hr for up to 1 year
Zoster:
IV (all ages): 30 mg/kg/24 hr or 1500 mg/m²/24 hr ÷ Q8 hr × 7–10 days
PO (≥12 yr): 4000 mg/24 hr ÷ 5×/24 hr × 5–7 days
Varicella:
IV(≥2 yr): 30 mg/kg/24 hr or 1500 mg/m²/24 hr ÷ Q8 hr × 7–10 days
PO (≥2 yr): 80 mg/kg/24 hr ÷ four times a day × 5 days (begin treatment at earliest signs/symptoms); **max. dose:** 3200 mg/24 hr
Max. dose of oral acyclovir in children = 80 mg/kg/24 hr.
IMMUNOCOMPROMISED:
HSV:
IV (all ages): 750–1500 mg/m²/24 hr ÷ Q8 hr × 7–14 days
PO (≥2 yr): 1000 mg/24 hr ÷ 3–5 times/24 hr × 7–14 days; **max. dose** for child: 80 mg/kg/24 hr
HSV prophylaxis:
IV (all ages): 750 mg/ m²/24 hr ÷ Q8 hr during risk period
PO (≥2 yr): 600–1000 mg/24 hr ÷ 3–5 times/24 hr during risk period; **max. dose** for child: 80 mg/kg/24 hr

Continued

ACYCLOVIR *continued*

Varicella or zoster:

IV (all ages): 1500 mg/m^2/24 hr ÷ Q8 hr × 7–10 days

PO (consider using valacyclovir or famciclovir for better absorption):

Infant and child: 20 mg/kg/dose (**max. dose:** 800 mg) Q6 hr × 7–10 days

Adolescent and adult: 20 mg/kg/dose (**max. dose:** 800 mg) 5 times daily × 7–10 days

Max. dose of oral acyclovir in children = 80 mg/kg/24 hr.

TOPICAL:

Apply 0.5-inch ribbon of 5% ointment for 4-inch square surface area 6 times a day × 7 days.

Contraindications: Hypersensitivity to acyclovir or any other of its components

Warnings/Precautions: Use with **caution** in patients with preexisting neurologic or renal impairment **(adjust dose; see Chapter 3)** or dehydration. **Do not** use topical product on the eye or for the prevention of recurrent HSV infections.

Resistant strains of HSV and VZV have been reported in **immunocompromised** patients (e.g., advanced HIV infection). See most recent edition of the *AAP Red Book* for additional information.

Use ideal body weight for obese patients when calculating dosages (see Chapter 3). Drug is removed by hemodialysis. Peritoneal dialysis and blood exchange transfusion **do not** appear to appreciably remove the drug. **Dose alteration is necessary in patients with impaired renal function (see Chapter 3).**

Adverse effects:

Systemic route: May cause renal impairment; has been infrequently associated with headache, vertigo, insomnia, encephalopathy, GI tract irritation, elevated liver function tests, rash, urticaria, arthralgia, fever, renal pain, and adverse hematologic effects. Inflammation/phlebitis at injection site is common with IV route.

Topical route: May cause a local pain and irritation.

Drug interactions: Probenecid decreases acyclovir renal clearance. Acyclovir may increase the concentration of tenofovir, and meperidine and its metabolite (normeperidine).

Drug administration: Maintain adequate hydration while on therapy.

IV: Slow (1 hr) IV administration at a concentration ≤7 mg/mL are essential to prevent crystallization in renal tubules and risk for phlebitis.

PO: Doses may be administered with or without food. Shake oral suspension well before each use.

ADEFOVIR DIPIVOXIL
Hepsera
Antiviral, reverse transcriptase inhibitor

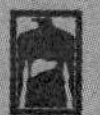
No
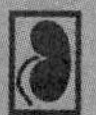
Yes
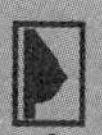
3
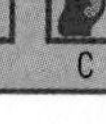
C

Tabs: 10 mg

Chronic hepatitis B infection (assess for treatment modification when serum hepatitis B virus DNA remains >1000 copies/mL with continued treatment; see remarks for additional pediatric data):

≥12 yr and adult: 10 mg PO once daily

Lamivudine-resistant hepatitis B infection: Use in combination with lamivudine to reduce risk for resistance.

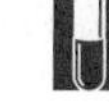

Contraindications: Hypersensitivity to adefovir or any other components in the formulation

Warnings/Precautions: Use with caution in patients with risk for liver disease and suspend treatment if lactic acidosis or hepatotoxicity develops. Severe acute exacerbation of hepatitis B may occur with therapy discontinuation (reinitiation of antihepatitis therapy may be required).

Continued

For explanation of icons, see p. 364.

ADEFOVIR DIPIVOXIL *continued*

May cause HIV resistance in patients with undiagnosed/untreated HIV (determine HIV status before initiation of therapy).

Pediatric pharmacokinetic data that mimic adult drug exposure suggest the following dosages for children 2 to 18 years old with a **maximum** dose of 10 mg/24 hr:

2–6 yr: 0.3 mg/kg/dose PO once daily

7–11 yr: 0.25 mg/kg/dose PO once daily

≥12 to <18 yr: 10 mg PO once daily

Phase 3 efficacy data in children after 48 weeks of therapy showed significant antiviral efficacy (similar to adult data) in 12- to 17-year-olds. However, therapy was less effective in children 2 to 11 years old. Adefovir was well tolerated across all pediatric age groups. (See Pediatr Infect Dis J 2012;31:578–582 for more information.)

Avoid use with tenofovir; see drug interactions below. Dose alteration is necessary in patients with impaired renal function (see Chapter 3).

Adverse effects: Asthenia, elevated serum creatinine and ALT/SGPT, and hepatitis exacerbation are common. Stevens–Johnson syndrome, TEN, nephrotoxicity, hepatomegaly with steatosis, pancreatitis, hypophosphatemia, and lactic acidosis have been reported. Fatal cases of lactic acidosis and severe hepatomegaly with steatosis have been reported with concurrent use of other antiretroviral agents. Myopathy and osteomalacia have been associated with proximal renal tubulopathy.

Drug interactions: Ganciclovir and valganciclovir may increase risk for hematologic side effects. Ribavirin may enhance hepatotoxicity (lactic acidosis may occur). Adefovir may decrease the effects (by reducing viral susceptibility of tenofovir) and increase serum concentrations of tenofovir (avoid this combination).

Drug administration: Doses may be administered with or without food.

ALBENDAZOLE
Albenza
Anthelmintic, benzimidazole derivative

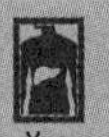
Yes
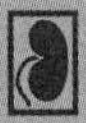
Yes
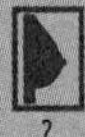
?
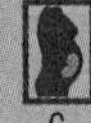
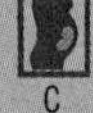
C

Tabs: 200 mg

Child and adult:

Hydatid disease (tapeworm,* Echinococcus granulosus*):

<60 kg: 15 mg/kg/24 hr ÷ BID PO (**max. dose:** 800 mg/24 hr) × 1–6 mo

≥60 kg: 400 mg BID PO × 1–6 mo

Neurocysticercosis (tapeworm,* Cysticercus cellulosae*; use with concurrent anticonvulsant and corticosteroid therapy):

<60 kg: 15 mg/kg/24 hr ÷ BID PO (**max. dose:** 800 mg/24 hr) × 8–30 days, may be repeated if necessary

≥60 kg: 400 mg BID PO × 8–30 days, may be repeated if necessary

Ancylostoma caninum (Eosinophilic enterocolitis), ***ascariasis (*Ascaris lumbricoides *or roundworm), hookworm (*Ancylstoma duodenale, Necator americanus*),*** **Trichostrongylus:** 400 mg PO × 1

Cutaneous larva migrans, trichuriasis (whipworm or* Trichuris trichiura*), gongylonemiasis (*Gongylonema *sp.): 400 mg once daily PO × 3 days

Visceral larva migrans (toxocariasis): 400 mg once daily PO × 5 days

Fluke (*Clonorchirs sinensis, *Chinese liver fluke): 10 mg/kg/dose PO once daily × 7 days

Enterobiusvermicularis (pinworm): 400 mg PO × 1, repeat × 1 in 2 wk

Continued

ALBENDAZOLE *continued*

Filariasis (**Mansonella perstans*****), capillariasis (*****Capillaria philippinensis*****; mebendazole is drug of choice):*** 400 mg once daily PO × 10 days
Gnathostomiasis (**Gnathostoma spinigerum*****):*** 400 mg BID PO × 21 days
Trichinellosis (**Trichinella spiralis*****; use steroids for severe symptoms):*** 400 mg BID PO × 8–14 days

Contraindications: Hypersensitivity to albendazole or benzimidazole products
Warnings/Precautions: Before initiating therapy for neurocysticercosis, assess for retinal lesions to weigh the risk/benefit of potential retinal damage caused by albendazole-induced changes to the existing retinal lesion. Patients treated for neurocysticercosis should receive appropriate steroid and anticonvulsant therapy to minimize cerebral hypertensive episodes. Preexisting neurocysticercosis may be uncovered in patients being treated for other conditions with albendazole.
Should not be used in pregnancy unless in circumstances where no alternative management is appropriate. Patients **should not** become pregnant at least 1 month after the cessation of therapy. Rare granulocytopenia/pancytopenia resulting in fatalities and hepatotoxicity have been reported; blood counts and LFTs should be monitored with prolonged regimens (before each 28-day cycle and every 2 weeks).
Extrahepatic obstruction increases the systemic availability of albendazole sulfoxide (prolonged rate of absorption/conversion and elimination).
Adverse effects: Gastrointestinal disturbances (abdominal pain, nausea, and vomiting) and headache are common. Rare but serious effects include acute renal failure, hepatotoxicity with increased LFTs, leukopenia, and thrombocytopenia.
Drug interactions: Dexamethasone and praziquantel may increase albendazole sulfoxide levels. Albendazole is an inducer of CYP 450 1A2 and a substrate for 3A4 (major) and 1A2 (minor).
Drug administration: Administer doses with meals; fatty meals enhance bioavailabilty.

AMANTADINE HYDROCHLORIDE
Symmetrel and others
Antiviral agent

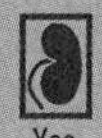
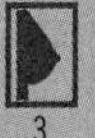
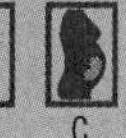

Yes Yes 3 C

Capsule: 100 mg
Tabs: 100 mg
Oral solution or syrup: 50 mg/5 mL (480 mL); may contain parabens

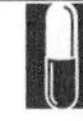

Influenza A prophylaxis and treatment (for treatment, it is best to initiate therapy immediately after the onset of symptoms; within 2 days):
- ***1–9 yr:*** 5 mg/kg/24 hr PO ÷ BID; **max. dose:** 150 mg/24 hr
- ***>9 yr:***
  - ***<40 kg:*** 5 mg/kg/24 hr PO ÷ BID; **max. dose:** 200 mg/24 hr
  - ***≥40 kg:*** 200 mg/24 hr PO ÷ BID

Alternative dosing for influenza A prophylaxis:
- ***Child >20 kg and adult:*** 100 mg/24 hr PO ÷ BID

Prophylaxis (duration of therapy):
- ***Single exposure:*** at least 10 days
- ***Repeated/uncontrolled exposure:*** up to 90 days
- ***Use with influenza A vaccine when possible***

Symptomatic treatment (duration of therapy):
Continue for 24–48 hr after disappearance of symptoms.

Continued

For explanation of icons, see p. 364.

AMANTADINE HYDROCHLORIDE *continued*

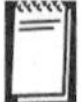

Contraindications: Hypersensitivity to amantadine or any of its components. **Do not** use in the first trimester of a pregnancy.

Warnings/Precautions: Individuals immunized with live attenuated influenza vaccine **should not** receive amantadine prophylaxis for 14 days after the vaccine. Chemoprophylaxis does not interfere with immune response to inactivated influenza vaccine. Use with **caution** in patients with liver disease, seizures, renal disease, congestive heart failure, peripheral edema, orthostatic hypotension, history of recurrent eczematoid rash, serious mental illness, and in those receiving CNS stimulants. Neuroleptic malignant syndrome has been reported with abrupt dose reduction or discontinuation (especially if patient is receiving neuroleptics).

Adjust dose in patients with renal insufficiency (see Chapter 3).

Adverse effects: May cause dizziness, anxiety, depression, mental status change, rash (livedo reticularis), nausea, orthostatic hypotension, edema, CHF, and urinary retention. Impulse control disorder has been reported.

Drug interactions: Anticholinergic drugs may potentiate the anticholinergic side effect of amantadine. Quinidine, quinine, triamterene, and trimethoprim may increase the effects/toxicity of amantadine. Use with CNS stimulants may enhance CNS stimulant effects.

Drug administration: Administer doses with meals to enhance absorption and decrease GI symptoms, and **do not** administer within 4 hours of bedtime to prevent insomnia.

AMINOSALICYLIC ACID

See *Para-aminosalicylic acid*

AMIKACIN SULFATE

Amikin and many generics

Antibiotic, aminoglycoside

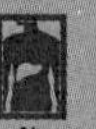
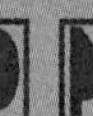
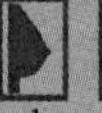
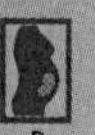

No Yes 1 D

Injection: 250 mg/mL; may contain sodium bisulfite

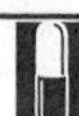

Initial empiric dosage; patient-specific dosage defined by therapeutic drug monitoring (see remarks).

Neonates: See the following table.

Postconceptional Age (wk)	Postnatal Age (days)	Dose (mg/kg/dose)	Interval (hr)
≤29*	0–7	18	48
	8–28	15	36
	>28	15	24
30–33	0–7	18	36
	>7	15	24
34–37	0–7	15	24
	>7	15	18–24†
≥38	0–7	15	24
	>7	15	12–18

*Or significant asphyxia, PDA, indomethacin use, poor cardiac output, reduced renal function.

†Use Q36 hr interval for HIE patients receiving whole-body therapeutic cooling.

Infant and child: 15–22.5 mg/kg/24 hr ÷ Q8 hr IV/IM; infants and patients requiring higher doses (e.g., cystic fibrosis) may receive initial doses of 30 mg/kg/24 hr ÷ Q8 hr IV/IM

Continued

AMIKACIN SULFATE *continued*

Cystic fibrosis (if available, use patient's previous therapeutic mg/kg dosage):
Conventional Q8 hr dosing: 30 mg/kg/24 hr ÷ Q8 hr IV
High-dose extended interval (once daily) dosing (limited data): 30–35 mg/kg/dose Q24 hr IV
Adult: 15 mg/kg/24 hr ÷ Q8–12 hr IV/IM
Initial **max. dose:** 1.5 g/24 hr, then monitor levels

Contraindications: Hypersensitivity to amikacin and aminoglycosides

Warnings/Precautions: Use with **caution** in preexisting renal, vestibular, or auditory impairment; concomitant anesthesia or neuromuscular blockers, neurotoxic; concomitant neurotoxic, ototoxic, or nephrotoxic drugs; sulfite sensitivity; and dehydration.

Adjust dosage in renal failure (see Chapter 3). Rapidly eliminated in patients with cystic fibrosis, burns, and in febrile neutropenic patients. Longer dosing intervals may be necessary for neonates receiving indomethacin for PDAs and for all patients with poor cardiac output.

Therapeutic levels (using conventional dosing): peak, 20 to 30 mg/L; trough 5 to 10 mg/L. Recommended serum sampling time at steady state: trough within 30 minutes before the third consecutive dose and peak 30 to 60 minutes after the administration of the third consecutive dose. Peak levels of 25 to 30 mg/L have been recommended for CNS, pulmonary, bone, life-threatening infections, and in febrile neutropenic patients.

Therapeutic levels for cystic fibrosis using high-dose extended interval (once daily) dosing: peak, 80 to 120 mg/L; trough, <10 mg/L. Recommended serum sampling time: trough within 30 minutes before the dose and peak 30 to 60 minutes after the administration of the dose.

For initial dosing in obese patients, use an adjusted body weight (see Chapter 3).

Adverse effects: May cause ototoxicity, nephrotoxicity, neuromuscular blockade, and rash.

Drug interactions: Loop diuretics may potentiate the ototoxicity of all aminoglycoside antibiotics. See Warnings/Precautions. β-Lactam antibiotics may inactivate aminoglycosides in vitro and in vivo in patients with severe renal failure. Degradation depends on β-lactam concentration, storage time, and temperature.

Drug administration: IM or IV infusion over 30 minutes at a concentration ≤10 mg/mL. **Do not** administer β-lactam antibiotics within 1 hour before or after amikacin dose.

AMOXICILLIN
Amoxil, Trimox, Wymox, Polymox, Moxatag, and other generics
Antibiotic, aminopenicillin

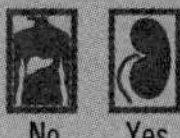
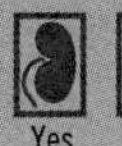
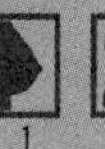
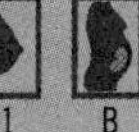

No Yes 1 B

Oral suspension: 125, 250 mg/5 mL (80, 100, 150 mL); and 200, 400 mg/5 mL (50, 75, 100 mL)
Caps: 250, 500 mg
Tablets: 500, 875 mg
Chewable tabs: 125, 200, 250, 400 mg; may contain phenylalanine
Extended-release tabs (Moxatag; see remarks): 775 mg

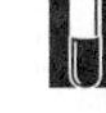

Neonate ≤3 mo: 20–30 mg/kg/24 hr ÷ Q12 hr PO
Child:
Standard dose: 25–50 mg/kg/24 hr ÷ Q8–12 hr PO
High-dose (resistant* Streptococcus pneumoniae*): 80–90 mg/kg/24 hr ÷ Q12 hr PO
Max. dose: 2–3 g/24 hr
Adult:
Mild/moderate infections: 250 mg/dose Q8 hr PO *or* 500 mg/dose Q12 hr PO
Severe infections: 500 mg/dose Q8 hr PO *or* 875 mg/dose Q12 hr PO
Max. dose: 2–3 g/24 hr

Continued

For explanation of icons, see p. 364.

AMOXICILLIN *continued*

Reccurent otitis media prophylaxis: 20 mg/kg/dose QHS PO
SBE prophylaxis:
Child: 50 mg/kg/dose × 1 PO 1 hr before procedure; **max. dose:** 2 g/dose
Adult: 2 g/dose × 1 PO 1 hr before procedure
Early Lyme disease:
Child: 50 mg/kg/24 hr ÷ Q8 hr PO × 14–21 days; **max. dose:** 1.5 g/24 hr
Adult: 500 mg/dose Q8 hr PO × 14–21 days

Contraindications: Hypersensitivity to penicillins
Warnings/Precautions: Epstein–Barr virus infection, acute lympocytic leukemia, or CMV infections may increase risk for amoxicillin-induced maculopapular rash. Chewable tablets may contain phenylalanine and **should not** be used by phenyketonurics.
High-dose regimen increasingly useful in respiratory infections, especially acute otitis media and sinusitis, because of increasing incidence of penicillin-resistant pneumococci. **Adjust dose in renal failure (see Chapter 3).**
Adverse effects: Rash, diarrhea, nausea, and vomiting
Drug interactions: Use with allopurinol increases risk for rash. Decreases the efficacy of oral contraceptives. Probenecid increases serum amoxicillin levels. May increase warfarin's effect by increasing INR.
Drug administration: Doses may be administered with or without food.

AMOXICILLIN WITH CLAVULANIC ACID
Augmentin, Amoclan, Augmentin ES-600, Augmentin XR, and various generic products
Antibiotic, aminopenicillin with β-lactmase inhibitor

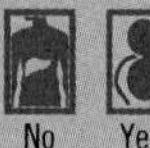
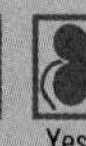
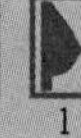
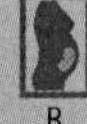

No Yes 1 B

Tabs:
For TID dosing: 250, 500 mg (with 125 mg clavulanate)
For BID dosing: 875 mg amoxicillin (with 125 mg clavulanate); Augmentin XR: 1 g amoxicillin (with 62.5 mg clavulanate)
Chewable tabs:
For BID dosing: 200, 400 mg amoxicillin (28.5 and 57 mg clavulanate, respectively); contains saccharin and aspartame
Oral suspension:
For TID dosing: 125, 250 mg amoxicillin/5 mL (31.25 and 62.5 mg clavulanate/5 mL, respectively) (75, 100, 150 mL); contains saccharin
For BID dosing: 200, 400 mg amoxicillin/5 mL (28.5 and 57 mg clavulanate/5 mL, respectively) (50, 75, 100 mL); 600 mg amoxicillin/5 mL (Augmentin ES-600; contains 42.9 mg clavulanate/5 mL) (50, 75, 100, 150 mL); contains saccharin and/or aspartame
Contains 0.63 mEq K^+ per 125 mg clavulanate (Augmentin ES-600 contains 0.23 mEq K^+ per 42.9 mg clavulanate)

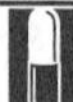

Dosage based on amoxicillin component (see remarks for resistant* Streptococcus pneumoniae*).
Infant 1 to <3 mo: 30 mg/kg/24 hr ÷ Q12 hr PO (recommended dosage form is 125 mg/5 mL suspension)
Child ≥3 mo:
TID dosing (see remarks):
20–40 mg/kg/24 hr ÷ Q8 hr PO

Continued

AMOXICILLIN WITH CLAVULANIC ACID *continued*

BID dosing (see remarks):
25–45 mg/kg/24 hr ÷ Q12 hr PO

Augmentin ES-600:
≥3 mo and <40 kg: 90 mg/kg/24 hr ÷ Q12 hr PO × 10 days

Adult: 250–500 mg/dose Q8 hr PO or 875 mg/dose Q12 hr PO for more severe and respiratory infections

Augmentin XR:
≥16 yr and adult: 2 g Q12 hr PO × 10 days for acute bacterial sinusitis or × 7–10 days for community-acquired pneumonia

Contraindications: Hypersensitivity to penicillins and patients with a history of cholestatic jaundice/hepatitic dysfunction associated with amoxicillin-clauvulanic acid. Augmentin XR is contraindicated in patients with CrCl <30 mL/min.

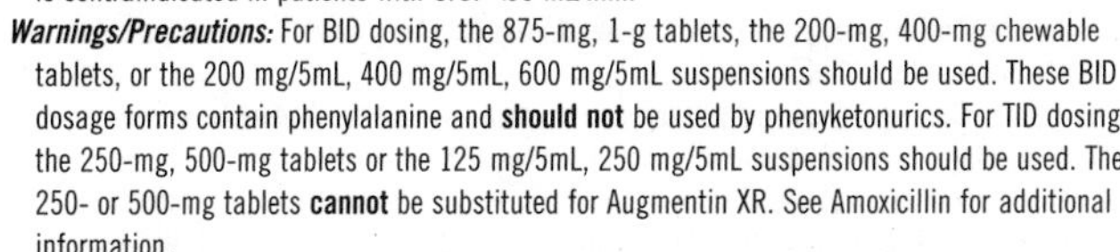

Warnings/Precautions: For BID dosing, the 875-mg, 1-g tablets, the 200-mg, 400-mg chewable tablets, or the 200 mg/5mL, 400 mg/5mL, 600 mg/5mL suspensions should be used. These BID dosage forms contain phenylalanine and **should not** be used by phenyketonurics. For TID dosing, the 250-mg, 500-mg tablets or the 125 mg/5mL, 250 mg/5mL suspensions should be used. The 250- or 500-mg tablets **cannot** be substituted for Augmentin XR. See Amoxicillin for additional information.

Higher doses of 80 to 90 mg/kg/24 hr (amoxicillin component) have been recommended for resistant strains of *Streptococcus pneumoniae* in acute otitis media (use BID formulations containing 7:1 ratio of amoxicillin to clavulanic acid or Augmentin ES-600). See Amoxicillin. **Adjust dose in renal failure (see Chapter 3).**

Adverse effects: Rash, urticaria, diarrhea (clavulanate increases risk), nausea, and vomiting are common. BID dosing schedule is associated with less diarrhea. Rare hepatoxicity has been reported.

Drug interactions: See Amoxicillin. May reduce mycofenolate levels.

Drug administration: May be administered without regard to meals; administering doses before meals may enhance absorption and minimize GI side effects. **Do not** administer with high-fat meals; may decrease absorption of clavulanate.

AMPHOTERICIN B (CONVENTIONAL)
Fungizone, Amphocin
Antifungal, polyene

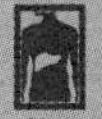
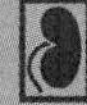
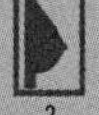
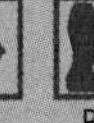

Yes Yes ? B

Injection: 50 mg vials

IV: See Drug Administration section.

Optional test dose: 0.1 mg/kg/dose IV up to **maximum** 1 mg (followed by remaining initial dose)

Initial dose: 0.5–1 mg/kg/24 hr; if test dose NOT used, infuse first dose over 6 hr and monitor frequently during the first several hours.

Increment: Increase as tolerated by 0.25–0.5 mg/kg/24 hr once daily or every other day. Use larger dosage increment (0.5 mg once daily) for critically ill patients.

Usual maintenance:
Once daily dosing: 0.5–1 mg/kg/24 hr once daily
Every other day dosing: 1.5 mg/kg/dose every other day

Max. dose: 1.5 mg/kg/24 hr

Intrathecal: 25–100 mcg Q48–72 hr. Increase to 500 mcg as tolerated.

Continued

For explanation of icons, see p. 364.

AMPHOTERICIN B (CONVENTIONAL) *continued*

Bladder irrigation for urinary tract mycosis: 5–15 mg in 100 mL sterile water for irrigation at 100–300 mL/24 hr. Instill solution into bladder, clamp catheter for 1 to 2 hr, then drain; repeat three to four times a day for 2 to 5 days.

Intranasal for aspergillus prophylaxis in neutropenic patients: 7 mg in 7 mL sterile water administered via a De Vilbiss atomizer intranasally four times a day

Contraindications: Hypersensitivity to any form of amphotericin B

Warnings/Precautions: Primarily used for severe, progressive, life-threatening fungal infections. Anaphylaxis has been reported. Avoid other nephrotoxic drugs. Monitor renal, hepatic, electrolyte, and hematologic status closely.

Approximately 66% of plasma concentrations detected in fluids from inflamed pleura, peritoneum, synovium, and aqueous humor. Good placenta penetration. Poor CSF (≤4% of serum concentration) and eye penetration. CNS/CSF levels are lower than amphotericin B, liposomal (AmBisome). **(For dosing information in renal failure, see Chapter 3.)** Use total body weight for obese patients when calculating dosages (see Chapter 3).

Adverse effects: Common infusion-related reactions include fever, chills, headache, hypotension, nausea, vomiting; may premedicate with acetaminophen and diphenhydramine 30 minutes before and 4 hours after infusion. Meperidine useful for chills. Hydrocortisone, 1 mg/mg amphotericin (**max. dose:** 25 mg), added to bottle may help prevent immediate adverse reactions. Hypercalciuria, hypokalemia, hypomagnesemia, RTA, renal failure (salt loading with 10–15 mL/kg NS infused before each dose may minimize risk, and maintaining sodium intake of >4 mEq/kg/24 hr may reduce risk in premature neonates), acute hepatic failure, hypotension, and phlebitis may occur.

Drug interactions: Nephrotoxic drugs such as aminoglycosides, chemotherapic agents, and cyclosporine may result in synergistic toxicity. May increase the toxicity of neuromuscular blocking agents and cardiac glycosides due to hypokalemia.

Drug administration: For IV route, mix with D_5W to concentration 0.1 mg/mL (peripheral administration) or 0.25 mg/mL (central line only). pH > 4.2. Infuse over 2 to 6 hours.

AMPHOTERICIN B CHOLESTERYL SULFATE
Amphotec, ABCD
Antifungal, polyene

Yes No ? B

Injection: 50, 100 mg vials

IV: See Drug Administration section.

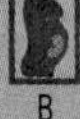

Start at 3–4 mg/kg/24 hr once daily; dose may be increased to 6 mg/kg/24 hr if necessary. A 10-mL test dose of the diluted solution administered over 15 to 30 minutes has been recommended. Doses of 3–6 mg/kg/24 hr have been used to treat invasive *Candida* or *Cryptococcus* infections in patients who have failed to respond to or could not tolerate conventional amphotericin B. Doses as high as 7.5 mg/kg/24 hr have been used to treat invasive fungal infections in BMT patients.

Contraindications: Hypersensitivity to any form of amphotericin B

Warnings/Precautions: Primarily used for severe, progressive, life-threatening fungal infections. Monitor renal, hepatic, electrolyte, and hematologic status closely.

In animal models, concentrations in the spleen, kidneys, lungs, heart, and brain are lower than conventional amphotericin B. CNS/CSF levels are lower than amphotericin B, liposomal (AmBisome). Pharmacokinetics in severe renal and hepatic impairment have not been studied.

Adverse effects: Common infusion-related reactions, including fever, chills, rigors, nausea, vomiting, hypotension, and headache, are more frequent with initial doses; may premedicate with acetaminophen, diphenhydramine, and meperidine (see Amphotericin B remarks).

Continued

AMPHOTERICIN B CHOLESTERYL SULFATE *continued*

Thrombocytopenia, anemia, leukopenia, tachycardia, hypokalemia, hypomagnesemia, hypocalcemia, hyperglycemia, diarrhea, dyspnea, back pain, nephrotoxicity, and increases in serum creatinine, aminotransferases, and bilirubin may occur.

Drug interactions: See Amphotericin B.

Drug administration: Mix with D_5W to concentration 0.16 to 0.83 mg/mL.

Infusion rate: Give first dose at 1 mg/kg/hr; if well tolerated, infusion time can be gradually shortened to a minimum of 2 hours. **Do not** use an inline filter.

AMPHOTERICIN B LIPID COMPLEX
Abelcet, ABLC
Antifungal, polyene

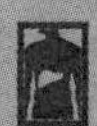
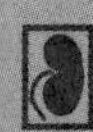
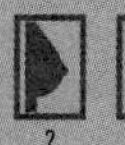
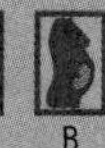

Yes No ? B

Injection: 5 mg/mL (20 mL)
(formulated as a 1 : 1 molar ratio of amphotericin B to lipid complex composed of dimyristoylphosphatidylcholine and dimyristoylphosphatidylglycerol)

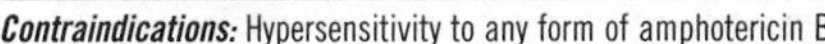

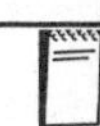

IV: See Drug Administration section.
2.5–5 mg/kg/24 hr once daily
For viseral leishmaniasis that failed to respond to or replased after treatment with antimony compound, a dosage of 1–3 mg/kg/24 hr once daily × 5 days has been used.

Contraindications: Hypersensitivity to any form of amphotericin B

Warnings/Precautions: Primarily used for severe, progressive, life-threatening fungal infections. Monitor renal, hepatic, electrolyte, and hematologic status closely.

Highest concentrations achieved in spleen, lung, and liver from human autopsy data from one heart transplant patient. CNS/CSF levels are lower than amphotericin B, liposomal (AmBisome). In animal models, concentrations are higher in the liver, spleen, and lungs, but the same in the kidneys when compared with conventional amphotericin B. Pharmacokinetics in renal and hepatic impairment have not been studied.

Adverse effects: Common infusion-related reactions include fever, chills, rigors, nausea, vomiting, hypotension, and headache; may premedicate with acetaminophen, diphenhydramine, and meperidine (see Amphotericin B remarks). Thrombocytopenia, anemia, leukopenia, hypokalemia, hypomagnesemia, diarrhea, respiratory failure, nephrotoxicity, skin rash, and increases in serum creatinine, liver enzymes, and bilirubin may occur.

Drug interactions: See Amphotericin B.

Drug administration: Mix with D_5W to concentration 1 or 2 mg/mL for fluid-restricted patients.

Infusion rate: 2.5 mg/kg/hr; shake the infusion bag every 2 hours if total infusion time exceeds 2 hours. **Do not** use an inline filter.

AMPHOTERICIN B, LIPOSOMAL
AmBisome
Antifungal, polyene

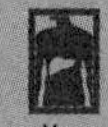
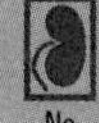
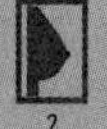
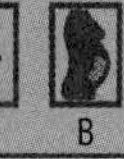

Yes No ? B

Injection: 50 mg (vials); contains soy, 900 mg sucrose
(formulated in liposomes composed of hydrogenated soy phosphatidylcholine, cholesterol, distearoylphosphatidylglycerol, and α-tocopherol)

Continued

For explanation of icons, see p. 364.

AMPHOTERICIN B, LIPOSOMAL *continued*

IV: See Drug Administration section.

Empiric therapy for febrile neutropenia: 3 mg/kg/24 hr once daily

Systemic fungal infections: 3–5 mg/kg/24 hr once daily; an upper dosage limit of 10 mg/kg/24 hr has been suggested based on pharmacokinetic end points and risk for hypokalemia. However, dosages as high as 15 mg/kg/24 hr have been used. Dosages as high as 10 mg/kg/24 hr have been used in patients with aspergillus.

Cryptococcal meningitis in HIV: 6 mg/kg/24 hr once daily

Leishmaniasis:

Immunocompetent patient: 3 mg/kg/24 hr on days 1 to 5, 14, and 21; a repeat course may be necessary if infection does not clear.

Immunocompromised patient: 4 mg/kg/24 hr on days 1 to 5, 10, 17, 24, 31, and 38; a repeat course may be necessary if infection does not clear.

Contraindications: Hypersensitivity to any form of amphotericin B

Warnings/Precautions: Primarily used for severe, progressive, life-threatening fungal infections. Monitor renal, hepatic, electrolyte, and hematologic status closely. Safety and effectiveness in neonates have not been established.

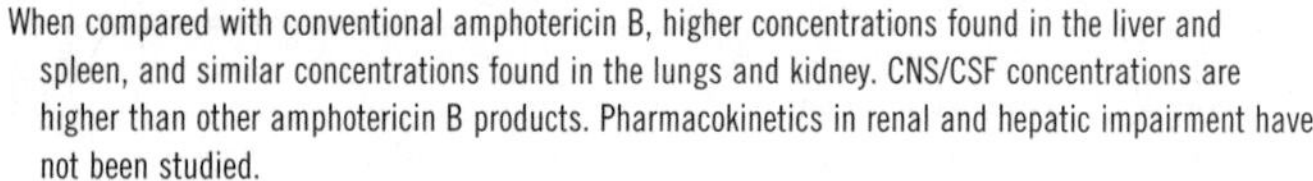

When compared with conventional amphotericin B, higher concentrations found in the liver and spleen, and similar concentrations found in the lungs and kidney. CNS/CSF concentrations are higher than other amphotericin B products. Pharmacokinetics in renal and hepatic impairment have not been studied.

Adverse effects: Common infusion-related reactions include fever, chills, rigors, nausea, vomiting, hypotension, and headache; may premedicate with acetaminophen, diphenhydramine, and meperidine (see Amphotericin B remarks). Thrombocytopenia, anemia, leukopenia, tachycardia, hypokalemia, hypomagnesemia, hypocalcemia, hyperglycemia, diarrhea, dyspnea, skin rash, low back pain, nephrotoxicity, and increases in serum creatinine, liver enzymes, and bilirubin may occur. Rhabdomyolysis has been reported.

Drug interactions: See amphotericin B. False elevations of serum phosphate have been reported with the PHOSm assay (used in Beckman Coulter analyzers).

Drug administration: Mix with D_5W to concentration 1 to 2 mg/mL (0.2–0.5 mg/mL may be used for infants and small children).

Infusion rate: Administer dose over 2 hours; infusion may be reduced to 1 hour if well tolerated. A ≥1 micron inline filter may be used.

AMPICILLIN

Omnipen, Principen, Totacillin, and others

Antibiotic, aminopenicillin

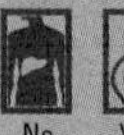
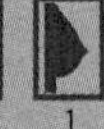
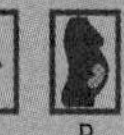

No Yes 1 B

Oral suspension: 125 mg/5 mL (100, 200 mL), 250 mg/5 mL (100, 200 mL)

Caps: 250, 500 mg

Injection: 250, 500 mg; 1, 2, 10 g

Contains 3 mEq Na/1 g IV drug

Neonate (IM/IV):

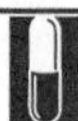

<7 days:

<2 kg: 50–100 mg/kg/24 hr ÷ Q12 hr

≥2 kg: 75–150 mg/kg/24 hr ÷ Q8 hr

Group B streptococcal meningitis: 200–300 mg/kg/24 hr ÷ Q8 hr

Continued

AMPICILLIN *continued*

≥7 days:

<1.2 kg: 50–100 mg/kg/24 hr ÷ Q12 hr

1.2–2 kg: 75–150 mg/kg/24 hr ÷ Q8 hr

>2 kg: 100–200 mg/kg/24 hr ÷ Q6 hr

Group B streptococcal meningitis: 300 mg/kg/24 hr ÷ Q4–6 hr

Infant/child:

Mild-to-moderate infections:

IM/IV: 100–200 mg/kg/24 hr ÷ Q6 hr

PO: 50–100 mg/kg/24 hr ÷ Q6 hr; **max. PO dose:** 2–3 g/24 hr

Severe infections: 200–400 mg/kg/24 hr ÷ Q4–6 hr IM/IV

Community-acquired pneumonia in a fully immunized patient:

Streptococcus pneumoniae ***penicillin MIC ≤2.0:*** 150–200 mg/kg/24 hr ÷ Q6 hr IV/IM

Streptococcus pneumoniae ***penicillin MIC ≥4.0:*** 300–400 mg/kg/24 hr ÷ Q6 hr IV/IM

Max. IV/IM dose: 12 g/24 hr

Adult:

IM/IV: 500–3000 mg Q4–6 hr

PO: 250–500 mg Q6 hr

Max. IV/IM dose: 14 g/24 hr

SBE prophylaxis:

Moderate-risk patients:

Child: 50 mg/kg/dose × 1 IV/IM 30 min before procedure; **max. dose:** 2 g/dose

Adult: 2 g/dose × 1 IV/IM 30 min before procedure

High-risk patients with GU and GI procedures: Above doses PLUS gentamicin 1.5 mg/kg × 1 (**max. dose:** 120 mg) IV within 30 min of starting procedure

Contraindications: Hypersensitivity to penicillins

Warnings/Precautions: Epstein–Barr virus (EBV) infection may increase risk for maculopapular rash. Use higher doses to treat CNS disease. **Adjust dose in renal failure (see Chapter 3).**

Adverse effects: Produces the same side effects as penicillin, with cross-reactivity. Rash commonly seen at 5 to 10 days, and rash may occur with concurrent EBV infection or allopurinol use. May cause interstitial nephritis, diarrhea, and pseudomembranous enterocolitis.

Drug interactions: Chloroquine reduces ampicillin's oral absorption. May decrease the effectiveness of estrogen-containing oral contraceptives.

Drug administration:

PO: Doses should be administered on an empty stomach; 1–2 hr before food.

IV: Doses may be given via IV push at a concentration ≤100 mg/mL over 3–5 min or via intermittent IV infusion at ≤30 mg/mL over 15–30 min. IV doses have a shorter stability when diluted in dextrose-containing solutions.

AMPICILLIN WITH SULBACTAM

Unasyn

Antibiotic, aminopenicillin with β-lactamase inhibitor

No Yes 1 B

Injection:

1.5 g = ampicillin 1 g + sulbactam 0.5 g

3 g = ampicillin 2 g + sulbactam 1 g

15 g = ampicillin 10 g + sulbactam 5 g

Contains 5 mEq Na per 1.5 g drug combination

Continued

For explanation of icons, see p. 364.

AMPICILLIN WITH SULBACTAM *continued*

Dosage based on ampicillin component:

Neonate:

Premature (based on pharmacokinetic data): 100 mg/kg/24 hr ÷ Q12 hr IM/IV

Full-term: 100 mg/kg/24 hr ÷ Q8 hr IM/IV

Infant ≥1 mo:

Mild-to-moderate infections: 100–150 mg/kg/24 hr ÷ Q6 hr IM/IV

Meningitis/severe infections: 200–300 mg/kg/24 hr ÷ Q6 hr IM/IV

Child:

Mild-to-moderate infections: 100–200 mg/kg/24 hr ÷ Q6 hr IM/IV

Meningitis/severe infections: 200–400 mg/kg/24 hr ÷ Q4–6 hr IM/IV

Adult: 1–2 g Q6–8 hr IM/IV

Max. dose: 8 g ampicillin/24 hr

Contraindications: Hypersensitivity to ampicillin, penicillin, or sulbactam products

Warnings/Precautions: See Ampicillin. Similar spectrum of antibacterial activity to ampicillin with the added coverage of β-lactamase–producing organisms. Total sulbactam dose **should not exceed** 4 g/24 hr.

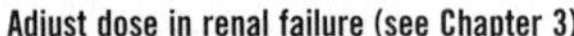

Adjust dose in renal failure (see Chapter 3).

Adverse effects: See Ampicillin.

Drug interactions: See Ampicillin.

Drug administration:

IV: Dilute medication at a concentration ≤30 mg/mL ampicillin and 15 mg/mL slubactam. IV solution stability is shorter when diluted in dextrose-containing solutions. For slow IV injection, give over 10 to 15 minutes. For intermittent IV injection give over 15 to 30 minutes.

IM: Administer at concentrations of 250 mg/mL ampicillin and 125 mg sulbactam. Drug may be diluted in sterile water for injection, or 0.5% or 2% lidocaine.

AMPRENAVIR

Agenerase, APV

Antiviral, protease inhibitor

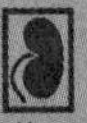

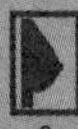

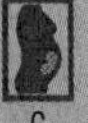

Yes Yes 3 C

Capsules: 50 mg; each capsule contains 19 mg propylene glycol and 36.3 IU vitamin E (d-α-tocopherol)

Oral solution: 15 mg/mL (240 mL); each 1 mL contains 46 IU vitamin E (d-α-tocopherol) and 550 mg propylene glycol

Use in combination with other HIV antiretroviral agents.

Child 4–12 yr and adolescent 13–16 yr <50 kg:

Oral solution: 22.5 mg/kg/dose PO BID or 17 mg/kg/dose PO TID up to a **max. dose** of 2800 mg/24 hr

Capsules: 20 mg/kg/dose PO BID or 15 mg/kg/dose PO TID up to a **max. dose** of 2400 mg/24 hr

Adolescent 13–16 yr ≥50 kg and adult:

Oral solution: 1400 mg PO BID; switch to capsules as soon as possible to lower the amount of propylene glycol and vitamin E content

Capsules: 1200 mg PO BID

Capsules in combination with efavirenz and ritonavir:

Adult: 1200 mg amprenavir PO BID + 600 mg efavirenz PO once daily + 200 mg ritonavir PO BID; only amprenavir boosted with ritonavir should be used in combination with efavirenz

Continued

AMPRENAVIR *continued*

In combination with ritonavir:

Adult: 600 mg amprenavir PO BID + 100 mg ritonavir PO BID, *or* 1200 mg amprenavir PO once daily + 200 mg ritonavir PO once daily

Contraindications: Hypersensitivity to amprenavir or any of its components. Oral solution is **contraindicated** in children younger than 4 years old, pregnant women, patients with hepatic or renal failure, and patients receiving metronidazole or disulfiram. **Do not** coadminister the following drugs: astemizole, terfenadine, cisapride, midazolam, triazolam, ergot derivatives, lipid-lowering agents (e.g., atorvastatin and cervistatin), and pimozide. Concomitant flecainide and propafenone are **contraindicated** when amprenavir is coadministered with ritonavir.

Warnings/Precautions: Drug contains significant amounts of vitamin E and propylene glycol. Therapeutic dosages of the oral solution will provide 1650 mg/kg/24 hr propylene glycol and 138 IU/kg/24 hr vitamin E. Use with **caution** in sulfonamide-allergic patients because the drug is a sulfonamide; potential risk for cross-sensitivity reactions is unknown. Oral solutions of amprenavir and ritonavir **should not** be used in combination because of significant of propylene glycol and alcohol, respectively. Oral liquid and capsules are not interchangeable on a milligram per milligram basis; oral solution is 14% less bioavailable. Noncompliance can quickly promote resistant HIV strains. There are many drug interactions (see Contraindications and Drug Interaction sections).

Consider toxicity, pill or liquid volume burden, adherence, and virologic and immunologic parameters when determining when to transition from pediatric to adult doses.

The following dosage adjustment for adults with hepatic insufficiency have been recommended:

Child–Pugh Score	Dose for Capsules	Dose for Solution
5–8	450 mg PO BID	513 mg PO BID
9–12	300 mg PO BID	342 mg PO BID

Adverse effects: Rash, hyperglycemia, hypertriglyceridemia, GI symptoms and discomfort, headache, and paresthesia may occur. Severe life-threatening rashes (~1% of patients) have been reported.

Drug interactions: Amprenavir is a substrate and inhibitor of CYP 450 3A4. Efavirenz, rifampin, rifabutin, anticonvulsants (e.g., Phenytoin), oral contraceptives, and St. John's wort can lower amprenavir levels. Always check the potential for other drug interactions when either initiating therapy or adding new drug onto an existing regimen. See Contraindications section.

Drug administration: Drug may be taken with or without food; **avoid** administering with high-fat meals. Administer drug 1 hour before or after antacid or didanosine use.

ANIDULAFUNGIN

Eraxis

Antifungal, echinocandin

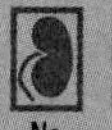

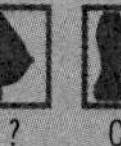

Yes No ? C

Injection: 50, 100 mg

Each 50 mg of drug contains 50 mg fructose, 250 mg mannitol, 125 mg polysorbate 80, and 5.6 mg tartaric acid.

Neonate and infant: Recommended dosages from a multidose safety and PK study in neonates 27 to 43 weeks postmenstrual age and infants 50 to 451 days old.

To mimic an adult dosage of 100 mg/24 hr: 1.5 mg/kg/dose IV once daily

Child: Recommended dosages based on steady-state pharmacokinetic data in immunocompromised children 2 to 17 years old. Efficacy data are incomplete.

To mimic an adult dosage of 50 mg/24 hr: 0.75 mg/kg/dose IV once daily

To mimic an adult dosage of 100 mg/24 hr: 1.5 mg/kg/dose IV once daily

Continued

For explanation of icons, see p. 364.

ANIDULAFUNGIN *continued*

An ongoing phase 3 trial in children (1 mo to 17 years old) with invasive candidasis is evaluating the following dosage: 3 mg/kg (**max. dose:** 200 mg) IV × 1 on day 1, then 1.5 mg/kg/dose (**max. dose:** 100 mg) IV once daily

Adult:

Candidal infections (excluding esophagitis): 200 mg IV × 1 on day 1, then 100 mg IV once daily for at least 14 days after the last positive culture

Candidal esophagitis: 100 mg IV × 1 on day 1, then 50 mg IV once daily for at least 14 days after the last positive culture

Contraindications: Hypersensitivity to andulafungin and any other components in the formulation or other echinocandins

Warnings/Precautions: Hepatic dysfunction and abnormal or worsening of liver function tests have occurred.

Adverse effects: Hypokalemia, bronchospasms, diarrhea, and abnormal liver function tests may occur. Histamine-mediated effects such as rash, urticaria, flushing, pruritus, dyspnea, and hypotension are minimized with IV infusion rates less than 1.1 mg/min.

Drug interactions: Drug is not metabolized by CYP 450 metabolizing enzymes.

Drug administration: Dilute dose with either D_5W or NS at a concentration ≤0.5 mg/mL. **Do not** infuse dose >1.1 mg/min.

ARTEMETHER WITH LUMEFANTRINE
Coartem
Antimalarial

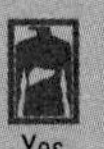
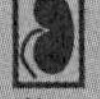
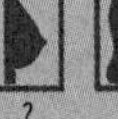
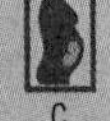

Yes Yes ? C

Tab: artemether 20 mg and lumefantrine 120 mg

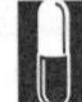

Acute uncomplicated malaria (**Plasmodium vivax** ***acquired in areas of chloroquine-resistant*** **P. vivax*****):***

Child (2 mo–16 yr): PO dosage at hour 0 and at hour 8 for day 1, followed by same PO dosage BID for days 2 and 3

5 to <15 kg: 1 tablet
15 to <25 kg: 2 tablets
25 to <35 kg: 3 tablets
≥35 kg: 4 tablets

Adolescent (>16 yr) and adult (≥35 kg): 4 tablets PO at hour 0 and at hour 8 for day 1, followed by 4 tablets PO BID for days 2 and 3. Use child dosage for adults <35 kg.

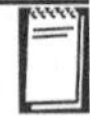

Contraindications: Hypersensitivity to artemether, lumefantrine, and any other component of the product; and first trimester of pregnancy (safety in second and third trimester is not known)

Warnings/Precautions: Avoid use in clinical situations with an increased risk for QT interval prolongation, electrolyte imbalances, and concomitant use of medications can prolong the QT interval (e.g., antipsychotics, antidepressants, macrolides, fluoroquinolones, triazole antifungals). **Avoid** use with concurrent medications that are metabolized by CYP2D6. Use with **caution** in hepatic and renal impairment (no specific dosage adjustments have been recommended with mild-to-moderate impairment). **Should not** be used for severe malaria or for prophylaxis therapy.

Adverse effects: Palpitations, abdominal pain, diarrhea, loss of appetite, nausea, vomiting, arthralgia, myalgia, asthenia, dizziness, headache, sleep disorders, cough, fatigue, fever, and shivering are common. Somnolence, involuntary muscle contractions, paresthesia, hypoesthesia, abnormal gait, and ataxia have been reported.

Continued

ARTEMETHER WITH LUMEFANTRINE *continued*

Drug interactions: Both drugs are substrates for CYP 450 3A4; use with **caution** with inhibitors, inducers, and substrates of CYP 450 3A4. See Warning/Precautions for additional drug interactions. Grapefruit juice may increase levels of artemether and/or lumefantrine, and also potentiate QT prolongation.

Drug administration: Doses are best administered with a full meal to assure absorption. Tablets may be crushed and mixed with 5 to 10 mL water per tablet for patients who are unable to swallow tablets.

ARTESUNATE

Antimalarial agent, artemisinin derivative

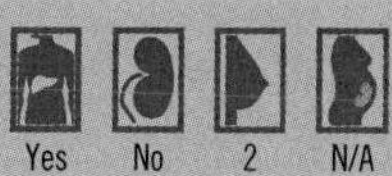
Yes No 2 N/A

Available from the U.S. Centers for Disease and Prevention (770-488-7788 Monday–Friday 8:00 a.m.–4:30 p.m. EST or 770-488-7100 evenings, weekends, or holidays, ask for CDC Malaria Branch clinician)

Injection powder for reconstitution: reconstitute with 11 mL of provided diluent for a final concentration of 10 mg/mL

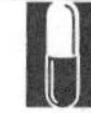

Severe malaria:

Child and adult: 2.4 mg/kg/dose IV × 1, followed by 2.4 mg/kg/dose IV at 12, 24, 48, and 72 hr after the first dose. Longer treatment duration may be required in severly ill patients or for patients unable to take oral therapies.

Contraindications: Hypersensitivity to artesunate, dihydroartemisinin, and first trimester of pregnancy

Warnings/Precautions: QT interval prolongation has been reported with medications in this class (artemisinin). Use with **caution** in hepatic disease (pharmacokinetic data not available), seizures/neurologic diseases, arrhythmias/conduction defects, cardiovascular diseases, and bone marrow suppression.

Adverse effects: Ataxia, slurred speech, GI discomfort, neurotoxicity, seizures, and QT interval prolongation may occur. Rash, hair loss, marrow suppression, elevated AST/ALT, and hypersensitivity reactions have been reported.

Drug administration: Dilute drug to a final concentration of 10 mg/mL and administer IV over 1–2 min through a 0.8-micron hydrophilic polyethersulfone filter.

ANTITOXIN, DIPHTHERIA

See *Diphtheria Antitoxin*

ATAZANAVIR

Reyataz, ATV

Antiviral, protease inhibitor

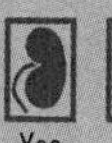
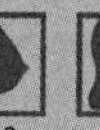
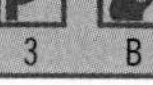
Yes Yes 3 B

Caps: 100, 150, 200, 300 mg

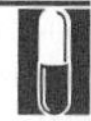

Child 6 to <18 yr (do not exceed adult maximum doses; see remarks):

Antiretroviral naïve:

Monotherapy (for those unable to tolerate ritonavir):

≥13 yr and ≥39 kg: 400 mg PO once daily

Continued

For explanation of icons, see p. 364.

ATAZANAVIR *continued*

In combination with ritonavir (preferred):
15 to <25 kg: atazanavir 150 mg and ritonavir 80 mg PO once daily
25–32 kg: atazanavir 200 mg and ritonavir 100 mg PO once daily
32–39 kg: atazanavir 250 mg and ritonavir 100 mg PO once daily
≥39 kg: atazanavir 300 mg and ritonavir 100 mg PO once daily
Antiretroviral experienced:
In combination with ritonavir (preferred):
25–32 kg: atazanavir 200 mg and ritonavir 100 mg PO once daily
32–39 kg: atazanavir 250 mg and ritonavir 100 mg PO once daily
≥39 kg: atazanavir 300 mg and ritonavir 100 mg PO once daily

Adult (see adult guidelines for maximum doses of concurrent H2 blockers and PPI use, and additional information; see remarks):
Antiretroviral naïve:
Monotherapy (for those unable to tolerate ritonavir): 400 mg PO once daily
In combination with ritonavir: atazanavir 300 mg plus ritonavir 100 mg PO once daily
In combination with tenofovir (must use ritonavir): atazanavir 300 mg plus ritonavir 100 mg PO and tenofovir 300 mg PO with food once daily
In combination with efavirenz (must use ritonavir): atazanavir 400 mg plus ritonavir 100 mg PO with food once daily and efavirenz 600 mg PO on an empty stomach QHS
Antiretroviral experienced:
In combination with ritonavir: atazanavir 300 mg plus ritonavir 100 mg PO once daily
In combination with tenofovir (must use ritonavir): atazanavir 300 mg plus ritonavir 100 mg PO and tenofovir 300 mg PO with food once daily

---

Contraindications: Hypersensitivity to atazanavir or any of its componenets. **Do not** coadminister the following drugs: astemizole, terfenadine, cisapride, midazolam, triazolam, alfuzosin, PDE5 inhibitors (e.g., sildenafil), ergot derivatives, lipid-lowering agents (e.g., atorvastatin and cervistatin), and pimozide. **Should not** be used in severe hepatic impairment (Child–Pugh class C).

Warnings/Precautions: There are many drug interactions, see Contraindications and Drug Interactions sections. Use with indinavir is not recommended because of increased risk for hyperbillirubinemia and jaundice; atazanavir is highly protein bound. Use with **caution** in mild-to-moderate hepatic impairment (dose reduction of 300 mg PO once daily has been recommended in patients with Child–Pugh class B), renal disease, preexisting cardiac conduction disorders, other drugs known to prolong PR interval (e.g., calcium channel blockers, β-blockers, and digoxin). Gastric acid–reducing medications (H2 blockers and PPIs) may decrease atazanavir levels; see adult guidelines for specific dosage limitations.

Patients with hepatitis B or C infections with elevated transaminases may be at risk for further elevations and hepatic decompensation.

Data currently insufficient for dosing in children younger than 6 years, monotherapy for younger than 13 years, and treatment-experienced children less than 25 kg.

Adverse effects: Hyperbilirubinemia, jaundice, headache, fever, arthralgia, depression, insomnia, dizziness, GI symptoms, and parasthesias are common.

Cardiac PR interval prolongation, AV block, rash (including Stevens–Johnson, erythemia multiforme, eosinophilia, and DRESS), hyperglycemia, serum transaminase elevation, spontaneous bleeding in hemophiliacs, fat redistribution, and lipid abnormalities have been reported.

Drug interactions: Atazanavir is substrate and inhibitor of CYP 450 3A. Also inhibits the glucoronidation enzyme UGT1A1, and CYP 450 1A2 and 2C9. Antacids, H2 antagonists, PPIs,

Continued

ATAZANAVIR *continued*

bosentan, rifampin, St. John's wort, nevirapine, tenofovir, and efavirenz decrease atazanavir levels/effects. Voriconazole and ritonavir may increase atazanavir levels/effects. Atazanavir may increase the effects/toxicity of inhaled β agonists (cardiovascular side effects) and colchicine. Always check the potential for other drug interactions when either initiating therapy or adding new drugs onto an existing regimen. See Contraindications and Warnings/Precautions sections.

Drug administration: Doses should be administered with food to enhance absorption. Administer doses 2 hours before and 1 hour after antacids and buffered formulations of didanosine or other medications. Administer at least 2 hours before and at least 10 hours after H2 antagonists, and at least 12 hour after PPIs. If used with ritonavir, take both medications simultaneously.

ATOVAQUONE ± PROGUANIL
Mepron; in combination with proguanil: Malarone Pediatric tablets, Malarone tablets
Antiprotozoal, antimalarial agent

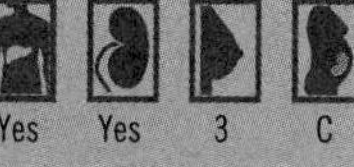

Oral suspension: 750 mg/5 mL (210 mL); contains benzyl alcohol
In combination with proguanil:
Malarone Pediatric tablets: 62.5 mg atovaquone and 25 mg proguanil
Malarone tablets: 250 mg atovaquone and 100 mg proguanil

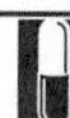

Atovaquone:
Pneumocystis *jiroveci (carinii) pneumonia (PCP):*
Treatment (210-day course):
Child: 30–40 mg/kg/24 hr PO ÷ BID with fatty foods; **max. dose:** 1500 mg/24 hr. Infants 3–24 mo may require higher doses of 45 mg/kg/24 hr PO ÷ BID
Adult: 750 mg/dose PO BID
Prophylaxis (first episode and recurrence):
Child 1–3 mo or >24 mo: 30 mg/kg/24 hr PO once daily; **max. dose:** 1500 mg/24 hr
Child 4–24 mo: 45 mg/kg/24 hr PO once daily; **max. dose:** 1500 mg/24 hr
Adult: 1500 mg/dose PO once daily
Toxoplasa gondii:
Child:
First episode prophylaxis and recurrence prophylaxis: Use PCP prophylaxis dosages ± pyrimethamine 1 mg/kg/dose (**max.** 25 mg/dose) PO once daily PLUS leucovorin 5 mg PO Q3 days.
Adult:
Treatment: 1500 mg/dose PO BID ± (sulfadiazine 1000–1500 mg PO Q6 hr or pyrimethamine PLUS leucovorin)
First episode prophylaxis: 1500 mg/dose PO once daily ± pyrimethamine 25 mg PO once daily PLUS leucovorin 10 mg PO once daily.
Recurrence prophylaxis: 750 mg/dose PO Q6–12 hr ± pyrimethamine 25 mg PO once daily PLUS leucovorin 10 mg PO once daily.
Baesiosis (duration of therapy: 7–10 days)
Child: 40 mg/kg/24 hr PO ÷ BID (**max. dose:** 1500 mg/24 hr) PLUS azithromycin 12 mg/kg/dose PO once daily × 7–10 days.
≥13 yr and adult: 750 mg/dose PO BID PLUS azithromycin 600 mg PO once daily × 7–10 days.

Continued

For explanation of icons, see p. 364.

ATOVAQUONE ± PROGUANIL *continued*

Atovaquone with proguanil (Malarone):

Malaria (chloroquine-resistant* Plasmodium falciparum*):

Treatment (use for a total of 3 days):

Treatment Dosages

Age	Daily Dosage (atovaquone/proguanil) ÷ once to twice daily PO
Child	
5–8 kg	125 mg/50 mg
9–10 kg	187.5 mg/75 mg
11–20 kg	250 mg/100 mg
21–30 kg	500 mg/200 mg
31–40 kg	750 mg/300 mg
>40 kg	1000 mg/400 mg
Adult	1000 mg/400 mg

Prophylaxis (initiate therapy 1–2 days before travel, during stay, and for 1 wk after leaving):

Prophylaxis Dosages

Age	Daily Dosage (atovaquone/proguanil) ÷ once daily PO
Child	
5–8 kg	31.25 mg/12.5 mg
9–10 kg	46.88 mg/18.75 mg
11–20 kg	62.5 mg/25 mg
21–30 kg	125 mg/50 mg
31–40 kg	187.5 mg/75 mg
>40 kg	250 mg/100 mg
Adult	250 mg/100 mg

Contraindications: Hypersensitivity to atovaquone, proguanil, or both. **Do not** use combination product for malaria prophylaxis in patients with severe renal impairment (<30 mL/min).

Warnings/Precautions: Atovaquone is not recommended in the treatment of severe PCP because of the lack of clinical data. Patients with GI disorders or severe vomiting and who **cannot** tolerate oral therapy should consider alternative IV therapies. Use the combination product with **caution** in severe hepatic impairment.

Adverse effects: Rash, pruritus, sweating, GI symptoms, LFT elevation, dizziness, headache, insomnia, anxiety, cough, and fever are common with both agents. Anemia, Stevens–Johnson syndrome, and hepatitis have been reported with atovaquone and rare anaphylaxis with the combination product.

Drug interactions:

Atovaquone: Metoclopramide, rifampin, rifabutin, and tetracycline may decrease atovaquone levels.

Proguanil: Inhibitors or substrates to CYP 450 2C19 may potentially decrease the conversion of cycloguanil. May increase anticoagulation effects of warfarin.

Drug administration:

Atovaquone: Shake oral suspension well before dispensing all doses. Take all doses with high-fat foods to maximize absorption.

Atovaquone + Proguanil: Take all doses with food or milky drink. If vomiting occurs within 1 hour of dosing, repeat dose.

AZITHROMYCIN
Zithromax, Zithromax TRI-PAK, Zithromax Z-PAK, Zmax (extended-release oral suspension), Azasite, and other generics
Antibiotic, macrolide

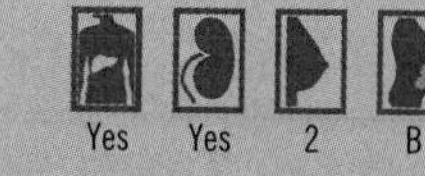

Tablets: 250, 500, 600 mg
TRI-PAK: 500 mg (3s as unit dose pack)
Z-PAK: 250 mg (6s as unit dose pack)
Oral suspension: 100 mg/5 mL (15 mL), 200 mg/5 mL (15, 22.5, 30 mL)
Oral powder (Sachet): 1 g (3s, 10s)
Extended-release oral suspension (microspheres):
Zmax: 2 g reconstituted with 60 mL water
Injection: 500 mg; contains 9.92 mEq Na/1 g drug
Ophthalmic solution (Azasite): 1% (2.5 mL)

Infant and child:
Otitis media (≥6 mo):
5-day regimen: 10 mg/kg PO day 1 (**max. dose:** 500 mg), followed by 5 mg/kg/24 hr PO once daily (**max. dose:** 250 mg/24 hr) on days 2–5
3-day regimen: 10 mg/kg/24 hr PO once daily × 3 days (**max. dose:** 500 mg/24 hr)
1-day regimen: 30 mg/kg/24 hr PO × 1 (**max. dose:** 1500 mg/24 hr)
Community-acquired pneumonia (≥6 mo):
Tablet or oral suspension: Use earlier otitis media 5-day regimen
Extended-release oral suspension: (Zmax): 60 mg/kg (**max. dose:** 1500 mg/24 hr)
Pharyngitis/tonsillitis (2–15 yr): 12 mg/kg/24 hr PO once daily × 5 days (**max. dose:** 500 mg/24 hr)
Acute sinusitis (≥6 mo): 10 mg/kg/dose (**max. dose:** 500 mg) PO once daily × 3 days
Pertussis:
Infant <6 mo: 10 mg/kg/dose PO once daily × 5 days
≥6 mo: 10 mg/kg/dose (**max. dose:** 500 mg) PO × 1, followed by 5 mg/kg (**max. dose:** 250 mg) PO once daily on days 2–5
Uncomplicated chlamydial cervicitis or urethritis:
<8 yr and <45 kg: 20 mg/kg/dose (**max. dose:** 1 g) × 1 PO
≥8 yr and ≥45 kg: 1 g × 1 PO
Chancroid: 20 mg/kg/dose (**max. dose:** 1 g) × 1 PO
Mycobacterium avium ***complex in HIV (see www.aidsinfo.nih.gov/guidelines for most current recommendations):***
Prophylaxis for first episode: 20 mg/kg/dose PO Q7 days (**max. dose:** 1200 mg/dose); alternatively, 5 mg/kg/24 hr PO once daily (**max. dose:** 250 mg/dose) with or without rifabutin
Prophylaxis for recurrence: 5 mg/kg/24 hr PO once daily (**max. dose:** 250 mg/dose), plus ethambutol 15 mg/kg/24 hr (**max. dose:** 900 mg/24 hr) PO once daily with or without rifabutin 5 mg/kg/24 hr (**max. dose:** 300 mg/24 hr)
Treatment: 10–12 mg/kg/24 hr PO once daily (**max. dose:** 500 mg/24 hr) × ≥1 mo, plus ethambutol 15–25 mg/kg/24 hr (**max. dose:** 1g/24 hr) PO once daily with or without rifabutin 10–20 mg/kg/24 hr (**max. dose:** 300 mg/24 hr)
Endocarditis prophylaxis: 15 mg/kg/dose (**max. dose:** 500 mg) × 1, 30–60 min before procedure
Anti-inflammatory agent in cystic fibrosis:
25–39 kg: 250 mg PO every Monday, Wednesday, and Friday
≥40 kg: 500 mg PO every Monday, Wednesday, and Friday

Continued

For explanation of icons, see p. 364.

AZITHROMYCIN *continued*

Adolescent and adult:

Pharyngitis, tonsillitis, pertussis, skin, and soft-tissue infection: 500 mg PO day 1, then 250 mg/24 hr PO once daily on days 2–5

Mild-to-moderate bacterial COPD exacerbation: above 5 day dosing regimen *or* 500 mg PO once daily × 3 days

Community-acquired pneumonia:

Tablets: 500 mg PO day 1, then 250 mg/24 hr PO once daily on days 2–5

Extended-release oral suspension (Zmax): Single dose 2 g PO

IV and tablet regimen: 500 mg IV once daily × 2 days followed by 500 mg PO once daily to complete a 7- to 10-day regimen (IV and PO)

Sinusitis:

Tablets: 500 mg PO once daily × 3 days

Extended-release oral suspension (Zmax): Single dose 2 g PO

Uncomplicated chlamydial cervicitis or urethritis: Single 1 g dose PO

Gonococcal cervicitis or urethritis: Single 2 g dose PO

Acute PID (chlamydia): 500 mg IV once daily × 1–2 days followed by 250 mg PO once daily to complete a 7-day regimen (IV and PO)

M. avium *complex in HIV (see www.aidsinfo.nih.gov/guidelines for most recent recommendations):*

Prophylaxis for first episode: 1200 mg PO Q7 days with or without rifabutin 300 mg PO once daily

Prophylaxis for recurrence: 500 mg PO once daily, plus ethambutol 15 mg/kg/dose PO once daily, with or without rifabutin 300 mg PO once daily

Treatment: 500–600 mg PO once daily with ethambutol 15 mg/kg/dose PO once daily with or without rifabutin 300 mg PO once daily

Endocarditis prophylaxis: 500 mg × 1, 30–60 min before procedure

Anti-inflammatory agent in cystic fibrosis: Use same dosing in children.

Ophthalmic:

≥1 yr and adult: Instill 1 drop into the affected eye(s) BID, 8–12 hr apart, × 2 days, followed by 1 drop once daily for the next 5 days.

Contraindications: Hypersensitivity to macrolides, ketolides, or any other components in the formulation; and history of cholestatic jaundice/hepatic dysfunction with prior use

Warnings/Precautions: Use with **caution** in impaired hepatic function, GFR <10 mL/min (limited data), and prolonged QT intervals (elderly patients are more susceptible). CNS penetration is poor. Discontinue use if signs and symptoms of hepatitis occur.

Adverse effects: Can cause increase in hepatic enzymes, cholestatic jaundice, GI discomfort, and pain at injection site (IV use). Vomiting, diarrhea, and nausea have been reported at higher frequency in otitis media with 1-day dosing regimen. Hepatic dysfunction, tongue discoloration, Stevens–Johnson syndrome, and TEN have been reported. Eye irritation is common with ophthalmic use.

Drug interactions: Compared with other macrolides, less risk for drug interactions. Nelfinavir may increase azithromycin levels; monitor for liver enzyme abnormalities and hearing impairment. Interaction studies have not been completed for the following medications by which macrolides may increase their effects/toxicity: digoxin, ergotamine, dihydroergotamine, cyclosporine, hexobarbital, and phenytoin. Despite not affecting prothrombin time to a single dose of warfarin, careful monitoring of prothrombin time is recommended with warfarin.

Drug administration:

PO: Oral dosage forms may be administered with or without food, but **do not** give simultaneously with aluminum- or magnesium-containing antacids.

IV: Dilute dose to 1–2 mg/mL and infuse dose over 60 min (**do not** infuse dose <60 min).

Ophthalmic drops: Apply finger pressure to lacrimal sac during and for 1–2 min after dose application. **Do not** touch the applicator tip, and **do not** wear contact lenses.

AZTREONAM
Azactam, Cayston
Antibiotic, monobactam

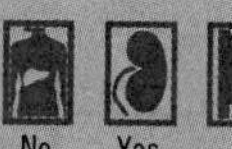
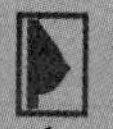
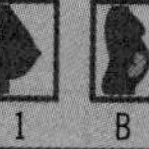
No Yes 1 B

Injection: 1, 2 g
Frozen inj: 1 g/50 mL 3.4% dextrose, 2 g/50 mL 1.4% dextrose (iso-osmotic solutions)
Each 1 g drug contains approximately 780 mg L-Arginine
Nebulizer solution *(Cayston):* 75 mg powder to be reconstituted with the supplied diluent of 1 mL 0.17% sodium chloride (28-day course contains 84 sterile vials of Caysten and 88 ampules of diluent)

Neonate:
30 mg/kg/dose:
<1.2 kg and 0–4 wk age: Q12 hr IV/IM
1.2–2 kg and 0–7 days: Q12 hr IV/IM
1.2–2 kg and >7 days: Q8 hr IV/IM
>2 kg and 0–7 days: Q8 hr IV/IM
>2 kg and >7 days: Q6 hr IV/IM
Child: 90–120 mg/kg/24 hr ÷ Q6–8 hr IV/IM
Cystic fibrosis: 150–200 mg/kg/24 hr ÷ Q6–8 hr IV/IM
Adult:
Moderate infections: 1–2 g/dose Q8–12 hr IV/IM
Severe infections: 2 g/dose Q6–8 hr IV/IM
Max. dose (all ages): 8 g/24 hr
Inhalation:
Cystic fibrosis prophylactic therapy:
≥7 yr and adult: 75 mg TID (minimum 4 hr between doses) administered in repeated cycles of 28 days on drug followed by 28 days off drug. Administer each dose with the Altera Nebulizer System.

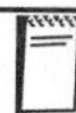

Contraindications: Hypersensitivity to aztreonam or any other of its components
Warnings/Precautions: Use with **caution** in arginase deficiency. Low cross-allergenicity between aztreonam and other β-lactams. Good CNS penetration. **Adjust dose in renal failure (see Chapter 3).**
Adverse effects:
Systemic use: Thrombophlebitis, eosinophilia, leukopenia, neutropenia, thrombocytopenia, liver enzyme elevation, hypotension, seizures, and confusion
Inhalation use: Cough, nasal congestion, wheezing, pharyngolaryngeal pain, pyrexia, chest discomfort, abdominal pain, and vomiting may occur. Bronchospasm has been reported.
Drug interactions: Probenecid and furosemide increases aztreonam levels.
Drug administration:
IV: Dose may be administered via IV push (**max. concentration** of 66 mg/mL over 3–5 min) or intermittent infusion (**max. concentration** of 20 mg/mL over 20–60 min).
IM: Administer into a large muscle such as the upper outer quadrant of the gluteus maximus or lateral part of the thigh. See package insert for recommended IM concentration.
Inhalation: Use the following order of administration: bronchodilator (first), chest physiotherapy, other inhaled medications (if indicated), and aztreonam last.

For explanation of icons, see p. 364.

BACITRACIN ± POLYMYXIN B
AK-Tracin Ophthalmic, Baciguent Topical, BACiiM, and others
In combination with polymyxin B: AK-Poly-Bac Ophthalmic, Polysporin Ophthalmic, Polysporin Topical, and others
Antibiotic, topical

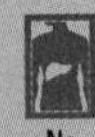
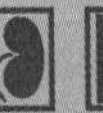
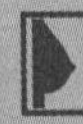
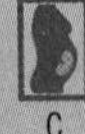

No Yes ? C

BACITRACIN:
- **Ophthalmic ointment:** 500 units/g (3.5 g)
- **Topical ointment [OTC]:** 500 units/g (15, 30 g)
- **Injection (BACiiM):** 50,000 units

BACITRACIN IN COMBINATION WITH POLYMYXIN B:
- **Ophthalmic ointment:** 500 units bacitracin + 10,000 units polymyxin B/g (3.5 g)
- **Topical ointment:** 500 units bacitracin + 10,000 units polymyxin B/g (15, 30 g)

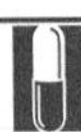

BACITRACIN
Child and adult:
Topical: Apply to affected area 1–5 times/24 hr.
Ophthalmic: Apply 0.25- to 0.5-inch ribbon into the conjunctival sac of the infected eye(s) Q3–12 hr; frequency depends on severity of infection. Administer Q3–4 hr × 7–10 days for mild-to-moderate infections.
Irrigation solution (use when less toxic alternatives are not effective): Using a 50- to 100-unit/mL solution diluted in NS, LR, or sterile water for irrigation, soak sponges in solution for topical compresses one to five times a day or PRN during surgical procedure.
IM (use when less toxic alternatives are not effective; see remarks):
Infant:
≤2.5 kg: 900 units/kg/24 hr ÷ BID–TID
>2.5 kg: 1000 units/kg/24 hr ÷ BID–TID
Child: 800–1200 units/kg/24 hr ÷ Q8 hr
Adult: 10,000–25,000 units/dose Q6 hr
Max. dose: 100,000 units/24 hr
Antibiotic-associated colitis:
Adult: 25,000 units PO Q6 hr × 7–10 days

BACITRACIN + POLYMYXIN B
Child and adult:
Topical: Apply ointment or powder to affected area once daily to TID.
Ophthalmic: Apply 0.25- to 0.5-inch ribbon into the conjunctival sac of the infected eye(s) Q3–12 hr; frequency depends on severity of infection. Administer Q3–4 hr × 7–10 days for mild-to-moderate infections.

Contraindications: Hypersensitivity to bacitracin and/or polymyxin B or any other components in the formulation.

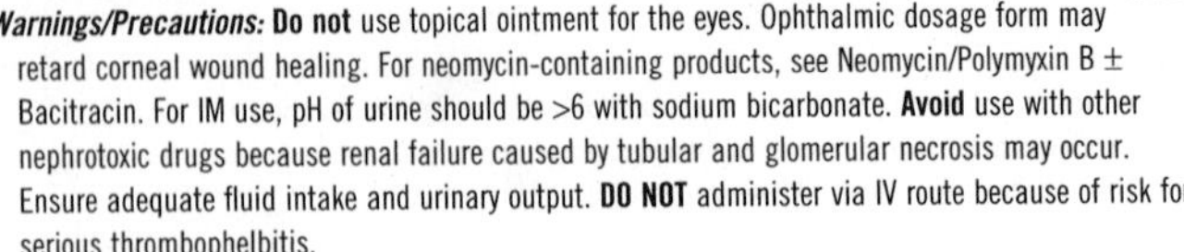

Warnings/Precautions: **Do not** use topical ointment for the eyes. Ophthalmic dosage form may retard corneal wound healing. For neomycin-containing products, see Neomycin/Polymyxin B ± Bacitracin. For IM use, pH of urine should be >6 with sodium bicarbonate. **Avoid** use with other nephrotoxic drugs because renal failure caused by tubular and glomerular necrosis may occur. Ensure adequate fluid intake and urinary output. **DO NOT** administer via IV route because of risk for serious thrombophelbitis.

Adverse effects: Topical dosage form may cause rash, itching, burning, edema, and contact dermatitis. Ophthalmic dosage form may cause temporary blurred vision.

Continued

BACITRACIN ± POLYMYXIN B *continued*

Drug administration:

Ophthalmic route: **Avoid** contact of ointment tube tip with skin or eye and apply dose into the conjuctival sac of the infected eye(s).

IM route: Dissolve in NS containing 2% procaine and administer into the upper outer quadrant of the buttocks (alternating sites); see earlier Warnings/Precautions section for additional information.

BENZYL ALCOHOL
Ulesfia
Antiparasitic agent, pediculocide

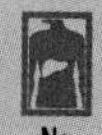 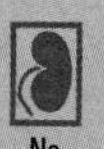 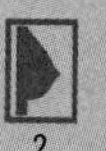 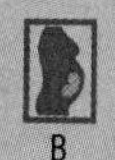
No No 2 B

Topical lotion: 5% (4, 8 ounces)

Head lice infestation:

≥6 mo and adult: Apply the following dosage volume by hair length to dry hair, saturate scalp completely, leave on for 10 min, and rinse thoroughly with water. May shampoo hair and use a lice comb to remove dead lice after application. Repeat dose in 7 days.

Hair Length (in.)	Dose (oz)
0–2	4–6
2–4	6–8
4–8	8–12
8–16	12–24
16–22	24–32
>22	32–48

Contraindications: Hypersensitivity to benzyl alcohol or any other of its components

Warnings/Precautions: Neonates may be at risk for developing a gasping syndrome; use is indicated for children ≥6 mo. Avoid contact with eyes. May cause allergic or contact dermatitis. Use in children should be supervised by an adult.

Adverse effects: Irritation, anesthesia and hypoesthesia to the application site, pain, pruritus, erythema, pyoderma, and ocular irritation are common. Application site dryness, excoriation, paraesthesia, dermatitis, excoriation, thermal burn, dandruff, rash and skin exfoliation have been reported.

Drug administration: See dosage information from above.

BESIFLOXACIN
Besivance
Antibiotic, quinolone

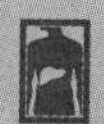 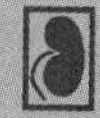 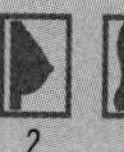 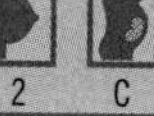
No No 2 C

Ophthalmic suspension: 0.6% (5 mL); contains benzalkonium chloride

Bacterial conjunctivitis:

≥1 yr and adult: Instill 1 drop into affected eye(s) TID (4–12 hr between doses) × 7 days.

Contraindications: Hypersensitivity to besifloxacin or any other of its components.

Warnings/Precautions: For topical ophthalmic use only. Avoid use of contact lenses while receiving medication. Prolonged use may increase risk for resistant organisms.

Adverse effects: Conjunctival redness, blurred vision, eye pain, eye irritation, eye puritis, and headache may occur.

Drug administration: Shake bottle once before each use. Avoid contact of the applicator tip with skin or affected eye.

For explanation of icons, see p. 364.

BOCEPREVIR
Victrelis
Antiviral, protease inhibitor

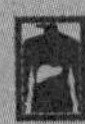
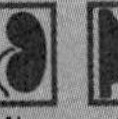
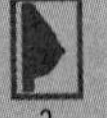
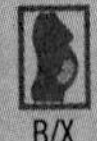
No No 3 B/X

Capsules: 200 mg

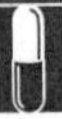

Chronic hepatitis C genotype 1, treatment naïve or previous partial responders or relapsers to interferon and ribavirin patients without cirrhosis: Use in combination with peginterferon alfa (SQ) and ribavirin (PO).

Adult:

Weeks 1–4: Peginterferon alfa and ribavirin only

Weeks ≥5: Add boceprevir 800 mg PO TID (every 7–9 hr) with peginterferon alfa and ribavirin. Therapy is dictated by assessing the patient's HCV RNA at treatment weeks 8, 12, and 24 as outlined in the following table:

	HCV RNA Results		
	Treatment Week 8	**Treatment Week 24***	**Recommendation**
Previously untreated patients	Undetectable	Undetectable	Complete three-medicine regimen through week 28.
	Detectable†	Undetectable	Continue all three medicines through week 36 followed by 12 additional weeks of peginterferon and ribavirin.
Previous partial responder or relapsers	Undetectable	Undetectable	Complete three-medicine regimen through week 36.
	Detectable†	Undetectable	Continue all three medicines through week 36 followed by 12 additional weeks of peginterferon and ribavirin.

*If HCV RNA is detectable at treatment week 24, discontinue all three medications.
†Reassess HCV RNA at treatment week 12; discontinue all three medications if HCV RNA is ≥100 IU/mL.

Patients with compensated cirrhosis should receive 4 weeks peginterferon alfa (SQ) and ribaviran (PO) followed by 44 weeks of boceprevir 800 mg PO TID (every 7–9 hr) with peginterferon alfa and ribavirin. See package insert dosing recommendations for additional clinical situations.

Contraindications: Hypersensitivity to besifloxacin or any other of its components; use with medications metabolized by the CYP 450 3A4 system for which increased levels are associated with serious/life-threatening effects (e.g., cisapride, ergot alkaloids, lovastatin/simvastatin, oral midazolam or triazolam, pimozide, sildenafil); pregnant women and men whose female partners are pregnant because of the required use of ribavirin.

Warnings/Precautions: Must not be used as monotherapy and in pregnancy. Should be used in combination with peginterferon and ribavirin. Use with ritonavir-boosted HIV protease inhibitor therapy is not recommended because hepatitis C efficacy may be reduced. Dosage adjustment is not required in hepatic (no data in decompensated cirrhosis) and renal impairment.

Adverse effects: Fatigue, anemia, rash, dry skin, GI disturbances, headache, and dysgeusia are common. Anemia with peginterferon and ribavirin may worsen with boceprevir. Neutropenia and thrombocytopenia may occur.

Drug interactions: Boceprevir is a substrate and strong inhibitor of CYP 450 3A4/5. See the earlier Contraindications and Warnings/Precautions sections for specific interactions.

Drug administration: Administer all doses with food. Doses should be spaced approximately every 7–9 hr.

BOTULINUM IMMUNE GLOBULIN INTRAVENOUS, HUMAN
BabyBIG, BIG-IV
Immune globulins, botulism

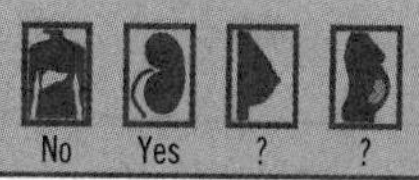

IV preparation in powder for reconstitution: 100 ± 20 mg vial of type A and B immunoglobulins; diluted with 2 mL sterile water for injection (each vial contains 1% albumin, 5% sucrose, 0.02 M sodium phosphate buffer, and trace amounts of IgA and IgM).

Product potency is ≥15 IU/mL anti-type A toxin and ≥4 IU/mL anti-type B toxin activities.

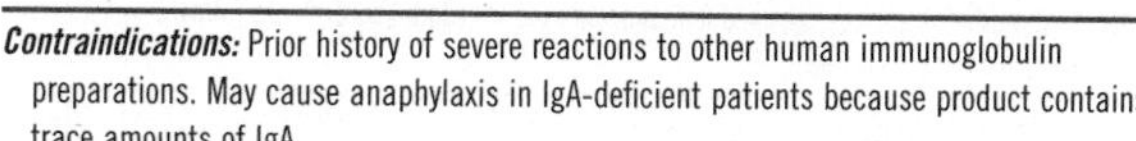

Infant botulism:

IV infusion: 75 mg/kg × 1 as soon as clinical diagnosis is made.

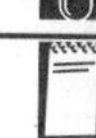

Contraindications: Prior history of severe reactions to other human immunoglobulin preparations. May cause anaphylaxis in IgA-deficient patients because product contains trace amounts of IgA.

Warnings/Precautions: Product contains sucrose; minimize risk for renal dysfunction by administering at the minimum concentration available and at the minimum rate of infusion (see later). Like other plasma products, the risk for transmission of unrecognized bloodborne viral agents may occur. Monitor vital signs during drug administration. Product has only been evaluated in children <1 yr old.

Adverse effects: Anaphylaxis or hypotension may occur; discontinue use and administer supportive care immediately. Chills, muscle cramps, back pain, fever, nausea, vomiting, and wheezing may occur; slow rate of infusion or temporarily interrupt the infusion. Erythematous rash, blood pressure changes, and other GI disturbances have also been reported.

Drug interactions: Defer administration of live virus vaccines approximately 5 mo after BIG-IV.

Drug administration: After initial reconstitution to 50 mg/mL, the solution should be infused within 4 hr. May be further diluted to a minimum concentration of 16.7 mg/mL. Administering with an 18-micron inline or syringe-tip sterile filter is recommended. Use this product only if it is colorless, free of particulate matter, and not turbid.

Initiate infusion at a rate of 25 mg/kg/hr (0.5 mL/kg/hr with a 50-mg/mL solution) for the first 15 minutes. If tolerated, increase rate to a **maximum** of 50 mg/kg/hr. Discontinue infusion and give epinephrine if anaphylaxis or significant hypotension occurs. Slow infusion rate or temporarily interrupt infusion if minor side effects (i.e., flushing, see earlier) occur.

BUTENAFINE
Mentax, Lotrimin Ultra
Antifungal, benzylamine

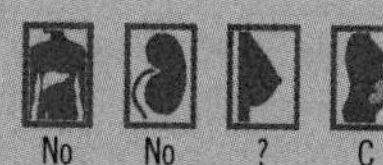

Cream: 1% (12, 15, 24, 30 g)

≥12 yr old:

Pityriasis versicolor, tinea corporis, tinea, cruris: Apply topically to affected areas once daily × 2 weeks

Tinea pedis, interdigital: Apply topically to affected areas BID × 7 days, or once daily × 4 weeks

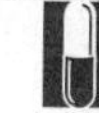

Contraindications: Hypersensitivity to butenafine products or any of its components

Warnings/Precautions: Use with **caution** in patients sensitive to allylamine antifungals. **Avoid** contact with eyes, nose, mouth, and mucous membranes. Safety and efficacy studies have not been conducted for children <12 yr old.

Adverse Effects: May cause burning/stinging, irritation, and itching. Contact dermatitis and exacerbation of fungal infection have been reported.

Drug Interactions: None identified.

Drug Administration: Apply to cover affected areas and immediately surrounding skin, avoiding the eyes, nose, mouth, and mucous membranes.

For explanation of icons, see p. 364.

CAPREOMYCIN
Capastat
Antituberculous agent

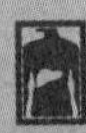 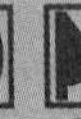 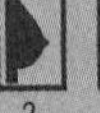 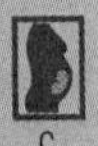
No Yes 2 C

Injection: 1 g

Infant and child <15 yr and ≤40 kg (IV/IM): 15–30 mg/kg/24 hr (**max. dose:** 1 g/24 hr) × 2–4 mo followed by 15–30 mg/kg/24 hr (**max. dose:** 1 g/24 hr) twice weekly
Child ≥15 yr and >40 kg (IV/IM): 15 mg/kg/24 hr (**max. dose:** 1 g/24 hr) × 2–4 mo followed by 15 mg/kg/24 hr (**max. dose:** 1 g/24 hr) 2–3 times/wk
Adult (IV/IM): 1 g/24 hr (**max. dose:** 20 mg/kg/24 hr) × 60–120 days followed by 1 g (**max. dose:** 20 mg/kg/24 hr) 2–3 times/wk; *or* 15 mg/kg/dose (**max. dose:** 1 g/dose) × 2–4 mo followed by 15 mg/kg/dose (**max. dose:** 1 g/dose) 2–3 times/wk

Contraindications: Hypersensitivity to any component of the formulation
Warnings/Precautions: Use with **caution** in preexisting auditory impairment and renal impairment; benefits should be weighed against risks. Adjust dose in patients with renal insufficiency (see Chapter 3).
Adverse effects: Ototoxicity, nephrotoxicity, and eosinophilia are common. Hypocalcemia, hypokalemia, hypomagnesemia, and acute renal tubular necrosis may occur.
Drug interactions: Capreomycin increases the neuromuscular blocking side effects of aminoglycosides, colistimethate, polymyxin B, and neuromuscular blocking agents, and decreases the effects of BCG.
Drug administration:
IM: Dilute with NS or sterile water for injection (see package insert for dilution volume and resultant final concentration) and administer by deep IM injection into a large muscle mass.
IV: Dilute in 100 mL NS and infuse over 60 minutes.

CASPOFUNGIN
Cancidas
Antifungal, echinocandin

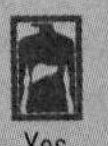 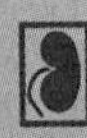 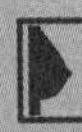 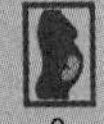
Yes No ? C

Injection: 50, 70 mg; contains sucrose (39 mg in 50-mg vial and 54 mg in 70-mg vial)

Preterm neonate to <3 mo infant (based on a small pharmacokinetic study, achieving similar plasma exposure as seen in adults receiving 50 mg/24 hr): 25 mg/m²/dose IV once daily. Alternatively, 1 mg/kg/dose IV once daily × 2 days followed by 2 mg/kg/dose IV once daily has been reported in a case series with microbiological results.
3 mo infant to 17 yr (see remarks): 70 mg/m²/dose IV loading dose on day 1 followed by 50 mg/m²/dose IV once-daily maintenance dose. Increase the maintenance dose to 70 mg/m²/dose if response is inadequate or if the patient is receiving an enzyme-inducing medication (see remarks).
Maximum loading and maintenance dose: 70 mg/dose
Adolescent and adult (see remarks):
Loading dose: 70 mg IV × 1
Maintenance dose:
Usual: 50 mg IV once daily. If tolerated and response is inadequate, or if patient is receiving an enzyme-inducing medication (see remarks), increase to 70 mg IV once daily.
Hepatic insufficiency (Child–Pugh score 7–9): 35 mg IV once daily

Contraindications: Hypersensitivity to caspofungin or any other components in the formulation
Warnings/Precautions: **Use with caution** in hepatic impairment and concomitant enzyme-inducing drugs. Higher maintenance doses (70 mg/m²/dose in children and 70 mg

Continued

CASPOFUNGIN *continued*

once daily in adults) are recommended for concomitant use of enzyme inducers such as carbamazepine, dexamethasone, phenytoin, nevirapine, efavirenz, or rifampin. In moderate hepatic impairment (Child–Pugh score 7–9), decrease dose by 30%.

Adverse effects: Fever, diarrhea, rash, elevated ALT/AST, hypokalemia, hypotension, and chills are common in children. Facial swelling, nausea/vomiting, headache, infusion site phlebitis, and LFT elevation may occur. Hepatobiliary adverse effects have been reported in children with serious underlying medical conditions.

Drug interactions: Cyclosporine may cause transient increase in LFTs and caspofungin level elevations. May decrease tacrolimus levels. See earlier Warnings/Precautions section.

Drug administration: Administer doses by slow IV infusion over 1 hour at a concentration ≤0.47 mg/mL. **Do not** mix or co-infuse with other medications and **avoid** using dextrose-containing diluents (e.g., D_5W).

CEFACLOR
Ceclor, Ceclor CD, Raniclor, and others
Antibiotic, cephalosporin (second generation)

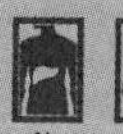 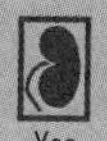 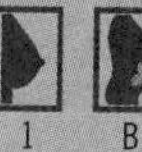
No Yes 1 B

Caps: 250, 500 mg
Extended-release tabs (Ceclor CD): 500 mg
Chewable tabs (Raniclor): 125, 187, 250, 375 mg; contains phenylalanine
Oral suspension: 125 mg/5 mL (75, 150 mL); 187 mg/5 mL (100 mL); 250 mg/5 mL (75, 150 mL); 375 mg/5 mL (100 mL)

Child >1 mo old (use regular release dosage forms): 20–40 mg/kg/24 hr PO ÷ Q8 hr; **max. dose:** 2 g/24 hr
Q12 hr dosage interval optional in otitis media (40 mg/kg/24 hr or pharyngitis 20 mg/kg/24 hr)

Adult: 250–500 mg/dose PO Q8 hr; **max. dose:** 4 g/24 hr
Extended-release tablets: 500 mg/dose PO Q12 hr

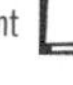

Contraindications: Hypersensitivity to cephalosporin antibiotics

Warnings/Precautions: Use with **caution** in patients with penicillin allergy or renal impairment **(adjust dose in renal failure; see Chapter 3)**. Extended-release tablets are **not recommended** for children.

Adverse effects: Elevated liver function tests, bone marrow suppression, and moniliasis. Serum sickness reactions have been reported in patients receiving multiple courses of cefaclor.

Drug interactions: Probenecid increases cefaclor concentration. May cause positive Coombs' test or false-positive test for urinary glucose.

Drug administration: Administer all doses on an empty stomach; 1 hour before or 2 hours after meals. **Do not** crush, cut, or chew extended-release tablets.

CEFADROXIL
Duricef and others
Antibiotic, cephalosporin (first generation)

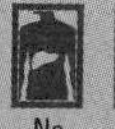 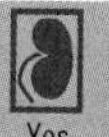 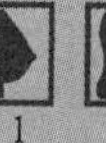
No Yes 1 B

Oral suspension: 250, 500 mg/5 mL (75, 100 mL)
Tabs: 1 g
Caps: 500 mg

Continued

For explanation of icons, see p. 364.

CEFADROXIL *continued*

Infant and child: 30 mg/kg/24 hr PO ÷ Q12 hr (daily dose may be administered once daily for group A β-hemolytic streptococci pharyngitis/tonsillitis); **max. dose:** 2 g/24 hr

Bacterial endocarditis prophylaxis for dental and upper airway procedures: 50 mg/kg/dose (**max. dose:** 2 g) × 1 PO 1 hr before procedure

Adolescent and adult: 1–2 g/24 hr PO ÷ Q12–24 hr (administer Q12 hr for complicated UTIs); **max. dose:** 2 g/24 hr

Bacterial endocarditis prophylaxis for dental and upper airway procedures: 2 g × 1 PO 1 hr before procedure

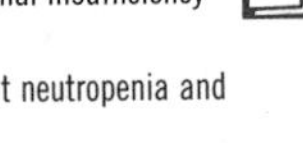

Contraindications: Hypersensitivity to cephalosporin antibiotics

Warnings/Precautions: Use with **caution** in penicillin-allergic patients and renal insufficiency **(adjust dose in renal failure; see Chapter 3)**.

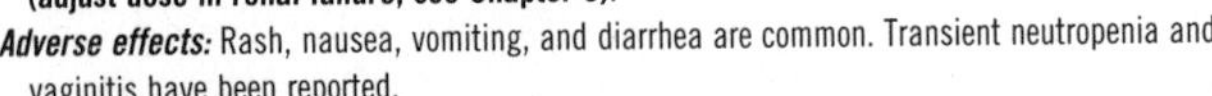

Adverse effects: Rash, nausea, vomiting, and diarrhea are common. Transient neutropenia and vaginitis have been reported.

Drug interactions: Probenecid increases serum cefadroxil levels. May cause false-positive urinary-reducing substances (Clinitest).

Drug administration: Doses may be given with or without food.

CEFAZOLIN

Ancef, Zolicef, and others

Antibiotic, cephalosporin (first generation)

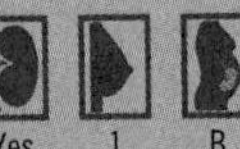
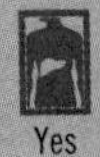
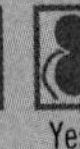
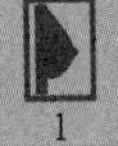
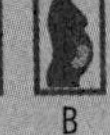

Yes Yes 1 B

Injection: 0.5, 1, 5, 10, 20 g

Frozen injection: 1 g/50 mL 5% dextrose (iso-osmotic solution)

Contains 2.1 mEq Na/g drug.

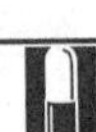

Neonate IM, IV:

Postnatal age ≤7 days: 40 mg/kg/24 hr ÷ Q12 hr

Postnatal age >7 days:

≤2000 g: 40 mg/kg/24 hr ÷ Q12 hr

>2000 g: 60 mg/kg/24 hr ÷ Q8 hr

Infant >1 mo and child: 50–100 mg/kg/24 hr ÷ Q6–8 hr IV/IM; **max. dose:** 6 g/24 hr

Adult: 2–6 g/24 hr ÷ Q6–8 hr IV/IM; **max. dose:** 12 g/24 hr

Bacterial endocarditis prophylaxis for dental and upper airway procedures:

Infant and child: 50 mg/kg/dose (**max. dose:** 1 g) IV/IM 30 min before procedure

Adult: 1 g IV/IM 30 min before procedure

Contraindications: Hypersensitivity to cephalosporin antibiotics

Warnings/Precautions: Use with **caution** in penicillin allergy, patients stabilized on anticoagulants, and hepatic or renal impairment **(adjust dose in renal failure; see Chapter 3)**. Does not penetrate well into CSF.

Adverse effects: GI disturbances are common. Leukopenia, thrombocytopenia, hepatotoxicity, and Stevens–Johnson syndrome have been reported.

Drug interactions: Probenecid increases serum cefazolin levels. May cause transient liver enzyme elevation, and false-positive urine-reducing substance (Clinitest) and Coombs' test.

Drug administration:

IV: IV push, infuse over 3–5 min at a concentration ≤100 mg/mL. For intermittent infusion, infuse over 10–60 min at a concentration of 20 mg/mL. Fluid-restricted patients have received 138 mg/mL via IV push.

IM: Dilute with sterile water to 225–330 mg/mL.

CEFDINIR
Omnicef
Antibiotic, cephalosporin (third generation)

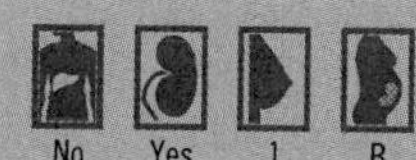

Caps: 300 mg
Oral suspension: 125 mg/5 mL (60, 100 mL), 250 mg/5 mL (60, 100 mL)

6 mo to 12 yr:
Otitis media, sinusitis, pharyngitis/tonsillitis: 14 mg/kg/24 hr PO ÷ Q12–24 hr; **max. dose:** 600 mg/24 hr
Uncomplicated skin infections (see remarks): 14 mg/kg/24 hr PO ÷ Q12 hr; **max. dose:** 600 mg/24 hr
≥13 yr and adult:
Bronchitis, sinusitis, pharyngitis/tonsillitis: 600 mg/24 hr PO ÷ Q12–24 hr
Community-acquired pneumonia, uncomplicated skin infections (see remarks): 600 mg/24 hr PO ÷ Q12 hr

Contraindications: Hypersensitivity to cephalosporin antibiotics
Warnings/Precautions: Use with **caution** in penicillin-allergic patients or in presence of renal impairment **(adjust dose in renal failure; see Chapter 3)**. Good gram-positive cocci activity. Once-daily dosing has not been evaluated in pneumonia and skin infections.
Adverse effects: Diarrhea (especially in children <2 years old), headache, and vaginitis are common. Eosinophilia and abnormal liver function tests have been reported with higher than usual doses.
Drug interactions: Iron-containing vitamins and antacids containing aluminum or magnesium may decrease the drug's absorption (space doses 2 hours apart). Probenecid increases serum cefdinir levels. May cause false-positive urine-reducing substance (Clinitest) and Coombs' test.
Drug administration: Doses may be taken without regard to food. Administer doses at least 2 hours before or after antacids (containing magnesium or aluminum) or iron supplements.

CEFDITOREN PIVOXIL
Spectracef
Antibiotic, cephalosporin (third generation)

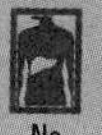
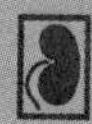
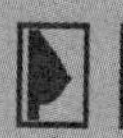
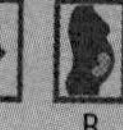
No Yes 1 B

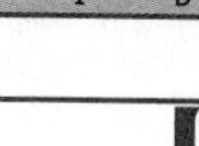

Tabs: 200, 400 mg; contains sodium caseinate

≥12 yr and adult:
Acute bacterial exacerbation in COPD: 400 mg BID PO × 10 days
Community-acquired pneumonia: 400 mg BID PO × 14 days
Pharyngitis, tonsillitis, or uncomplicated skin and skin structure infections: 200 mg PO BID PO × 10 days

Contraindications: Hypersensitivities to cephalosporins or milk protein (tablet contains sodium caseinate). Carnitine deficiency or inborn errors of metabolism that may result in clinical significant carnitine deficiency (pivalate component causes carnitine renal excretion).

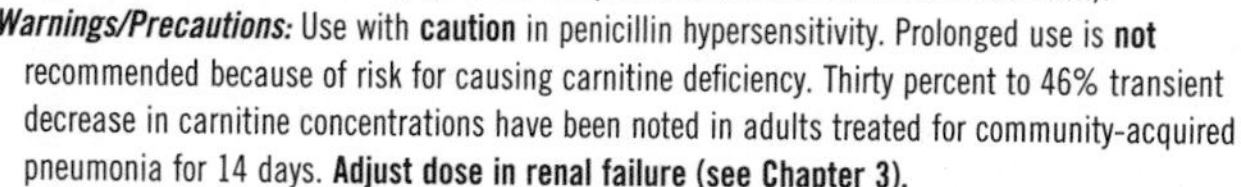

Warnings/Precautions: Use with **caution** in penicillin hypersensitivity. Prolonged use is **not** recommended because of risk for causing carnitine deficiency. Thirty percent to 46% transient decrease in carnitine concentrations have been noted in adults treated for community-acquired pneumonia for 14 days. **Adjust dose in renal failure (see Chapter 3).**
Adverse effects: Diarrhea, nausea, headache, abdominal pain, vaginal moniliasis, dyspepsia, and vomiting may occur.
Drug interactions: Probenecid increases cefditoren levels and antacids (aluminum/magnesium containing) decreases cefditoren absorption.
Drug administration: Doses may be administered with or without food. Administer doses at least 2 hours before or after antacids (containing magnesium or aluminum) or iron supplements.

For explanation of icons, see p. 364.

CEFEPIME
Maxipime and others
Antibiotic, cephalosporin (fourth generation)

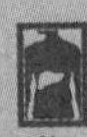 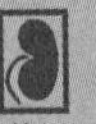 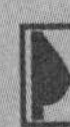 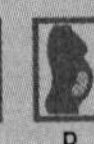 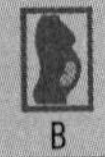
No Yes 1 B

Injection: 0.5, 1, 2 g
Premixed injection: 1 g/50 mL, 2 g/100 mL (iso-osmotic dextrose solution)
Each 1 g drug contains 725 mg L-arginine

Neonate:
<14 days: 60 mg/kg/24 hr ÷ Q12 hr IV/IM
≥14 days: 100 mg/kg/24 hr ÷ Q12 hr IV/IM. For meningitis or *Pseudomonas* infections, use 150 mg/kg/24 hr ÷ Q8 hr IV/IM
Child ≥2 mo: 100 mg/kg/24 hr ÷ Q12 hr IV/IM
Meningitis, fever, and neutropenia, or serious infections: 150 mg/kg/24 hr ÷ Q8 hr IV/IM
Max. dose: 6 g/24 hr
Cystic fibrosis: 150 mg/kg/24 hr ÷ Q8 hr IV/IM, up to a **max. dose** of 6 g/24 hr
Adult: 1–4 g/24 hr ÷ Q12 hr IV/IM
Severe infections: 6 g/24 hr ÷ Q8 hr IV/IM
Max. dose: 6 g/24 hr

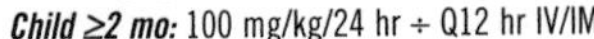

Contraindications: Hypersensitivity to cephalosporin antibiotics
Warnings/Precautions: Use with **caution** in patients with penicillin allergy or renal impairment **(adjust dose in renal failure; see Chapter 3)**. Good activity against *Pseudomonas aeruginosa* and other gram-negative bacteria plus most gram-positive bacteria *(Staphylococcus aureus)*.
Adverse effects: Rash, GI discomfort, and headache are common. May cause thrombophlebitis and transient increases in liver enzymes.
Drug interactions: Probenecid increases serum cefepime levels. May cause false-positive urine-reducing substance (Clinitest) and Coombs' test. Encephalopathy, myoclonus, seizures, transient leukopenia, neutropenia, agranulocytosis, and thrombocytopenia have been reported.
Drug administration:
IV: For IV push, infuse over 3–5 min at a concentration of 100 mg/mL. For intermittent infusion, infuse over 20–30 min at a concentration ≤40 mg/mL.
IM: Dilute with sterile water, D_5W, NS, or lidocaine (0.5% or 1%) to 280 mg/mL. Assess the potential risk/benefit for using lidocaine as a diluent.

CEFIXIME
Suprax
Antibiotic, cephalosporin (third generation)

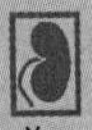 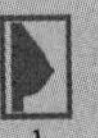 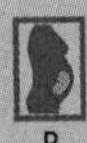
No Yes 1 B

Oral suspension: 100 mg/5 mL (50, 75 mL)
Tabs: 400 mg

Infant (>6 mo) and child: 8 mg/kg/24 hr ÷ Q12–24 hr PO; **max. dose:** 400 mg/24 hr
Acute UTI: 16 mg/kg/24 hr ÷ Q12 hr on day 1, followed by 8 mg/kg/24 hr Q24 hr PO × 13 days; **max. dose:** 400 mg/24 hr
Sexual victimization prophylaxis: 8 mg/kg PO × 1 (**max. dose:** 400 mg) **PLUS** azithromycin 20 mg/kg PO × 1 (**max. dose:** 1 g)
Adolescent and adult: 400 mg/24 hr ÷ Q12–24 hr PO
Uncomplicated cervical, urethral, or rectal infections caused by Neisseria gonorrhoeae: 400 mg × 1 PO **PLUS** azithromycin 1 g × 1 PO or doxycycline 100 mg PO BID × 7 days

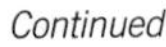
Continued

CEFIXIME *continued*

Sexual victimization prophylaxis: 400 mg PO × 1, **PLUS** azithromycin 1 g PO × 1 or doxycycline 100 mg BID PO × 7 days, **PLUS** metronidazole 2 g PO × 1, **PLUS** hepatitis B vaccine (if not immunized)

Contraindications: Hypersensitivity to cephalosporin antibiotics

Warnings/Precautions: Use with **caution** in patients with penicillin allergy or renal failure **(adjust dose in renal failure; see Chapter 3). Do not** use tablet dosage form for the treatment of otitis media because of reduced bioavailability. Drug is excreted unchanged in urine (50%) and bile (5%–10%).

Adverse effects: Diarrhea, abdominal pain, nausea, and rash

Drug interactions: Probenecid increases serum cefixime levels. May increase carbamazepine serum concentrations. May cause false-positive urine-reducing substance (Clinitest), Coombs' test, and nitroprusside test for ketones.

Drug administration: Doses may be given with or without food.

CEFOTAXIME
Claforan and others
Antibiotic, cephalosporin (third generation)

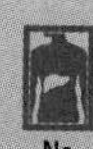
No
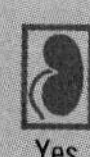
Yes
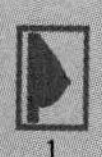
1
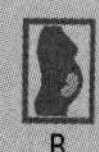
B

Injection: 0.5, 1, 2, 10 g
Frozen injection: 1 g/50 mL 3.4% dextrose, 2 g/50 mL 1.4% dextrose (iso-osmotic solutions)
Contains 2.2 mEq Na/g drug.

Neonate: IV/IM:
Postnatal age ≤7 days:
<2000 g: 100 mg/kg/24 hr ÷ Q12 hr
≥2000 g: 100–150 mg/kg/24 hr ÷ Q8–12 hr
Postnatal age >7 days:
<1200 g: 100 mg/kg/24 hr ÷ Q12 hr
1200–2000 g: 150 mg/kg/24 hr ÷ Q8 hr
>2000 g: 150–200 mg/kg/24 hr ÷ Q6–8 hr

Infant and child (1 mo to 12 yr and <50 kg): 100–200 mg/kg/24 hr ÷ Q6–8 hr IV/IM. Higher doses of 150–225 mg/kg/24 hr ÷ Q6–8 hr have been recommended for infections outside the CSF because of penicillin-resistant pneumococci.
Meningitis: 200 mg/kg/24 hr ÷ Q6 hr IV/IM. Higher doses of 225–300 mg/kg/24 hr ÷ Q6–8 hr, in combination with vancomycin (dosed at CNS target levels), have been recommended for meningitis because of penicillin-resistant pneumococci.
Max. dose: 12 g/24 hr

Child (>12 yr or ≥50 kg) and adult: 1–2 g/dose Q6–8 hr IV/IM
Severe infection: 2 g/dose Q4–6 hr IV/IM
Max. dose: 12 g/24 hr
Uncomplicated gonorrhea: 0.5–1 g × 1 IM

Contraindications: Hypersensitivity to cephalosporin antibiotics

Warnings/Precautions: Use with **caution** in penicillin allergy and renal impairment **(adjust dose in renal failure; see Chapter 3)**. Good CNS penetration.

Adverse effects: Injection-site pain and phlebitis, and GI disturbances are common. Stevens–Johnson syndrome, agranulocytosis, and transient elevations in liver function tests have been reported.

Continued

For explanation of icons, see p. 364.

CEFOTAXIME *continued*

Drug interactions: Probenecid increases serum cefotaxime levels. May cause false-positive urine-reducing substance (Clinitest) and Coombs' test, elevated BUN, creatinine, and liver enzymes.

Drug administration:

IV: For IV push, infuse over 3–5 min at a concentration ≤ 100 mg/mL. For intermittent infusion, infuse over 15–30 min at a concentration 20–60 mg/mL. For fluid restricted patients, 150 mg/mL may be administered via IV push over 3–5 min.

IM: Dilute with sterile water to 230–330 mg/mL.

CEFOTETAN

Cefotan

Antibiotic, cephalosporin (second generation)

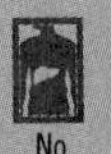 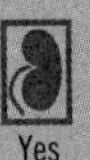 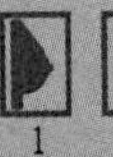 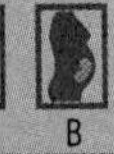

No Yes 1 B

Injection: 1, 2, 10 g

Frozen injection: 1 g/50 mL 3.8% dextrose, 2 g/50 mL 2.2% dextrose (iso-osmotic solutions)

Contains 3.5 mEq Na/g drug.

Infant and child (limited data): 40–80 mg/kg/24 hr ÷ Q12 hr IV/IM

Adolescent and adult: 2–4 g/24 hr ÷ Q12 hr IV/IM

PID: 2 g Q12 hr IV × 24–48 hr after clinical improvement with 100 mg doxycycline Q12 hr PO/IV × 14 days

Max. dose (all ages): 6 g/24 hr

Preoperative prophylaxis (30–60 min before procedure):

Child: 40 mg/kg/dose (**max. dose:** 2 g/dose) IV

Adult: 1–2 g IV

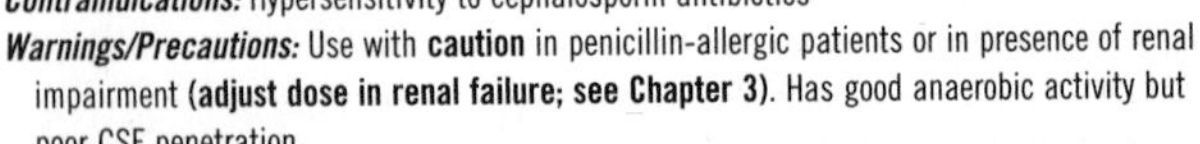

Contraindications: Hypersensitivity to cephalosporin antibiotics

Warnings/Precautions: Use with **caution** in penicillin-allergic patients or in presence of renal impairment **(adjust dose in renal failure; see Chapter 3)**. Has good anaerobic activity but poor CSF penetration.

Adverse effects: Injection-site pain and thrombophlebitis, and diarrhea are common. Hemolytic anemia has been reported.

Drug interactions: Disulfiram-like reaction may occur when taken with ethanol. May increase effects/toxicities of anticoagulants. May cause false-positive urine-reducing substance (Clinitest), and false elevations of serum and urine creatinine (Jaffe method).

Drug administration:

IV: For IV push, infuse over 3–5 min at a concentration of 97–180 mg/mL. For intermittent infusion, infuse over 20–60 min at a concentration 10–40 mg/mL.

IM: Dilute with sterile water or lidocaine (0.5% or 1%) to 375 or 472 mg/mL. Assess the potential risk/benefit for using lidocaine as a diluent.

CEFOXITIN

Mefoxin

Antibiotic, cephalosporin (second generation)

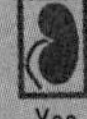 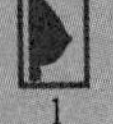 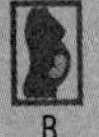

No Yes 1 B

Injection: 1, 2, 10 g

Frozen injection: 1 g/50 mL 4% dextrose, 2 g/50 mL 2.2% dextrose (iso-osmotic solutions)

Contains 2.3 mEq Na/g drug.

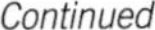

Continued

CEFOXITIN *continued*

Neonate: 90–100 mg/kg/24 hr ÷ Q8 hr IV/IM.

Infant and child:

Mild-to-moderate infections: 80–100 mg/kg/24 hr ÷ Q6–8 hr IM/IV

Severe infections: 100–160 mg/kg/24 hr ÷ Q4–6 hr IM/IV

Adult: 1–2 g/dose Q6–8 hr IM/IV

PID: 2 g IV Q6 hr × 24–48 hr after clinical improvement with 100 mg doxycycline Q12 hr PO/IV × 14 days at the same time

Max. dose (all ages): 12 g/24 hr

Contraindications: Hypersensitivity to cephalosporin antibiotics

Warnings/Precautions: Use with **caution** in penicillin-allergic patients or in presence of renal impairment **(adjust dose in renal failure; see Chapter 3)**. Has good anaerobic activity but poor CSF penetration.

Adverse effects: Injection-site pain, thrombophlebitis, rash, and diarrhea may occur. Immunologic allergic reactions have been reported.

Drug interactions: Probenecid increases serum cefoxitin levels. May cause false-positive urine-reducing substance (Clinitest and other copper reduction method tests), and false elevations of serum and urine creatinine (Jaffe and KDA methods).

Drug administration:

IV: For IV push, infuse over 3–5 min at a concentration ≤200 mg/mL. For intermittent infusion, infuse over 10–60 min at a concentration ≤40 mg/mL.

IM: Dilute with sterile water or lidocaine (0.5 or 1%) to 400 mg/mL. Assess the potential risk/benefit for using lidocaine as a diluent.

CEFPODOXIME PROXETIL
Vantin and others
Antibiotic, cephalosporin (third generation)

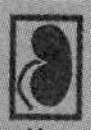
No

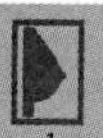
Yes

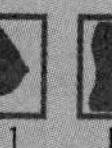
1

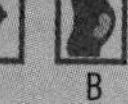
B

Tabs: 100, 200 mg

Oral suspension: 50, 100 mg/5 mL (50, 100 mL)

2 mo to 12 yr:

Otitis media: 10 mg/kg/24 hr PO ÷ Q12–24 hr × 5 days; **max. dose:** 400 mg/24 hr

Pharyngitis/tonsillitis: 10 mg/kg/24 hr PO ÷ Q12 hr × 5–10 days; **max. dose:** 200 mg/24 hr

Acute maxillary sinusitis: 10 mg/kg/24 hr PO ÷ Q12 hr × 10 days; **max. dose:** 400 mg/24 hr

≥13 yr to adult: 200–800 mg/24 hr PO ÷ Q12 hr

Uncomplicated gonorrhea: 200 mg PO × 1

Contraindications: Hypersensitivity to cephalosporin antibiotics

Warnings/Precautions: Use with **caution** in penicillin-allergic patients or in presence of renal impairment **(adjust dose in renal failure; see Chapter 3)**.

Adverse effects: May cause diarrhea, nausea, vomiting, and vaginal candidiasis.

Drug interactions: Probenecid increases serum cefpodoxime levels. High doses of antacids or H2 blockers may reduce absorption. May cause false-positive Coombs' test.

Drug administration: Tablets should be administered with food to enhance absorption. Suspension may be administered without regard to food.

For explanation of icons, see p. 364.

CEFPROZIL
Cefzil and others
Antibiotic, cephalosporin (second generation)

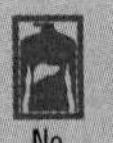 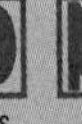 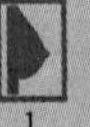 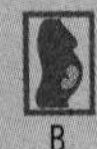
No Yes 1 B

Tabs: 250, 500 mg
Oral suspension: 125 mg/5 mL, 250 mg/5 mL (50, 75, 100 mL) (contains aspartame and phenylalanine)

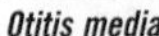

Otitis media:
6 mo to 12 yr: 30 mg/kg/24 hr PO ÷ Q12 hr
Pharyngitis/tonsillitis:
2–12 yr: 15 mg/kg/24 hr PO ÷ Q12 hr
Acute sinusitis:
6 mo to 12 yr: 15–30 mg/kg/24 hr PO ÷ Q12–24 hr
Uncomplicated skin infections:
2–12 yr: 20 mg/kg/24 hr PO Q24 hr
Other:
≥12 yr and adult: 500–1000 mg/24 hr PO ÷ Q12 hr or 500 mg/dose PO Q24 hr
Max. dose (all ages): 1 g/24 hr

Contraindications: Hypersensitivity to cephalosporin antibiotics
Warnings/Precautions: Use with **caution** in penicillin-allergic patients or in presence of renal impairment **(adjust dose in renal failure; see Chapter 3)**. Oral suspension contains aspartame and phenylalanine, and should not be used by phenylketonurics.
Adverse effects: May cause nausea, vomiting, diarrhea, liver enzyme elevations, rash, and vaginitis. Immunologic reactions such as erythema multiforme and Stevens–Johnson syndrome have been reported.
Drug interactions: Probenecid increases serum cefprozil levels. May cause false-positive urine-reducing substance (Clinitest and other copper reduction method tests) and Coombs' test.
Drug administration: Doses may be administered with or without food.

CEFTAROLINE FOSAMIL
Teflaro
Antibiotic, cephalosporin, (fifth generation)

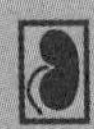 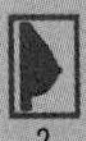 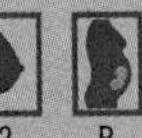
No Yes 2 B

Injection: 400, 600 mg; contains L-arginine

Child: Current clinical trials are investigating the following indications and doses; see www.clinicaltrials.gov for updated information:
Complicated skin infections and community-acquired bacteria pneumonia:
2–6 mo: 8 mg/kg/dose IV Q8 hr
6 mo–<18 yr:
≤33 kg: 12 mg/kg/dose IV Q8 hr
>33 kg: 400 mg/dose IV Q8 hr
Adult: 600 mg IV Q12 hr with the following duration of therapy
Community-acquired pneumonia: 5–7 days
Skin and skin structure infections: 5–14 days

Continued

C

CEFTAROLINE FOSAMIL *continued*

Contraindications: Hypersensitivity to cephalosporin antibiotics

Warnings/Precautions: Use with **caution** in penicillin-allergic patients or in presence of renal impairment (**adult renal dosage adjustment:** CrCl 31–50 mL/min: 400 mg Q12 hr; CrCl 15–30 mL/min: 300 mg Q12 hr; CrCl <15 with hemodialysis: 200 mg Q12 hr and administer dose after dialysis)

Adverse effects: Diarrhea, nausea, and rash are common. May cause constipation, vomiting, phlebitis, increased transaminases.

Drug interactions: Probenecid increases serum ceftaroline levels. Direct Coombs' test seroconversion has been reported with use.

Drug administration: Intermittent IV infusion over 60 min. Adult dosages have been further diluted with 50–250 mL NS, D_5W, dextrose 2.5%, or 0.45% sodium chloride. A maximum concentration of 12 mg/mL has been suggested.

CEFTAZIDIME

Fortaz, Tazidime, Tazicef, Ceptaz (arginine salt)

Antibiotic, cephalosporin (third generation)

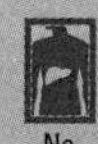
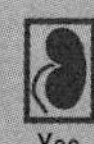
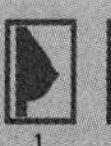
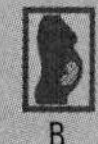

No Yes 1 B

Injection: 0.5, 1, 2, 6 g
Frozen injection: 1g/50 mL 4.4% dextrose, 2 g/50 mL 3.2% dextrose (iso-osmotic solutions)
(Fortaz, Tazicef, Tazidime contains 2.3 mEq Na/g drug)
(Ceptaz contains 349 mg L-arginine/g drug)

Neonate:
IV/IM:
Postnatal age ≤7 days:
<2000 g: 100 mg/kg/24 hr ÷ Q12 hr
≥2000 g: 100–150 mg/kg/24 hr ÷ Q8–12 hr
Postnatal age >7 days:
<1200 g: 100 mg/kg/24 hr ÷ Q12 hr
≥1200 g: 150 mg/kg/24 hr ÷ Q8 hr

Infant (>1 mo) and child: 100–150 mg/kg/24 hr ÷ Q8 hr IV/IM; **max. dose:** 6 g/24 hr
Cystic fibrosis and meningitis: 150 mg/kg/24 hr ÷ Q8 hr IV/IM; **max. dose:** 6 g/24 hr

Adult: 1–2 g/dose Q8–12 hr IV/IM; **max. dose:** 6 g/24 hr

Contraindications: Hypersensitivity to cephalosporin antibiotics

Warnings/Precautions: Use with **caution** in penicillin-allergic patients or in presence of renal impairment **(adjust dose in renal failure; see Chapter 3)**. Good *Pseudomonas* coverage and CSF penetration.

Adverse effects: May cause diarrhea, phlebitis, injection-site pain, rash, and liver enzyme elevations.

Drug interactions: Probenecid increases serum ceftazidime levels. May cause false-positive urine-reducing substance (Clinitest and other copper reduction method tests) and Coombs' test.

Drug administration:
IV: For IV push, infuse over 3–5 min at a concentration ≤180 mg/mL. For intermittent infusion, infuse over 15–30 min at a concentration ≤40 mg/mL.
IM: Dilute with sterile water or lidocaine (0.5% or 1%) to 280 mg/mL. Assess the potential risk/benefit for using lidocaine as a diluent.

For explanation of icons, see p. 364.

CEFTIBUTEN
Cedax
Antibiotic, cephalosporin (third generation)

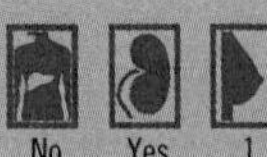
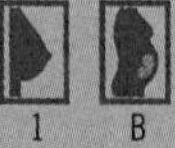
No Yes 1 B

Oral suspension: 90 mg/5 mL (60, 90, 120 mL), 180 mg/5 mL (60 mL); contains sodium benzoate
Caps: 400 mg

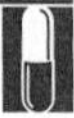

Child (>6 mo):
Otitis media and pharyngitis/tonsillitis: 9 mg/kg/24 hr (**max. dose:** 400 mg/24 hr) PO once daily × 10 days
≥12 yr and adult: 400 mg PO once daily; **max. dose:** 400 mg/24 hr × 10 days

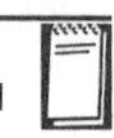

Contraindications: Hypersensitivity to cephalosporin antibiotics
Warnings/Precautions: Use with **caution** in penicillin-allergic patients or in presence of renal impairment **(adjust dose in renal failure; see Chapter 3)**.
Adverse effects: May cause GI symptoms, headache, and transient elevations in liver function tests, eosinophils, and BUN. Stevens–Johnson syndrome has been reported.
Drug interactions: Gastric acid–lowering medications (e.g., ranitidine and omeprazole) may enhance bioavailability of ceftibuten.
Drug administration: Oral suspension should be administered 2 hours before or 1 hour after a meal. Capsules may be administered with or without food.

CEFTRIAXONE
Rocephin and others
Antibiotic, cephalosporin (third generation)

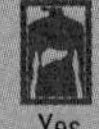
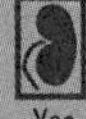
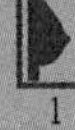
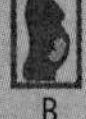
Yes Yes 1 B

Injection: 0.25, 0.5, 1, 2, 10 g
Frozen injection: 1 g/50 mL 3.8% dextrose, 2 g/50 mL 2.4% dextrose (iso-osmotic solutions)
Contains 3.6 mEq Na/g drug.

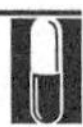

Neonate:
Gonococcal ophthalmia or prophylaxis: 25–50 mg/kg/dose IM/IV × 1; **max. dose:** 125 mg/dose
Infant (>1 mo) and child:
Mild and moderate infections: 50–75 mg/kg/24 hr ÷ Q12–24 hr IM/IV; **max. dose:** 2 g/24 hr
Meningitis (including penicillin-resistant pneumococci) and severe infections: 100 mg/kg/24 hr IM/IV ÷ Q12 hr; **max. dose:** 2 g/dose and 4 g/24 hr
Penicillin-resistant pneumococci outside of the CSF: 80–100 mg/kg/24 hr ÷ Q12–24 hr (**max. dose:** 2 g/dose and 4 g/24 hr)
Acute otitis media: 50 mg/kg IM × 1; **max. dose:** 1 g
Adult: 1–2 g/dose Q12–24 hr IV/IM; **max. dose:** 2 g/dose and 4 g/24 hr
Uncomplicated gonorrhea or chancroid: 250 mg IM × 1
Bacterial endocarditis prophylaxis for dental and upper respiratory procedures:
Infant and child: 50 mg/kg IV/IM (**max. dose:** 1 g) 30 min before procedure
Adult: 1 g IV/IM 30 min before procedure

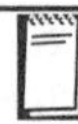

Contraindications: Hypersensitivity to cephalosporin antibiotics and neonates with hyperbilirubinemia. **Do not** administer with IV calcium-containing solutions or products (mixed or administered simultaneously via different lines) in neonates (<28 days old) because of risk for precipitation of ceftriaxone-calcium salt (see later). **Do not** administer simultaneously with IV calcium-containing solutions via a Y-site for any age group. IV

Continued

CEFTRIAXONE *continued*

calcium-containing products may be administered sequentially only when the infusion lines are thoroughly flushed between infusions with a compatible fluid.

Warnings/Precautions: Use with **caution** in penicillin allergy; patients with gallbladder, biliary tract, liver, or pancreatic disease; presence of renal impairment; or in neonates with continuous dosing (risk for hyperbilirubinemia). In neonates, consider using an alternative third generation cephalosporin with similar activity. Unlike other cephalosporins, ceftriaxone is significantly cleared by the biliary route (35%–45%).

Cases of fatal reactions with calcium-ceftriaxone precipitates in lung and kidneys in term and preterm neonates have been reported.

Adverse effects: Rash, injection-site pain, diarrhea, and transient increase in liver enzymes are common. May cause reversible cholelithiasis, sludging in gallbladder, and jaundice. Immune-mediated hemolytic anemia has been reported.

Drug interactions: High-dose probenecid increases serum ceftriaxone levels. May interfere with serum and urine creatinine assays (Jaffe method), and cause false-positive urinary protein and urinary-reducing substances (Clinitest).

Drug administration:

IV: For IV push, infuse over 2–4 min at a concentration ≤40 mg/mL. For intermittent infusion, infuse over 10–30 min at a concentration ≤40 mg/mL.

IM: Dilute drug with either sterile water for injection or 1% lidocaine to a concentration of 250 or 350 mg/mL (250 mg/mL has lower incidence of injection-site reactions). Assess the potential risk/benefit for using lidocaine as a diluent.

CEFUROXIME (IV, IM)/CEFUROXIME AXETIL (PO)
CEFUROXIME AXETIL (PO)
IV: Zinacef and others; PO: Ceftin and others
Antibiotic, cephalosporin (second generation)

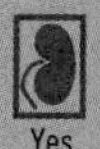
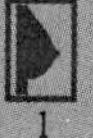
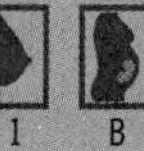

No Yes 1 B

Injection: 0.75, 1.5, 7.5 g
Frozen injection: 750 mg/50 mL 2.8% dextrose, 1.5 g/50 mL water (iso-osmotic solutions)
Injectable dosage forms contain 2.4 mEq Na/g drug.
Tabs: 250, 500 mg
Oral suspension: 125 mg/5 mL, 250 mg/5 mL (50, 100 mL)

IM/IV:

Neonate: 50–100 mg/kg/24 hr ÷ Q12 hr
Infant (>3 mo)/child: 75–150 mg/kg/24 hr ÷ Q8 hr
Adult: 750–1500 mg/dose Q8 hr
Max. dose: 9 g/24 hr

PO (see remarks):

Child (3 mo to 12 yr):

Pharyngitis and tonsillitis:
Oral suspension: 20 mg/kg/24 hr ÷ Q12 hr; **max. dose:** 500 mg/24 hr
Tab: 125 mg Q12 hr

Otitis media, impetigo, and maxillary sinusitis:
Oral suspension: 30 mg/kg/24 hr ÷ Q12 hr; **max. dose:** 1 g/24 hr
Tab: 250 mg Q12 hr

Lyme disease (alternative to doxycycline or amoxicillin):
Oral suspension: 30 mg/kg/24 hr ÷ Q12 hr; **max. dose:** 500 mg/24 hr × 14–28 days

Continued

For explanation of icons, see p. 364.

CEFUROXIME (IV, IM)/CEFUROXIME AXETIL (PO)
CEFUROXIME AXETIL (PO) *continued*

Child (≥13 yr):
Sinusitis, otitis media, pharyngitis, and tonsillitis:
Tab: 250 mg Q12 hr
Adult: 250–500 mg BID
Max. dose: 1 g/24 hr

Contraindications: Hypersensitivity to cephalosporin antibiotics
Warnings/Precautions: Use with **caution** in penicillin-allergic patients or in presence of renal impairment **(adjust dose in renal failure; see Chapter 3). Not recommended for meningitis;** use appropriate third generation cephalosporin instead. Tablets and suspension are **NOT** bioequivalent and are **NOT** substitutable on a mg/mg basis.
Adverse effects: May cause GI discomfort; transient increase in liver enzymes; and thrombophlebitis at the infusion site (IV use).
Drug interactions: Concurrent use of antacids, H2 blockers, and proton pump inhibitors may decrease oral absorption. May cause false-positive urine-reducing substance (Clinitest and other copper-reduction method tests) and Coombs' test; and may interfere with serum and urine creatinine determinations by the alkaline picrate method.
Drug administration:
IV: For IV push, infuse over 3–5 min at a concentration ≤100 mg/mL. For intermittent infusion, infuse over 15–30 min at a concentration ≤30 mg/mL (137 mg/mL concentration may be used in fluid-restricted patients).
IM: Dilute with sterile water to 200–220 mg/mL.
PO: Administer suspension with food. Tablets may be administered with or without food. Avoid crushing tablets because of its bitter taste.

CEPHALEXIN
Keflex and others
Antibiotic, cephalosporin (first generation)

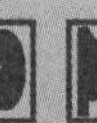
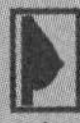
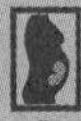
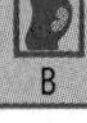
No Yes 1 B

Caps: 250, 500, 750 mg
Tabs: 250, 500 mg
Oral suspension: 125 mg/5 mL, 250 mg/5 mL (100, 200 mL)

Infant and child: 25–100 mg/kg/24 hr PO ÷ Q6 hr. Less frequent dosing (Q8–12 hr) can be used for uncomplicated infections.
Otitis media: 75–100 mg/kg/24 hr PO ÷ Q6 hr
Streptococcal pharyngitis and skin structure infections: 25–50 mg/kg/24 hr PO ÷ Q6–12 hr. Total daily dose may be divided Q12 hr for streptococcal pharyngitis (>1 yr).
Adult: 1–4 g/24 hr PO ÷ Q6 hr
Max. dose (all ages): 4 g/24 hr
Bacterial endocarditis prophylaxis for dental and upper airway procedures:
Infant and child: 50 mg/kg/dose (**max. dose:** 2 g) × 1 PO 1 hr before procedure
Adult: 2 g × 1 PO 1 hr before procedure

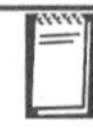

Contraindications: Hypersensitivity to cephalosporin antibiotics
Warnings/Precautions: Some cross-reactivity with penicillins. Use with **caution** in renal insufficiency **(adjust dose in renal failure; see Chapter 3).**

Continued

CEPHALEXIN *continued*

Adverse effects: May cause GI discomfort and transient elevation of liver enzymes.

Drug interactions: May increase the effects of metformin. Probenecid increases serum cephalexin levels, and concomitant administration with cholestyramine may reduce cephalexin absorption. May cause false-positive urine-reducing substance (Clinitest and other copper reduction method tests) and Coombs' test; false elevation of serum theophylline levels (HPLC method); and false urinary protein test.

Drug administration: Administer doses on an empty stomach, 2 hours before or 1 hour after meals.

CHLORAMPHENICOL
Chloromycetin and others
Antibiotic

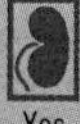
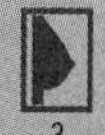
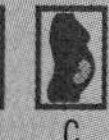

Yes Yes 3 C

Injection: 1 g
Contains 2.25 mEq Na/g drug.

Neonate IV:
- ***Loading dose:*** 20 mg/kg
- ***Maintenance dose (first dose should be given 12 hours after loading dose):***
  - ***≤7 days:*** 25 mg/kg/24 hr Q24 hr
  - ***>7 days:***
    - ***≤2 kg:*** 25 mg/kg/24 hr Q24 hr
    - ***>2 kg:*** 50 mg/kg/24 hr ÷ Q12 hr

Infant, child, and adult: 50–75 mg/kg/24 hr IV ÷ Q6 hr
- ***Meningitis:*** 75–100 mg/kg/24 hr IV ÷ Q6 hr
- **Max. dose (all ages):** 4 g/24 hr

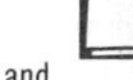

Contraindications: Hypersensitivity to chloramphenicol or any other components in the formulation

Warnings/Precautions: Use with **caution** in G6PD deficiency, renal or hepatic dysfunction, and neonates.

Dose recommendations are just guidelines for therapy; monitoring of blood levels is essential in neonates and infants. Follow hematologic status for dose-related or idiosyncratic marrow suppression. "Gray baby" syndrome may be seen with levels greater than 50 mg/L.

Therapeutic levels: 15–25 mg/L for meningitis; 10–20 mg/L for other infections. Trough: 5–15 mg/L for meningitis; 5–10 mg/L for other infections. Recommended serum sampling time: trough (IV/PO) within 30 min before next dose; peak (IV) 30 min after the end of infusion; peak (PO) 2 hr after oral administration. Time to achieve steady state: 2–3 days for newborns; 12–24 hr for children and adults. *Note:* Higher serum levels may be achieved using the oral, rather than the IV, route.

Adverse effects: Headache, confusion, neurotoxicity, delirium, and depression may occur.

Drug interactions: Concomitant use of phenobarbital and rifampin may decrease chloramphenicol serum levels. Phenytoin may increase chloramphenicol serum levels. Chloramphenicol may increase the effects/toxicity of phenytoin, chlorpropamide, cyclosporin, tacrolimus, and oral anticoagulants, and decrease absorption of vitamin B_{12}. Chloramphenicol is an inhibitor of CYP 450 2C9.

Drug administration: For IV push, infuse over 5 minutes at a concentration ≤100 mg/mL. For intermittent infusion, infuse over 15 to 30 minutes at a concentration ≤20 mg/mL. IM administration is not recommended because it may be less effective by this route.

For explanation of icons, see p. 364.

CHLORHEXIDINE GLUCONATE
Peridex, PerioGard, Dyna-Hex, Betasept, Hibiclens, Avagard, Bactoshield
Topical antibacterial, oral antibiotic rinse

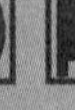
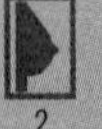
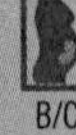

No No 2 B/C

Oral liquid rinse (Peridex, PerioGard [OTC]): 0.12% (15, 118, 480, 1893 mL); contains 11.6% ethanol
Topical liquid (Dyna-Hex [OTC], Betasept [OTC], Hibiclens [OTC]): 2% (120, 480, 960, 3840 mL), 4% (15, 118, 236, 473, 946, 3840 mL); contains isopropyl alcohol
Topical lotion (Avagard [OTC]): 1% (500 mL); contains 61% ethanol
Topical solution (Bactoshield [OTC]): 2% (120, 480, 750, 960, 3840 mL), 4% (120, 473, 960, 3840 mL); contains isopropyl alcohol

Oral rinse (use Peridex or PerioGard):
Adult: 15 mL rinse for 30 sec PO BID after brushing teeth
Topical cleanser (use topical dosage forms):
Child and adult:
Scrub or hand wash: Apply 5 mL per application.

Contraindications: Hypersensitivity to chlorhexidine or any other components in the formulation. **Do not** use as a preoperative skin prep for the face or head because irreversible eye injury has been reported when chlorhexidine is in contact with the eyes during surgery.
Warnings/Precautions: Cases of anaphylaxis have been reported with all products. Tooth staining with the oral rinse may be permanent. Bradycardic episodes have been reported from a breast-fed infant whose mother had used chlorhexidine topically on her breasts to prevent mastitis. Deafness has been reported with direct instillation into the middle ear through a perforated eardrum; and corneal injury has been associated with contact with the eyes.
Use extra **caution** with the topical dosage forms in premature infants or infants younger than 2 months. Topical products that contain alcohol are flammable. Safety and efficacy of the oral rinse have not been determined in children younger than 18 years. Pregnancy category is listed as B or C depending on specific manufacturer.
Adverse effects:
Oral rinse: Tooth staining and taste alteration are common. Irritation and local allergic symptoms have been reported.
Topical cleanser: Irritation/chemical burns, sensitization, and general allergic reactions have been reported (especially in the genital areas).
Drug interactions: None identified.
Drug administration:
Oral rinse: Administer undiluted after brushing teeth and expectorate mouthwash after rinsing for 30 seconds. **Do not** rinse with water or other mouthwashes, or brush teeth after each dose. **Do not** eat for 2 to 3 hours after each application.
Topical cleanser: For surgical scrub, scrub cleanser (without adding water) for 3 minutes and rinse thoroughly, then scrub for 3 more minutes. For hand wash, wash for 15 seconds and rinse.

CHLOROQUINE PHOSPHATE
Aralen and others
Amebicide, antimalarial

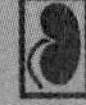

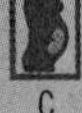

Yes Yes 1 C

Tabs: 250, 500 mg as phosphate (150, 300 mg base, respectively)
Oral suspension: 16.67 mg/mL as phosphate (10 mg/mL base), 15 mg/mL as phosphate (9 mg/mL base)

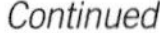

Continued

CHLOROQUINE PHOSPHATE *continued*

Doses expressed in milligrams of chloroquine base:
Malaria prophylaxis (start 1 week before exposure and continue for 4 weeks after leaving endemic area):

Infant and child: 5 mg/kg/dose PO every wk; **max. dose:** 300 mg/dose
Adult: 300 mg/dose PO every wk

Malaria treatment (chloroquine-sensitive strains):
For treatment for malaria, consult with ID specialist or see the latest edition of the *AAP Red Book.*

Infant and child: 10 mg/kg/dose (**max. dose:** 600 mg/dose) PO × 1; followed by 5 mg/kg/dose (**max. dose:** 300 mg/dose) 6 hr later and then once daily for 2 days
Adult: 600 mg/dose PO × 1; followed by 300 mg/dose 6 hr later and then once daily for 2 days

Contraindications: Hypersensitivity to 4-aminoquinoline compounds and retinal/visual changes
Warnings/Precautions: Use with **caution** in liver disease, preexisting auditory damage or seizures, G6PD deficiency, psoriasis, porphyria, or concomitant hepatotoxic drugs. **Adjust dose in renal failure (see Chapter 3).**

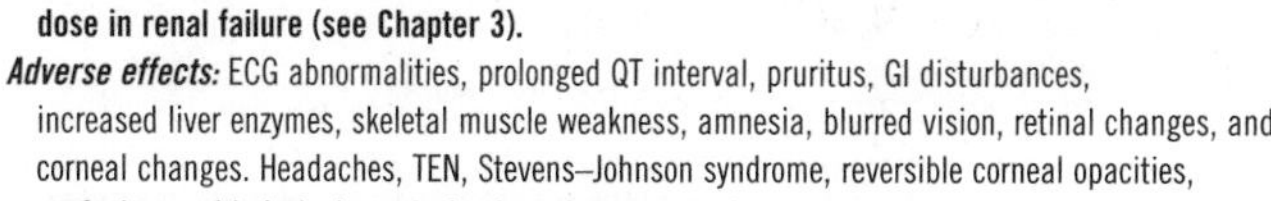

Adverse effects: ECG abnormalities, prolonged QT interval, pruritus, GI disturbances, increased liver enzymes, skeletal muscle weakness, amnesia, blurred vision, retinal changes, and corneal changes. Headaches, TEN, Stevens–Johnson syndrome, reversible corneal opacities, confusion, and hair depigmentation have been reported.
Drug interactions: Chloroquine is a substrate for CYP 450 2D6 and 3A4, and inhibitor of CYP 2D6. Antacids, ampicillin, and kaolin may decrease the absorption of chloroquine (allow 4-hour interval between these drugs and chloroquine). May increase serum cyclosporine levels. Cimetidine may increase effects/toxicity of chloroquine. May increase cyclosporine levels. Use with mefloquine may increase risk for convulsions. May reduce the antibody response to intradermal human diploid-cell rabies vaccine.
Drug administration: Administer oral doses with meals to reduce GI complications. Mixing tablets with chocolate syrup or placing tablets in capsules may be used to mask bitter-tasting tablets.

CICLOPIROX/CICLOPIROX OLAMINE
Loprox, Penlac, Ciclodan, Ciclopirox olamine
Antifungal, synthetic

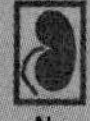
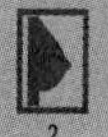
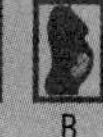

No No ? B

Shampoo: 1% (120 mL)
Topical gel: 0.77% (30, 45, 100 g)
Topical suspension: 0.77% (30, 60 mL)
Topical nail lacquer solution: 8% (3.3, 6.6 mL); contains isopropyl alcohol
Topical cream (Ciclopirox olamine): 0.77% (15, 30, 90 g); contains 1% benzyl alcohol

(See remarks for pediatric [age] considerations):
Tinea pedis, tinea cruris, tinea corporis, cutaneous candidiasis and tinea versicolor:

Topical suspension, gel, cream, or lotion: Apply to affected area BID × 4 wk.

Seborrheic dermatitis of scalp:

Gel: Apply to affected scalp areas BID × 4 wk.
Shampoo: Wet hair and apply 5 mL (up to 10 mL for long hair) to the scalp. Lather, leave on for 3 min, then rinse. Repeat twice weekly for 4 wk with at least 3 days between applications.

Onychomycosis (fingernails or toenails):

Nail lacquer solution: Apply lacquer once daily (preferably QHS or 8 hr before washing) to affected nails, including under nail plate (if free of the nail bed). Daily dose applications should be made

Continued

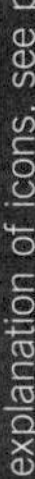

CICLOPIROX/CICLOPIROX OLAMINE *continued*

over the previous coat and removed with alcohol every 7 days. Also file away loose nail material and trim nails as needed when removing the previous coat. Therapy may last up to 48 weeks.

Contraindications: Hypersensitivity to ciclopirox or any other components in the formulation

Warnings/Precautions: **Not** for ophthalmic, oral, or intravaginal use. Discontinue use of shampoo or nail lacquer form with sensitivity reactions or irritation. **Pediatric studies have not been completed** for the cream and lotion forms (<10 years old), gel and shampoo forms (<16 years old), and nail lacquer solution (<12 years old). Nail lacquer solution is flammable.

Adverse effects: Itching, burning, and erythremia may occur with all dosage forms. Nail disorders have been reported with the use of the nail lacquer product. Hair discoloration has been reported with shampoo.

Drug administration: **Avoid** contact with eyes and mucous membranes.

Shampoo, gel (seborrheic dermatitis), and nail lacquer: See respective dosage section.

Topical suspension, gel, cream, or lotion: Apply to affected areas and surrounding skin. Occlusive dressing should not be used.

CIDOFOVIR
Vistide
Antiviral

No Yes 3 C

Injection: 75 mg/mL (5 mL); preservative free

Safety and efficacy has not been established in children.

CMV retinitis:

Adult:

Induction: 5 mg/kg IV once weekly × 2 with probenecid and hydration

Maintenance: 5 mg/kg IV Q2wk with probenecid and hydration

Adenovirus infection in immunocompromised oncology patients (limited data; see remarks):

Child: 5 mg/kg/dose IV once weekly until PCR negative. Administer oral probenecid 1–1.25 g/m²/dose (rounded to the nearest 250-mg interval) 3 hr before and 1 and 8 hr after each dose of cidofovir. Also give IV normal saline at 3 times maintenance fluid 1 hr before and 1 hr after cidofovir, followed by 2 times maintenance fluid for an additional 2 hr. For patients with renal dysfunction (see remarks), give 1 mg/kg/dose IV 3 times weekly until PCR negative.

BK virus hemorrhagic cystitis (limited data): 1 mg/kg/dose IV once weekly without probenecid

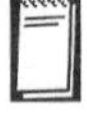

Contraindications: Hypersensitivity to probenecid or sulfa-containing drugs; sCr >1.5 mg/dL, CrCl ≤55 mL/min, urine protein ≥100 mg/dL (2+ proteinuria), direct intraocular injection of cidofovir, and concomitant nephrotoxic drugs

Warnings/Precautions: Monitor renal function and neutrophil counts during therapy. IV NS prehydration and probenecid must be used (unless not indicated) to reduce risk for nephrotoxicity. A reported criteria for defining renal dysfunction in children include a sCr >1.5 mg/dL, GFR <90 mL/min/1.73 m², and >2+ proteinuria.

Modify dose in changing renal function. For adults, reduce maintenance dose to 3 mg/kg if sCr increases 0.3 to 0.4 mg/dL from baseline. Discontinue therapy if sCr increases >0.5 mg/dL from baseline or development of >3+ proteinuria.

Adverse effects: **Renal impairment is the major dose-limiting toxicity.** May also cause nausea, vomiting, headache, rash, metabolic acidosis, uveitis, decreased intraocular pressure, and neutropenia.

Continued

CIDOFOVIR *continued*

Drug interactions: Nephrotoxic medications (e.g., aminoglycosides, amphotericin B) increase risk for toxicity and is contraindicated. Consider drug interactions of probenecid; increases effects/toxicity of zidovudine.

Drug administration: IV infusion over 1 hour at a concentration ≤8 mg/mL.

CIPROFLOXACIN

Cipro, Cipro XR, Ciloxan ophthalmic, Cetraxal, Ciprodex, Cipro HC Otic, and others

Antibiotic, quinolone

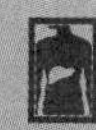
No

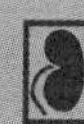
Yes

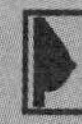
2

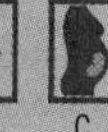
C

Tabs: 100, 250, 500, 750 mg
Extended-release tabs (Cipro XR): 500, 1000 mg
Oral suspension: 250 mg/5 mL (100 mL), 500 mg/5 mL (100 mL)
Injection: 10 mg/mL (40 mL)
Premixed injection: 200 mg/100 mL 5% dextrose, 400 mg/100 mL 5% dextrose (iso-osmotic solutions)
Ophthalmic solution: 3.5 mg/mL (2.5, 5, 10 mL)
Ophthalmic ointment: 3.3 mg/g (3.5 g)
Otic suspension:
Cetraxal: 0.5 mg/0.25 mL (14s)
With dexamethasone (Ciprodex): 3 mg/mL ciprofloxacin + 1 mg/mL dexamethasone (7.5 mL); contains benzalkonium chloride
With hydrocortisone (Cipro HC Otic): 2 mg/mL ciprofloxacin + 10 mg/mL hydrocortisone (10 mL); contains benzyl alcohol

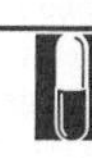

Child:
PO: 20–30 mg/kg/24 hr ÷ Q12 hr; **max. dose:** 1.5 g/24 hr
IV: 20–30 mg/kg/24 hr ÷ Q12 hr; **max. dose:** 800 mg/24 hr
Complicated UTI or pyelonephritis (× 10–21 days):
PO: 20–40 mg/kg/24 hr ÷ Q12 hr; **max. dose:** 1.5 g/24 hr
IV: 18–30 mg/kg/24 hr ÷ Q8 hr; **max. dose:** 1.2 g/24 hr
Cystic fibrosis:
PO: 40 mg/kg/24 hr ÷ Q12 hr; **max. dose:** 2 g/24 hr
IV: 30 mg/kg/24 hr ÷ Q8 hr; **max. dose:** 1.2 g/24 hr
Anthrax (see remarks):
Inhalational/systemic/cutaneous: Start with 20–30 mg/kg/24 hr ÷ Q12 hr IV (**max. dose:** 800 mg/24 hr) and convert to oral dosing with clinical improvement at 20–30 mg/kg/24 hr ÷ Q12 hr PO (**max. dose:** 1 g/24 hr). Duration of therapy: 60 days (IV and PO combined).
Postexposure prophylaxis: 20–30 mg/kg/24 hr ÷ Q12 hr PO × 60 days; **max. dose:** 1 g/24 hr

Adult:
PO:
Immediate release: 250–750 mg/dose Q12 hr
Extended release (Cipro XR):
Uncomplicated UTI/cystitis: 500 mg/dose Q24 hr
Complicated UTI/uncomplicated pyelonephritis: 1000 mg/dose Q24 hr
IV: 200–400 mg/dose Q12 hr; 400 mg/dose Q8 hr for more severe/complicated infections

Continued

For explanation of icons, see p. 364.

CIPROFLOXACIN *continued*

Anthrax (see remarks):

Inhalational/systemic/cutaneous: Start with 400 mg/dose Q12 hr IV and convert to oral dosing with clinical improvement at 500 mg/dose Q12 hr PO. Duration of therapy: 60 days (IV and PO combined).

Postexposure prophylaxis: 500 mg/dose Q12 hr PO × 60 days

Ophthalmic solution: 1–2 drops Q2 hr while awake × 2 days, then 1–2 gtt Q4 hr while awake × 5 days

Ophthalmic ointment: Apply 0.5-inch ribbon TID × 2, then BID × 5 days

Otic:

Cetraxal:

Acute otitis externa (≥1 yr and adult): 0.25 mL to affected ear(s) BID × 7 days

Ciprodex:

Acute otitis media with tympanostomy tubes or acute otitis externa (≥6 mo and adult): 4 drops to affected ear(s) BID × 7 days

Cipro HC Otic:

Otitis externa (≥1 yr and adult): 3 drops to affected ear(s) BID × 7 days

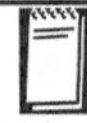

Contraindications: Hypersensitivity to ciprofloxacin, fluoroquinolones, or any other components in the formulation. Concomitant use with tizanidine may result in excessive sedation and dangerous hypotension. Otic formulation should not be used with viral infections of the external ear canal.

Warnings/Precautions: Use with **caution** in children younger than 18 years (like other quinolones, tendon rupture can occur during or after therapy, especially with concomitant corticosteroid use), alkalinized urine (crystalluria), seizures, excessive sunlight (photosensitivity), and renal dysfunction **(adjust dose in renal failure; see Chapter 3)**. Avoid use in myasthenia gravis; may exacerbate muscle weakness. **Not recommended** for gonorrhea because of potential resistance. **Do not** use Cipro HC otic suspension with perforated tympanic membranes.

Combinational antimicrobial therapy is recommended for anthrax. For penicillin-susceptible strains, consider changing to high-dose amoxicillin (25–35 mg/kg/dose TID PO). See www.bt.cdc.gov for the latest information.

Extended-release tablets are formulated as combination of immediate (~35%) and sustained (~65%) release components. See Chapter 3 for dosing in obese patients.

Adverse effects:

Systemic: GI symptoms, headache, restlessness, and rash are common. Tendinitis, rupture tendon (concomitant corticosteroid use and in elderly), photosensitivity, renal failure, psychosis, and seizures have been reported.

Ophthalmic: Burning and discomfort are common. Lid crusting, foreign body sensation, and conjunctival hyperemia may occur.

Otic: Altered taste sense, headache, and otalgia may occur.

Drug interactions: Inhibits CYP 450 1A2. Ciprofloxacin can increase effects and/or toxicity of caffeine, methotrexate, theophylline, tizanidine, warfarin, and cyclosporine. Ciprofloxacin may reduce mycophenolate levels. Probenecid increases serum ciprofloxacin levels.

Drug administration:

IV: For intermittent infusion, infuse over 60 minutes at a concentration ≤2 mg/mL.

PO: All oral dosage forms may be administered with or without food. **Do not administer** antacids, other divalent salts (including dairy products), or sucralfate. Administer ciprofloxacin 2 hours before or 6 hours after taking aforementioned products. **Do not administer** oral suspension through a feeding tube because suspension adheres to tube.

Continued

CIPROFLOXACIN *continued*

Ophthalmic:

Drops: Apply finger pressure to lacrimal sac during and for 1 to 2 minutes after dose application.

Ointment: Instill ointment in lower conjunctival sac by avoiding contact of ointment tip with eye or skin.

Otic:

AOM with tympanostomy tube: Instill drops by having patient lie with affected ear upward. Pump tragus five times by pushing inward to facilitate penetration of drops to middle ear and remain in the same position for 1 minute.

Otitis external: Patient should lie with the affected ear upward while instilling drops. Remain in this position for 1 minute after dosing.

CLARITHROMYCIN

Biaxin, Biaxin XL, and others

Antibiotic, macrolide

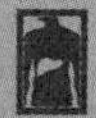
Yes
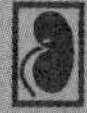
Yes
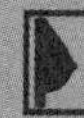
2
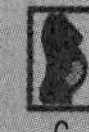
C

Film tablets: 250, 500 mg
Extended-release tablets (Biaxin XL): 500 mg
Granules for oral suspension: 125 mg/5 mL, 250 mg/5 mL (50, 100 mL)

Infant and child:

Acute otitis media, pharyngitis/tonsillitis, pneumonia, acute maxillary sinusitis, or uncomplicated skin infections: 15 mg/kg/24 hr PO ÷ Q12 hr

Pertussis (≥1 mo): 15 mg/kg/24 hr PO ÷ Q12 hr × 7 days; **max. dose:** 1 g/24 hr

Bacterial endocarditis prophylaxis: 15 mg/kg (**max. dose:** 500 mg) PO 1 hr before procedure

Mycobacterium avium ***complex:***

Prophylaxis (first episode and recurrence): 15 mg/kg/24 hr PO ÷ Q12 hr

Treatment: 15 mg/kg/24 hr PO ÷ Q12 hr with other antimycobacterial drugs

Max. dose: 1 g/24 hr

Adolescent and adult:

Pharyngitis/tonsillitis, acute maxillary sinusitis, bronchitis, pneumonia, or uncomplicated skin infections:

Immediate release: 250–500 mg/dose Q12 hr PO

Extended release (Biaxin XL): 1000 mg Q24 hr PO (currently not indicated for pharyngitis/tonsillitis or uncomplicated skin infections)

Adult:

Pertussis: 500 mg (immediate release)/dose Q12 hr PO × 7 days

Bacterial endocarditis prophylaxis: 500 mg PO 1 hr before procedure

M. avium ***complex:***

Prophylaxis (first episode and recurrence): 500 mg/dose Q12 hr PO

Treatment: 500 mg Q12 hr PO with other antimycobacterial drugs

Helicobacter pylori ***GI infection:*** 250 mg Q12 hr to 500 mg Q8 hr PO with omeprazole or ranitidine bismuth; or amoxicillin and omeprazole or lansoprazole

Contraindications: Hypersensitivity to macrolide antibiotics (e.g., erythromycin). Concomitant cisapride, pimozide, astemizole, terfenadine, ergotamine, or dihydroergotamine may result in QT interval prolongation. History of cholestatic jaundice/hepatic dysfunction associated with prior clarithromycin use.

Continued

For explanation of icons, see p. 364.

CLARITHROMYCIN *continued*

Warnings/Precautions: As with other macrolides, clarithromycin has been associated with QT prolongation and ventricular arrhythmias, including ventricular tachycardia and torsades de pointes. Exacerbation of myasthenia gravis symptoms has been reported.

Adjust dose in renal failure (see Chapter 3).

Adverse effects: Diarrhea, nausea, abnormal taste, dyspepsia, abdominal discomfort (less than erythromycin but greater than azithromycin), and headache. Rare cases of anaphylaxis, hepatic dysfunction, Stevens–Johnson syndrome, and toxic epidermal necrolysis have been reported.

Drug interactions: Substrate and inhibitor of CYP 450 3A4; and inhibitor of CYP 1A2. May increase effects/toxicity of carbamazepine, theophylline, cyclosporine, digoxin, ergot alkaloids, fluconazole, tacrolimus, triazolam, and warfarin.

Drug administration: Extended-release tablets must be administered with food. All other dosage forms may be administered with or without food.

CLINDAMYCIN
Cleocin, Cleocin-T, and many others
Antibiotic, lincomycin derivative

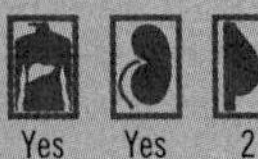
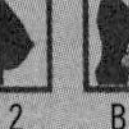
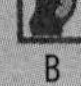

Yes Yes 2 B

Caps: 75, 150, 300 mg
Oral solution: 75 mg/5 mL (100 mL)
Injection: 150 mg/mL (contains 9.45 mg/mL benzyl alcohol)
Solution, topical (Cleocin-T): 1% (30, 60 mL); may contain 50% isopropyl alcohol
Gel, topical (Cleocin-T): 1% (30, 60 g); may contain methylparaben
Lotion, topical (Cleocin-T): 1% (60 mL); may contain methylparaben
Foam, topical: 1% (50, 100 g); contains 58% ethanol
Vaginal cream: 2% (40 g); may contain benzyl alcohol
Vaginal suppository: 100 mg (3s)

Neonate:
IV/IM: 5 mg/kg/dose with following dosage intervals:

≤7 days:
≤2 kg: Q12 hr
>2 kg: Q8 hr
>7 days:
<1.2 kg: Q12 hr
1.2–2 kg: Q8 hr
>2 kg: Q6 hr

Child:
PO: 10–30 mg/kg/24 hr ÷ Q6–8 hr; **max. dose:** 1.8 g/24 hr
IM/IV: 25–40 mg/kg/24 hr ÷ Q6–8 hr; **max. dose:** 4.8 g/24 hr
Bacterial endocarditis prophylaxis: 20 mg/kg (**max. dose:** 600 mg) 1 hr before procedure with PO route and 30 min before procedure with IV route

Adult:
PO: 150–450 mg/dose Q6–8 hr; **max. dose:** 1.8 g/24 hr
IM/IV: 1200–1800 mg/24 hr IM/IV ÷ Q6–12 hr; **max. dose:** 4.8 g/24 hr
Bacterial endocarditis prophylaxis: 600 mg 1 hr before procedure with PO route and 30 min before procedure with IV route

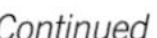
Continued

CLINDAMYCIN *continued*

Topical (≥12 yr and adult): Apply to affected area BID.
Bacterial vaginosis (adolescent and adult):
Suppositories: 100 mg/dose QHS × 3 days
Vaginal cream (2%): 1 applicator dose (5 g) QHS for 3 or 7 days in nonpregnant patients and for 7 days in pregnant patients in second and third trimesters

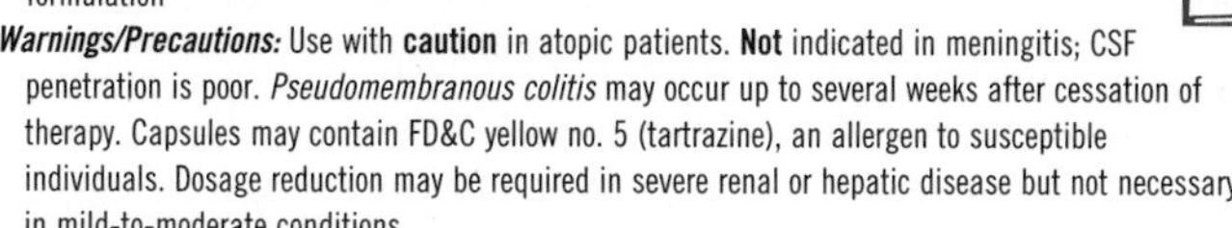

Contraindications: Hypersensitivity to clindamycin, lincomycin, or any other components in the formulation
Warnings/Precautions: Use with **caution** in atopic patients. **Not** indicated in meningitis; CSF penetration is poor. *Pseudomembranous colitis* may occur up to several weeks after cessation of therapy. Capsules may contain FD&C yellow no. 5 (tartrazine), an allergen to susceptible individuals. Dosage reduction may be required in severe renal or hepatic disease but not necessary in mild-to-moderate conditions.
Adverse effects:
Systemic use: Diarrhea, rash, Stevens–Johnson syndrome, granulocytopenia, thrombocytopenia, or sterile abscess at injection site have been reported.
Topical use: Itching, burning, dryness and irritation of the skin, headache, and allergic reactions (including anaphylaxis) have been reported.
Vaginal use: Pruritus, fungal infections, vaginal pain, and headache have been reported.
Drug interactions: Clindamycin may increase the neuromuscular blocking effects of tubocurarine, pancuronium.
Drug administration:
IV: For intermittent infusion, infuse over 10–60 min at a rate ≤30 mg/min (hypotension and cardiac arrest have been reported with rapid infusions) and at a concentration ≤18 mg/mL.
IM: Use 150 mg/mL injectable solution. **Do not exceed** 600 mg per IM dose.
PO: All dosage forms may be administered with or without meals. Take capsules with a glassful of water. Oral liquid preparation is not palatable; consider use of oral capsules as a sprinkle onto applesauce or pudding.
Topical gel, cream, and lotion: **Do not** use intravaginally, in the eye, or orally.

CLOFAZIMINE
Lamprene
Leprostatic agent

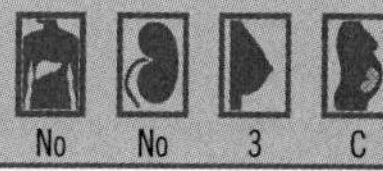

Caps: 50, 100 mg
Drug is available under an IND held by National Hansen's Disease Programs. Prescribers must call (225) 578-9861 or (800) 642-2477 to obtain drug.

Multibacillary leprosy (≥6 patches):
Child: 7.5 mg/kg/24 hr (**max. dose:** 50 mg) once daily PO, *with* rifampin 10 mg/kg/24 hr (**max. dose:** 600 mg) once daily PO and dapsone 1 mg/kg/dose (**max. dose:** 100 mg) once daily PO × 24 mo
Adult: 50 mg once daily PO, *with* rifampin 600 mg/24 hr once daily PO and dapsone 100 mg once daily PO × 24 mo
Erythema nodosum leprosum:
Adult: 100–200 mg once daily PO up to 3 mo to facilitate steroid dose reduction or elimination, then taper dose to 100 mg as soon as reactive episode is controlled.

Continued

For explanation of icons, see p. 364.

CLOFAZIMINE *continued*

Contraindications: Hypersensitivity to clofazimine products

Warnings/Precautions: Several GI effects (bowel obstruction, GI hemorrhage, splenic infarction), some fatal, have been reported rarely. Pink to brownish black skin discoloration side effect may take months to years to reverse. Dosages are generally well tolerated when ≤100 mg/24 hr. *AAP Red Book* does not recommend use for treatment of MAC infections because of poor efficacy.

Adverse effects: Skin discoloration, dry skin, rash, GI disturbances, conjunctival/corneal pigmentation, and abnormal body fluid color. Depression related to skin discoloration has been reported.

Drug interactions: Concurrent administration with antacids containing aluminum/magnesium and orange juice will reduce clofazimine absorption. May reduce phenytoin levels. Use with isoniazid may increase plasma and urinary concentration, and decrease skin concentrations.

Drug administration: Administer doses with meals.

CLOTRIMAZOLE
Lotrimin AF, Cruex, Gyne-Lotrimin 3, Gyne-Lotrimin 7, Mycelex, Mycelex-7, and others
Antifungal, imidazole

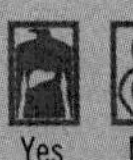
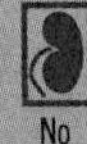
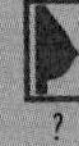
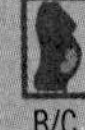
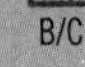

Yes No ? B/C

Oral troche: 10 mg
Cream, topical (OTC): 1% (15, 30, 45 g); contains benzyl alcohol
Solution, topical (OTC): 1% (10, 30 mL)
Lotion, topical (OTC): 1% (20 mL); contains benzyl alcohol
Vaginal suppository (OTC): 200 mg
Vaginal cream (OTC): 1% (45 g), 2% (21 g)

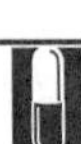

Topical: Apply to skin BID × 4–8 wk

Vaginal candidiasis (>12 yr and adult):

Vaginal suppositories (may be used in combination with a vaginal cream applied onto the vulva once or twice daily):
100 mg/dose QHS × 7 days, or
200 mg/dose QHS × 3 days

Vaginal cream:
1 applicator dose (5 g) of 1% cream intravaginally QHS × 7–14 days, or
1 applicator dose of 2% cream intravaginally QHS × 3 days

Thrush:

>3 yr to adult: Dissolve slowly (15–30 min) one troche in the mouth 5 times/24 hr ×14 days

Contraindications: Hypersensitivity to clotrimazole or any other components in the formulation

Warnings/Precautions: **Avoid** use of condoms and diaphragms with vaginal cream or suppository because latex can be weakened. **Do not use** troches for systemic infections. Pregnancy code is a "B" for topical and vaginal dosage forms, and "C" for troches.

Adverse effects: May cause erythema, blistering, or urticaria with topical use. Liver enzyme elevation, nausea, and vomiting may occur with troches.

Drug administration:

PO: Troches should be dissolved slowly in the mouth over 15 to 30 minutes.

Topical: **Avoid** contact with eyes.

Vaginal: Wash hands before using. Remain lying down for 30 minutes after application of cream or suppository. Wash applicator after every use. **Do not use** tampons until therapy is completed.

COLISTIMETHATE SODIUM
Coly-Mycin M Parenteral, colistin, colistin sodium methanesulfonate
Antibiotic, polypeptide

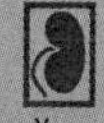
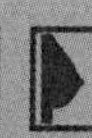
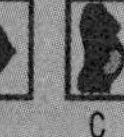
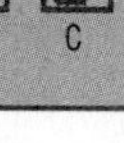
No Yes ? C

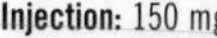

Injection: 150 mg
1 mg pure colistin is equivalent to 30,000 units
Nebulizer solution: 75 mg/3 mL, 150 mg/4 mL (mixed in 0.25% NS, preservative free 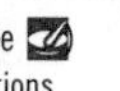
For otic preparation (Cortisporin-TC Otic), see *Neomycin/Hydrocortisone* Otic Preparations

Dosages are expressed in terms of milligrams colistin.
Neonate:
<7 days: 5 mg/kg/24 hr IM ÷ Q12 hr
≥7 days: 7.5 mg/kg/24 hr IM ÷ Q8 hr
Child and adult: 2.5–5 mg/kg/24 hr IV/IM ÷ Q6–12 hr; **max. dose:** 7 mg/kg/24 hr ÷ Q8 hr
Cystic fibrosis: 5–8 mg/kg/24 hr IV ÷ Q8 hr; **max. dose:** 100 mg/dose
Inhalation:
Cystic fibrosis prophylaxis therapy:
Use with conventional nebulizer (e.g., PARI LC Plus): 150 mg Q12 hr administered in repeated cycles of 28 days on drug followed by 28 days off drug
Use with eFlow nebulizer: 75 mg Q12 hr administered in repeated cycles of 28 days on drug followed by 28 days off drug

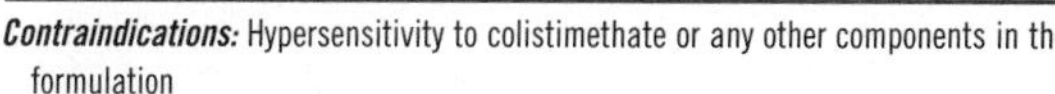
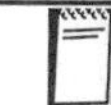
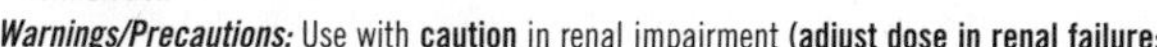

Contraindications: Hypersensitivity to colistimethate or any other components in the formulation
Warnings/Precautions: Use with **caution** in renal impairment **(adjust dose in renal failure; see Chapter 3)** and with neuromuscular blocking agents. Dose-dependent nephrotoxicity may occur. Use ideal body weight for obese patients when calculating dosages.
Do not use premixed unit dose vials for inhalation. Premixing colistimethate (a prodrug) into an aqueous solution and storing it will increase concentrations of the more active and toxic product, colistin. Inhaled colistin has been shown to cause massive inflammation in rats and dogs.
Adverse effects: GI disturbances, rash, and transient neurologic symptoms (circumoral paresthesias, tingling of extremities or tongue). Respiratory distress and nephrotoxicity have been reported. Bronchospasm may occur with nebulized route, especially those with CF or asthma.
Drug interactions: Aminoglycosides, muscle relaxants (e.g., Tubocurarine), polymyxin, succinylcholine, gallamine, decamethonium, and sodium citrate may potentiate neuromuscular blockade. Cephalothin may enhance nephrotoxicity.
Drug administration:
IV: For intermittent infusion, infuse over 3–5 min at a convenient concentration. For continuous infusion, infuse half of the total daily dose over 3–5 min, give remainder of dose over 22–23 hr by diluting to a convenient concentration with compatible IV fluid (D5W, NS, and others).
IM: Dilute to 75 mg/mL concentration with sterile water.
Inhalation:
Conventional nebulizer: If using PARI LC Plus nebulizer, use a DeVilbiss Pulmo-Aide compressor. Treatment period is usually over 15 min.
eFlow nebulizer: Dose may be diluted with NS up to a total volume of 4 mL. Treatment period is usually over 10–12 min.

COLISTIN

See *Colistimethate sodium*

For explanation of icons, see p. 364.

CO-TRIMOXAZOLE

See *Sulfamethoxazole and Trimethoprim*

CYCLOSERINE
Seromycin
Antituberculosis agent

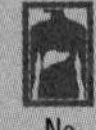
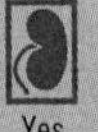
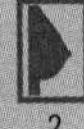
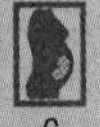

No Yes 2 C

Caps: 250 mg

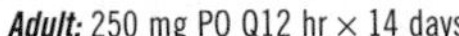

Mycobacterium avium *complex and tuberculosis:*
Child: 10–20 mg/kg/24 hr PO ÷ Q12 hr; **max. dose:** 1 g/24 hr
Adult: 250 mg Q12 hr PO × 14 days, then as tolerated to 250 mg Q6–8 hr; **max. dose:** 1 g/24 hr
UTI:
Adult: 250 mg PO Q12 hr × 14 days

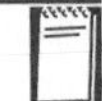

Contraindications: Hypersensitivity to cycloserine, epilepsy, depression, anxiety, psychosis, and alcohol abuse
Warnings/Precautions: **Adjust dose in renal impairment (see Chapter 3).** Should be given as part of a multidrug regimen.
Therapeutic peak serum levels: 20–35 mg/L; recommended serum sampling time at steady state: 2 hr postdose after 3–4 days of continuous dosing
Adverse effects: Confusion, dizziness, headache, and somnolence are common. Seizures have been reported.
Drug interactions: Increases effects/toxicity of phenytoin. Alcohol increases risk for seizures. Ethionamide and isoniazid may increase neurotoxicity.
Drug administration: Should be given on an empty stomach for maximum absorption.

CYTOMEGALOVIRUS IMMUNE GLOBULIN
CytoGam
Immune globulin, CMV (high titer)

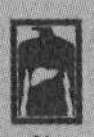
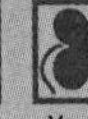
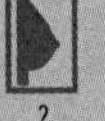
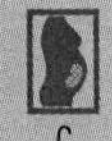

No Yes ? C

Injection: 50 mg/mL (20, 50 mL); each 1 mL contains 50 mg sucrose, 10 mg albumin; 20–30 mEq/L sodium; and trace amounts of IgA and IgM

Child and adult:
CMV prophylaxis after transplant (IV):
Kidney: 150 mg/kg/dose × 1 within 72 hr before transplant, then 100 mg/kg/dose at 2, 4, 6, and 8 wk after transplant, followed by 50 mg/kg/dose at 12 and 16 wk after transplant
Liver, pancreas, lung, or heart (for CMV-negative recipient receiving organ from CMV-positive donor; consider concomitant use of ganciclovir) (IV): 150 mg/kg/dose within 72 hr before transplant and on 2, 4, 6, and 8 wk after transplant, followed by 100 mg/kg/dose at 12 and 16 wk after transplant
Bone marrow transplantation (IV): 200 mg/kg/dose at 6 and 8 days before transplant and on days 1, 7, 14, 21, 28, 42, 56, and 70 after transplant

Contraindications: History of a prior severe reaction associated with any immunoglobulin preparation; IgA deficiency
Warnings/Precautions: Use with **caution** in preexisting or predisposition to renal insufficiency; formulation contains sucrose. Defer administration of live virus vaccines approximately 3 months after CMV-Ig; revaccination may be necessary if vaccines were administered after CMV-Ig.

Continued

CYTOMEGALOVIRUS IMMUNE GLOBULIN *continued*

Adverse effects: Flushing, shivering, GI disturbances, arthralgia, back pain, cramping, hypotension, wheezing, and fever are common and most often infusion related. Anaphylaxis and aseptic meningitis have been reported.

Drug interactions: Live virus vaccines (e.g., MMR, varicella); see earlier Warnings/Precautions.

Drug administration: Administer via IV infusion at a concentration 16.7–50 mg/mL (not >1 : 2 dilution) at the following rates:

Initial dose: 15 mg/kg/hr; if no adverse reaction after 30 min, increase to 30 mg/kg/hr. If no adverse reaction after 30 min, increase to **maximum** rate of 60 mg/kg/hr.

Subsequent doses: 30 mg/kg/hr; if no adverse reaction after 15 min, increase to maximum rate of 60 mg/kg/hr.

Maximum infusion rate: 75 mL/hr of 50 mg/mL concentration or 3750 mg/hr.

DAPSONE
Aczone, diaminodiphenylsulfone, DDS, and others
Antibiotic, sulfone derivative

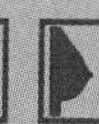
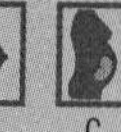

No Yes 2 C

Tabs: 25, 100 mg
Oral suspension: 2 mg/mL
Topical gel (Aczone): 5% (30, 60 g)

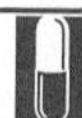

Pneumocystis jiroveci ***(formerly*** **carinii*****) treatment:***

Child and adult: 2 mg/kg/24 hr PO once daily; **max. dose:** 100 mg/24 hr with trimethoprim 15 mg/kg/24 hr PO ÷ TID

Pneumocystis jiroveci ***(formerly*** **carinii*****) prophylaxis (first episode and recurrence):***

Child ≥ 1 mo: 2 mg/kg/24 hr PO once daily; **max. dose:** 100 mg/24 hr. Alternative weekly dosing, 4 mg/kg/dose PO Q7 days; **max. dose:** 200 mg/dose.

Adult: 100 mg/24 hr PO ÷ once to twice daily with or without pyrimethamine 50 mg PO Q7 days and leucovorin 25 mg PO Q7 days; other combination regimens with pyrimethamine and leucovorin can be used (see http://www.hivatis.org)

Toxoplasma gondii ***prophylaxis (prevent first episode):***

Child ≥ 1 mo: 2 mg/kg/24 hr PO once daily; **max. dose:** 25 mg/24 hr with 1 mg/kg/24 hr pyrimethamine (**max. dose:** 25 mg/dose) PO once daily and 5 mg leucovorin PO Q3 days

Adult: 50 mg PO once daily with 50 mg pyrimethamine PO Q7 days and 25 mg leucovorin PO weekly; other combination regimens with pyrimethamine and leucovorin can be used (see http://www.hivatis.org)

Leprosy (see www.who.int/lep/disease/disease.htm for latest recommendations including combination regimens such as rifampin ± clofazimine):

Child: 1–2 mg/kg/24 hr PO once daily; **max. dose:** 100 mg/24 hr

Adult: 50–100 mg PO once daily

Acne vulgaris (topical gel, Aczone):

≥12 yr: Apply small amount of topical gel onto clean, acne-affected areas BID.

Contraindications: Hypersensitivity to dapsone products or any other components in the formulation

Warnings/Precautions: Patients with HIV, glutathione deficiency, or G6PD deficiency may be at increased risk for development of methemoglobinemia. Skin discoloration leading to depression and suicide has been reported. Oral suspension may not be absorbed as well as tablets.

Adverse effects: Adverse effects include hemolytic anemia (dose related), agranulocytosis, methemoglobinemia, aplastic anemia, nausea, vomiting, hyperbilirubinemia, headache, nephrotic

Continued

For explanation of icons, see p. 364.

DAPSONE *continued*

syndrome, and hypersensitivity reaction (sulfone syndrome). Cholestatic jaundice, peripheral neuropathy, and suicidal intent have been reported.

Drug interactions: Didanosine, rifabutin, and rifampin decreases dapsone levels. Trimethoprim increases dapsone levels. Pyrimethamine, nitrofurantoin, primaquine, and zidovudine increase risk for hematologic side effects. Topical dapsone use in combination with benzoyl peroxide may result in an orange–brown discoloration of the skin.

Drug administration:

PO: Doses may be administered with or without food.

Topical: Gently wash skin and pat dry before use. Apply pea-sized amount in thin layer and rub in completely.

DAPTOMYCIN
Cubicin
Antibiotic, lipopeptide

No Yes 2 B

Injection: 500 mg

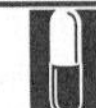

Child: Current clinical trials are investigating the following indications and doses; see www.clinicaltrials.gov for updated information (see remarks for adpharmacokinetic data):

Skin and skin structure infections:

2–6 yr: 9 mg/kg/dose IV Q24 hr
7–11 yr: 7 mg/kg/dose IV Q24 hr
12–17 yr: 5 mg/kg/dose IV Q24 hr

Adult:

Complicated skin and skin structure infections: 4 mg/kg/dose IV Q24 hr × 7–14 days

Staphylococcus aureus ***bacteremia, including those with right-sided endocarditis:*** 6 mg/kg/dose IV Q24 hr for a minimum of 2–6 wk

Contraindications: Hypersensitivity to daptomycin

Warnings/Precautions: **Do not** use for treatment of pneumonia. Use with **caution** in renal insufficiency **(adjust dose in renal failure; see Chapter 3)**. Concomitant use of HMG-CoA reductase inhibitors (e.g., atorvastatin) increases risk for myopathy.

Pediatric pharmacokinetics (PK) data from a single 4 mg/kg dose revealed similar healthy adult PK profile for adolescents 12 to 17 years old. Younger children had lower drug exposures; an inverse linear correlation between plasma clearance and age was observed (~2-fold increase in clearance for children 2–6 years old). Additional pediatric studies are needed.

Adverse effects: GI disturbances, rash, pruritus, increase in creatine kinase levels, headache, insomnia, pain, dizziness, and dyspnea are common. Jaundice, abnormal LFTs, eosinophilic pneumonia, rhabdomyolysis, and renal failure have been reported.

Drug interactions: See earlier Warnings/Precautions.

Drug administration: Dilute drug with NS to a convenient volume and infuse over 30 minutes.

DARUNAVIR
Prezista, DRV, TMC 114
Antiviral agent, protease inhibitor

Yes No 3 C

Tabs: 75, 150, 400, 600 mg
Oral suspension: 100 mg/mL

Continued

DARUNAVIR *continued*

Use in combination with other HIV antiretroviral agents.

Child ≥3 to <18 yr:

10 to <15 kg: 20 mg/kg/dose PO BID with 3 mg/kg/dose ritonavir PO BID or by the following table with the oral liquid dosage forms of darunavir and ritonavir:

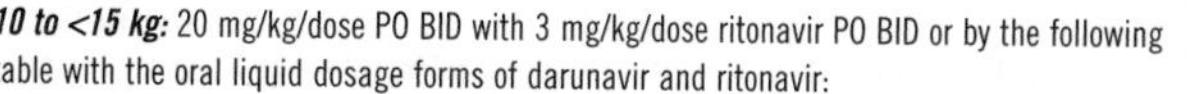

Weight (kg)	Darunavir PO BID	Ritonavir (80 mg/mL) PO BID
10 to <11	200 mg (2 mL)	32 mg (0.4 mL)
11 to <12	220 mg (2.2 mL)	32 mg (0.4 mL)
12 to <13	240 mg (2.4 mL)	40 mg (0.5 mL)
13 to <14	260 mg (2.6 mL)	40 mg (0.5 mL)
14 to <15	280 mg (2.8 mL)	48 mg (0.6 mL)

≥15 kg:

Oral tablet dosage form with ritonavir:

Weight (kg)	Darunavir PO BID	Ritonavir PO BID
≥15 to <30	375 mg	50 mg (0.6 mL)*
≥30 to <40	450 mg	60 mg (0.75 mL)*
≥40	600 mg	100 mg†

*Ritonavir oral liquid 80 mg/mL.

†Ritonavir oral tablet or capsule.

Oral liquid dosage forms for patients unable to swallow tablets:

Weight (kg)	Darunavir PO BID	Ritonavir (80 mg/mL) PO BID
≥15 to <30	375 mg (3.8 mL)	50 mg (0.6 mL)
≥30 to <40	450 mg (4.6 mL, rounded dose)	60 mg (0.75 mL)
≥40	600 mg (6 mL)	100 mg (1.25 mL)

≥18 yr and adult:

Therapy naïve and experienced without darunavir resistance: 800 mg PO once daily with 100 mg ritonavir PO once daily

Therapy experienced with ≥1 darunavir resistance: 600 mg PO BID with 100 mg ritonavir PO BID

Contraindications: Hypersensitivity to darunavir or other components of the formulation. Concomitant administration with drugs that are highly dependent on CYP 3A clearance such as alfuzosin, astemizole, cisapride, ergot derivatives, midazolam, pimozide, St. John's wort, sildenafil, rifampin, lovastatin, simvastatin, and triazolam.

Warnings/Precautions: Potential cross-sensitivity with sulfa-allergic patients. Coadministration with carbamazepine, pheonbarbital, phenytoin, rifampin, lopinavir/ritonavir or saquinavir, and St. John's wort is **not recommended** because of reducing darunavir levels. Also **not recommended** in combination with lovastatin, simvastatin, and other HMG-CoA reductase inhibitors because of risk for myopathy and rhabdomyolysis. **Use with caution** in hepatic impairment (primary route of metabolism; no dose reduction recommendations available), hemophilia type A or B, and diabetes or hyperglycemia. Increased monitoring of AST/ALT has been recommended in patients with

Continued

For explanation of icons, see p. 364.

DARUNAVIR *continued*

underlying chronic hepatitis, cirrhosis, or with elevated transaminases. **Darunavir should always be administered in combination with ritonavir.**

Adverse effects: GI disturbances, abdominal pain, headache, and fatigue are common. Skin rash (including erythema multiforme, TEN, and Stevens–Johnson syndrome), fever, immune reconstitution syndrome, elevated hepatic transaminases, drug-induced hepatitis, and lipid abnormalities have been reported. Diarrhea, vomitting, and rash were common in pediatric studies.

Drug interactions: Substrate and inhibitor of cytochrome P450 3A. Ritonavir boosts darunavir levels and is also a substrate and inhibitor of CYP P450 3A. See earlier Contraindications and Warnings/Precautions sections. Always check the potential for other drug interactions when either initiating therapy or adding new drugs onto an existing regimen.

Drug administration: Drug is always given in combination with ritonavir. Administer all doses with food.

DELAVIRDINE
Rescriptor, DLV
Antiviral, nonnucleoside reverse transcriptase inhibitor

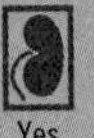 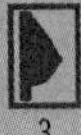 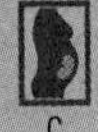

Yes Yes 3 C

Tablets: 100, 200 mg

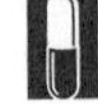

Use in combination with other HIV antiretroviral agents.
≥16 yr and adult: 400 mg PO TID

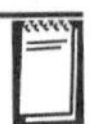

Contraindications: Hypersensitivity to delavirdine or any components in the formulation. Do not administer with CYP 3A substrates with a low therapeutic index (e.g., alprazolam, midazolam, triazolam, cisapride, calcium channel blockers, ergot alkaloid dervatives, amphetamines, cisapride, and sildenafil); increased risk for toxicity of these drugs.

Warnings/Precautions: Use with caution in hepatic disease. Metabolized primarily via CYP 450 3A4 (*N*-dealkylation andpyridine hydroxylation). CYP 450 2D6, 2C9, and 2C19 may also play a role. Hepatic and renal impairment pharmacokinetics have not been evaluated.

Adverse effects: Incidence rate of rash has been reported as high as 50% and occurs within 1 to 3 weeks after initiation of therapy. Dose titration does not significantly reduce the incidence of rash. Other major negative side effects include headache, fatigue, increased transaminase levels, and gastrointestinal complaints. Hepatic failure, hemolytic anemia, rhabdomyolysis, and acute kidney failure have been reported.

Drug interactions: See Contraindications section for serious interactions. Delavirdine inhibits the CYP450 3A4 and 2C9 drug-metabolizing isoenzymes. Antacids, didanosine, H2 antagonists, rifabutin, rifampin, carbamazepine, phenytoin/fosphenytoin, phenobarbital, and saquinavir may decrease delavirdine's efficacy. Ketoconazole, fluoxetine, and clarithromycin may increase delavirdine levels and effects. When administered with protease inhibitors, delavirdine can increase the effects of amprenavir, saquinavir, and indinivir. May increase the effects of warfarin. Carefully review the patients' drug profile for other drug interactions each time delavirdine is initiated or when a new drug is added to a regimen containing delavirdine.

Drug administration: Doses may be administered with or without food. Doses of antacids and didanosine should be administered 1 hour before or 1 hour after taking delavirdine. Only the 100-mg tablets can be dissolved in water (four 100-mg tablets in ≥3 oz water) to make a dispersion to be taken immediately. The 200-mg tablets do not dissolve well in water.

DEMECLOCYCLINE
Declomycin, Declostatin, and others
Antibiotic, tetracycline derivative

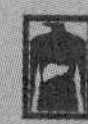
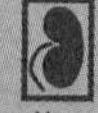
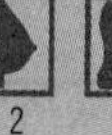
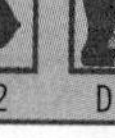

Yes Yes 2 D

Tablets: 150, 300 mg

Child >8 yr:

Severe acne (adjunct), bacterial infections, anthrax (when penicillin is contraindicated), bartonellosis, brucellosis, chancroid, cholera, plague, and Mycoplasma pneumonia: 8–12 mg/kg/24 hr ÷ Q6–12 hr PO; **max. dose:** 600 mg/24 hr

Adult:

Severe acne (adjunct), bacterial infections, anthrax (when penicillin is contraindicated), bartonellosis, brucellosis, chancroid, cholera, plague, UTI, tuaremia, and Mycoplasma pneumonia: 600 mg/24 hr ÷ Q6 hr or Q12 hr PO

Uncomplicated gonorrhea: 600 mg × 1 PO, followed by 300 mg Q12 hr × 4 days PO (3 g total)

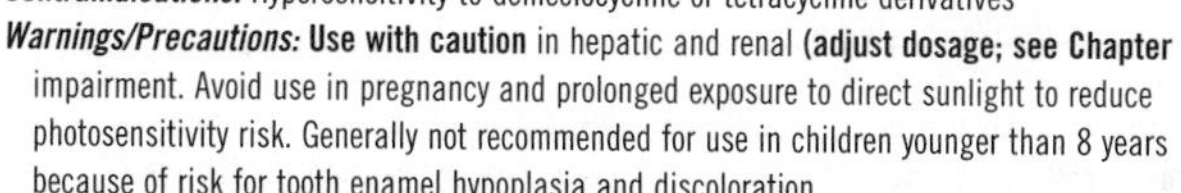

Contraindications: Hypersensitivity to demeclocycline or tetracycline derivatives

Warnings/Precautions: **Use with caution** in hepatic and renal **(adjust dosage; see Chapter 3)** impairment. Avoid use in pregnancy and prolonged exposure to direct sunlight to reduce photosensitivity risk. Generally not recommended for use in children younger than 8 years because of risk for tooth enamel hypoplasia and discoloration.

Adverse effects: GI symptoms and photosensitivity may occur. Increased intracranial pressure (pseudotumor cerebri), nephrogenic DI, hepatitis/hepatotoxicity, anaphylaxis, and acute renal failure have been reported.

Drug interactions: Bile acid salts and penicillins may decrease demeclocycline's effects. Demeclocycline may enhance the effects of warfarin and neuromuscular blocking agents, and decrease the effects of BCG vaccine and desmopressin. See Tetracycline for additional drug/food interactions and comments.

Drug administration: Administer with plenty of fluids to reduce risk for esophageal ulceration or irritation. Avoid divalent cations (e.g., antacids, dairy products/calcium salts, magnesium, iron), bismuth, and sucralfate for 1 hour before or 2 hours after administration.

DICLOXACILLIN SODIUM
Dycill, Pathocil, and others
Antibiotic, penicillin (penicillinase resistant)

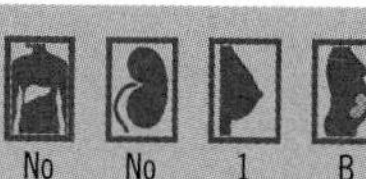

No No 1 B

Caps: 250, 500 mg; contains 0.6 mEq Na/250 mg

Child (<40 kg; see remarks):

Mild-to-moderate infections: 12.5–25 mg/kg/24 hr PO ÷ Q6 hr
Severe infections: 50–100 mg/kg/24 hr PO ÷ Q6 hr
Max. dose: 2 g/24 hr

Child (≥40 kg) and adult: 125–500 mg/dose PO Q6 hr; **max. dose:** 2 g/24 hr

Contraindications: History of penicillin allergy

Warnings/Precautions: Use with caution in cephalosporin hypersensitivity. Limited experience in neonates and very young infants. Higher doses (50–100 mg/kg/24 hr) are indicated after IV therapy for osteomyelitis.

Adverse effects: Nausea, vomiting, and diarrhea are common. Immune hypersensitivity has been reported.

Drug interactions: May decrease the effects of oral contraceptives and warfarin.

Drug administration: Administer 1 hour before meals or 2 hours after meals.

For explanation of icons, see p. 364.

DIDANOSINE

Videx, Videx EC, Dideoxyinosine, ddI

Antiviral agent, nucleoside analogue reverse transcriptase inhibitor

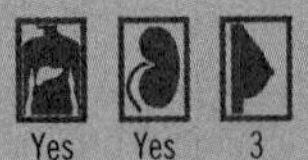
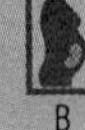
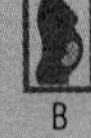

Tabs (buffered, chewable/dispersable): 25, 50, 100, 150, 200 mg; contains 11.5 mEq sodium, 15.7 mEq magnesium, and phenylalanine per tablet

Capsules (delayed-release, enteric-coated beadlets):

- **Videx EC:** 125, 200, 250, 400 mg
- **Generic:** 200, 250, 400 mg

Oral pediatric powder (10 mg/mL solution reconstituted with antacid solution): 2 g (4 oz), 4 g (8 oz)

Powder (buffered) for oral solution in single-dose packets: 100, 167, 250 mg

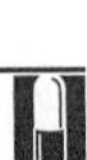

Neonate and infant:

- ***2 wk to 4 mo:*** 100 mg/m²/24 hr ÷ Q12 hr PO
- ***>4–8 mo:*** 200 mg/m²/24 hr ÷ Q12 hr PO

Child >8 mo:

- ***Usual dose (in combination with other antiretrovirals):*** 240 mg/m²/24 hr ÷ Q12 hr PO
- ***Dose range:*** 180–300 mg/m²/24 hr ÷ Q12 hr; higher dose may be required for CNS disease

Child 6–18 yr:

- ***Delayed-release capsules:***
  - ***20 to <25 kg:*** 200 mg PO once daily
  - ***25 to <60 kg:*** 250 mg PO once daily
  - ***≥60 kg:*** 400 mg PO once daily

Adolescent/adult (see remarks for additional adolescent dosing information):

- ***<60 kg:***
  - ***Tabs:*** 250 mg/24 hr ÷ Q12–24 hr PO; Q12 hr dosing interval is preferred for efficacy, but Q24 hr dosing my improve compliance.
  - ***Caps (delayed-release, enteric-coated beadlets):*** 250 mg Q24 hr PO
- ***≥60 kg:***
  - ***Tabs:*** 400 mg/24 hr ÷ Q12–24 hr PO; Q12 hr dosing interval is preferred for efficacy, but Q24 hr dosing my improve compliance.
  - ***Caps (delayed-release, enteric-coated beadlets):*** 400 mg Q24 hr PO

Combination therapy with tenofovir:

- ***Adult:***
  - ***<60 kg:*** 200 mg Q24 hr PO using the delayed-release capsules
  - ***≥60 kg:*** 250 mg Q24 hr PO using the delayed-release capsules

Contraindications: Hypersensitivity to didanosine or any other components contained in the formulation

Warnings/Precautions: Pancreatitis has occurred during therapy in treatment-naïve and -experienced patients regardless of level of immunosuppression. Fatal lactic acidosis has been reported in pregnant women taking didanosine in combination with stavudine.

Use with caution in patients on sodium restriction or with phenylketonuria (buffered tablet contains 11.5 mEq Na/tablet and phenylketonuria), and in combination with other drugs associated with peripheral neuropathy (e.g., chloramphenicol, cisplatin, dapsone, ethambutol, ethionamide, metronidazole). **Reduce dose in renal impairment (see Chapter 3).** Pharmacokinetics in impaired hepatic function is incomplete. Delayed-release capsules should not be used for patients smaller than 60 kg with GFR less than 10 mL/min.

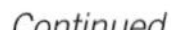

Continued

DIDANOSINE *continued*

Adverse effects: Adverse effects include headaches, diarrhea, abdominal pain, nausea, vomiting, peripheral neuropathy (dose related), electrolyte abnormalities, hyperuricemia, increased liver enzymes, retinal depigmentation, CNS depression, rash/pruritus, myalgia, and pancreatitis (dose related, more in adults when used with tenofovir). Lactic acidosis, noncirrhotic portal hypertension, and severe hepatomegaly with steatosis have been reported.

Drug interactions: Impairs absorption of drugs requiring an acidic environment and drugs that have impaired absorption in the presence of divalent ions (e.g., ketoconazole and fluoroquinolones, respectively). Didanosine mitochondrial toxicity is enhanced with ribavirin. Use with stavudine or zalcitabine increases risk for lactic acidosis or pancreatitis. Tenofivir may increase didanosine levels.

Drug administration: Administer all doses on empty stomach (30 minutes before and 2 hours after a meal). Videx EC should be swallowed intact. Separate dosing when used in combination with the following drugs: 1 hour before or after ddI (indinavir); 2 hours before or after ddI (delavirdine, ritonavir, lopinavir/ritonavir, fluoroquinolones, ketoconazole, itraconazole, tetracyclines, and dapsone). To ensure adequate buffering capacity with the chewable tablet dosage form, administer at least two of the appropriate-strength tablets (e.g., if the dose is 50 mg, give two 25-mg tablets and not one 50-mg tablet). Consult package insert for additional details.

DIETHYLCARBAMAZINE
Hetrazan, carbamazine, diethylcarbamazine citrate, DEC
Anthelmintic

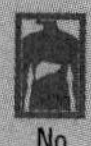
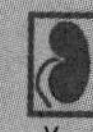
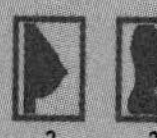
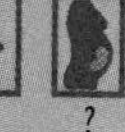

No Yes ? ?

AVAILABLE FROM THE U.S. CENTERS FOR DISEASE CONTROL AND PREVENTION (404-639-3670 Monday–Friday 8:00 AM–4:30 PM EST or 770-488-7100 for all other times)
Tabs: 50 mg

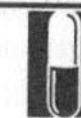

Filariasis (**Wuchereria bancrofti, Brugia malayi,** ***or*** **Brugia timori** ***infections):***

Child ≥18 yr and adult (PO): 6 mg/kg/24 hr ÷ TID PO × 12 days; concurrent corticosteroids may be needed to reduce secondary reactions from therapy

Loa loa (use with caution in heavy infestations because occular problems or encephalopathy may occur):

Child ≥18 yr (PO): Start with 1 mg/kg/dose on day 1, then 1 mg/kg/dose TID on day 2, then 1–2 mg/kg/dose TID on day 3, followed by 9 mg/kg/24 hr ÷ TID on days 4–21

Adult (PO): Start with 50 mg on day 1, then 50 mg TID on day 2, then 100 mg TID on day 3, followed by 9 mg/kg/24 hr ÷ TID on days 4–21

Onchocerciasis (alternative to ivermectin; therapy should be followed by suramin IV):

Child ≥18 mo (PO): Start with 0.5 mg/kg/dose TID (**max. dose:** 25 mg/24 hr) × 3 days, then 1 mg/kg/dose TID (**max. dose:** 50 mg/24 hr) for 3–4 additional days, then 1.5 mg/kg/dose TID (**max. dose:** 100 mg/24 hr) for 3–4 additional days, followed by maintenance doses of 2 mg/kg/dose TID × 14–21 days

Adult (PO): Start with 25 mg/24 hr once daily × 3 days, then 50 mg/24 hr once daily for 5 additional days, then 100 mg/24 hr ÷ BID for 3 additional days, followed by maintenance doses of 150 mg/24 hr ÷ TID × 12 days

Tropical pulmonary eosinophilia:

Child ≥18 mo and adult (PO): 6 mg/kg/24 hr ÷ TID PO × 14–21 days

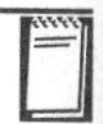

Contraindications: Hypersensitivity to diethylcarbamazine and its components

Warnings/Precautions: Should not be used for *Onchocerca volvulus* because of risk for increased ocular adverse effects, including blindness. Dose reductions are indicated in

Continued

For explanation of icons, see p. 364.

DIETHYLCARBAMAZINE *continued*

patients with renal insufficiency (>50% drug excreted unchanged in urine), alkaline urine (renal elimination reduced to <10%), or eating a vegitarian diet (alkaline diet). In pregnancy, use of drug is recommended after delivery; some consider use in pregnancy as a contraindication. Crosses the blood–brain barrier.

Adverse effects: GI disturbances and drowsiness are common; frequency is proportional with dosage. Headache, lassitude, weakness, general malaise, and skin rash have been reported in the treatment of *Wuchereria bancrofti.* Mazzotti reaction, facial edema, or pruritus (especially occular) have been reported in the treatment of onchocerciasis. Giddiness, GI disturbances, and malaise have been reported in children treated for ascariasis.

Drug administration: Administer doses after meals.

DIIODOHYDROXYQUIN

See Iodoquinol.

DIPHTHERIA ANTITOXIN (EQUINE)
Antitoxin

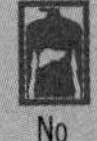
No
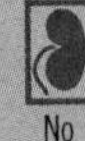
No
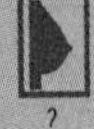
?
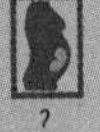
?

AVAILABLE FROM THE U.S. CENTERS FOR DISEASE CONTROL AND PREVENTION (404-639-8257 or 770-488-7100)

Injection: 10,000 units

Child and adult:

Diphtheria treatment (in combination with appropriate antibiotic therapy):

Pharyngeal or laryngeal symptoms of 48-hour duration: 20,000–40,000 units IV/IM × 1

Nasopharngeal symptoms: 40,000–60,000 units IV/IM × 1

Extensive illness of >3 days or in patients with brawny neck swelling: 80,000–120,000 units IV/IM × 1

Diphtheria prophylaxis (in combination with appropriate antibiotic therapy for 7–10 days and active immunization with diphtheria toxoid absorbed): 5,000–10,000 units IM × 1

Serum-sensitivity testing (intradermal or scratch skin test and a conjunctival test should be performed):

Intradermal skin test: Intradermal injection of 0.1 mL of a 1 : 100 dilution in NS × 1; skin test is read 20 min after injection. Use 0.05 mL of a 1 : 1000 dilution in NS for patients with allergy history. Administer with NS control test. A positive intradermal skin test reaction consists of an urticarial wheal, with or without pseudopods, surrounded by a zone of erythema.

Scratch skin test: Place 1 drop of a 1 : 100 dilution on the skin followed by making a 0.25-inch scratch through the drop. Test is read after 20 minutes. An NS control test should be used to facilitate interpretation. A positive scratch skin test reaction consists of an urticarial wheal, with or without pseudopods, surrounded by a zone of erythema.

Conjunctival test: Place 1 drop of a 1 : 10 dilution into the lower conjunctival sac of one eye. Test is read after 15 min. An NS control test is used in the other eye. Positive conjunctival test reaction consists of itching, burning, redness, and lacrimation; these signs and symptoms can be relieved by placing 1 drop of an ophthalmic solution of epinephrine on the affected eye.

Continued

DIPHTHERIA ANTITOXIN (EQUINE) *continued*

Desensitization: Subcutaneous injection of the following dosages and concentrations at 15-min intervals. In the event of an immediate sensitivity reaction at any time, apply a tourniquet proximal to the sites of injection and administer epinephrine proximal to the tourniquet. Continue the procedure 1 hour after using the last dose of antitoxin that did not produce a reaction.

Dose 1: 0.05 mL of a 1 : 20 dilution
Dose 2: 0.1 mL of a 1 : 10 dilution
Dose 3: 0.3 mL of a 1 : 10 dilution
Dose 4: 0.1 mL undiluted diphtheria antitoxin
Dose 5: 0.2 mL undiluted diphtheria antitoxin
Dose 6: 0.5 mL undiluted diphtheria antitoxin

After successsfully completing dose 6, the remaining usual dose may be administered IV or IM.

Contraindications: Hypersensitivity to horse serum
Warnings/Precautions: Test for sensitivity to horse serum before administering any doses. **Use with extreme caution** with history of allergic disorders and asthma.
When the skin or conjunctival test is positive or a doubtful reaction occurs, the risk of administering diphtheria antitoxin should be weighed against the risk of withholding it; if diphtheria antitoxin must be used, desensitization should be performed.
Adverse effects: Dermatologic wheal and flare; pain, erythema, urticaria at site of injection; and immediate hypersensitivity reactions may occur. Serum sickness has been reported.
Drug interactions: If being given with diphtheria and tetanus toxiod, administer at separate sites.
Drug administration: Warm drug vial to 90°F to 95°F.
IV: Dilute dose to an appropriate volume of NS or D_5W to provide a 1 : 20 dilution of antitoxin and infuse slowly at a rate not exceeding 1 mL/min.

DOCOSANOL
Abreva, behenyl alcohol
Antiviral, topical

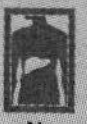
No
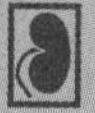
No
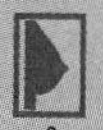
?
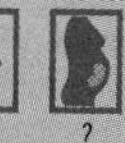
?

Cream: 10% (2 g) [OTC]

Herpes labialis:
≥12 yr and adult: Apply to lesions 5 times a day until lesions heal up to a maximum of 10 days.

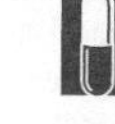

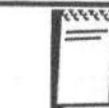

Contraindications: History of hypersensitivity to docosanol or any other components in the formulation
Warnings/Precautions: Use is intended for the symptomatic treatment of herpes labialis in immunocompentent patients. **Do not use** for localized herpes zoster or any other cutaneous or mucocutaneous conditions.
Adverse effects: Headache and secondary bacterial infection have been reported.
Drug interactions: None identified.
Drug administration: Use a separate applicator (e.g., cotton swab) each time to prevent the spread of HSV infection. Apply topically to affected areas of the lips and surrounding skin by rubbing gently and completely. Do not apply in or near the eyes or inside the mouth. For best results, remove cosmetics before applying dose; cosmetics may be applied after application of docosanol.

For explanation of icons, see p. 364.

DORIPENEM

Doribax

Carbapenem antibiotic

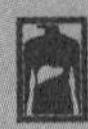 No 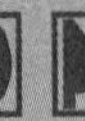 Yes 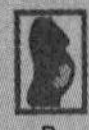 ? 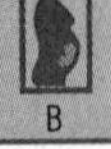 B

Injection: 250, 500 mg

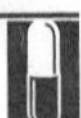

≥18 yr and adult: 500 mg IV Q8 hr with the following recommended duration of therapy:

Complicated intraabdominal infection: 5–14 days (minimum of 3 days IV with possible switch to appropriate PO therapy)

Complicated UTI and pyelonephritis: 10 days (may be extended up to 14 days in patients with concurrent bacteremia)

IV catheter-related bloodstream infection and health care/ventilator-associated pneumonia: 7–14 days

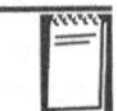

Contraindications: Patients sensitive to carbapenems or with a history of anaphylaxis to β-lactam antibiotics

Warnings/Precautions: **Use with caution** in renal impairment **(adjust dose; see Chapter 3).** Drug penetrates well into peritoneal and retroperitoneal fluids and tissues.

Adverse effects: Diarrhea, nausea, headache, rash, and phlebitis are common. Dermatologic reactions, including Stevens–Johnson and TEN, neutropenia, *Clostridium difficile* colitis, anemia, neutropenia/leukopenia, and hypersensitivity reactions have been reported.

Drug interactions: Probenecid may increase serum doripenem levels. May reduce valproic acid levels.

Drug administration: Infuse dose over 1 hour at a concentration ≤4.5 mg/mL. Reconstituted IV solutions have short stability times; consult with a pharmacist.

DOXYCYCLINE

Vibramycin, Periostat, and others

Antibiotic, tetracycline derivative

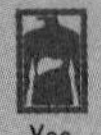 Yes 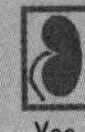 Yes 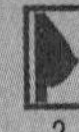 2 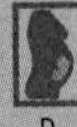 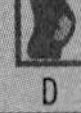 D

Caps: 20 (Periostat), 50, 75, 100 mg
Tabs: 20 (Periostat), 50, 75, 100 mg
Syrup: 50 mg/5 mL (60 mL)
Oral suspension: 25 mg/5 mL (60 mL)
Injection: 100, 200 mg

Initial:

≤45 kg: 2.2 mg/kg/dose BID PO/IV × 1 day to **max. dose** of 200 mg/24 hr

>45 kg: 100 mg/dose BID PO/IV × 1 day

Maintenance:

≤45 kg: 2.2–4.4 mg/kg/24 hr once to twice daily PO/IV

>45 kg: 100–200 mg/24 hr ÷ once to twice daily PO/IV

Max. dose: 200 mg/24 hr

PID:

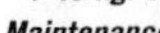

Inpatient: 100 mg IV/PO Q12 hr with cefotetan, cefoxitin, or ampicillin/sulbactam. Convert to oral therapy 24 hr after patient improves on IV to complete a 14-day total course (IV and PO).

Outpatient: 100 mg PO Q12 hr × 14 days with ceftriaxone, cefoxitin + probenecid, or other parenteral third generation cephalosporin ± metronidazole

Anthrax (inhalation/systemic/cutaneous; see remarks): Initiate therapy with IV route and convert to PO route when clinically appropriate. Duration of therapy is 60 days (IV and PO combined):

≤8 yr or ≤45 kg: 2.2 mg/kg/dose BID IV/PO; **max. dose:** 200 mg/24 hr

>8 yrs and >45 kg: 100 mg/dose BID IV/PO

Continued

DOXYCYCLINE *continued*

Malaria prophylaxis (start 1–2 days before exposure and continue for 4 weeks after leaving edemic area):

>8 yr: 2 mg/kg/24 hr PO once daily; **max. dose:** 100 mg/24 hr

Adult: 100 mg PO once daily

Periodontitis:

Adult: 20 mg BID PO × ≤9 mo

Contraindications: Hypersensitivity to doxycycline or tetracycline products

Warnings/Precautions: **Use with caution** in hepatic and renal disease, and in patients with a history of candidal infections. Avoid prolonged exposure to direct sunlight to reduce photosensitivity risk. Generally not recommended for use in children younger than 8 years because of risk for tooth enamel hypoplasia and discoloration. However, the *AAP Red Book* recommends doxycycline as the drug of choice for rickettsial disease regardless of age.

Doxycycline is approved for the treatment of anthrax *(Bacillus anthracis)* in combination with one or two other antimicrobials. If meningitis is suspected, consider using an alternative agent because of poor CNS penetration. Consider changing to high-dose amoxicillin (25–35 mg/kg/dose TID PO) for penicillin-susceptible strains. See www.bt.cdc.gov for the latest information.

Adverse effects: GI symptoms, photosensitivity, hemolytic anemia, rash, and hypersensitivity reactions may occur. Increased intracranial pressure, TEN, erythema multiforme, and Stevens–Johnson syndrome have been reported.

Drug interactions: Rifampin, barbiturates, phenytoin, and carbamazepine may increase clearance of doxycycline. Doxycycline may enhance the hypoprothrombinemic effect of warfarin. See Tetracycline for additional drug/food interactions and comments.

Drug administration:

IV: Infuse over 1 to 4 hours at a concentration of 0.1 to 1 mg/mL.

PO: Fluid intake should accompany oral administration to reduce risk for esophageal ulceration or irritation. Avoid divalent cations (e.g., antacids, dairy products, iron) for 1 hour before or 2 hours after administration. Doses may be administered with food to decrease GI upset. For periodontitis, take capsules ≥1 hour before meals, and take tablets ≥1 hour before or 2 hours after meals.

ECONAZOLE NITRATE

Spectazole and various generics

Antifungal, imidazole

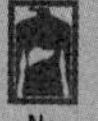
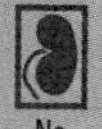
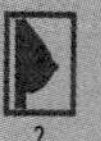
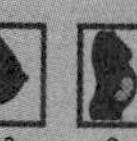

No No ? C

Topical cream: 1% (15, 30, 85 g); contains mineral oil

Tinea pedis, tinea cruris, tinea corporis, and tinea versicolor (see remarks): Apply to affected areas once daily.

Duration of therapy:

Tinea cruris and tinea corporis: 2 wk

Tinea pedis: 1 mo

Cutaneous candidiasis: Apply to affected areas BID (morning and evening) × 2 wk.

Contraindications: Hypersensitivity to econazole or any other components in the formulation

Warnings/Precautions: **Not for ophthalmic use.** If no clinical improvement is seen after the treatment period, consider alternative diagnosis. Clinical and mycologic response for tinea versicolor is usually seen after 2 weeks of therapy.

Adverse effects: Burning, itching, stinging, and erythema may occur.

Drug interactions: Econazole, an azole antifungal agent, can inhibit CYP 450 3A4 and may potentially increase the effects of 3A4 substrates (e.g., Fentanyl).

Drug administration: Apply to cover affected areas. **Avoid** contact with eyes.

For explanation of icons, see p. 364.

EFAVIRENZ

Sustiva, DMP-266

Antiviral agent, nonnucleoside reverse transcriptase inhibitor

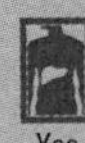 Yes 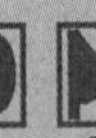 No 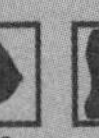 3 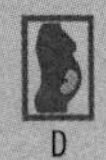 D

Caps: 50, 200 mg
Tabs: 600 mg
Oral solution: Available as an expanded access compassionate use program via Bristol-Myers Squibb (877-372-7097).
In combination with emtricitabine and tenofovir as Atripla:
Tabs: 600 mg efavirenz, 200 mg emtricitabine, and 300 mg tenofovir

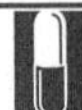

Administer with other antiretroviral agents.
Child ≥3 yr and weighing ≥10 kg: Daily PO dose administered once daily (see following table)

Body Weight (kg)	Dose (mg)
10 to <15	200
15 to <20	250
20 to <25	300
25 to <32.5	350
32.5 to <40	400
≥40	600

Adolescent and adult (see remarks): 600 mg/dose PO once daily
If coadministered with rifampin and patient weighing >50 kg: 800 mg/dose efavirenz PO once daily
If coadministered with voriconazole: 300 mg efavirenz (one 200-mg cap and two 50-mg caps, *or* six 50-mg caps)/dose PO once daily and 400 mg voriconazole PO Q12 hr
Atripla:
Adult (GFRs ≥50 mL/min): 1 tablet PO once daily on an empty stomach

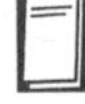

Contraindications: Hypersensitivity to efavirenz or any other components in the formulation; should not be used with astemizole, cisapride, triazolam, midazolam, ergot derivatives, and voriconazole.

Warnings/Precautions: **Do not** use as a single agent for HIV or added on as a sole agent to a failing regimen. Therapy should always be initiated in combination with at least one other antiretroviral agent to which the patient has not been previously exposed. **Avoid** use in pregnancy; meningomyelocele and Dandy–Walker malformation have been reported in infants. Pharmacokinetics in hepatic or renal impairment have not been adequately evaluated. Use in moderate/severe hepatic impairment is not recommended. Consider alternative therapy for patients who have had a history of life-threatening cutaneous reactions (e.g., Stevens–Johnson syndrome).

Adverse effects: Dizziness, somnolence, insomnia, hallucinations, and euphoria are common side effects. Skin rashes (usually mild-to-moderate maculopapular eruptions) may occur within the first 2 weeks of initiating therapy and usually resolve (with continuing the drug) within 1 month. Rash is more common in children and more often of greater severity. Discontinue therapy in patients developing severe rash associated with blistering, desquamation, mucosal involvement, or fever. Diarrhea, fever, cough, nausea, vomiting, pancreatitis, vertigo, and elevations in liver enzymes and serum lipids have been reported.

Drug interactions: Drug is a substrate and inducer of CYP 450 3A4, and may also inhibit other CYP 450 isoenzymes (2C9, 2C19, and 3A4). Monitor effect/serum levels of drugs metabolized by the aforementioned CYP 450 isoenzymes (e.g., warfarin, rifampin). Increases serum levels of nelfinavir

Continued

EFAVIRENZ *continued*

and ritonavir, and decreases levels of indinavir and saquinavir. See earlier Contraindications. May cause false-positive urinary cannabinoid test (CEDIA DAU Multi-Level THC assay).

Drug administration: Doses should be administered on an empty stomach. **Avoid** high-fat meals (increases absorption). Capsules may be opened and added to liquids or foods but has a peppery taste; grape jelly may be used to disguise taste. Initiate dosing at bedtime for the first 2 to 4 weeks to reduce central nervous system side effects.

EMTRICITABINE
Emtriva, FTC
Antiviral agent, nucleoside analogue reverse transcriptase inhibitor

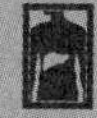
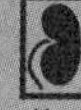
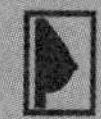
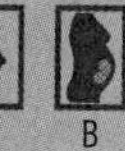

Yes Yes 3 B

Caps: 200 mg
Oral solution: 10 mg/mL
In combination with tenofovir as Truvada:
Tabs: 200 mg emtricitabine and 300 mg tenofovir disoproxil fumarate
In combination with emtricitabine and tenofovir as Atripla:
Tabs: 600 mg efavirenz, 200 mg emtricitabine, and 300 mg tenofovir

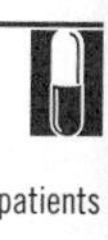

Use in combination with other HIV antiretroviral agents.
Child:
<3 mo: 3 mg/kg/24 hr PO once daily
3 mo to 17 yr: 6 mg/kg/24 hr PO once daily; **max. dose:** 240 mg/24 hr or 200 mg/24 hr for patients >33 kg using capsule dosage form
Adult (≥18 yr):
Caps: 200 mg PO once daily
Oral solution: 240 mg PO once daily
Truvada (GFR ≥30 mL/min and not receiving hemodialysis):
Child ≥12 yr and ≥35 kg and adult: 1 tab PO once daily with or without food
Atripla (GFR ≥50 mL/min):
Adult: 1 tab PO once daily on an empty stomach (QHS administration has been recommended to minimize CNS symptoms)

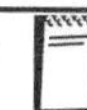

Contraindications: Hypersensitivity to emtricitabine or any other components contained in the formulation.

Warnings/Precautions: Lactic acidosis and severe hepatomegaly with steatosis, including fatal cases, have been reported. Emtricitabine is not approved for the treatment of hepatitis B; some HIV patients with hepatitis B treated with emtricitabine experience hepatitis B exacerbations with liver decompensation and liver failure. Patients co-infected with HIV and HBV should be monitored closely for hepatitis several months after stopping treatment with emtricitabine. Oral solution dosage form is less bioequivalent than the oral capsule. **Adjust dosage in renal impairment (see Chapter 3).**

Adverse effects: Headache, dizziness, insomnia, fever, diarrhea, nausea, abnormal dreams, rash, and hyperpigmentation on palms and/or soles (primarily seen in non-white patients) are common. Neutropenia, anemia, lactic acidosis, and severe hepatomegaly with steatosis have been reported. Upper respiratory infections, pneumonia, and other infections have been reported in children. Hepatitis exacerbations in patients co-infected with HIV and HBV have occurred after discontinuing emtricitabine.

Continued

For explanation of icons, see p. 364.

EMTRICITABINE *continued*

Drug interactions: Potential interactions may occur with drugs that are eliminated via tubular secretion. **Do not** use with lamivudine because of similar resistance profile and no additional additive benefit. May enhance the hematologic toxicity and hepatotoxic effects of emtricitabine when used with ganciclovir/valganciclovir and ribavirin, respectively.

Drug administration: Doses may be administered with or without food.

ENFUVIRTIDE

Fuzeon, T-20

Antiviral agent, fusion inhibitor

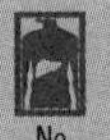
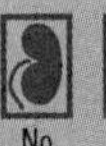
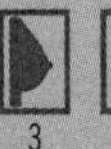
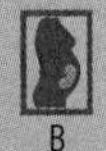

No No 3 B

Injection: 108 mg; delivers 90 mg/L following reconstitution with 1.1 mL sterile water for injection (available in a Convenience Kit containing 60 single-use vials with sterile water diluent, syringes, and alcohol wipes)

Child 6–16 yr: 2 mg/kg/dose SQ BID; **max. dose:** 90 mg/kg/dose BID
≥16 yr to adult: 90 mg SQ BID

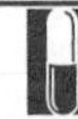

Contraindications: Hypersensitivity to enfuvirtide or any other components in the formulation

Warnings/Precautions: Currently **not recommended** for antiretroviral-naïve patients because of lack of data. Patients with history of lung disease, low CD4 counts, high initial viral load, IV drug use, or smoking may be at greater risk for bacterial pneumonia. A theoretical production of anti-enfuvirtide antibodies may cross-react with HIV-1 gp41 to potentially cause false-positive ELISA test in noninfected HIV individuals. Currently, no information on dosing recommendations for patients with GFR less than 35 mL/min or with hepatic impairment is available.

Adverse effects: Local injection-site reactions are extremely high (98%), which are usually mild/moderate in severity. Duration of reaction usually 3 to 7 days but have been more than 7 days in about 24% of patients. Hypersensitivity reactions, GI disturbances, fever, chills, rigors, hypotension, and elevated liver transaminases have been reported.

Drug interactions: May increase serum concentration of protease inhibitors; tipranavir trough concentrations have been reported to be ~45% higher in phase 3 trials. Protease inhibitors may increase serum concentration of enfuvirtide.

Drug administration: Inject SQ into the upper arm, anterior thigh, or abdomen; **avoid** scar tissue, moles, bruises, the naval, or a site experiencing an injection-site reaction. Reconstituted vials must be used within 24 hours; the dosage form is preservative free.

ENTECAVIR

Baraclude

Antiviral agent, nucleoside reverse transcriptase inhibitor

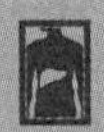
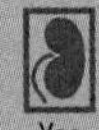
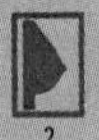
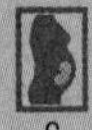
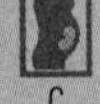

Yes Yes ? C

Oral solution: 0.05 mg/mL (210 mL)
Tabs: 0.5, 1 mg

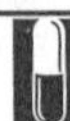

Chronic hepatitis B:
Compensated liver disease (≥16 yr and adult):
Nucleoside naïve: 0.5 mg PO once daily
History of hepatitis B viremia while receiving lamivudine; or unknown lamivudine or telbivudine resistance mutations rtM204I/V ± rtL180M, rTL80I/v or rtV173L: 1 mg PO once daily
Decompensated liver disease (adult): 1 mg PO once daily

Continued

ENTECAVIR *continued*

Contraindications: Hypersensitivity to entecavir or any component of the formulation

Warnings/Precautions: Severe acute exacerbations of hepatitis B have been reported in patients who have discontinued antihepatitis B therapy; monitor hepatic function for several months after decontinuation. Use not recommended for patients with HIV and hepatitis B receiving HAART because of the potential for development of HIV resistance to nucleoside reverse transcriptase inhibitors. Lactic acidosis and severe hepatomegaly with steatosis have been reported with this class of antiviral agents.

Use with caution in renal impairment **(adjust dose; see Chapter 3).** No dosage adjustment is necessary in hepatic impairment. Oral solution and tablet are bioequivalent.

Adverse effects: Headache, fatigue, pyrexia, peripheral edema, ascites, dizziness, and nausea are common. See Warnings/Precautions section for other adverse effects. Alopecia, rash, increase transaminases, lactic acidosis, and anaphylaxis have been reported.

Drug interactions: Ganciclovir/valganciclovir and ribavirin may increase toxicity of entecavir.

Drug administration: Administer on an empty stomach, 2 hours before or after a meal. Do not mix or dilute oral solution dosage form with water or other beverages.

ERTAPENEM
Invanz
Antibiotic, carbapenem

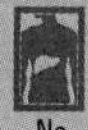
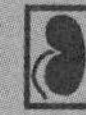
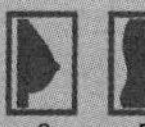
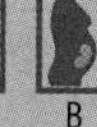

No Yes 2 B

Injection: 1 g
Contains ~6 mEq Na/g drug.

3 mo to 12 yr: 15 mg/kg/dose IV/IM Q12 hr; **max. dose:** 1 g/24 hr
Adolescent and adult: 1 g IV/IM Q24 hr
Recommended duration of therapy (all ages):
Complicated intraabdominal infection: 5–14 days
Complicated skin/subcutaneous tissue infections: 7–14 days
Diabetic foot infection without osteomyelitis: up to 28 days
Community-acquired pneumonia, complicated UTI/pyelonephritis: 10–14 days
Acute pelvic infection: 3–10 days
Surgical-site prophylaxis for colorectal surgery: 1 g IV 1 hr before procedure

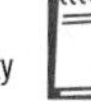

Contraindications: Hypersensitivity to ertapenem and other carbapenems (e.g., imipenem, meropenem), and prior anaphylactic reaction to β-lactams; for IM injection, hypersensitivity to amide-type anesthetics (e.g., lidocaine)

Warnings/Precautions: **Do not** use in meningitis because of poor CSF penetration. **Use with caution** with CNS disorders, including seizures. Adjust dosage in renal impairment by decreasing dose by 50% when GFR less than 30 mL/min. Ertapenem has poor activity against *Pseudomonas aeruginosa, Acinetobacter, MRSA,* and *Enterococcus faecalis.*

Adverse effects: Diarrhea, infusion complications, nausea, headache, vaginitis, phlebitis/thrombophlebitis, and vomiting are common. Seizures have been reported primarily in renal insufficiency and/or CNS disorders such as brain lesions or seizures. Muscle weakness, gait disturbance, abnormal coordination, altered mental status, and DRESS syndrome have been reported.

Drug interactions: Probenecid may increase ertapenem levels. May decrease valproic acid levels.

Drug administration:

IV: For intermittent infusion, infuse over 30 minutes at a concentration ≤20 mg/mL. **Do not** mix with dextrose-containing solutions. Reconstituted drug is stable for 6 hours at room temperature.

IM: Reconstitute 1-g vial with 3.2 mL of 1% lidocaine without epinephrine (~280 mg/mL) and use within 1 hour of preparation. Administer by deep IM injection into large muscle mass such as the gluteal muscles or lateral part of thigh.

For explanation of icons, see p. 364.

ERYTHROMYCIN ETHYLSUCCINATE AND ACETYLSULFISOXAZOLE
Pediazole, Eryzole, and others
Antibiotic, macrolide + sulfonamide derivative

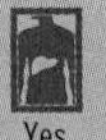
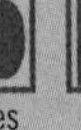
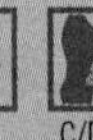
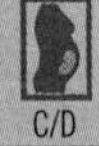

Yes Yes 2 C/D

Oral suspension: 200 mg erythromycin and 600 mg sulfa/5 mL (100, 150, 200, 250 mL)

Otitis media:
Child ≥2 mo: 50 mg/kg/24 hr (as erythromycin) and 150 mg/kg/24 hr (as sulfa) ÷ Q6 hr PO, or give 1.25 mL/kg/24 hr ÷ Q6 hr PO
Max. dose: 2 g erythromycin, 6 g sulfisoxazole/24 hr
Adult: 400 mg erythromycin and 1200 mg sulfisoxazole Q6 hr PO

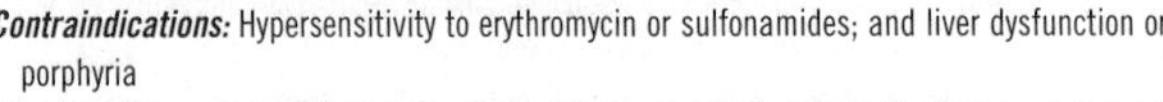

Contraindications: Hypersensitivity to erythromycin or sulfonamides; and liver dysfunction or porphyria
Warnings/Precautions: **Not** recommended in infants younger than 2 months. **Do not** use in renal impairment because dosage adjustments are inconsistent for sulfisoxazole and erythromycin. Pregnancy category changes to "D" if administered near term. See Erythromycin for additional information.
Adverse effects: Fever, rash, photosensitivity, GI disturbances, hepatitis, SLE-like syndrome, vasculitis, bone marrow suppression, hemolysis (patients with G6PD deficiency), and Stevens–Johnson syndrome may occur. See Erythromycin for additional information.
Drug interactions: May cause increased effects of warfarin, methotrexate, thiazide diuretics, uricosuric agents and sulfonylureas. Large quantities of vitamin C or acidifying agents (e.g., cranberry juice) may cause crystalluria. Interferes with folate absorption. See Erythromycin for additional information.
Drug administration: May be administered with or without food.

ERYTHROMYCIN PREPARATIONS
Erythrocin, Pediamycin, E-Mycin, Ery-Ped, and others
Ophthalmic ointment: Ilotycin, Romycin, and others
Antibiotic, macrolide

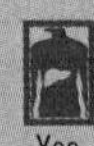
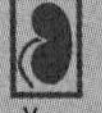
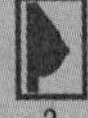
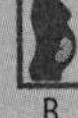

Yes Yes 2 B

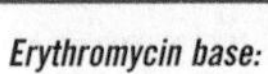

Erythromycin base:
Tabs: 250, 500 mg
Delayed-release tabs: 250, 333, 500 mg
Delayed-release caps: 250 mg
Topical ointment: 2% (25 g)
Topical gel: 2% (30, 60 g); contains alcohol 92%
Topical solution: 2% (60 mL); may contain 44%–66% alcohol
Topical pad/swab: 2% (60s)
Ophthalmic ointment: 0.5% (1, 3.5 g)
Erythromycin ethyl succinate (EES):
Oral suspension: 200 mg/5 mL (100, 200 mL), 400 mg/5 mL (100 mL)
Tabs: 400 mg
Erythromycin stearate:
Tabs: 250 mg
Erythromycin lactobionate:
Injection: 500, 1000 mg; may contain benzyl alcohol

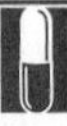

Oral:
Neonate:
<1.2 kg: 20 mg/kg/24 hr ÷ Q12 hr PO

Continued

ERYTHROMYCIN PREPARATIONS *continued*

≥1.2 kg:

0–7 days: 20 mg/kg/24 hr ÷ Q12 hr PO

>7 days:

1.2–2 kg: 30 mg/kg/24 hr ÷ Q8 hr PO

≥2 kg: 30–40 mg/kg/24 hr ÷ Q6–8 hr PO

Chlamydial conjunctivitis and pneumonia: 50 mg/kg/24 hr ÷ Q6 hr PO × 14 days; **max. dose:** 2 g/24 hr.

Child (use base or EES preparations): 30–50 mg/kg/24 hr ÷ Q6–8 hr PO; **max. dose:** 2 g/24 hr for base preparations and 3.2 g/24 hr for EES preparations

Pertussis: 40–50 mg/kg/24 hr ÷ Q6 hr PO × 14 days (**max. dose:** 2 g/24 hr); use azithromycin for infants <1 mo old

Adult: 1–4 g/24 hr ÷ Q6 hr PO; **max. dose:** 4 g/24 hr

Parenteral:

Child: 20–50 mg/kg/24 hr ÷ Q6 hr IV

Adult: 15–20 mg/kg/24 hr ÷ Q6 hr IV

Max. dose: 4 g/24 hr

Rheumatic fever prophylaxis: 500 mg/24 hr ÷ Q12 hr PO

Ophthalmic: Apply 0.5-inch ribbon to affected eye BID–QID. Apply as a one-time dose for prophylaxis of neonatal gonococcal ophthalmia.

Preoperative bowel prep: 20 mg/kg/dose PO erythromycin base × 3 doses, with neomycin, 1 day before surgery

Prokinetic agent:

Infant and child: 10–20 mg/kg/24 hr PO ÷ TID–QID (QAC or QAC and QHS)

Contraindications: Hypersensitivity to erythromycin or any other components in the formulation. **Avoid** use with astemizole, cisapride, pimozide, or terfenadine.

Warnings/Precautions: Hypertrophic pyloric stenosis in neonates receiving prophylactic therapy for pertussis, and life-threatening episodes of ventricular tachycardia associated with prolonged QTc interval have been reported. **Avoid** in patients with known prolongation of QT interval, proarrhythmic conditions (e.g., hypokalemia, hypomagnesemia, significant bradycardia), and receiving class IA or class III antiarrhythmic agents. **Use with caution** in liver disease. **Adjust dose in renal failure (see Chapter 3).** Use ideal body weight for obese patients when calculating doses.

Formulations of IV lactobionate dosage form may contain benzyl alcohol. Because of different absorption characteristics, higher oral doses of EES are needed to achieve therapeutic effects. Oral therapy should replace IV as soon as possible. **Avoid** IM route (pain, necrosis).

Adverse effects: Nausea, vomiting, and abdominal cramps are common. Estolate dosage form may cause cholestatic jaundice, although hepatotoxicity is uncommon (2% of reported cases). Cardiac dysrhythmia, anaphylaxis, interstitial nephritis, and hearing loss have been reported. See Warnings/Precautions section for additional adverse effects. May produce false-positive urinary catecholamines.

Drug interactions: Inhibits CYP 450 1A2, 3A3/4 isoenzymes. May produce elevated digoxin, theophylline, carbamazepine, clozapine, cyclosporine, and methylprednisolone levels. May produce false-positive urinary catecholamines, 17-hydroxycorticosteroids, and 17-ketosteroids.

Drug administration:

PO: Administer doses after meal to reduce GI upset. **Avoid** acidic beverages and milk 1 hour before and after dose. Swallow delayed-release or enteric-coated dosage forms whole.

IV: For intermittent infusion, infuse over 20–60 min at a concentration 1–2.5 mg/mL (**max.** 5 mg/mL). For continuous infusion (recommended for decreasing cardiotoxic effects), infuse at a concentration ≤1 mg/mL. **Avoid** IM route (pain, necrosis).

Ophthalmic ointment: Instill 0.5–1 cm ointment in lower conjunctival sac by avoiding contact of ointment tip with eye or skin.

For explanation of icons, see p. 364.

ETHAMBUTOL HCL
Myambutol and others
Antituberculosis drug

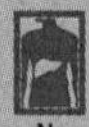 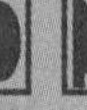 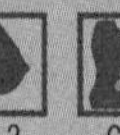 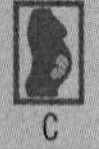
No Yes 2 C

Tabs: 100, 400 mg

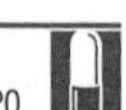

Tuberculosis:

Infant, child, adolescent, and adult: 15–25 mg/kg/dose PO once daily or 50 mg/kg/dose PO twice weekly

Max. dose: 2.5 g/24 hr

Nontuberculous mycobacterial infection, and* Mycobacterium avium *complex in AIDS (recurrence prophylaxis or treatment; use in combination with other medications):

Infant, child, adolescent, and adult: 15–25 mg/kg/24 hr PO; **max. dose:** 2.5 g/24 hr

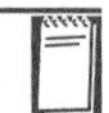

Contraindications: Hypersensitivity to ethambutol products or any other components in the formulation. **Do not use** in optic neuritis (unless clinically necessary) and in children whose visual acuity cannot be assessed.

Warnings/Precautions: Obtain baseline ophthalmologic studies before beginning therapy and then monthly. Follow visual acuity, visual fields, and (red–green) color vision. Discontinue if any visual deterioration occurs. Monitor uric acid, liver function, heme status, and renal function. **Adjust dose with renal failure (see Chapter 3).**

Adverse effects: Hyperuricemia, nausea, vomiting, and mania are common. May cause reversible optic neuritis, especially with larger doses. Erythema multiforme, thrombocytopenia, neutropenia, and peripheral neuropathy have been reported.

Drug interactions: Coadministration with aluminum hydroxide–containing antacids may reduce ethambutol's absorption; space administration by 4 hours.

Drug administration: Doses may be administered with food; especially with GI symptoms.

ETHIONAMIDE
Trecator
Antituberculosis drug

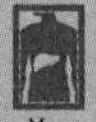 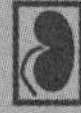  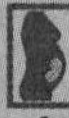 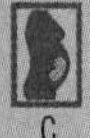
Yes Yes ? C

Tabs: 250 mg

Tuberculosis (as part of combination therapy):

Infant, child, and adolescent: 15–20 mg/kg/24 hr PO ÷ BID–TID; **max. dose:** 1 g/24 hr

Adult: 15–20 mg/kg/24 hr (usually 500–750 mg/24 hr) PO ÷ once to twice daily; **max. dose:** 1 g/24 hr (Initiate dose at 250 mg/24 hr × 1–2 days, then increase to 250 mg BID × 1–2 days with gradual increase to the highest tolerated dose.)

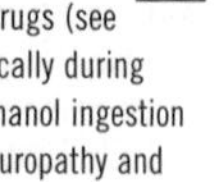

Contraindications: Hypersensitivity to ethionamide or any other components in the formulation; severe hepatic impairment

Warnings/Precautions: May potentiate the adverse effects of other anti-tuberculous drugs (see Drug Interactions). Ophthalmologic examinations should be done before and periodically during therapy. Use with **caution** in diabetes; may cause hypoglycemia. **Avoid** excessive ethanol ingestion because of potential psychotic reaction; **avoid** drugs that could cause peripheral neuropathy and optic neuritis. Adjust dose in renal insufficiency by administering 50% of normal dose when GFR less than 10 mL/min.

Adverse effects: GI disturbances, transient metallic taste, and anorexia are common and may be minimized by dose reduction, drug administration time change, or use of an antiemetic. Orthostatic hypotension, gynecomastia, impotence, acne, hypoglycemia, hypothyroidism, drowsiness, and transient increases in bilirubin, SGOT, and SGPT have been reported.

Continued

ETHIONAMIDE *continued*

Drug interactions: May increase the effects/toxicity of isoniazid. Seizures have been reported with cycloserine. Increased hepatic side effects may occur with rifampin, pyrazinamide, and ethambutol. See Warnings/Precautions.

Drug administration: Administer doses with meals.

ETRAVIRINE

Intelence, TMC 125

Antiviral agent, nonnucleoside reverse transcriptase inhibitor

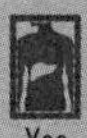
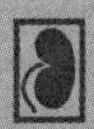
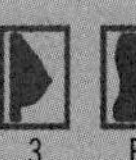

Yes No 3 B

Tabs: 25, 100, 200 mg

Use in combination with other HIV antiretroviral agents.

Child 6 to <18 yr:

16 to <20 kg: 100 mg PO BID

20 to <25 kg: 125 mg PO BID

25 to <30 kg: 150 mg PO BID

≥30 kg: 200 mg PO BID

Adult: 200 mg PO BID

Contraindications: Hypersensitivity to any component of the formulation

Warnings/Precautions: **Do not** use in treatment-naïve or treatment-experienced patients who do not have viral mutation testing of NNRTI and PI resistance. Many potential drug interactions may require dosage adjustments, cautious use, or avoidance of use; see later Drug Interactions section. Severe skin and hypersensitivity reactions, fat redistribution, and immune reconstitution syndrome have been reported.

Despite being metabolized primarily by the liver, similar pharmacokinetic parameters were observed in patients with mild and moderate hepatic impairment (Child–Pugh class A and B) and normal hepatic function. Has not been evaluated in severe hepatic impairment and renal impairment.

Adverse effects: Increase in serum cholesterol and triglycerides, nausea, diarrhea, elevated liver function tests, and increased serum creatinine may occur.

Rash and diarrhea are common in children; rash and peripheral neuropathy are common in adults. Stevens–Johnson syndrome, erythema multiforme, rhabdomyolysis, hepatic failure, and hypersensitivity reactions have been reported.

Drug interactions: Etravirine is a major substrate of CYP 450 2C19, 2C9, and 3A4. Inhibits CYP 2C19 and 2C9, and P-gp; and induces CYP 3A4. May increase the effects/toxicity of diazepam and warfarin; may decrease the effects of amiodarone, clarithromycin, and clopidogrel. Azole antifungal agents (fluconazole, itraconazole, ketoconazole, posaconazole, voriconazole) may increase etravirine levels. Carbamazepine, phenobarbital, phenytoin, clarithromycin, rifampin, rifapentine, rifabutin, dexamethasone, and St. John's wort may decrease etravirine levels/effects. Always check the potential for other drug interactions when either initiating therapy or adding new drugs onto an existing regimen. Many interactions with combination antiretroviral therapies exist (check for specific combinations); efavirenz, nevirapine, and ritonavir may decrease etravirine levels.

Drug administration: Administer each dose after meals. Patients who are unable to swallow tablets may dissolve tablet(s) in a glass with enough water to cover the medication; stir well until water looks milky, add more water or orange juice or milk (water is always first used to dissolve the tablets). **Avoid** using grapefruit juice, carbonated, or warm (>40°C) beverages. Rinse the glass several times with water, orange juice, or milk, and completely swallow the rinse each time to assure complete dose administration.

For explanation of icons, see p. 364.

FAMCICLOVIR
Famvir and others
Antiviral

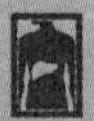 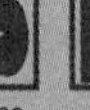 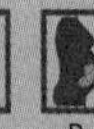 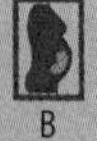
Yes Yes ? B

Tabs: 125, 250, 500 mg

Adult:

Herpes zoster: 500 mg Q8 hr PO × 7 days; initiate therapy promptly as soon as diagnosis is made (initiation within 48 hr after rash onset is ideal; currently, no data for starting treatment >72 hr after rash onset).

Genital herpes (first episode): 250 mg Q8 hr PO × 7–10 days

Recurrent genital herpes:

Immunocompetent: 1000 mg Q12 hr PO × 1 day or 125 mg Q12 hr PO × 5 days; initiate therapy at first sign or symptom. Efficacy has not been established when treatment is initiated >6 hr after onset of symptoms or lesions.

Immunocompromised: 500 mg Q8 hr PO × 7 days

Suppression of recurrent genital herpes (immunocompetent): 250 mg Q12 hr PO up to 1 year, then reassess for HSV infection recurrence.

Recurrent herpes labialis:

Immunocompetent: 1500 mg PO × 1

Immunocompromised: 500 mg PO Q8 hr PO × 7 days

Recurrent mucocutaneous herpes in HIV: 500 mg Q12 hr PO × 7 days

Contraindications: Hypersensitivity to famciclovir, penciclovir, or any other components in the formulation

Warnings/Precautions: Drug is converted to its active form (penciclovir). Hepatic impairment may impair/reduce the conversion of famciclovir to penciclovir. Better absorption than PO acyclovir. **Reduce dose in renal impairment (see Chapter 3).** Safety and efficacy in suppression of recurrent genital herpes have not been established beyond 1 year.

Adverse effects: Headache, diarrhea, nausea, and abdominal pain are common. Serious skin reactions (e.g., TEN and Stevens–Johnson), cholestatic jaundice, angioedema, and abnormal LFTs have been reported.

Drug interactions: Concomitant use with probenecid and other drugs eliminated by active tubular secretion may result in decreased penciclovir (active metabolite) clearance.

Drug administration: May be given with or without food.

FIDAXOMICIN
Dificid
Antibiotic, macrolide

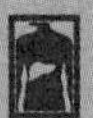  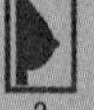 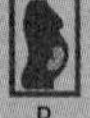
No No 2 B

Tabs: 200 mg; contains soy lecithin

C. difficile*–associated diarrhea:*

Child: Current Phase 2A clinical trial evaluating the safety, tolerability, and pharmacokinetics of fidaxomicin in children uses the following dosage (see www.clinicaltrials.gov for updated information):

6 mo to 5 yr (investigational oral suspension): 32 mg/kg/24 hr (max. 400 mg/24 hr) ÷ BID PO × 10 days

6 to <18 yr (oral tablets): 200 mg BID PO × 10 days

Adult: 200 mg BID PO × 10 days

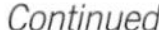

Continued

FIDAXOMICIN *continued*

Contraindications: Have not been determined

Warnings/Precautions: Should not be used for systemic infections because fidaxomicin is minimally absorbed. Only use fidaxomicin for infection proved or strongly suspected to be caused by *Clostridium difficile*.

Adverse effects: Nausea, vomiting, abdominal pain and GI hemorrhage, anemia, and neutropenia are common.

Drug interactions: Fidaxomicin and its major metabolite, OP-118, are substrates of P-gp efflux transporter of the intestinal tract. Cyclosporin, a P-gp inhibitor, may increase systemic absorption of fidaxomicin and OP-118, and reduce their concentrations at the desired site of action.

Drug administration: Doses may be administered with or without food.

FLUCONAZOLE
Diflucan and others
Antifungal agent

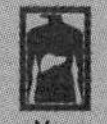
Yes
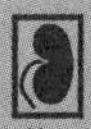
Yes
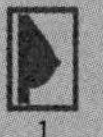
1
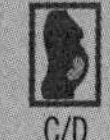
C/D

Tabs: 50, 100, 150, 200 mg
Injection: 2 mg/mL (100, 200 mL); contains 9 mEq Na/2 mg drug
Premixed injection:
Diluted in iso-osmotic dextrose: 200 mg in 100 mL, 400 mg in 200 mL
Diluted in iso-osmotic sodium chloride: 100 mg in 50 mL, 200 mg in 100 mL, and 400 mg in 200 mL; 200 and 400 mg solutions are also available as preservative free
Oral suspension: 10 mg/mL (35 mL), 40 mg/mL (35 mL)

Neonate:

Loading dose: 12–25 mg/kg IV/PO

Maintenance dose: 6–12 mg/kg IV/PO with the following dosing intervals (see following table); use higher doses for severe infections of *Candida* strains with MICs >4–8 mcg/mL.

Postconceptional Age (wk)	Postnatal Age (days)	Dosing Interval (hr) and Time (hr) to Start First Maintenance Dose after Load
≤29	0–14	48
	>14	24
≥30	0–7	48
	>7	24

Child (IV/PO):

Indication	Loading Dose	Maintenance Dose (Q24 hr) to Begin 24 hr after Loading Dose
Oropharyngeal candidiasis	6 mg/kg	3 mg/kg
Esophageal candidiasis	12 mg/kg	6 mg/kg
Invasive systemic candidiasis and cryptococcal meningitis	12 mg/kg	6–12 mg/kg
Suppressive therapy for HIV-infected with cryptococcal meningitis	6 mg/kg	6 mg/kg

Max. dose: 12 mg/kg/24 hr

Continued

For explanation of icons, see p. 364.

FLUCONAZOLE *continued*

Adult:

Oropharyngeal and esophageal candidiasis: Loading dose of 200 mg PO/IV followed by 100 mg Q24 hr (24 hr after load); doses up to **max. dose** of 400 mg/24 hr should be used for esophageal candidiasis

Systemic candidiasis and cryptococcal meningitis: Loading dose of 400 mg PO/IV, followed by 200–800 mg Q24 hr (24 hr after load)

Bone marrow transplant prophylaxis: 400 mg PO/IV Q24 hr

Suppressive therapy for HIV infected with cryptococcal meningitis: 200 mg PO/IV Q24 hr

Vaginal candidiasis: 150 mg PO × 1

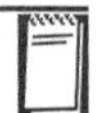

Contraindications: Concomitant administration of fluconazole with cisapride is **contraindicated;** arrhythmias may occur. Hypersensitivity to fluconazole or any other components in the formulation.

Warnings/Precautions: **Use with caution** in patients with proarrhythmic conditions and impaired hepatic or renal function. **Adjust dose in renal failure (see Chapter 3).** Pediatric to adult dose equivalency: every 3 mg/kg pediatric dosage is equal to 100 mg adult dosage. Consider using higher doses in morbidly obese patients.

Pregnancy category is "C" for single-dose vaginal candidiasis indication and is "D" for all other indications.

Adverse effects: May cause nausea, headache, rash, vomiting, abdominal pain, hepatitis, liver enzyme elevation, cholestasis, and diarrhea. Neutropenia, agranulocytosis, and thrombocytopenia have been reported.

Drug interactions: Inhibits CYP 450 2C9/10 and CYP 450 3A3/4 (weak inhibitor). May increase effects, toxicity, or levels of cyclosporine, midazolam, phenytoin, rifabutin, tacrolimus, theophylline, warfarin, oral hypoglycemics, and AZT. Rifampin increases fluconazole metabolism.

Drug administration:

IV: For intermittent infusion, infuse over 1–2 hr (not to exceed 200 mg/hr) at a concentration of 2 mg/mL. Administer doses ≥6 mg/kg/24 hr over 2 hr.

PO: Doses may be given with or without food.

FLUCYTOSINE

Ancobon, 5-FC, 5-Fluorocytosine, and others

Antifungal agent

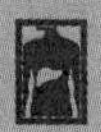
No

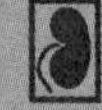
Yes

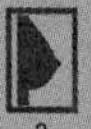
3

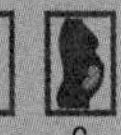
C

Caps: 250, 500 mg

Oral liquid: 10 mg/mL

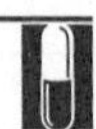

Neonate: 80–160 mg/kg/24 hr ÷ Q6 hr PO

Child and adult: 50–150 mg/kg/24 hr ÷ Q6 hr PO

Contraindications: Hypersensitivity to flucytosine or any other components in the formulation. Use is **contraindicated** in the first trimester of pregnancy.

Warnings/Precautions: **Use extreme caution in renal impairment (adjust dose in renal failure; see Chapter 3).** Monitor CBC, BUN, serum creatinine, alkaline phosphatase, AST, and ALT.

Therapeutic levels: 25–100 mg/L. Recommended serum sampling time at steady state: Obtain peak level 2–4 hr after oral dose following 4 days of continuous dosing. Peak levels of 40–60 mg/L have been recommended for systemic candidiasis. Maintain trough leves >25 mg/L.

Continued

FLUCYTOSINE *continued*

Prolonged levels >100 mg/L can increase risk for bone marrow suppression. Bone marrow suppression in immunosuppressed patients can be irreversible and fatal.

Adverse effects: Nausea, vomiting, diarrhea, rash, and CNS disturbance are common. Cardiotoxicity, anemia, leukopenia, and thrombocytopenia have been reported.

Drug interactions: Amphotericin may increase efficacy and toxicity (enterocolitis, myelosuppression); use with caution. Cytarabine may decrease flucytosine activity. Flucytosine interferes with creatinine assay tests using the dry-slide enzymatic method (Kodak Ektachem analyzer: Eastman-Kodak, Rochester, NY).

Drug administration: Administer dose with food over a 15-min period to decrease nausea and vomiting.

FOSAMPRENAVIR
Lexiva, f-APV
Antiretroviral, protease inhibitor

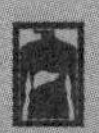

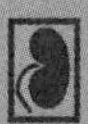

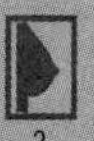

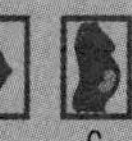

Oral suspension: 50 mg/mL equvalent to 43 mg/mL amprenavir (225 mL); contains propylene glycol
Tabs: 700 mg; equivalent to 600 mg amprenavir

Doses based on milligrams of fosamprenavir (fosamprenavir tablets may be used for pediatric patients ≥39 kg and ritonavir capsules for ≥33 kg; see Warnings/Precautions).

Child (see remarks):

Antiretroviral naïve:

Regimens with ritonavir (≥4 wk to 18 yr):

Weight (kg)	Fosamprenavir dose PO BID	Ritonavir dose PO BID
<11	45 mg/kg	7 mg/kg
11 to <15	30 mg/kg	3 mg/kg
15 to <20	23 mg/kg	3 mg/kg
≥20	18 mg/kg	3 mg/kg

Max. dose: 700 mg fosamprenavir BID and 100 mg ritonavir BID

Regimens without ritonavir (≥2–18 yr): 30 mg/kg/dose PO BID; **max. dose:** 1400 mg BID

Therapy experienced:

≥6 mo to 18 yr:

Regimens with ritonavir: Follow dosing recommendation table for antiretroviral naïve with ritonavir from above. **Max. dose:** 700 mg fosamprenavir BID and 100 mg ritonavir BID.

Regimens without ritonavir (≥47 kg): 1400 mg (as tablets) PO BID

Adolescent and adult:

Antiretroviral naïve:

Regimens without ritonavir: 1400 mg PO BID

Regimens containing ritonavir:

Once-daily regimen: 1400 mg fosamprenavir PO once daily with 200 mg ritonavir PO once daily

Twice-daily regimen: 700 mg fosamprenavir PO BID with 100 mg ritonavir PO BID

Protease inhibitor experienced: 700 mg fosamprenavir PO BID with 100 mg ritonavir PO BID; add an additional 100 mg/24 hr ritonavir when efavirenz is included in the regimen. Once-daily regimen is not recommended for these patients.

Continued

For explanation of icons, see p. 364.

FOSAMPRENAVIR *continued*

Adult:

In combination with efavirenz (should be boosted with ritonavir):

Once-daily regimen: 1400 mg fosamprenavir PO once daily with 300 mg ritonavir PO once daily and 600 mg efavirenz PO once daily

Twice-daily regimen: 700 mg fosamprenavir PO BID with 100 mg ritonavir PO BID and 600 mg efavirenz PO once daily

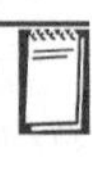

Contraindications: Hypersensitivity to fosamprenavir or amprenavir and any of its components. **Do not use** with agents highly dependent on cytochrome P450 3A4 for clearance (e.g., astemizole, terfenadine, cisapride, midazolam, triazolam, ergot derivatives, lipid-lowering agents such as atorvastatin and cervistatin, pimozide and triazolam) and antiarrhythmic agents (e.g., flecainide and propafenone).

Warnings/Precautions: **Use with caution** with sulfanamide allergy, hepatic impairment (should not be used in severe hepatic disease), and hemophilia (reports of spontaneous bleeding). Autoimmune disorders (e.g., Graves disease, polymyositis, and Guillain–Barre syndrome) may occur in the setting of immune reconstitution. Patients with hepatitis B or C, or marked elevations in transaminases before therapy may develop transaminase elevations.

Dosing in hepatic impairment:

Mild/Moderate impairment (Child–Pugh score 5–8) recommended adult regimens:

Treatment naïve: 700 mg fosamprenavir PO BID without ritonavir, or 450 mg fosamprenavir PO BID with ritonavir 100 mg PO once daily

PI therapy experienced: 450 mg fosamprenavir PO BID with ritonavir 100 mg PO once daily

Severe impairment (Child–Pugh score 9–12) recommended adult regimen:

Treatment naïve: 350 mg fosamprenair PO BID without ritonavir

Fosamprenavir is a prodrug of amprenavir and is rapidly hydrolyzed to the amprenavir in the GI tract. Should be administered to infants born ≥38 weeks' gestation with a postnatal age of ≥28 days. For children 2 to 5 years old, data are currently insufficient to recommend once-daily dosing.

Adverse effects: GI disturbances, perioral paresthesias, headache, rash, and lipid abnormalities are common. Life-threatening rash (e.g., Steven–Johnson), fat redistribution, nephrolithiasis, angioedema, neutropenia, hyperglycemia, hemolytic anemia, and elevations in serum transaminases and creatinine kinase have been reported.

Drug interactions: Amprenavir is a substrate and inhibitor of CYP 450 3A4. Efavirenz, rifampin, rifabutin, anticonvulsants, oral contraceptives, and St. John's wort can lower amprenavir levels. Always check the potential for other drug interactions when either initiating therapy or adding new drug onto an existing regimen. See Contraindications section.

Drug administration: Doses may be administered with or without food. Administer doses 1 hour before or after any antacids or buffered medications (e.g., didanosine).

FOSCARNET
Foscavir and others
Antiviral agent

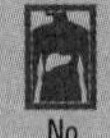
No
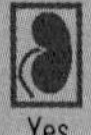
Yes
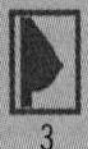
3
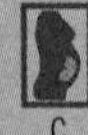
C

Injection: 24 mg/mL (250, 500 mL)

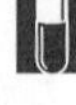

IV route (HIV positive or exposed):

CMV disease:

Infant and child:

Induction: 180 mg/kg/24 hr ÷ Q8 hr in combination with ganciclovir, continue until symptom improvement and convert to maintenance therapy

Maintenance: 90–120 mg/kg/dose Q24 hr

Continued

FOSCARNET *continued*

CMV retinitis (disseminated disease):

Infant and child:

Induction: 180 mg/kg/24 hr ÷ Q8 hr × 14–21 days with or without ganciclovir

Maintenance: 90–120 mg/kg/24 hr once daily

Adolescent and adult:

Induction: 180 mg/kg/24 hr ÷ Q8–12 hr × 14–21 days

Maintenance: 90–120 mg/kg/24 hr once daily

Acyclovir-resistant herpes simplex:

Infant and child: 40 mg/kg/dose Q8 hr or 60 mg/kg/dose Q12 hr for up to 3 wk or until lesions heal

Adolescent and adult: 40 mg/kg/dose Q8–12 hr × 14–21 days or until lesions heal

Varicella zoster unresponsive to acyclovir:

Infant and child: 40–60 mg/kg/dose Q8 hr × 7–10 days

Adolescent: 90 mg/kg/dose Q12 hr

Varicella zoster, progressive outer retinal necrosis:

Infant and child: 90 mg/kg/dose Q12 hr in combination with ganciclovir IV and intravitreal foscarnet with or without ganciclovir

Adolescent: 90 mg/kg/dose Q12 hr in combination with IV ganciclovir and intravitreal foscarnet and/or ganciclovir

Intravitreal route for progressive outer retinal necrosis (HIV positive or exposed):

Child and adolescent: 1.2 mg/0.05 mL per dose twice weekly in combination with IV foscarnet and ganciclovir and/or intravitreal ganciclovir

---

Contraindications: Hypersensitivity to foscarnet or any other components in the formulation

Warnings/Precautions: **Use with caution** in patients with renal insufficiency. **Discontinue** use in adults if serum Cr ≥2.9 mg/dL. **Adjust dose in renal failure (see Chapter 3).** Monitor renal function and plasma minerals and electrolytes (especially calcium and those with neurologic and cardiac conditions) are recommended. Adequate fluid hydration should be maintained during therapy to reduce nephrotoxicity risk.

Adverse effects: GI disturbances, anemia, headache, and fever are common. May cause peripheral neuropathy, seizures, hallucinations, increased LFTs, hypertension, chest pain, ECG abnormalities, coughing, dyspnea, bronchospasm, and renal failure (adequate hydration and avoiding nephrotoxic medications may reduce risk). Hypocalcemia (increased risk if given with pentamidine), hypokalemia, and hypomagnesemia may also occur.

Drug interactions: Nephrotoxic medications (e.g., ampotericin, aminoglycosides) increase risk for nephrotoxicity. Ciprofloxacin may increase risk for seizures.

Drug administration: For intermittent infusion, infuse at a rate **not exceeding** 60 mg/kg/dose over 1 hr or 120 mg/kg/dose over 2 hr at a concentration of ≤12 mg/mL for peripheral line administration or ≤24 mg/mL for central line administration.

FOSFOMYCIN TROMETHAMINE
Monurol
Antibacterial, phosponic acid derivative

No No ? B

Oral powder for solution: 3 g single-dose sachet

Uncomplicated UTI (acute cystitis):

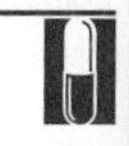

Child: 2 g PO × 1; 1 g PO × 1 has been suggested for infants <1 year old

Adult: 3 g PO × 1

Continued

For explanation of icons, see p. 364.

FOSFOMYCIN TROMETHAMINE *continued*

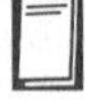

Contraindications: Hypersensitivity to fosfomycin or any other components in the formulation

Warnings/Precautions: Multiple daily doses over 2 to 3 days do not offer any advantage over a single-dose regimen and can increase incidence of adverse events.

Adverse effects: GI disturbances, headache, vaginitis, and rhinitis are common. Although rare, angioedema, aplastic anemia, jaundice, hepatic necrosis, and toxic megacolon have been reported.

Drug interactions: Drugs that increase GI motility (e.g., metoclopramide and erythromycin) may lower serum concentrations by decreasing fosfomycin's absorption.

Drug administration: All doses should be dissolved in 3 to 4 ounces of water (not hot water) and administered immediately. Doses may be given with or without food.

GANCICLOVIR
Cytovene, Vitrasert, Zirgan, and others
Antiviral agent

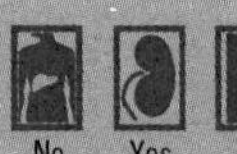
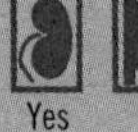
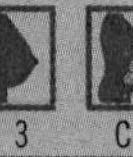

Injection: 500 mg; contains 4 mEq Na per 1 g drug
Intravitreal implant (sustained release over 5–8 mo):
Vitrasert: 4.5 mg
Ophthalmic gel (drops):
Zirgan: 0.15% (5 g); contains benzalkonium chloride

Cytomegalovirus (CMV) infections:

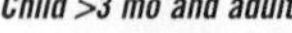

Neonate (congenital CMV): 12 mg/kg/24 hr ÷ Q12 hr IV ≥6 wk

Child >3 mo and adult:

Induction therapy (duration 14–21 days): 10 mg/kg/24 hr ÷ Q12 hr IV

IV maintenance therapy: 5 mg/kg/dose once daily IV ≥7 days/wk or 6 mg/kg/dose once daily IV for 5 days/wk

Prevention of CMV in transplant recipients:

Child and adult:

Induction therapy (duration 7–14 days): 10 mg/kg/24 hr ÷ Q12 hr IV

IV maintenance therapy: 5 mg/kg/dose once daily IV for 7 days/wk or 6 mg/kg/dose once daily IV for 5 days/wk for 100–120 days after transplant

Prevention of CMV in HIV-infected individuals (see www.hivatis.org for latest recommendations and guidelines for CMV treatment as well):

Infant, child, adolescent, and adult:

Recurrence prophylaxis: 5 mg/kg/dose IV once daily. Consider valganciclovir as an oral alternative.

CMV retinitis (intravitreal implant):

≥9 yr and adult: One implant lasts for 5–8 mo period. As drug is depleted from the implant, retinitis will progress; the implant may be removed and replaced.

Herpetic keratitis (ophthalmic gel/drops):

≥2 yr and adult: Apply 1 drop onto affected eye(s) 5 times a day (~Q3 hr while awake) until cornial ulcer is healed, then 1 drop TID × 7 days.

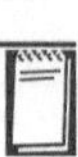

Contraindications: Hypersensitivity to ganciclovir/acyclovir products or any of its components, or severe neutropenia (ANC <500/microliter) or severe thrombocytopenia (platelets <25,000/microliter). Any occular surgery contraindication (infection or severe thrombocytopenia) for the intravitreal implant dosage form.

Continued

GANCICLOVIR *continued*

Warnings/Precautions: Limited experience with use in children younger than 12 years. Use with extreme caution. **Reduce dose in renal failure (see Chapter 3).** May impair male and female infertility. For oral route of administration, see Valganciclovir.

Adverse effects:

IV: Neutropenia, thrombocytopenia, anemia, fever, and phlebitis are common. Drug reactions alleviated with dose reduction or temporary interruption.

Intravitreal implant: Visual acuity loss of ≥3 lines during the first 2 mo after implantation. Cataract formation, macular abnormalities, intraocular pressure spikes, optic disk/nerve changes, hyphemas, and uveitis have occurred.

Ophthalmic gel: Blurred vision, irritation, conjuntival hyperemia, and punctate keratitis

Drug interactions: Immunosuppressive agents may increase hematologic toxicities. Amphotericin B, cyclosporine, and tacrolimus increase risk for nephrotoxicity. May increase the risk for seizures with imipenem/cilastatin, and increase didanosine and zidovudine levels. Probenecid, didanosine, and zidovudine may decrease ganciclovir levels.

Drug administration: Use proper procedures for handling and disposal; drug is potentially carcinogenic and mutagenic.

IV: For intermittent infusion, infuse ≥1 hr at a concentration ≤10 mg/mL. IM and SC administration are **contraindicated** because of high pH (pH = 11).

Intravitreal implant: Maintain aseptic technique at all times before and during surgical implantation procedure.

Ophthalmic gel/drop: **Avoid** contamination with applicator tip and **do not** wear contact lenses while using this medication.

GATIFLOXACIN

Zymaxid

Ophthalmic antibiotic, quinolone

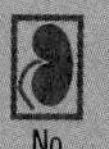
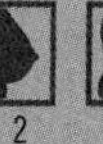
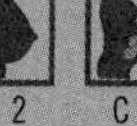

No No 2 C

Ophthalmic drops: 0.5% (2.5 mL); contains benzalkonium chloride

≥1 yr and adult: Instill 1 drop into affected eye(s) Q2 hr while awake (**max. dose:** 8 times/24 hr) × 1 day, followed by 1 drop to affected eye(s) BID–QID while awake × 6 days.

Contraindications: Hypersensitivity to gatifloxacin, fluoroquinolones, or any other components in the formulation

Warnings/Precautions: Indicated for the treatment of bacterial conjunctivitis caused by susceptible strains of *Haemophilus influenzae, Staphylococcus aureus, Staphylococcus epidermidis, Streptococcus mitis group, Streptococcus oralis,* and *Streptococcus pneumonia.*

For topical ophthalmic use only (**do not** inject into eye). Fungal or bacterial superinfection may occur with prolonged use.

Adverse effects: Worsening of conjunctivitis, eye irritation, dysgeusia, and eye pain are common. Chemosis, conjunctival hemorrhage, dry eye, eye discharge, eyelid edema, headache, increased lactrimation, keratititis, papillary conjunctivitis, and reduced visual acuity have been reported.

Drug interactions: No interaction studies have been conducted.

Drug administration: **Avoid** contaminating the applicator tip while using. **Do not** wear contact lenses while receiving therapy. Apply finger pressure to lacrimal sac during and for 1 to 2 minutes after dose application.

For explanation of icons, see p. 364.

GEMIFLOXACIN
Factive
Antibiotic, quinolone

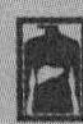 No 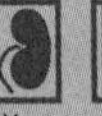 Yes 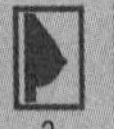 2 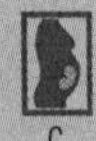 C

Tabs: 320 mg (scored)

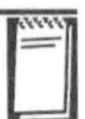

Adult: 320 mg PO once daily with the following duration of therapy:
Chronic bronchitis acute exacerbation: 5 days
Community-acquired pneumonia: 5–7 days

Contraindications: Hypersensitivity to gemifloxacin, fluoroquinolones, or any other components in the formulation

Warnings/Precautions: **Avoid use** in patients with history of QTc prolongation, uncorrected hypokalemia, hypomagnesemia, or administration with other medications that can prolong QTc interval. Like other quinolones, tendon rupture can occur during or after therapy, especially with concomitant corticosteroid use, organ transplant recipients, and age older than 60 years. **Avoid use** in myasthenia gravis; may exacerbate muscle weakness. Convulsions, increased intracranial pressure, and toxic psychosis have been reported with other fluoroquinolones.

Use with caution in renal impairment (see Chapter 3).

Adverse effects: Diarrhea, rash, nausea, headache, abdominal pain, vomiting, and dizziness are common.

Hyperglycemia; increases in ALT, AST, alkaline phosphatase, and creatine phosphokinase; insomnia; leukopenia; taste abnormalities; and vaginitis may occur. Hypersensitivity reactions have been reported with fluoroquinolones, including gemifloxacin.

Drug interactions: Antacids containing aluminum and/or magnesium, and sucralfate may decrease the absorption of gemifloxacin (see Drug Administration). Probenecid may increase levels and toxicity of gemifloxacin. May increase the effects/toxicity of warfarin.

Drug administration: May be administered with or without food, milk, or calcium supplements. Should be administered 3 hours before or 2 hours after taking sucralfate, multivitamins, and other divalent/trivalent salts (e.g., alluminum, iron, zinc, or magnesium).

GENTAMICIN
Garamycin and many others
Antibiotic, aminoglycoside

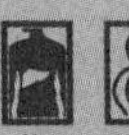 No 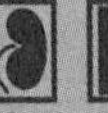 Yes 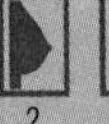 2 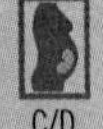 C/D

Injection: 10 mg/mL (2 mL), 40 mg/mL (2, 20 mL); some products may contain sodium metabisulfite
Premixed injection in NS: 40 mg (50 mL), 60 mg (50 mL), 70 mg (50 mL), 80 mg (50, 100 mL), 90 mg (100 mL), 100 mg (50, 100 mL), 120 mg (50, 100 mL)
Ophthalmic ointment: 0.3% (3.5 g)
Ophthalmic drops: 0.3% (5, 15 mL)
Topical ointment: 0.1% (15, 30 g)
Topical cream: 0.1% (15, 30 g)

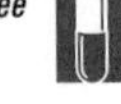

Initial empiric dosage; patient-specific dosage defined by therapeutic drug monitoring (see remarks):
Parenteral (IM or IV):

Continued

GENTAMICIN *continued*

Neonate/Infant (see following table):

Postconceptional Age (wk)	Postnatal Age (days)	Dose (mg/kg/dose)	Interval (hr)
≤29*	0–7	5	48
	8–28	4	36
	>28	4	24
30–33	0–7	4.5	36
	>7	4	24
34–37	0–7	4	24
	>7	4	18–24
≥38	0–7	4	24†
	>7	4	12–18

*Or significant asphyxia, PDA, indomethacin use, poor cardiac output, and reduced renal function.
†Use Q36 hr interval for HIE patients receiving whole-body therapeutic cooling.

Child: 7.5 mg/kg/24 hr ÷ Q8 hr
Adult: 3–6 mg/kg/24 hr ÷ Q8 hr
Cystic fibrosis: 7.5–10.5 mg/kg/24 hr ÷ Q8 hr
Intrathecal/intraventricular (use preservative-free product only):
Newborn: 1 mg once daily
>3 mo: 1–2 mg once daily
Adult: 4–8 mg once daily
Ophthalmic ointment: apply Q8–12 hr
Ophthalmic drops: 1–2 drops Q2–4 hr

Contraindications: Hypersensitivity to aminoglycosides or any other components in the formulation

Warnings/Precautions: **Use with caution** in combination with neurotoxic, ototoxic, or nephrotoxic drugs; anesthetics or neuromuscular blocking agents; preexisting renal, vestibular, or auditory impairment; and in patients with neuromuscular disorders. Pregnancy category is a "C" for ophthalmic use and "D" with IV use.

Eliminated more quickly in patients with cystic fibrosis, neutropenia, and burns. **Adjust dose in renal failure (see Chapter 3).** Monitor peak and trough levels.

Therapeutic peak levels with conventional Q8 hr dosing:
6–10 mg/L general
8–10 mg/L in pulmonary infections, neutropenia, osteomyelitis, and severe sepsis

An individualized peak concentration to target a peak/MIC ratio of 8–10 : 1 may be applied to maximize bacterialcidal effects.

Therapeutic trough levels with conventional Q8 hr dosing: <2 mg/L. Recommended serum sampling time at steady state: trough within 30 min before the third consecutive dose and peak 30–60 min after the administration of the third consecutive dose.

For initial dosing in obese patients, use adjusted body weight (ABW), ABW = ideal body weight + 0.4 (total body weight – ideal body weight); see Chapter 3 for additional information.

Adverse effects: May cause nephrotoxicity, ototoxicity, and neuromuscular blockade.

Drug interactions: Ototoxicity may be potentiated with the use of loop diuretics. See Warnings/Precautions section.

Drug administration:

IV: Infuse over 30 to 60 minutes at a concentration ≤10 mg/mL. Administer β-lactam antibiotics at least 1 hour before or after gentamicin.

IM: Use either undiluted commercial products of 10 or 40 mg/mL.

Continued

For explanation of icons, see p. 364.

GENTAMICIN *continued*

Intrathecal/intraventricular: Use the preservative-free 10 mg/mL product.

Ophthalmic:

Drops: Apply finger pressure to lacrimal sac during and for 1 to 2 minutes after dose application.

Ointment: Instill ointment in lower conjunctival sac by **avoiding** contact of ointment tip with eye or skin.

GENTIAN VIOLET
Various generic products
Antifungal agent

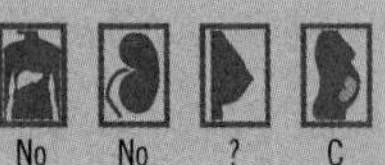
No No ? C

Topical solution: 1%, 2% (30 mL); contains 10% ethyl alcohol

Topical:

Child and adult: Apply to lesions BID–TID × 3 days. A 0.25% or 0.5% solution is as effective and may be less irritating than 1%–2% solutions.

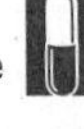

Contraindications: Hypersensitivity to gentian violet or any other components in the formulation; porphyria; and use on ulcerative lesions or open wounds

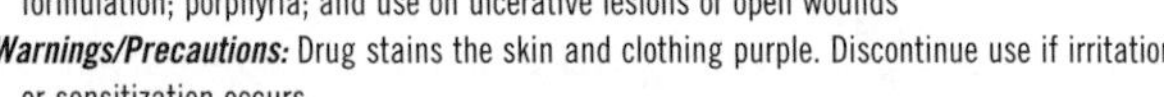

Warnings/Precautions: Drug stains the skin and clothing purple. Discontinue use if irritation or sensitization occurs.

Adverse effects: Pruritus, skin irritation, skin ulcer, and skin staining (permanent with granulation tissue) are common.

Drug interactions: None identified.

Drug administration: For topical administration, apply to lesion with cotton and **avoid** application to ulcerative lesions. **Avoid** contact with eyes, skin, and clothing.

GRISEOFULVIN
Grifulvin V, Griseofulvin Microsize, Grisactin, Gris-PEG, and others
Antifungal agent

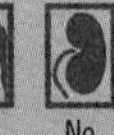
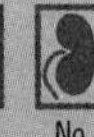
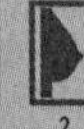
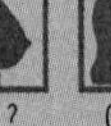
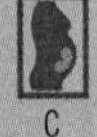
Yes No ? C

Microsize:

Tabs (Grifulvin V): 500 mg

Oral suspension (Griseofulvin Microsize): 125 mg/5 mL (120 mL); contains 0.2% alcohol, parabens, and propylene glycol

Ultramicrosize (250 mg ultramicrosize is approximately 500 mg microsize):

Tabs (Gris-PEG): 125, 250 mg

Microsize:

Child >2 yr: 10–20 mg/kg/24 hr PO ÷ once to twice daily; give with milk, eggs, or fatty foods. Some have recommended a higher dose of 20–25 mg/kg/24 hr PO for tinea capitis to improve efficacy because of relative resistance of the organism.

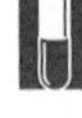

Adult: 500–1000 mg/24 hr PO ÷ once to twice daily

Max. dose: 1 g/24 hr

Ultramicrosize:

Child >2 yr: 10–15 mg/kg/24 hr PO ÷ once to twice daily

Adult: 330–750 mg/24 hr PO ÷ once to twice daily

Max. dose (all ages): 750 mg/24 hr

Contraindications: Hypersensitivity to griseofulvin products or any other components in the formulation; porphyria and hepatic disease; and pregnancy or intention to become pregnant within 1 month after stopping therapy

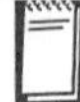

Continued

GRISEOFULVIN *continued*

Warnings/Precautions: Monitor hematologic, renal, and hepatic function. Possible cross-reactivity in penicillin-allergic patients. Usual treatment period is 8 weeks for tinea capitis and 4 to 6 months for tinea unguium.

Adverse effects: May cause leukopenia, rash, headache, photosensitivity, paresthesias, and GI symptoms. Severe skin reactions (e.g., Stevens–Johnson, TEN), erythema multiforme, LFT elevations (AST, ALT, bilirubin), and jaundice have been reported.

Drug interactions: May reduce effectiveness or decrease level of oral contraceptives, warfarin, and cyclosporine; potentiate the effects of alcohol (flushing and tachycardia). Induces CYP 450 1A2 isoenzyme. Phenobarbital may enhance clearance of griseofulvin.

Drug administration: Administer with fatty meals to increase the drug's absorption.

HEPATITIS B IMMUNE GLOBULIN
HyperHEP B S/D, Nabi-HB, HepaGam B, HBIG
Hyperimmune globulin, hepatitis B

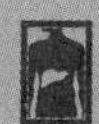
No
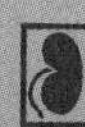
No
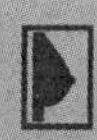
?
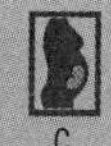
C

Injection:
HyperHEP B S/D: contains ≥220 IU/mL
Syringe: 0.5, 1 mL
Vials: 1, 5 mL
Nabi-HB: contains >312 IU/mL and 0.15 M glycine
Vials: 1, 5 mL; contains polysorbate 80
HepaGam B: contains >312 IU/mL and 10% maltose and 0.03% polysorbate 80
Vials: 1, 5 mL
Contains 4%–18% protein (of which not <80% is IgG) and trace amounts of IgA.

Prophylaxis of newborns (along with hepatitis B vaccine series initiated within 12 hours after birth):
HBsAg-positive mothers: 0.5 mL IM × 1 within 12 hr after birth
Unknown maternal HBsAg status:
<2 kg: 0.5 mL IM × 1 within 12 hr after birth, if unable to determine maternal HBsAg status within 12 hr
≥2 kg: 0.5 mL IM × 1 within 7 days after birth (pending results of maternal HBsAg status)

Postexposure prophylaxis (within 24 hours of needlestick, ocular, or mucosal exposure, or within 14 days of sexual exposure):
<1 yr with <2 hepatitis B vaccine doses administered: 0.5 mL IM × 1 with completed hepatits B vaccine series
≥1 yr and adult: 0.06 mL/kg/dose IM × 1 with completed hepatitis B vaccine series; a second HBIG dose may be given 1 month later for individuals refusing hepatitis B vaccine or are known nonresponders to the vaccine

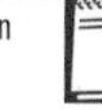

Contraindications: Anaphylactic or severe systematic reactions to parenteral human globulin products and IgA deficiency

Warnings/Precautions: IM administration only; IV administration may result in serious reactions. Defer administration of live virus vaccines approximately 3 months after HBIG; revaccination may be necessary if vaccines were administered after HBIG. See *AAP Red Book* for additional information.

Use of HepaGam B product may falsely increase glucose levels with the glucose dehydrogenase pyrroloquinequinone (GDH-PDQ) method.

Continued

For explanation of icons, see p. 364.

HEPATITIS B IMMUNE GLOBULIN *continued*

Adverse effects: Injection site pain and erythema, GI disturbances, myalgia, headache and malaise are common and generally mild. Mild leukopenia and elevations in alkaline phosphate, AST/SGOT, and serum creatinine have been reported.

Drug interactions: Live virus vaccines (e.g., MMR, varicella); see Warnings/Precautions.

Drug administration: Preferred IM injection sites include the anterolateral aspect of the upper thigh and deltoid muscle. If the buttock is used, use the upper, outer quadrant and avoid the central region.

HEXACHLOROPHENE
pHisoHex
Topical antibacterial

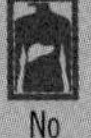
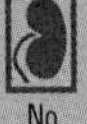
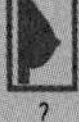
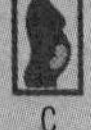

No No ? C

Topical liquid: 3% (150, 480 mL); contains sodium benzoate

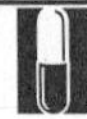

Skin-cleansing procedure or disease caused by gram-positive bacteria:

Child and adult: Apply 5 mL with small amounts of water to the area to be cleansed. Lather and rinse thoroughly with running water.

Surgical scrub prep:

Adult: Work 5 mL with small amounts of water into a lather on the skin for 3 minutes, then rinse thoroughly with water and repeat cleansing once.

Contraindications: Hypersensitivity to hexachlorophene or any component of the formulation. **Do not** use on mucous membranes, burned or denuded skin (neurotoxicity and death have occurred when applied to burned skin), routine total body bathing, with individuals with light sensitivity to halogenated phenol derivatives, and as an occlusive dressing, wet pack, or lotion.

Warnings/Precautions: Rinse thoroughly after each use. **Do not** use for bathing infants. **Avoid** use in premature and low-birth-weight infants because increased percutaneous absorption has resulted in generalized clonic muscle contractions, rigidity, brain lesions, apnea, seizures, agitation, and coma.

Adverse effects: Dermatitis and photosensitivity are common. Delirium and seizures have been reported.

Drug interactions: None identified.

Drug administration: **Avoid** prolonged contact with skin. Rinse thoroughly after each washing.

HYDROGEN PEROXIDE
Various generics
Topical antibacterial

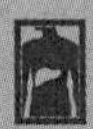
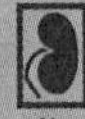
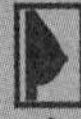
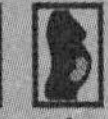

No No ? ?

Oral gel: 1.5% (15 g)

Topical solution:

3% (120, 480 mL)

30.5% concentrate (480 mL); should not be used undiluted

Cleansing or minor wounds or minor gum inflammation in the mouth

Child and adult: dosed once daily to QID (after meals and QHS)

Topical solution (3%): Dilute 3% solution with equal parts of water, swish around in the mouth over affected area for at least 1 minute, then expectorate.

Oral gel (1.5%): Apply a small amount to affected area for at least 1 minute, then expectorate.

Topical wound cleansing:

Child and adult: Use 1.5%–3% topical solution.

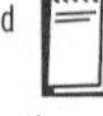

Contraindications: **Do not** use on abscesses or any closed body cavities for which the released oxygen is unable to be released.

Continued

HYDROGEN PEROXIDE *continued*

Warnings/Precautions: Repeated use of mouthwash may produce irritation of the buccal mucous membrane. The more concentrated 30% solution is caustic and should not be used undiluted.

Adverse effects: May cause irritation and burning with all routes of administration. Hypertrophy of the tongue papilae may occur with prolonged use as a mouthwash.

Drug interactions: None identified.

Drug administration: **Avoid** applying bandages too quickly after topical wound cleansing.

HYDROXYCHLOROQUINE
Plaquenil and others
Antimalarial, antirheumatic agent

Yes Yes 2 C

Tabs: 200 mg (155 mg base)
Oral suspension: 25 mg/mL (19.375 mg/mL base)

Doses expressed in milligrams of hydroxychloroquine base.

Malaria prophylaxis (start 2 wk before exposure and continue for 4 wk after leaving endemic area):

Child: 5 mg/kg/dose PO once weekly; **max. dose:** 310 mg
Adult: 310 mg PO once weekly

Malaria treatment (acute uncomplicated cases):

For treatment of malaria, consult with ID specialist or see the latest edition of the *AAP Red Book.*
Child: 10 mg/kg/dose (**max. dose:** 620 mg) PO × 1 followed by 5 mg/kg/dose (**max. dose:** 310 mg) 6 hr later. Then 5 mg/kg/dose (**max. dose:** 310 mg) Q24 hr × 2 doses starting 24 hr after the first dose.
Adult: 620 mg PO × 1 followed by 310 mg 6 hr later. Then 310 mg Q24 hr × 2 doses starting 24 hr after the first dose.

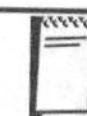

Contraindications: Hypersensitivity to hydroxychloroquine and 4-aminoquinoline; retinal or visual field changes from prior use; individuals with psoriasis or porphyria; and longer term use in children

Warnings/Precautions: **Use with caution** in liver disease, G6PD deficiency, concomitant hepatic toxic drugs, renal impairment, and metabolic acidosis or hematologic disorders.

Adverse effects: May cause headaches, skeletal muscle myopathy, GI distubances, skin and mucosal pigmentation, agranulocytosis, and visual disturbances.

Drug interactions: May increase digoxin serum levels. Use with aurothioglucose may increase risk for blood dyscrasias.

Drug administration: Administer doses with food or milk to reduce GI symptoms.

IMIPENEM-CILASTATIN
Primaxin IV and others
Antibiotic, carbapenem

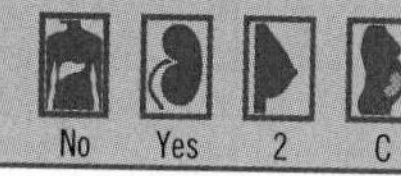

Injection: 250, 500 mg; contains 3.2 mEq Na/g drug
Each 1 mg drug contains 1 mg imipenem and 1 mg cilastatin

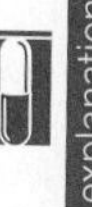

Neonate:

0–4 wk old and birth weight <1.2 kg: 50 mg/kg/24 hr ÷ Q12 hr IV
<1 wk old and birth weight ≥1.2 kg: 50 mg/kg/24 hr ÷ Q12 hr IV
≥1 wk old and birth weight ≥1.2 kg: 75 mg/kg/24 hr ÷ Q8 hr IV

Continued

For explanation of icons, see p. 364.

IMIPENEM-CILASTATIN *continued*

Child (4 wk to 3 mo): 100 mg/kg/24 hr ÷ Q6 hr IV
Child (>3 mo): 60–100 mg/kg/24 hr ÷ Q6 hr IV; **max. dose:** 4 g/24 hr
Cystic fibrosis: 90 mg/kg/24 hr ÷ Q6 hr IV; **max. dose:** 4 g/24 hr
Adult:
IV: 250–1000 mg/dose Q6–8 hr; **max. dose:** 4 g/24 hr or 50 mg/kg/24 hr, whichever is less
IM: 500–750 mg/dose Q12 hr

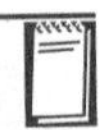

Contraindications: Hypersensitivity to imipenem or cilastatin or any other components in the formulation; amide local anesthetics hypersensitivity and severe shock or heart block with the **IM preparation** containing lidocaine

Warnings/Precautions: Greater risk for seizures may occur with CNS infections, concomitant use with ganciclovir, higher doses, and renal impairment. **Use with caution** in penicillin, cephalosporin, and other β-lactam–allergic patients and renal insufficiency **(adjust dose in renal failure; see Chapter 3)**. CSF penetration is variable but best with inflamed meninges.

Adverse effects: Injection-site pain, GI disturbances, thrombophlebitis, pruritus, urticaria, dizziness, hypotension, elevated LFTs, and blood dyscrasias may occur. See Warnings/Precautions. Nausea may be caused by the rapid rate of drug infusion; slowing infusion rate may reduce severity. Nausea and vomiting may be more common at doses exceeding 2 g/24 hr.

Drug interactions: **Do not administer** with probenecid (increases imipenem/cilastatin levels) and ganciclovir (increases seizure risk). May significantly reduce valproic acid levels.

Drug administration:
IV: For intermittent IV infusion, infuse over 30 to 60 minutes at a concentration ≤5 mg/mL.
IM: Dilute with 1% lidocaine without epinephrine to a concentration of 250 mg/mL and use within 1 hour of preparation. Assess the potential risk/benefit for using lidocaine as a diluent.

IMIQUIMOD
Aldara
Immunomodulator, topical

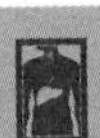
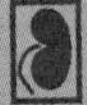
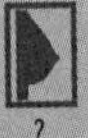
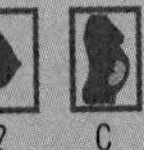

No No ? C

Topical cream: 5% (250 mg single-dose packets in a box of 12 packets); contains benzyl alcohol and parabens

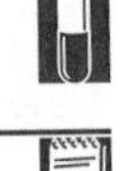

Condyloma acuminatum:
≥12 yr and adult: Apply to affected areas at bedtime 3 times/wk (avoid consecutive day dosing) for up to a **maximum** of 16 wk. Leave application on for 6–10 hr.

Contraindications: Hypersensitivity to imiquimod or any other components in the formulation

Warnings/Precautions: May exacerbate inflammatory conditions of the skin. **Use with caution** with preexisting autoimmune conditions. Delay use of imiquimod until genital/perianal tissue is healed from any previous drug or surgical treatment. **Avoid** excessive sunlight exposure including sunlamps. Safety and efficacy for condyloma acuminatum has not been established for children younger than 12 yr.

Severe vulvar swelling leading to urinary retention may occur from local inflammatory reactions of the vaginal area; interrupt/discontinue therapy if severe vulvar swelling occurs.

Adverse effects: Erythema is common; a rest period of several days may be taken to relieve patient discomfort or severe local skin reaction. Skin ulceration/peeling and edema may occur.

Drug administration: Apply a thin layer to affected areas; rub area until cream is no longer visible. Avoid contact to eyes, lips, and nostrils, and **do not** use occlusive dressings. Wash hands before and after administration.

IMMUNE GLOBULIN
Immune globulins

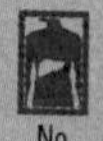
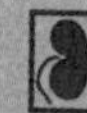
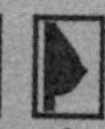
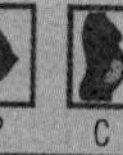
No Yes ? C

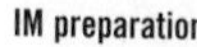

IM preparation:

GamaSTAN S/D: 150–180 mg/mL (2, 10 mL); contains 0.21–0.32 M glycine; preservative free

IV preparations in solution:

Flebogamma DIF: 5% (50 mg/mL) (10, 50, 100, 200, 400 mL), 10% (100 mg/mL) (50, 100, 200 mL); contains 50 mg/mL sorbitol and ≤6 mg/mL polyethylene glycol; sucrose free

Gamunex-C: 10% (100 mg/mL) (10, 25, 50, 100, 200 mL); contains 0.16–0.24 M glycine; sucrose free

Gammagard liquid: 10% (100 mg/mL) (10, 25, 50, 100, 200 mL); contains 0.25 M glycine; sucrose free

GammaKed: 10% (100 mg/mL) (10, 25, 50, 100, 200 mL); contains 0.16–0.24 M glycine; sucrose free

Gammaplex: 5% (50 mg/mL) (50, 100, 200 mL); contains 50 mg/mL sorbitol, 6 mg/mL glycine, and 0.05 mg/mL polysorbate 80; sucrose free

Octagam: 5% (50 mg/mL) (20, 50, 100, 200, 500 mL); contains 100 mg/mL maltose; sucrose free

Privagen: 10% (100 mg/mL) (50, 100, 200 mL); contains 210–290 mmol/L L-proline; sucrose free

IV preparations in powder for reconstitution:

Carimune NF: 3, 6, 12 g (contains 1.67 g sucrose and <20 mg NaCl per 1 g Ig); dilute to 3%, 6%, 9%, or 12%

Gammagard S/D: 2.5, 5, 10 g (contains 3 mg/mL albumin, 22.5 mg/mL glycine, 20 mg/mL glucose, 2 mg/mL polyethylene glycol, 1 mcg/mL tri-n-butyl phosphate, 1 mcg/mL octoxynol 9, and 100 mcg/mL polysorbate 80); dilute to 5% or 10%

Subcutaneous (SC) preparation:

Hizentra: 20% (200 mg/mL) (5, 10, 20 mL); contains 210–290 mmol/L L-proline, 10–30 mg/L polysorbate 80; sucrose free

---

IM preparation:

Hepatitis A, prophylaxis:

Preexposure to endemic areas:

≤3 mo length of stay: 0.02 mL/kg/dose IM × 1

>3 mo length of stay: 0.06 mL/kg/dose IM every 4–6 mo

Postexposure prophylaxis: 0.02 mL/kg/dose IM × 1 administered within 14 days of exposure

Measles, postexposure prophylaxis (administered within 6 days of exposure):

Immunocompetent: 0.25 mL/kg/dose IM × 1; **max. dose:** 15 mL

Immunodeficient: 0.5 mL/kg/dose IM × 1; **max. dose:** 15 mL

Rubella, postexposure prophylaxis: 0.55 mL/kg/dose IM × 1 administered within 72 hr of exposure

IV preparation:

Replacement therapy for antibody-deficient disorders: 400–600 mg/kg/dose IV every month; adjust dosing to maintain trough IgG level of at least 500 mg/dL.

Idiopathic thrombocytopenia: 400–1000 mg/kg/dose IV once daily × 2–5 days, then repeat dose every 3–6 wk based on clinical response and platelet count. May use Rh (D) immunoglobulin in Rh-positive patients.

Kawasaki disease: 2 g/kg/dose IV × 1 administered over 10–12 hr and initiated within the first 10 days of symptoms. Repeat dose of 2 g/kg × 1 may be considered if signs and symptoms persist.

Continued

For explanation of icons, see p. 364.

IMMUNE GLOBULIN *continued*

Pediatric HIV:

Hypogammaglobulinemia (<250 mg/dL), recurrent serious bacterial infections (>2 in 1 yr), failure to form antibodies to common antigens, or measles prophylaxis: 400 mg/kg/dose IV every 28 days

HIV-associated thrombocytopenia: 500–1000 mg/kg/dose IV once daily × 3–5 days

SQ preparation:

Converting to SQ route from previous IV dosage for patients receiving IV immune globulin (IVIg) infusions at regular intervals for at least 3 mo (≥2 yr):

Initial weekly dose (start 1 wk after last IV dose):

Dose in grams (g) = 1.53 × previous IVIG dose in grams (g) ÷ number of weeks between IVIG doses

To convert the above dose from grams to milliliters of drug, multiply dose (g) by 5.

Adjust dose over time by clinical response and serum IgG trough levels. Obtain a previous trough level from IVIG therapy before SQ conversion and repeat trough level 2–3 mo after initiating the SQ route. A goal trough with the SQ route of ~290 mg/dL higher than a trough with the IV route has been recommended.

Contraindications: History of severe systemic allergic reaction to human immunoglobulin products or its components (e.g., polysorbate 80). Select IgA deficiency; may cause **anaphylaxis** because of varied amounts of IgA in preparation. Some IV products are IgA depleted; consult a pharmacist. IV or intradermal use and severe thrombocytopenia or any coagulation disorder with the **IM preparation**. Hyperprolinemia with products containing L-proline.

Warnings/Precautions: These products are derived from human plasma and may contain infectious viruses. Risk for viral infections are reduced by screening donors and testing and/or inactivating certain viruses.

IV preparations containing sucrose **should not be infused** at a rate such that the amount of sucrose exceeds 3 mg/kg/min to decrease risk for renal dysfunction, including acute renal failure.

Adverse effects: Flushing, chills, fever, headache, and hypotension are common. Aseptic meningitis, acute renal failure (IV forms containing sucrose, see earlier), acute lung injury with pulmonary edema 1 to 6 hours after IV infusion, and hepatitis have been reported.

Severe hemolysis-related renal dysfunction/failure or disseminated intravascular coagulation have been reported after infusion with the Privigen product used in a variety of indications. Risk factors for hemolysis include doses ≥2 g/kg and non-O blood group.

Hypersensitivity reaction may occur when IV form is administered rapidly (see later Drug Administration). Injection-site reactions, urticaria, and angioedema may occur with the IM form.

Local reactions, headache, diarrhea, fatigue, back pain, nausea, pain in extremity, cough, rash, pruritus, vomiting, upper abdominal pain, migraine, and pain are common with SQ form.

Drug interactions:

IM: Delay live virus vaccines (e.g., MMR and varicella) for at least 3 mo for hepatitis A prophylaxis, for at least 5 mo for immunocompetent measles prophylaxis, and for at least 6 mo for immunodeficient measles prophylaxis.

IV and SQ: Delay live virus vaccines after IVIg administration (see latest edition of the *AAP Red Book* for details).

Drug administration:

IM: **Use IM product only.** Anterolateral aspects of the upper thigh and deltoid muscle of the upper arm are preferred injection sites. **Do not** use the gluteal region routinely because of risk for sciatic nerve injury. Limit single-injection volume to 1 to 3 mL for infants and small children, and 5 mL for large children and adolescents.

Continued

IMMUNE GLOBULIN *continued*

IV: **Use IV products only.** Refer to specific product's package insert. If infusion-related adverse reactions occur, stop infusion until adverse effects subside and may restart at a rate previously tolerated.

SQ: Injection sites include the abdomen, thigh, upper arm, and/or lateral hip.
Max. simultaneous injection sites: 4
Max. infusion rate:
First infusion: 15 mL/hr per infusion site
Subsequent infusion: 25 mL/hr per infusion site (max. 50 mL/hr for all simultaneous sites combined)
Max. infusion volume:
First infusion: 15 mL per infusion site (4 infusions)
Subsequent infusions: 20–25 mL per infusion site

IMMUNE GLOBULIN, BOTULINUM

See *Botulinum Immune Globulin Intravenous*

IMMUNE GLOBULIN, CYTOMEGALOVIRUS

See *Cytomegalovirus Immune Globulin*

INTRAVENOUS (HUMAN) IMMUNE GLOBULIN, HEPATITIS B

See *Hepatitis B Immune Globulin Intravenous (Human)*

IMMUNE GLOBULIN, RABIES

See *Rabies Immune Globulin Intravenous (Human)*

IMMUNE GLOBULIN, TETANUS

See *Tetanus Immune Globulin Intravenous (Human)*

IMMUNE GLOBULIN, VARICELLA ZOSTER

See *Varicella Zoster Immune Globulin (Human)*

INDINAVIR

Crixivan, IDV
Antiviral agent, protease inhibitor

Yes No 3 C

Caps: 100, 200, 400 mg

Child (investigational dose):

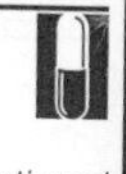

Unboosted therapy: 500–600 mg/m²/dose PO Q8 hr; **max. dose:** 800 mg/dose. This dose has resulted in slightly higher AUC and lower trough levels when compared with adults.

Continued

FORMULARY

For explanation of icons, see p. 364.

INDINAVIR *continued*

Ritonavir boosted: 400 mg/m^2/dose indinavir with 100–125 mg/m^2/dose ritonavir PO Q12 hr; **max. dose:** 800 mg/dose indinavir and 100 mg/dose ritonavir. This dose has resulted in AUCs approximating adult values with a considerable interindividual variability and high rates of toxicity.

Adolescent and adult:

Usual dose:

Unboosted: 800 mg PO Q8 hr

Ritonavir boosted: 800 mg indinavir with 100 or 200 mg ritonavir PO Q12 hr

Needlestick prophylaxis: 800 mg/dose PO TID × 28 days. Use in combination with zidovudine (AZT) 200 mg/dose PO TID or 300 mg/dose PO BID, and lamivudine 150 mg/dose PO BID × 28 days.

Adult:

In combination with efavirenz or nevirapine: 1000 mg PO Q8 hr

In combination with lopinavir/ritonavir (Kaletra): 600 mg PO Q12 hr

In combination with nelfinavir: 1200 mg PO Q12 hr

In combination with delavirdine: 600 mg PO Q8 hr with 400 mg delavirdine PO tid

In combination with itraconazole or ketoconazole, or dosing in mild-to-moderate hepatic impairment: 600 mg PO Q8 hr

In combination with rifabutin: 1000 mg PO Q8 hr and decrease standard rifabutin dose by 50%

Contraindications: Hypersensitivity to indinavir or any other components in the formulation. Concomitant use with astemizole, terfenadine, cisapride, HMG-CoA reductase inhibitors (e.g., lovastatin, simvastatin), ergot alkaloid derivatives, sildenafil, alfuzosin, pimozide, triazolam, and/or midazolam.

Warnings/Precautions: **Should not** be used in neonates because of risk for hyperbilirubinemia/ kernicterus, and in pregnancy. Reduce dose in mild-to-moderate hepatic impairment. Autoimmune disorders, such as Graves disease, polymyositites, and Guillain-Barré syndrome, have been reported in the setting of immune reconstitution with variable time to onset.

Should not be used with salmeterol. Dosage adjustments for bosentan, tadalafil, and colchicine are recommended when used in combination with indinavir; see respective package insert for specific dosage.

Adverse effects: GI discomfort, headache, metallic taste, hyperbilirubinemia, dizziness, and lipid abnormalities are common. Nephrolithiasis (children > adults, caused by poor hydration), hyperglycemia, hepatitis, spontaneous bleeding in hemophiliacs, tubulointerstitial nephritis, immune reconstitution syndrome, and body fat redistribution have been reported.

Drug interactions: Like other protease inhibitors, indinavir inhibits the cytochrome P450–3A4 isoenzyme to increase the effects or toxicities of many drugs. Rifampin, rifabutin, efavirenz, and nevirapine can decrease indinavir levels, whereas ketoconazole and itraconazole can increase levels. See the earlier Contraindications and Warnings/Precautions. **Carefully review the patients' medication profile for potential interactions!**

Drug administration: Administer doses on an empty stomach (1 hour before or 2 hours after meals) with adequate hydration (48 oz/24 hr in adults). If didanosine is included in the regimen, space 1 hour apart on an empty stomach. Capsules are sensitive to moisture and should be stored with a desiccant. **Noncompliance can quickly promote resistant HIV strains.**

IODOQUINOL
Yodoxin, Diquinol, diiodohydroxyquin, diiodohydroxyquinoline
Intestinal amebicide, topical antibacterial/antifungal

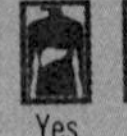
Yes
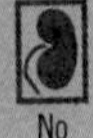
No
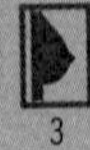
3
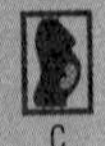
C

Tabs: 210, 650 mg
Contains approximately 64% iodine.

Continued

IODOQUINOL *continued*

Amebiasis, balantidiasis, and dientamoeba fragilis:

Child: 30–40 mg/kg/24 hr PO ÷ TID × 20 days; **max. dose:** 1.95 g/24 hr. Use 40 mg/kg/24 hr for balantidiasis.

Adult: 650 mg PO TID × 20 days; **max. dose:** 2 g/24 hr

Contraindications: Hypersensitivity to iodine and 8-hydroxyquinolones, and hepatic impairment

Warnings/Precautions: **Use with caution** in thyroid disease and neurologic disorders. **Avoid** long-term use because of risk for optic neuritis, optic atrophy, and peripheral neuropathy. **Should not** be used to treat nonspecific diarrhea.

Adverse effects: Pruritus, urticaria, GI disturbances, headache, fever, and shivering are common. Dose-related neurologic and ocular toxicities are the most serious adverse effect; see earlier Warnings/Precautions.

Drug interactions: May increase iodine levels and interfere with thyroid function tests (may persist up to 6 months after stopping therapy).

Drug administration: Take doses after meals. Tablets may be crushed and mixed with applesauce or chocolate syrup for better palatability.

ISONIAZID

INH, Nydrazid, Laniazid, and others
In combination with rifampin: Rifamate, IsonaRif
In combination with rifampin and pyrazinamide: Rifater
Antituberculous agent

Yes Yes 1 C

Tabs: 100, 300 mg
Syrup: 50 mg/5 mL (473 mL)
Injection: 100 mg/mL (10 mL); contains 0.25% chlorobutanol
In combination with rifampin:
Caps (Rifamate, IsonaRif): 150 mg isoniazid + 300 mg rifampin
In combination with rifampin and pyrazinamide:
Caps (Rifater): 50 mg isoniazid + 120 mg rifampin + 300 mg pyrazinamide

See most recent edition of the* AAP Red Book *for details and length of therapy.

Prophylaxis:

Infant and child: 10 mg/kg (**max. dose:** 300 mg) PO once daily. After 1 month of daily therapy and in cases where daily compliance cannot be assured, may change to 20–40 mg/kg (**max. dose:** 900 mg) per dose PO, given twice weekly.

Adult: 300 mg PO once daily

Treatment:

Infant and child: 10–15 mg/kg (**max. dose:** 300 mg) PO once daily or 20–30 mg/kg (**max. dose:** 900 mg) per dose twice weekly with rifampin for uncomplicated pulmonary tuberculosis in compliant patients. Additional drugs are necessary in complicated disease.

Adult: 5 mg/kg (**max. dose:** 300 mg) PO once daily or 15 mg/kg (**max. dose:** 900 mg) per dose twice weekly with rifampin. Additional drugs are necessary in complicated disease.

For INH-resistant TB: Discuss with Health Department or consult ID specialist.

Contraindications: Acute liver disease and previous isoniazid-associated hepatitis.

Warnings/Precautions: **Use with caution** in chronic liver disease and severe renal impairment. **Should not be used alone for treatment. Avoid** daily alcohol use to reduce risk for isoniazid-induced hepatitis. Follow LFTs monthly. Supplemental pyridoxine (1–2 mg/kg/24 hr) is recommended.

Continued

For explanation of icons, see p. 364.

ISONIAZID *continued*

Adverse effects: Peripheral neuropathy, optic neuritis, seizures, encephalopathy, and psychosis may occur. Hepatic side effects may occur with higher doses, especially in combination with rifampin. Drug-induced hepatitis risk also increases with age. Agranulocytosis, anemia, thrombocytopenia, and SLE have been reported. Severe liver injury has been reported in children and adults treated for latent TB. Oral liquid dosage form may cause diarrhea.

Drug interactions: Inhibits CYP 450 1A2, 2C9, 2C19, and 3A3/4 microsomal enzymes; decrease dose of carbamazepine, diazepam, valproic acid, and phenytoin. Aluminum salts may decrease absorption. Prednisone may decrease isoniazid's effects. Also a substrate and inducer of CYP 450 2E1 and may potentiate acetaminophen hepatotoxicity. May cause false-positive urine glucose test.

Drug administration:

PO: Administer 1 hour before and 2 hours after meals.

IM: May be given IM (same as oral doses) when oral therapy is not possible.

ITRACONAZOLE
Sporanox and others
Antifungal agent, triazole

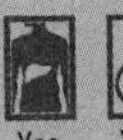
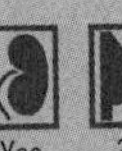
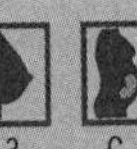
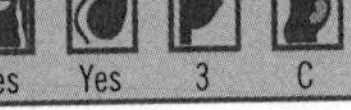

Caps: 100 mg
Oral solution: 10 mg/mL (150 mL); contains propylene glycol, saccharin, sorbitol, and hydroxypropyl-beta-cyclodextrin

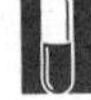

Neonate (limited data in full-term neonates treated for tinea capitis): 5 mg/kg/24 hr PO once daily × 6 wk

Child (limited data): 3–5 mg/kg/24 hr PO ÷ once to twice daily; dosages as high as 5–10 mg/kg/24 hr have been used for aspergillus prophylaxis in chronic granulomatous disease. Population pharmacokinetics data in pediatric cystic fibrosis and bone marrow transplant patients suggest an oral liquid dosage of 10 mg/kg/24 hr PO ÷ BID or oral capsule dosage of 20 mg/kg/24 hr ÷ BID to be more reliable for achieving trough plasma concentrations between 500 and 2000 ng/mL.

Prophylaxis for recurrence of opportunistic disease in HIV:

Coccidioides *spp.*: 2–5 mg/kg/dose PO Q12 hr; **max. dose:** 400 mg/24 hr

Cryptococcus neoformans: 5 mg/kg/dose PO Q24 hr; **max. dose:** 200 mg/24 hr

Histoplasma capsulatum: 5 mg/kg/dose PO Q12 hr; **max. dose:** 400 mg/24 hr

Treatment of opportunistic disease in HIV:

Candidiasis: 5 mg/kg/24 hr PO ÷ Q12–24 hr; **max. dose:** 400 mg/24 hr

Coccidioides *spp.*: 5–10 mg/kg/dose PO BID × 3 days, followed by 2–5 mg/kg/dose PO BID; **max. dose:** 400 mg/24 hr

Cryptococcus neoformans: 2.5–5 mg/kg/dose (**max. dose:** 200 mg/dose) PO TID × 3 days, followed by 5–10 mg/kg/24 hr (**max. dose:** 400 mg/24 hr) ÷ once to twice daily for a minimum of 8 wk

Histoplasma capsulatum: 2–5 mg/kg/dose (**max. dose:** 200 mg/dose) PO TID × 3 days, followed by 2–5 mg/kg/dose (**max. dose:** 200 mg/dose) PO BID × 12 mo

Adult:

Blastomycosis and nonmeningeal histoplasmosis: 200 mg PO once daily up to a **max. dose** of 400 mg/24 hr ÷ BID (**max. dose:** 200 mg/dose)

Aspergillosis and severe infections: 600 mg/24 hr PO ÷ TID × 3–4 days, followed by 200–400 mg/24 hr ÷ BID; **max. dose:** 600 mg/24 hr ÷ TID

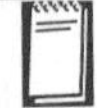

Contraindications: Coadministration of cisapride, dofetilide, felodipine, nisoldipine, pimozide, quinidine, triazolam, lovastatin, methadone (life-threatening cardiac dysrhythmias and/or

Continued

ITRACONAZOLE *continued*

sudden death have been reported), simvastatin, ergot derivatives, and oral midazolam are **contraindicated.** History of itraconazole hypersensitivity.

Warnings/Precautions: **Use with caution** in hepatic impairment, hypersensitivity to other azole antifungals, and with active/prior congestive heart failure. Oral solution and capsule dosage form **should NOT** be used interchangeably; oral solution is more bioavailable. Achlorhydria reduces absorption of the drug. Only the oral solution has been demonstrated effective for oral or esophageal candidiasis, or both.

Oral liquid dosage form **should not** be used in patients with GFR less than 30 mL/min because the hydroxypropyl-beta-cyclodextrin excipient has reduced clearance in patients with renal failure.

Steady-state trough serum concentrations of more than 250 ng/mL itraconazole and more than 1000 ng/mL hydroxyitraconazole (metabolite) have been recommended. Recommended serum sampling time at steady state: trough level after 2 wk after continuous dosing.

Adverse effects: May cause GI symptoms, headaches, rash, liver enzyme elevation, hepatitis, and hypokalemia. Congestive heart failure, Stevens–Johnson syndrome, pancreatitis, and anaphylaxis have been reported.

Drug interactions: Like ketoconazole, it inhibits the activity of the cytochrome P-450 3A4 drug metabolizing isoenzyme. See earlier Contraindications section. Grapefruit juice decreases itraconazole oral absorption, whereas cola beverage increases oral absorption. See remarks in ketoconazole for additional drug interaction information.

Drug administration: Administer oral solution on an empty stomach, but administer capsules with food. **Avoid** grapefruit juice.

IVERMECTIN

Stromectol, Sklice

Antihelmintic

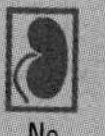
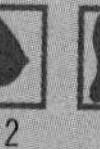
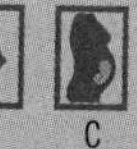

No No 2 C

Tab (Stromectol): 3 mg

Topical lotion (Sklice): 0.5% (117 g); each gram of lotion contains 5 mg ivermectin

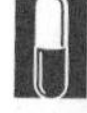

Cutaneous larva migrans or strongyloidiasis: 0.2 mg/kg/dose PO once daily × 1–2 days; dosing by body weight (see first table below):

Scabies: 0.2 mg/kg/dose PO × 1, may repeat in 10–14 days; dosing by body weight as follows:

Weight (kg)	Oral Dose
15–24	3 mg
25–35	6 mg
36–50	9 mg
51–65	12 mg
66–79	15 mg
≥80	0.2 mg/kg

Onchocerciasis: 0.15 mg/kg PO × 1, may repeat dose every 6–12 mo until asymptomatic; dosing by body weight as follows:

Weight (kg)	Single Oral Dose
15–25	3 mg
26–44	6 mg
45–64	9 mg
65–84	12 mg
≥85	0.15 mg/kg

Continued

For explanation of icons, see p. 364.

IVERMECTIN *continued*

Head lice infestation (topical therapy):
≥6 mo to adult: Apply lotion to dry hair in sufficient amounts (up to one full tube) to thoroughly coat the hair and scalp for 10 min. Then rinse off with water.

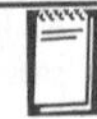

Contraindications: Hypersensitivity to ivermectin or any other components in the formulation
Warnings/Precautions:
PO: Rare fatal encephalopathy may occur in onchocerciasis with a concurrent heavy Loa loa infection.
Topical: Safety and efficacy have not been determined for children younger than 6 months. Topical lotion has not been evaluated in nursing mothers. Use of lotion for children should be supervised by an adult to avoid oral ingestion.
Adverse effects:
PO: Reactions experienced in strongyloidiasis include diarrhea, nausea, vomiting, pruritus, rash, dizziness, and drowsiness. Adverse reactions experienced in onchocerciasis include cutaneous or systemic allergic/inflammatory reactions of varying severity (Mazzotti reaction) and ophthalmologic reactions. Specific reactions may include arthralgia/synovitis, lymph node enlargement and tenderness, pruritus, edema, fever, orthostatic hypotension, and tachycardia. Therapy for postural hypotension may include oral hydration, recumbency, IV normal saline, and/or IV steroids. Antihistamines or aspirin, or both, have been used for most mild-to-moderate cases.
Topical: Conjunctivitis, ocular hyperemia, eye irritation, dandruff, dry skin, and skin-burning sensation are common.
Drug interaction:
PO: May increase the effects/toxicity of warfarin.
Topical: None identified.
Drug administration:
PO route: Take doses on an empty stomach with water.
Topical route: Apply topically to hair and scalp to thoroughly coat hair and scalp for 10 minutes. Then rinse off with water. Discard any unused portion. Lotion is not for PO, ophthalmic, or intravaginal use.

KANAMYCIN
Kantrex and others
Antibiotic, aminoglycoside

No Yes 2 D

Injection: 333 mg/mL; may contain sulfites

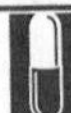

Neonate IV/IM administration (see following table):

Birth Weight (kg)	<7 days	≥7 days
<2 kg	15 mg/kg/24 hr ÷ Q12 hr	22.5 mg/kg/24 hr ÷ Q8 hr
≥2 kg	20 mg/kg/24 hr ÷ Q12 hr	30 mg/kg/24 hr ÷ Q8 hr

Infant and child: IM/IV: 15–30 mg/kg/24 hr ÷ Q8–12 hr
Adult: IV/IM: 15 mg/kg/24 hr ÷ Q8–12 hr
PO administration for GI bacterial overgrowth: 150–250 mg/kg/24 hr ÷ Q6 hr; **max. dose:** 4 g/24 hr

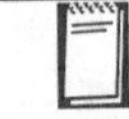

Contraindications: Hypersensitivity to kanamycin or other aminoglycosides, or any other components in the formulation; for oral route, patients with intestinal obstructions

Continued

KANAMYCIN *continued*

Warnings/Precautions: **Use with caution** in neuromuscular disorders (e.g., infant botulism, myasthenia gravis), anesthesia and muscle-relaxant medication use, and hypermagnesemia (may result in respiratory arrest). Renal toxicity and ototoxicity may occur. **Reduce dosage frequency with renal impairment (see Chapter 3).** Poorly absorbed orally, which is used to treat GI bacterial overgrowth.

Therapeutic levels: peak: 15–30 mg/L; trough: <5–10 mg/L. Recommended serum sampling time at steady state: trough within 30 minutes before the third consecutive dose and peak 30 to 60 minutes after the administration of the third consecutive dose.

Adverse effects:

IM/IV: Nephrotoxcity is common. Ototoxicity may occur with the following predisposing factors and may be irreversible: preexisting renal impairment, high serum drug levels, prolonged use of drug, preexisting hearing loss, and prior exposure to ototoxic drugs.

PO: GI disturbances are common. Prolonged use with oral route has induced intestinal malabsorption.

Drug interactions: Other ototoxic and nephrotoxic medications may increase risk for toxicities. Loop diuretics (e.g., furosemide) may increase risk for ototoxicity and should be **avoided**. Anesthesia and muscle-relaxant medications may result in neuromuscular blockade with respiratory paralysis.

Drug administration:

IV: For intermittent IV infusion, infuse over 30–60 min at a concentration 2.5–5 mg/mL.

KETOCONAZOLE
Nizoral, Nizoral A-D, Xolegel, Extina, and others
Antifungal agent, imidazole

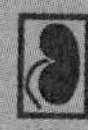
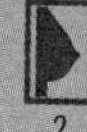
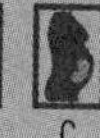

Yes No 2 C

Tabs: 200 mg
Oral suspension: 100 mg/5 mL
Cream: 2% (15, 30, 60 g); contains sulfites
Gel: 2% [Xolegel] (45 g); contains 34% alcohol
Shampoo: 1% [Nizoral A-D, OTC] (120, 210 mL), 2% (120 mL)
Foam: 2% [Extina] (50, 100 g)

Oral:

Child ≥2 yr: 3.3–6.6 mg/kg/24 hr once daily
Adult: 200–400 mg/24 hr once daily
Max. dose: 800 mg/24 hr ÷ BID

Topical: 1–2 applications/24 hr

Shampoo (dandruff): Twice weekly with at least 3 days between applications for up to 8 weeks, PRN. Thereafter, intermittently as needed to maintain control.

Suppressive therapy against mucocutaneous candidiasis in HIV:

Child: 5–10 mg/kg/24 hr ÷ once to twice daily PO; **max. dose:** 800 mg/24 hr ÷ BID
Adolescent and adult: 200 mg/dose once daily PO

Contraindications: Hypersensitivity to ketoconazole products or any other components in the formulation. Cardiac arrhythmias may occur when used with cisapride, mefolquine, terfinadine, quinidine, and pimozide; and excessive sedation and prolonged hypnotic effects with triazolam. Concomitant administration of ketoconazole with any of these drugs is **contraindicated.**

Warnings/Precautions: Achlorhydria or drugs that decrease gastric acidity will decrease oral absorption. Monitor LFTs in long-term use because hepatotoxicity (some fatal) has been reported; **use with caution** in hepatic impairment. Hypersensitivity reactions, including anaphylaxis, has been reported with systemic and topical use.

Continued

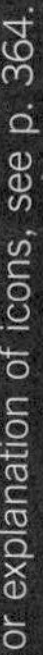
For explanation of icons, see p. 364.

KETOCONAZOLE *continued*

Adverse effects:

PO: Nausea, vomiting, rash, headache, pruritus, and fever are common. Gynecomastia and hepatotoxicity have been reported.

Topical: Pruritus and stinging may occur.

Drug interactions: Inhibits CYP 450 3A4. May increase levels/effects of phenytoin, digoxin, cyclosporin, corticosteroids, nevirapine, protease inhibitors, and warfarin. May increase risk for skeletal muscle toxicity (e.g., rhabdomyolysis) with HMG-CoA reductase inhibitors (e.g., lovastatin, simvastatin, atorvastatin). Phenobarbital, rifampin, isoniazid, H2 blockers, antacids, and omeprazole can decrease levels of ketoconazole. See earlier Contraindications section.

Drug administration:

PO: Administer doses with food or acidic beverages and 2 hr before antacids to increase absorption.

Shampoo: Wet hair and scalp with water; apply sufficient amount to scalp and gently massage for about 1 minute. Rinse hair thoroughly, reapply shampoo, and leave on the scalp for an additional 3 minutes; then rinse.

Topical: Apply sufficient amount and rub gently into affected and surrounding area.

KUNECATECHINS
Veregen, Sinecatechins
Keratolytic, sinecatechins

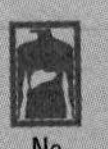 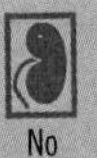 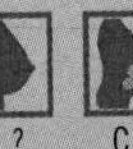 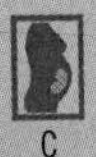

No No ? C

Ointment: 15% (15 g); approximately 2.5% of the product contains caffeine, theobromine, and gallic acid

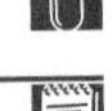

Condyloma acuminatum:

Adult: Apply a 0.5-cm strand of ointment TID to each external genital and perianal wart. Continue therapy until complete clearance of warts, but no longer than 16 weeks.

Contraindications: Hypersensitivity to any component of the product

Warnings/Precautions: **For external use only;** not for intra-anal, ophthalmic, or intravaginal use. Ointment may weaken condoms and vaginal diaphragms. **Avoid** use on open wounds and exposure of treated areas to sunlight and ultraviolet light. Has not been evaluated for treatment of urethral, intravaginal, cervical, rectal, or intra-anal human papilloma viral disease.

Adverse effects: Burning sensation, edema, erythema, skin induration pruritus, vesicular rash, and superficial skin ulcer are common.

Drug interactions: None identified.

Drug administration: Ointment may stain clothing or bedding. Use fingers to apply ointment to affected area and ensure complete coverage by applying a thin layer of ointment. Wash hands well before and after each application.

LAMIVUDINE
Epivir, Epivir-HBV, 3TC, and others
Antiviral agent, nucleoside analogue reverse transcriptase inhibitor

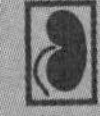 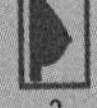 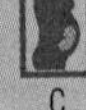

No Yes 3 C

Tabs: 100 mg (Epivir-HBV), 150, 300 mg

Oral solution: 5 mg/mL (Epivir-HBV), 10 mg/mL; both concentrations contain propylene glycol

In combination with zidovudine (AZT) as Combivir:

Tabs: 150 mg lamivudine + 300 mg zidovudine

In combination with abacavir as Epzicom:

Tabs: 300 mg lamivudine + 600 mg abacavir

Continued

LAMIVUDINE *continued*

In combination with abacavir and zidovudine (AZT) as Trizivir:
Tabs: 150 mg lamivudine + 300 mg abacavir + 300 mg zidovudine

HIV:

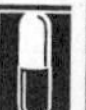

Neonate (<30 days):

Treatment: 2 mg/kg/dose PO BID

Prevention of maternal–fetal transmission to reduce nevirapine resistance (for infants born to mothers with no antiretroviral therapy before labor or during labor, infants born to mothers with only intrapartum antiretroviral therapy, infants born to mothers with suboptimal viral suppression at delivery, or infants born to mothers with known antiretroviral drug resistance): 2 mg/kg/dose PO BID × 7 days from birth to 7 days old

Child (1 mo to 16 yr): 4 mg/kg/dose PO BID; **max. dose:** 150 mg/dose

Adolescent (≥16 yr) and adult:

<50 kg: 4 mg/kg/dose PO BID; **max. dose:** 150 mg/dose

≥50 kg: 300 mg/24 hr PO ÷ once to twice daily

Needlestick prophylaxis: 150 mg/dose PO BID × 28 days. Use in combination with zidovudine (AZT), tenofovir, stavudine, or didanosine; with or without a protease inhibitor (depending on risk) for 28 days.

Combivir:

≥12 yr to adult: 1 tablet PO BID

Epzicom:

Adult: 1 tablet PO once daily

Trizivir:

Adolescent (≥40 kg) to adult: 1 tablet PO BID

Chronic hepatitis B (see remarks):

2–17 yr: 3 mg/kg/dose PO once daily up to a **max. dose** of 100 mg/dose

Adults: 100 mg/dose PO once daily

Contraindications: Hypersensitivity to lamivudine or any other component contained in the formulation

Warnings/Precautions: Lactic acidosis, severe hepatomegaly with steatosis, posttreatment exacerbations of hepatitis B and ALT elevations, pancreatitis, and emergence of resistant viral strains have been reported. Autoimmune disorders (e.g., Graves disease, polymyositis, and Guillain–Barré syndrome) have been reported in the setting of immune reconstitution syndrome. **Use with caution in renal impairment; adjust dose in renal impairment (see Chapter 3).** For use of any of the combination products (Combivir, Epzicom, and Trizivir), **do not use** in patients with creatinine clearance <50 mL/min.

CHRONIC HEPATITIS B: Use Epivir-HBV product for this indication. Safety and effectiveness beyond 1 year have not been determined. Patients with both HIV and hepatitis B should use the higher HIV doses together with an appropriate combination regimen. Rapid emergence of HIV resistance is likely to occur in patients with HBV with unrecognized or untreated HIV infection.

Adverse effects: Headache, fatigue, nausea, decreased appetite, diarrhea, skin rash, and abdominal pain are common. Pancreatitis (primarily in advanced disease), peripheral neuropathy, anemia, neutropenia, liver enzyme elevation, and fat redistribution may occur. See Warnings/Precautions for other serious side effects.

Drug interactions: Concomitant use with cotrimoxazole (TMP/SMX) may result in increased lamivudine levels. Should **not** be used in combination with zalcitabine or emtricitabine because it may inhibit intracellular phosphorylation of one another or share similar resistance profiles (no additive benefit), respectively.

Drug administration: Doses may be administered with or without food.

For explanation of icons, see p. 364.

LEVOFLOXACIN
Levaquin, Quixin, Iquix, and others
Antibiotic, quinolone

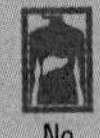 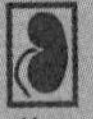 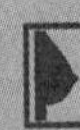 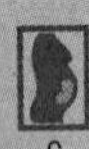
No Yes 2 C

Tabs: 250, 500, 750 mg
Oral solution: 25 mg/mL (100, 200, 480 mL)
Injection: 25 mg/mL (20, 30 mL)
Prediluted injection in D_5W: 250 mg/50 mL, 500 mg/100 mL, 750 mg/150 mL
Ophthalmic drops:
- **Quixin:** 0.5% (5 mL)
- **Iquix:** 1.5% (5 mL)

Child:

<5 yr: 10 mg/kg/dose IV/PO Q12 hr; **max. dose:** 500 mg/24 hr
≥5 yr: 10 mg/kg/dose IV/PO Q24 hr; **max. dose:** 500 mg/24 hr
Recurrent or persistent acute otitis media (6 mo to <5 yr): 10 mg/kg/dose PO Q12 hr × 10 days; **max. dose:** 500 mg/24 hr
Community-acquired pneumonia (IDSA/Pediatric Infectious Diseases Society):
- ***6 mo to <5 yr:*** 8–10 mg/kg/dose PO/IV Q12 hr; **max. dose:** 750 mg/24 hr
- ***5–12 yr:*** 8–10 mg/kg/dose PO/IV Q24 hr; **max. dose:** 750 mg/24 hr

Inhalational anthrax (postexposure) and plague:
- ***≥6 mo and <50 kg:*** 8 mg/kg/dose PO/IV Q12 hr; **max. dose:** 500 mg/24 hr
- ***>50 kg:*** 500 mg PO/IV once daily
- ***Duration of therapy:***
  - ***Inhalational anthrax (postexposure):*** 60 days
  - ***Plague:*** 10–14 days

Adult:

Community-acquired pneumonia: 500 mg PO/IV Q24 hr × 7–14 days, *or* 750 mg PO/IV Q24 hr × 5 days
Complicated UTI/acute pyelonephritis: 250 mg PO/IV Q24 hr × 10 days, *or* 750 mg PO/IV Q24 hr × 5 days
Uncomplicated UTI: 250 mg PO/IV Q24 hr × 3 days
Uncomplicated skin/skin structure infection: 500 mg PO/IV Q24 hr × 7–10 days
Acute bacterial sinusitis: 500 mg PO/IV Q24 hr × 10–14 days, *or* 750 mg PO/IV Q24 hr × 5 days
Inhalational anthrax (postexposure) and plague: 500 mg PO/IV Q24 hr; duration of therapy: inhalation anthrax: 60 days; and plague: 10–14 days

Conjunctivitis:

≥1 yr and adult: Instill 1–2 drops of the 0.5% solution to affected eye(s) Q2 hr up to 8 times/24 hr while awake for the first 2 days, then Q4 hr up to 4 times/24 hr while awake for the next 5 days.

Corneal ulcer:

≥6 yr and adult: Instill 1–2 drops of the 1.5% solution to affected eye(s) Q30 min–2 hr while awake and 4 and 6 hr after retiring for the first 3 days, then Q1–4 hr while awake.

Contraindications: Hypersensitivity to levofloxacin and to other quinolones
Warnings/Precautions: **Avoid** in patients with history of QTc prolongation or taking QTc-prolonging drugs, and excessive sunlight exposure. **Use with caution** in diabetes, seizures, children younger than 18 years, and renal impairment **(adjust dose in renal failure; see Chapter 3). Avoid use** in myasthenia gravis; may exacerbate muscle weakness. **Not** recommended for gonorrhea because of potential resistance.

Continued

LEVOFLOXACIN *continued*

Adverse effects: May cause GI disturbances, headache, and blurred vision with the ophthalmic solution. Musculoskeletal disorders (e.g., arthralgia, arthritis, tendinopathy, and gait abnormality) may occur. Like other quinolones, tendon rupture can occur during or after therapy. Safety in pediatric patients treated for more than 14 days has not been evaluated.

Drug interactions: Antacids containing aluminum, magnesium and/or calcium, sucralfate, metal cations (e.g., zinc, iron, copper, and magnesium), and didanosine may decrease levofloxacin oral absorption. May enhance the effects of warfarin. Use with corticosteroids may increase risk for tendon rupture and use with nonsteroidal anti-inflammatory drugs may increase risk for CNS stimulation and seizures. May cause false-positive opiate immunoassay urine screening tests.

Drug administration:

IV: Infuse IV over 1 to 1.5 hours at a concentration ≥5 mg/mL. **Avoid** IV push or rapid infusion because of risk for hypotension.

PO: **Do not** administer antacids or other divalent salts with or within 2 hours of oral levofloxacin dose; otherwise, may be administer with or without food.

Ophthalmic drops: Apply finger pressure to lacrimal sac during and for 1 to 2 minutes after dose application.

LINDANE
Various brands, Gamma benzene hexachloride
Scabicidal agent, pediculicide

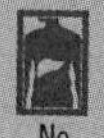
No
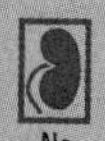
No
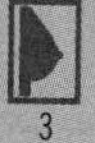
3
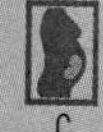
C

Shampoo: 1% (60 mL)
Lotion: 1% (60 mL)

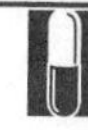

Child and adult (see remarks):

Scabies: Apply thin layer of lotion to skin. Bathe and rinse off medication in adults after 8–12 hr; children 6–8 hr. May repeat × 1 in 7 days PRN.

Pediculosis capitis: Apply 15–30 mL shampoo, lather for 4–5 min, rinse hair and comb with fine comb to remove nits. May repeat × 1 in 7 days PRN.

Pediculosis pubis: May use lotion or shampoo (applied locally) as above.

Contraindications: Premature infants and seizure disorders

Warnings/Precautions: Lindane is considered second-line therapy because of risk for adverse effects. Lindane is systemically absorbed. Risk for toxic effects is greater in young children; use other agents (permethrin) in infants, young children (<2 years), and during pregnancy.

For scabies, change clothing and bedsheets after starting treatment and treat family members. For pediculosis pubis, treat sexual contacts. Itching may occur after the successful killing of scabies and is not necessarily an indication for retreatment with lindane.

Adverse effects: May cause a rash; rarely may cause seizures or aplastic anemia.

Drug interactions: **Use with caution** with drugs that lower seizure threshold (e.g., antipsychotics, antidepressants, theophylline, cyclosporine).

Drug administration: **Avoid** contact with face, eyes, urethral meatus, damaged skin, open cuts, extensive excoriations, or mucous membranes. Use of rubber gloves for administration is recommended, especially when applying to more than one person. **Do not wash** skin with any lotion, cream, or oil; certain ingredients may enhance lindane systemic absorption. **Do not use** any covering (e.g., plastic lining or clothing) over the applied lindane that does not breathe.

For explanation of icons, see p. 364.

LINEZOLID
Zyvox
Antibiotic, oxazolidinone

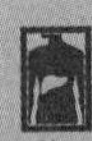 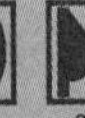 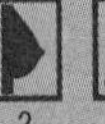 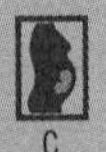
No No 2 C

Tabs: 400, 600 mg; contains ~0.45 mEq Na per 200 mg drug
Oral suspension: 100 mg/5 mL (150 mL); contains phenylalanine, sodium benzoate, and 0.8 mEq Na per 200 mg drug
Injection, premixed: 200 mg in 100 mL, 400 mg in 200 mL, 600 mg in 300 mL; contains 1.7 mEq Na per 200 mg drug

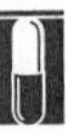

Neonate <7 days: 10 mg/kg/dose IV/PO Q12 hr; if response is suboptimal, increase dose to 10 mg/kg/dose Q8 hr
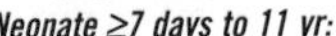
Neonate ≥7 days to 11 yr:
Pneumonia, bacteremia, complicated skin/skin structure infections, vancomycin-resistant **Enterococcus faecium** ***(VRE):*** 10 mg/kg/dose IV/PO Q8 hr. Duration of therapy: 10–14 days, except for VRE (14–28 days).
Uncomplicated skin/skin structure infections:
<5 yr: 10 mg/kg/dose PO Q8 hr × 10–14 days
5–11 yr: 10 mg/kg/dose PO Q12 hr × 10–14 days
≥12 yr and adult:
MRSA infections: 600 mg Q12 hr IV/PO
VRE: 600 mg Q12 hr IV/PO × 14–28 days
Community-acquired and nosocomial pneumonia, and bacteremia: 600 mg Q12 hr IV/PO × 10–14 days
Uncomplicated skin infections:
≥12 yr and adolescent: 600 mg Q12 hr PO × 10–14 days
Adult: 400 mg Q12 hr PO × 10–14 days

Contraindications: Hypersensitivity to linezolid or any other components in the formulation
Warnings/Precautions: **Do not use** with SSRIs (e.g., fluoxetine, paroxetine), tricyclic antidepressants, venlafaxine, and trazodone; may cause serotonin syndrome. **Avoid use** with monoamine oxidase inhibitors (e.g., phenelzine), amphetamines, and methylphenidate, and in patients with uncontrolled hypertension, pheochromocytoma, thyrotoxicosis, and taking sympathomimetics or vasopressive agents (may elevate blood pressure). **Use with caution** in consuming large amounts of foods and beverages containing tyramine; may increase blood pressure. Dosing information in severe hepatic failure with multiple doses has not been completed. **Use with caution** in neonates and the oral suspension dosage form because it contains sodium benzoate.
Adverse effects: Diarrhea, headache, and nausea are common. Anemia, leukopenia, pancytopenia, and thrombocytopenia may occur in patients who are at risk for myelosuppression and who receive regimens longer than 2 weeks. Complete blood count monitoring is recommended in these individuals. Pseudomembranous colitis and neuropathy (peripheral and optic) have also been reported.
Drug interactions: Reversible inhibitor of monoamine oxidase; see earlier Warnings/Precautions section.
Drug administration: Protect all dosage forms from light and moisture.
IV: Infuse over 30 to 120 minutes at the ready-to-use concentration of 2 mg/mL. **Do not** further dilute or mix/infuse with other medications.
PO: Oral suspension product must be gently mixed by inverting the bottle three to five times before each use **(do not shake).** All oral doses may be administered with or without food.

LOPINAVIR WITH RITONAVIR
Kaletra, LPV/RTV
Antiviral, protease inhibitor combination

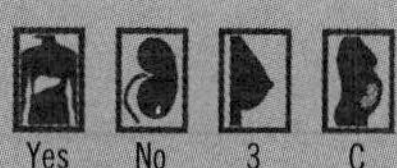

Tabs: 100 mg lopinavir and 25 mg ritonavir, 200 mg lopinavir and 50 mg ritonavir
Oral solution: 80 mg lopinavir and 20 mg ritonavir/1 mL; contains 42.4% alcohol, 15.3% propylene glycol and saccharin (160 mL)

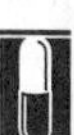

14 days postnatal age with postmenstrual age of ≥42 weeks to 6 mo (do not administer with efavirenz, nevirapine, amprenavir, or nelfinavir because of the absence of data): 300 mg/m²/dose lopinavir and 75 mg/m²/dose ritonavir BID PO; or 16 mg/kg/dose lopinavir and 4 mg/kg/dose ritonavir BID PO

6 mo to 18 yr (administer all doses with food and see remarks):

NOT in combination with nelfinavir, nevirapine, efavirenz, or amprenavir: 230 mg/m²/dose lopinavir and 57.5 mg/m²/dose ritonavir BID PO up to a **maximum** of 400 mg lopinavir and 100 mg ritonavir/dose, *or* use the following doses by weight:

Weight (kg)	Dose (Lopinavir and Ritonavir) BID PO
<15	12 mg/kg/dose and 3 mg/kg/dose (oral liquid)
15–25	10 mg/kg/dose and 2.5 mg/kg/dose (oral liquid); *or* 200 mg and 50 mg (tablets)
>25–35	10 mg/kg/dose and 2.5 mg/kg/dose (oral liquid); *or* 300 mg and 75 mg (tablets)
>35	400 mg and 100 mg (tablets or oral liquid)

In combination with nelfinavir, nevirapine, efavirenz, or amprenavir: 300 mg/m²/dose lopinavir and 75 mg/m²/dose ritonavir BID PO up to a **maximum** of 533 mg lopinavir and 133 mg ritonavir/dose; *or* use the following doses by weight:

Weight (kg)	Dose (Lopinavir and Ritonavir) BID PO
<15	13 mg/kg/dose and 3.25 mg/kg/dose (oral solution)
15–20	11 mg/kg/dose and 2.75 mg/kg/dose (oral solution), *or* 200 mg and 50 mg (tablets)
>20–30	11 mg/kg/dose and 2.75 mg/kg/dose (oral solution), *or* 300 mg and 75 mg (tablets)
>30–45	11 mg/kg/dose and 2.75 mg/kg/dose (oral solution), *or* 400 mg and 100 mg (tablets)
>45	500 mg and 125 mg (tablets), *or* 533 mg and 133 mg (6.5 mL oral solution)

Adult (administer all doses with food):

NOT in combination with nelfinavir, nevirapine, efavirenz, or amprenavir: 400 mg lopinavir and 100 mg ritonavir BID PO; once-daily dose of 800 mg lopinavir and 200 mg ritonavir PO may be used in patients with <3 lopinavir resistance-associated substitutions

In combination with nevirapine, efavirenz, amprenavir, or nelfinavir (once-daily regimen is not recommended):

Tabs: 500 mg lopinavir and 125 mg ritonavir (two 200-mg/50-mg tablets and one 100-mg/25-mg tablet) BID PO

Oral liquid: 533 mg lopinavir and 133 mg ritonavir BID PO

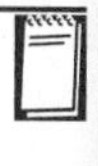

Contraindications: Hypersensitivity to lopinavir, ritonavir, or any other components in the formulation. **Do not administer** with alfuzosin, astemizole, cisapride, flecainide, lovastatin, propafenone, ergot alkaloids, pimozide, midazolam (PO), sildenafil, simvastatin, terfenadine, and triazolam; may result in serious/life-threatening events.

Continued

For explanation of icons, see p. 364.

LOPINAVIR WITH RITONAVIR *continued*

Warnings/Precautions: **Use with caution** in hepatic impairment (no dose adjustment information currently available), history of pancreatitis, diabetes, and hemophilia. Fatal cardiogenic shock has been reported in an infant receiving a 10-fold accidental overdose. Autoimmune disorders such as Graves disease, polymyositis, and Guillain–Barré syndrome have been reported in the presence of an immune reconstitution syndrome.

BSA dosing in children provides similar AUC as seen in adults but with lower trough levels; some clinicians may initiate therapy with higher LPV/RTV doses in PI-experienced pediatric patients who may have reduced PI susceptibility.

Should not be administered in neonates younger than 42 weeks' postmenstrual age and postnatal age younger than 14 days. Use oral solution with caution in infants and young children because of its alcohol and propylene glycol content.

Adverse effects: May cause diarrhea, headache, asthenia, nausea, vomiting, increase in serum lipids, and rash (in combination with other antiretroviral agents). Toxic epidermal necrolysis has been reported.

Drug interactions: Ritonavir is combined with lopinavir as an adjuvant for boosting lopinavir levels and not for its antiretroviral properties. Lopinavir/ritonavir is metabolized by CYP P450 3A and also inhibits the same enzyme. Efavirenz, amprenavir, and nevirapine induce metabolism of lopinavir; higher doses of lopinavir/ritonavir are necessary. Carbamazepine, dexamethasone, phenobarbital, phenytoin, rifampin, and St. John's wort may decrease lopinavir levels. Lopinavir/ritonavir may increase effects or toxicity of atorvastatin, cerivastatin, clarithromycin, fentanyl, rifabutin, lidocaine, quinidine, amiodarone, cyclosporine, tacrolimus, rapamycin, rosuvastatin, calcium channel blockers, ketoconazole, itraconazole, and metronidazole. Lopinavir can decrease the effectiveness of methadone, atovaquone, and birth control pills containing ethinyl estradiol (use alternative methods). Always check the potential for other drug interactions when either initiating therapy or adding new drugs onto an existing regimen.

Drug administration: Administer oral solution with food for better absorption. Tablets should be taken whole, with or without food. If didanosine is included in the regimen, administer didanosine 1 hour before or 2 hours after lopinavir/ritonavir. High-fat meal increases absorption (especially with liquid dosage form).

MALARONE

See *Atovaquone ± Proguanil*

MALATHION

Ovide and others

Pediculicide, organophosphate

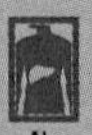
No
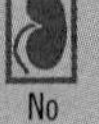
No
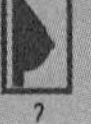
?
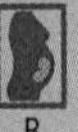
B

Lotion: 0.5% (59 mL); contains 78% isopropyl alcohol, terpineol, dipentene, and pine needle oil

Pediculosis capitis:

≥6 yr and adult: Sprinkle sufficient amounts of lotion onto dry hair and rub gently until the scalp is fully wet (pay special attention to the back of head and neck). Allow the hair to dry naturally; **do not** use hair dryer. After 8–12 hr, wash the hair with a nonmedicated shampoo, rinse, and use a fine-toothed comb to remove dead lice and eggs. If lice are still present, a second dose may be administered in 7–9 days.

Continued

MALATHION *continued*

Contraindications: Neonates and infants; hypersensitivity to malathion or any other ingredient in the vehicle

Warnings/Precautions: Use only under the direct supervision of an adult. If skin irritation occurs, discontinue use until resolution; then reapply lotion and discontinue use if irritation reoccurs.

Adverse effects: Contact hypersensitivity reaction and skin and scalp irritation are common. Chemical burns, including second-degree burns, have been reported.

Drug Interactions: None identified.

Drug administration: **For external use only.** Launder bedding and clothing. **Avoid** contact with eyes; flush eyes immediately with water if accidental exposure. **DO NOT** expose lotion and wet hair to open flame or electric heat, including hair dyers, because it contains flammable ingredients.

MARAVIROC

Selzentry

Antiviral agent, CCR5 coreceptor antagonist

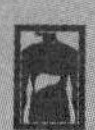
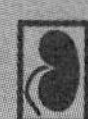
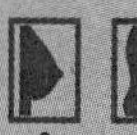
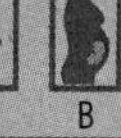

Yes Yes 3 B

Tabs: 150, 300 mg

≥17 and adult:

In combination with strong CYP 3A inhibitors (with or without CYP 3A inducers) including protease inhibitors (except tipranavir/ritonavir), delavirdine, ketoconazole, itraconazole, clarithromycin, nefazodone, and telithromycin): 150 mg PO BID

In combination with weak or non-CYP 3A inducers or inhibitors (including tipranavir/ritonavir, nevirapine, all nucleoside reverse transcriptase inhibitors, and enfuvirtide): 300 mg PO BID

In combination with CYP 3A inducers (without a strong CYP 3A inhibitor; including efavirenz, etravirine, rifampin, carbamazepine, phenobarbital, phenytoin, and others): 600 mg PO BID

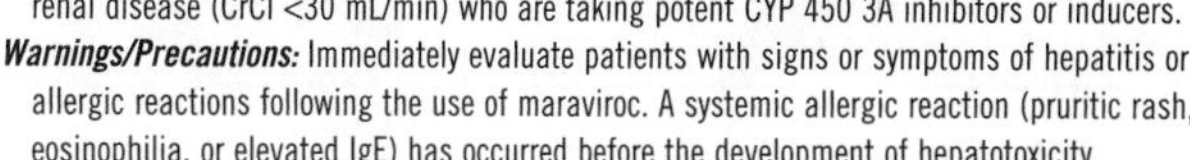

Contraindications: Should not be used in patients with severe renal impairment or end-stage renal disease (CrCl <30 mL/min) who are taking potent CYP 450 3A inhibitors or inducers.

Warnings/Precautions: Immediately evaluate patients with signs or symptoms of hepatitis or allergic reactions following the use of maraviroc. A systemic allergic reaction (pruritic rash, eosinophilia, or elevated IgE) has occurred before the development of hepatotoxicity.

Use caution with preexisting liver dysfunction, hepatitis B or C, or in patients with increased risk for cardiovascular events (more cardiovascular events including myocardial ischemia/infarction were observed in patients receiving the medication). Immune reconstitution syndrome with subsequent autoimmune disorders (e.g., Graves disease, polymyositis, and Guillain–Barré syndrome) have been reported.

Pharmacokinetics, safety, and efficacy have not been evaluated in severe hepatic impairment.

Adjust dose in renal impairment (see Chapter 3). Patients with impaired renal function may have cardiovascular comorbidities and could be at increased risk for cardiovascular adverse events triggered by postural hypotension (from increased maraviroc exposure in some patients).

Adverse effects: Rash, abdominal pain, cough, pyrexia, upper respiratory infections, musculoskeletal symptoms, and dizziness are common. Myocardial infarction/ischemia, cholestatic jaundice, liver cirrhosis, and hepatotoxicity (including failure) have been reported.

Drug interactions: Maraviroc is a substrate of CYP 450 3A isoenzyme and P-gp transporter. Drug levels are likely to be altered by inhibitors and inducers of the aforementioned systems. Efavirenz decreases maraviroc levels, whereas lopinavir/ritonavir increases maraviroc levels.

Drug administration: May be taken with or without food.

For explanation of icons, see p. 364.

MEBENDAZOLE
Vermox and others
Anthelmintic

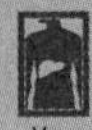 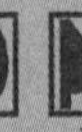 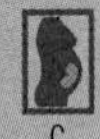 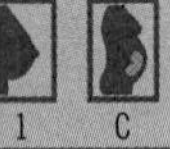
Yes No 1 C

Chewable tabs: 100 mg (may be swallowed whole or chewed) (boxes of 12)

Child (>2 yr) and adult:
***Pinworms* (Enterobius):** 100 mg PO × 1, repeat in 2 wk if not cured
***Hookworms, roundworms* (Ascaris), *and whipworm* (Trichuris):** 100 mg PO BID × 3 days. Repeat in 3–4 wk if not cured. Alternatively, may administer 500 mg PO × 1.
Capillariasis: 200 mg PO BID × 20 days
***Visceral larva migrans* (Toxocariasis):** 100–200 mg PO BID × 5 days
***Trichinellosis* (Trichinella spiralis):** 200–400 mg PO TID × 3 days, then 400–500 mg PO TID × 10 days; use with steroids for severe symptoms
Ancylostoma caninum *(Eosinophilic enterocolitis):* 100 mg PO BID × 3 days
See latest edition of the* AAP Red Book *for additional information.

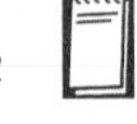

Contraindications: Hypersensitivity to mebendazole products
Warnings/Precautions: Ineffective in hydatid disease. Experience in children younger than 2 years and pregnancy is limited. Family may need to be treated as a group.
Adverse effects: Rash, GI disturbances, and headache are common. May cause diarrhea and abdominal cramping in cases of massive infection. LFT elevations and hepatitis have been reported with prolonged courses; monitor hepatic function with prolonged therapy.
Drug interactions: Therapeutic effect may be decreased if administered with aminoquinolines, carbamazepine, or phenytoin. Cimetidine may increase the effects/toxicity of mebendazole. Mebendazole may increase the adverse effects of metronidazole.
Drug administration: Administer doses with food. Tablets may crushed and mixed with food, swallowed whole, or chewed.

MEFLOQUINE HCL
Lariam and others
Antimalarial

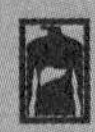 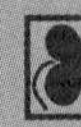  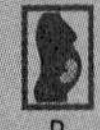 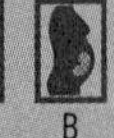
Yes No 2 B

Tabs: 250 mg (228 mg base)

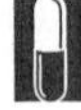

Doses expressed in milligrams mefloquine HCl salt
Malaria prophylaxis (start 1 week before exposure and continue for 4 weeks after leaving endemic area):
Child (PO, administered Q weekly):
<10 kg: 5 mg/kg
10–19 kg: 62.5 mg (1/4 tablet)
20–30 kg: 125 mg (1/2 tablet)
31–45 kg: 187.5 mg (3/4 tablet)
>45 kg: 250 mg (1 tablet)
Adult: 250 mg PO weekly
Malaria treatment (uncomplicated/mild infection, chloroquine-resistant* Plasmodium vivax*):
Child ≥6 mo and >5 kg: 15 mg/kg × 1 PO followed by 10 mg/kg × 1 PO 12 hr later (**max. total dose:** 1250 mg)
Adult: 750 mg × 1 PO followed by 500 mg × 1 PO 12 hr later
See latest edition of the* AAP Red Book *for additional information.

Continued

MEFLOQUINE HCL *continued*

Contraindications: Active or recent history of depression, anxiety disorders, psychosis or schizophrenia, seizures, or hypersensitivity to mefloquine, quinine, or quinidine.

Warnings/Precautions: **Use with caution** in cardiac dysrhythmias and neurologic disease. May cause psychiatric symptoms, ranging from anxiety, paranoia, and depression to hallucinations and psychotic behavior. ECG abnormalities may occur when used in combination with quinine, quinidine, chloroquine, halofantrine, and β-blockers. If any of the aforementioned antimalarial drugs are used in the initial treatment of severe malaria, initiate mefloquine at least 12 hours after the last dose of any of these drugs. **Do not** initiate halofantrine or ketoconazole within 15 days of the last dose of mefloquine because of the risk for fatal QTc interval prolongation. Monitor liver enzymes and ocular examinations for therapies longer than 1 year.

Adverse effects: GI disturbances, dizziness, somnolence, extrasystole, and bradycardia are common. May cause headache, syncope, seizures, ocular abnormalities, GI symptoms, leukopenia, and thrombocytopenia. Mood swings, memory impairment, irregular heartbeats, and hyperhidrosis have been reported. See Warnings/Precautions section.

Drug interactions: Mefloquine is a substrate and inhibitor of P-glycoprotein. Coadministration with chloroquine may increase risk for seizures. May reduce valproic acid levels. Rifampin may decrease mefloquine levels. See Warnings/Precautions section.

Drug administration: **Do not** take on an empty stomach. Administer with at least 240 mL (8 oz) water. Treatment failures in children may be related to vomiting of administered dose. If vomiting occurs less than 30 minutes after the dose, administer a second full dose. If vomiting occurs 30 to 60 minutes after the dose, administer an additional half dose. If vomiting continues, monitor patient closely and consider alternative therapy.

MELARSOPROL

Arsobal, Mel B, Melarsen Oxide-BAL

Antiprotozoal agent, trypanosomicidal agent

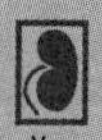
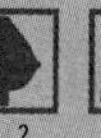
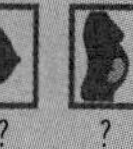

Yes Yes ? ?

AVAILABLE FROM THE U.S. CENTERS FOR DISEASE CONTROL AND PREVENTION (404-639-3670 Monday–Friday 8:00 AM–4:30 PM EST or 404-639-2888 evenings, weekends, or holidays)

Injection: 180 mg/5 mL; contains propylene glycol

African trypanosomiasis:

Child: Total dose of 18–25 mg/kg IV administered over a 1-month period as follows: start at 0.36 mg/kg/24 hr once daily, gradually increasing to a **maximum** of 3.6 mg/kg/24 hr at intervals of 1–5 days for a total of 9 or 10 doses

Adult: 3.6 mg/kg/dose IV once daily × 3 days; **max. dose:** 180–200 mg/24 hr. This regimen can be repeated 3–4 times with a 1-wk interval between treatment courses.

Contraindications: Hypersensitivity to melarsoprol

Warnings/Precautions: **Use with caution** in G6PD deficiency, renal (primary renal excretion; no dosing recommendation available) or hepatic insufficiency, and leprosy. Use during febrile episodes has been associated with a reactive arsenical encephalopathy; use during influenza epidemics is considered **contraindicated.**

Crosses the blood–brain barrier; CSF concentration is ~50-fold lower than serum.

Adverse effects: Jarisch–Herxheimer–like reaction, peripheral neuropathy, phlebitis, reactive arsenical encephalopathy, and local swelling at injection site are common. Hepatic dysfunction, hypertension, arrhythmias, myocardial damage, allergic reactions, exfoliative dermatitis, and renal dysfunction have been reported.

Continued

For explanation of icons, see p. 364.

MELARSOPROL *continued*

Drug administration: Have patient in the supine, fasting state during and several hours after dose. Administer dose by slow IV injection. Drug is incompatible with water. To reduce incidence of reactive encephalopathy, administer 1 mg/kg/dose prednisolone PO once daily (**max. dose:** 40 mg) starting the day before the first dose and continued through the second course. Taper prednisolone over 3 days after the second course. Reinitiate the same initial dose on the day before the third course and discontinue over 3 days.

MEROPENEM
Merrem and others
Carbapenem antibiotic

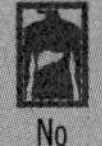
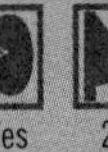
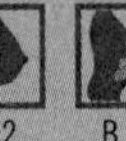

Injection: 0.5, 1 g
Contains 3.92 mEq Na/g drug.

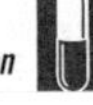

Neonate (IV)
Non-CNS intraabdominal infections with meropenem MIC <4 mcg/mL based on population PK modeling:
<32 wk gestation:
<14 days old: 20 mg/kg/dose Q12 hr
≥14 days old: 20 mg/kg/dose Q8 hr
≥32 wk gestation:
<14 days old: 20 mg/kg/dose Q8 hr
≥14 days old: 30 mg/kg/dose Q8 hr
Non-CNS infection with meropenem MIC 4–8 mcg/mL (moderately resistant) from a single-dose PK simulation study:
>30 wk gestation and >7 days old: 40 mg/kg/dose Q8 hr

Infant ≥1–3 mo (IV):
Non-CNS intraabdominal infections with meropenem MIC <4 mcg/mL based on population PK modeling: 20–30 mg/kg/dose Q8 hr
Meningitis (recommended dose from 2004 IDSA Meningitis practice guidelines): 40 mg/kg/dose Q8 hr

Infant ≥3 mo and adolescent (IV):
Skin and subcutaneous tissue infections: 30 mg/kg/24 hr ÷ Q8 hr; **max. dose:** 1.5 g/24 hr
Intraabdominal and mild-to-moderate infections; and fever/neutropenia empiric therapy: 60 mg/kg/24 hr ÷ Q8 hr; **max. dose:** 3 g/24 hr
Meningitis, severe infections, and cystic fibrosis pulmonary exacerbations: 120 mg/kg/24 hr ÷ Q8 hr; **max. dose:** 6 g/24 hr

Adult (IV):
Skin and subcutaneous tissue infections: 1.5 g/24 hr ÷ Q8 hr
Intraabdominal and mild-to-moderate infections; and fever/neutropenia empiric therapy: 3 g/24 hr ÷ Q8 hr
Meningitis and severe infections: 6 g/24 hr ÷ Q8 hr

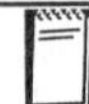

Contraindications: Patients sensitive to carbapenems or with a history of anaphylaxis to β-lactam antibiotics

Warnings/Precautions: **Use with caution** in meningitis, CNS disorders (may cause seizures), and renal impairment **(adjust dose; see Chapter 3).** Drug penetrates well into the CSF.

Adverse effects: Diarrhea, nausea, headache, and injection-site inflammation are common. Dermatologic reactions, including Stevens–Johnson and TEN, neutropenia, leukopenia, hepatic

Continued

MEROPENEM *continued*

enzyme and bilirubin elevation, and angioedema have been reported. Thrombocytopenia has been reported in patients with renal dysfunction.

Drug interactions: Probenecid may increase serum meropenem levels. May reduce valproic acid levels.

Drug administration: For IV push, infuse over 3 to 5 minutes at a concentration of 50 mg/mL. For intermittent infusion, infuse over 15 to 30 minutes at a concentration ≤50 mg/mL. Reconstituted IV solutions have short stability times; consult with a pharmacist.

METHENAMINE PREPARATIONS

Methenamine hippurate, Hiprex, Urex, Methenamine mandelate, Uroqid#2, and others

Note: Many methenamine combination products are also available.

Urinary germicide

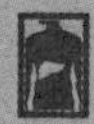
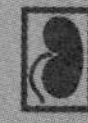
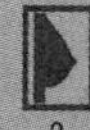
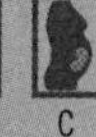

Yes Yes 2 C

Methenamine hippurate (Hiprex, Urex):
 Tabs: 1 g (Hiprex contains tartrazine)
Methenamine mandelate (Uroqid#2):
 Tabs: 0.5, 1 g

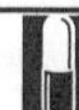

For recurrent UTIs (see remarks):

Methenamine hippurate:

Child (6–12 yr): 500–1000 mg/dose PO BID

>12 yr to adult: 1000 mg/dose PO BID

Methenamine mandelate:

Child (2–12 yr): 50–75 mg/kg/24 hr PO ÷ Q6 hr (**max. dose:** 4 g/24 hr); 500 mg/dose PO QID has been recommended for children 6–12 yr

≥12 yr–adult: 1000 mg/dose PO QID

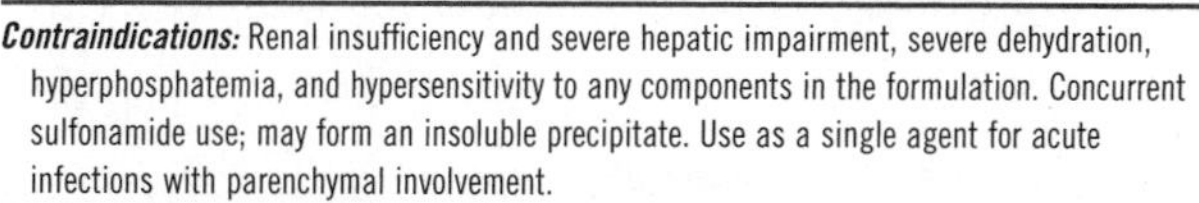

Contraindications: Renal insufficiency and severe hepatic impairment, severe dehydration, hyperphosphatemia, and hypersensitivity to any components in the formulation. Concurrent sulfonamide use; may form an insoluble precipitate. Use as a single agent for acute infections with parenchymal involvement.

Warnings/Precautions: Methenamine is hydrolyzed by acidic urine to form bactericidal formaldehyde and ammonia. *Proteus* or *Pseudomonas* (urea-splitting organisms) may be resistant to methenamine by inhibiting the release of formaldehyde; acidification of urine is essential.

Use only after eradication of urinary tract infection by other appropriate antimicrobial agents. Large doses have caused bladder irritation, painful and frequent micturition, proteinuria, and gross hematuria. **Use with caution** in gout (may cause urate crystals in urine) and preexisting liver disease (worsened by increased ammonia production).

Adverse effects: Nausea, upset stomach, dysuria, and rash are common. GI disturbances may be transient or severe enough to discontinue therapy or reduce the dosage. Headache, dyspnea, bladder irritation, and pruritus have been reported.

Drug interactions: Urinary alkalinizers and sulfonamides may decrease methenamine's effects. May falsely increase urinary levels of 17-hydroxycorticosteroids, catecholamines, and vanillylmandelic acid, and falsely decrease urinary tests for 5-hydroxyindoleacetic acid and certain pregnancy tests.

Drug administration: Take with food to minimize GI upset. Acidification of the urine with ascorbic acid or cranberry juice is recommended to enhance the drug's effect. **Avoid** excessive intake of alkalinizing foods and medications such as milk products, bicarbonate, and acetazolamide.

For explanation of icons, see p. 364.

METRONIDAZOLE
Flagyl, Flagyl ER, Protostat, MetroGel, MetroLotion, MetroCream, Noritate, MetroGel-Vaginal, and others
Antibiotic, antiprotozoal

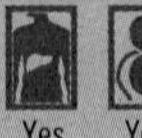
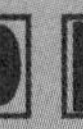
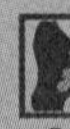
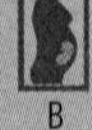
Yes Yes 3 B

Tabs: 250, 500 mg
Tabs, extended release (Flagyl ER): 750 mg
Caps: 375 mg
Oral suspension: 10 mg/mL or 50 mg/mL
Oral syrup: 5 mg/mL
Injection: 500 mg; contains 830 mg mannitol/g drug
Ready-to-use injection: 5 mg/mL (100 mL); contains 28 mEq Na/g drug
Gel, topical (MetroGel): 0.75% (28, 60 g)
Lotion (MetroLotion): 0.75% (60 mL); contains benzyl alcohol
Cream, topical:
 MetroCream: 0.75% (45 g); contains benzyl alcohol
 Noritate: 1% (30 g)
Gel, vaginal (MetroGel-Vaginal): 0.75% (70 g with 5 applicators)

Amebiasis:
 Child: 35–50 mg/kg/24 hr PO ÷ TID × 10 days
 Adult: 500–750 mg/dose PO TID × 10 days
Anaerobic infection:
 Neonate:
  PO/IV:
   <7 days:
    <1.2 kg: 7.5 mg/kg/dose Q48 hr
    1.2–2 kg: 7.5 mg/kg/dose Q24 hr
   ≥2 kg: 15 mg/kg/24 hr ÷ Q12 hr
  ≥7 days:
   <1.2 kg: 7.5 mg/kg Q24 hr
   1.2–2 kg: 15 mg/kg/24 hr ÷ Q12 hr
   ≥2 kg: 30 mg/kg/24 hr ÷ Q12 hr
 Infant/child/adult:
  IV/PO: 30 mg/kg/24 hr ÷ Q6 hr; **max. dose:** 4 g/24 hr
Other parasitic infections:
 Infant/child: 15–30 mg/kg/24 hr PO ÷ Q8 hr
 Adult: 250 mg PO Q8 hr or 2 g PO × 1
Bacterial vaginosis:
 Adolescent and adult:
  PO:
   Immediate-release tabs: 500 mg BID × 7 days
   Extended-release tabs: 750 mg once daily × 7 days
  Vaginal: 5 g (1 applicator full) BID × 5 days
Giardiasis:
 Child: 15 mg/kg/24 hr PO ÷ TID × 5 days; **max. dose:** 750 mg/24 hr
 Adult: 250 mg PO TID × 5 days
Trichomoniasis: Treat sexual contacts.
 Child: 15 mg/kg/24 hr PO ÷ TID × 7 days
 Adolescent/adult: 2 g PO × 1 or 250 mg PO TID or 375 mg PO BID × 7 days

Continued

METRONIDAZOLE *continued*

Clostridium difficile ***infection (IV may be less efficacious):***
Child: 30 mg/kg/24 hr ÷ Q6 hr PO/IV × 10 days
Adult: 250–500 mg TID–QID PO × 10–14 days, or 500 mg Q8 hr IV × 10–14 days
Helicobacter pylori ***infection (use in combination with amoxicillin and bismuth subsalicylate):***
Child: 15–20 mg/kg/24 hr ÷ BID PO × 4 wk
Adult: 250–500 mg TID PO × 14 days
Inflammatory bowel disease (as alternative to sulfasalazine):
Adult: 400 mg BID PO
Topical use: Apply and rub a thin film to affected areas at the following frequencies specific to product concentration:
0.75% cream: BID
1% cream: once daily

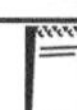

Contraindications: **Avoid** use in first-trimester pregnancy. Hypersensitivity to metronidazole or any other components in the formulation.

Warnings/Precautions: **Use with caution** in patients with CNS disease, blood dyscrasias, severe liver or renal disease (GFR <10 mL/min); **see Chapter 3.** Patients should **not** ingest alcohol for 24 to 48 hours after dose (disulfiram-type reaction).
For IV use in all ages, some references recommend a 15 mg/kg loading dose. If using single 2 g dose in a breast-feeding mother, discontinue breast-feeding for 12 to 24 hours to allow excretion of the drug. Single-dose oral regimen no longer recommended in bacterial vaginosis because of poor efficacy.

Adverse effects: Nausea, vomiting, diarrhea, ataxia, dizziness, headache, worsening of candidiasis, metallic taste, and peripheral neuropathy are common. May discolor urine. Leukopenia, thrombocytopenia, ototoxicity, encephalopathy, aseptic meningitis, optic neuropathy, Stevens–Johnson syndrome, and toxic epidermal necrolysis have been reported.

Drug interactions: May increase levels or toxicity of phenytoin, lithium, and warfarin. Phenobarbital and rifampin may increase metronidazole metabolism. Alcohol may cause disulfiram-like reactions.

Drug administration:
PO: Give on an empty stomach but may be given with food if GI upset occurs. **Do not** crush extended-release tablets.
IV: For intermittent infusion, infuse over 60 min at a concentration of 5–8 mg/mL.
Intravaginal: Use vaginal gel product only and **do not** apply to the eye.
Topical: Treated areas should be cleansed before drug application.

MICAFUNGIN SODIUM
Mycamine
Antifungal, echinocandin

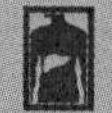
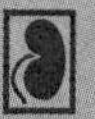
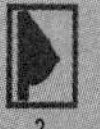
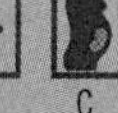

Yes Yes ? C

Injection: 50, 100 mg; contains lactose

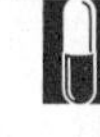

Invasive candidiasis (see remarks):
Neonate and infant (based on a multidose pharmacokinetic and safety trial in 13 neonates/infants >48 hr and <120 days old with suspected or invasive candidiasis; minimum of 4–5 days of therapy):
<1 kg: 10 mg/kg/dose IV once daily; additional data from another multidose trial in 12 preterm neonates (median birth weight: 775 g, 27 wk gestation) suggest 15 mg/kg/dose IV once daily will provide similar AUC drug exposure of ~5 mg/kg/dose in adults
≥1 kg: 7 mg/kg/dose IV once daily

Continued

For explanation of icons, see p. 364.

MICAFUNGIN SODIUM *continued*

Child and adolescent: 3–4 mg/kg/dose IV once daily; **max. dose:** 200 mg/dose
Adult: 100–150 mg IV once daily

Esophageal candidiasis (see remarks):

Child and adult:

<50 kg: 3–4 mg/kg/dose IV once daily; **max. dose:** 200 mg/dose
≥50 kg: 150 mg IV once daily; mean duration for successful therapy was 15 days (range: 10–30 days)

Candida prophylaxis in hematopoietic stem cell transplant:

Child and adult:

<50 kg: 1 mg/kg/dose IV once daily; **max. dose:** 50 mg/dose
≥50 kg: 50 mg IV once daily; mean duration 19 days (range: 6–51 days)

Invasive aspergillosis (see remarks; doses under investigation):

Child and adult:

<50 kg: 3–4 mg/kg/dose IV once daily; dosages as high as 7.5 mg/kg/24 hr have been tolerated
≥50 kg: 150 mg IV once daily

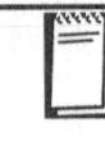

Contraindications: Hypersensitivity to micafungin or to any component of the product

Warnings/Precautions: Prior hypersensitivity to other echinocandins (anidulafungin, caspofungin) increases risk. Serious reactions such as anaphylactoid reactions and anaphylaxis with shock have been reported.

Use with caution in hepatic and renal impairment.

No dosing adjustments are required based on race or sex, or in patients with severe renal dysfunction or mild-to-moderate hepatic function impairment. Effect of severe hepatic function impairment on micafungin pharmacokinetics has not been evaluated. Higher dosage requirements in premature and young infants may be attributed to the faster drug clearance because of lower protein binding. Higher treatment doses in infants and children have been reported at 8.6 to 12 mg/kg/dose IV once daily.

Adverse effects: GI disturbances, phlebitis, rash, hyperbilirubinemia, LFT elevation, headache, fever, and rigor are common. Anemia, leukopenia, neutropenia, thrombocytopenia, hemolysis, Stevens–Johnson syndrome, toxic epidermal necrolysis, and disseminated intravascular coagulation have been reported.

Drug interactions: Micafungin is CYP450 3A isoenzyme substrate and weak inhibitor. May increase the effects/toxicity of nifedipine and sirolimus.

Drug administration:

IV: Flush line with NS before IV administration. Infuse over 1 hr at a concentration of 0.5–1.5 mg/mL in NS or D_5W.

MICONAZOLE
Topical products: Micatin, Lotrimin AF, and others
Vaginal products: Monistat, Vagistat-3, and others
Antifungal, imidazole

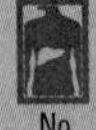

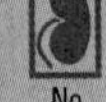

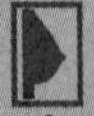

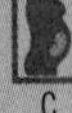

Cream (OTC): 2% (15, 30, 90 g)
Lotion (OTC): 2% (30, 60 mL)
Ointment (OTC): 2% (28.4 g)
Solution (OTC): 2% with alcohol (30.3 mL)
Gel (OTC): 2% with alcohol (24 g)
Topical solution (OTC): 2% with alcohol (30.3 mL)

Continued

MICONAZOLE *continued*

Powder (OTC): 2% (70, 90 g)
Spray, liquid (OTC): 2% (105 mL); contains alcohol
Spray, powder (OTC): 2% (85, 90, 100 g); contains alcohol
Vaginal cream (OTC): 2% (15, 25, 45 g), 4% (15, 25 g)
Vaginal suppository (OTC): 100 mg (7s), 200 mg (3s)
Vaginal combination packs:
Monistat 1 Combination Pack (OTC): 1200 mg suppository (1) and 2% cream (9 g)
Monistat 3, Vagistat-3 (OTC): 200 mg suppository (3s) and 2% cream (9 g)
Monistat 7 (OTC): 100 mg suppository (7s) and 2% cream (9 g)

Topical: Apply BID × 2–4 wk
Vaginal:
7-day regimen: 1 applicator full of 2% cream or 100-mg suppository QHS × 7 days
3-day regimen: 1 applicator full of 4% cream or 200-mg suppository QHS × 3 days
Monistat 1: 1200-mg suppository × 1 at bedtime or during the day

Contraindications: Hypersensitivity to miconazole or any other components in the formulation
Warnings/Precautions: **Use with caution** in hypersensitivity to other imidazole antifungal agents (e.g., clotrimazole, ketoconazole). Vegetable oil base in vaginal suppositories may interact with latex products (e.g., condoms and diaphragms); consider switching to the vaginal cream. **Avoid** contact with the eyes.
Adverse effects: Pruritus, rash, burning, phlebitis, headaches, and pelvic cramps
Drug interactions: Drug is a substrate and inhibitor of the CYP 450 3A3/4 isoenzymes. Vaginal use with concomitant warfarin use has also been reported to increase warfarin's effect.
Drug administration:
Topical: Apply sparingly to cleansed and dry affected area. For intertriginous areas, rub cream gently into the skin.
Vaginal: Wash hands before use. Gently insert suppository or applicator full of cream high into the vagina at bedtime. Remain lying down for 30 minutes after administration. Wash applicator with soap and water after each use.

MINOCYCLINE
Minocin, Dynacin, Arestin, Solodyn, and others
Antibiotic, tetracycline derivative

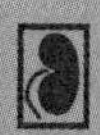
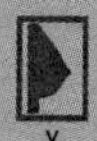
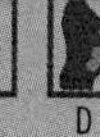

Yes Yes X D

Tabs: 50, 75, 100 mg
Caps: 50, 75, 100 mg
Extended-release tabs (Solodyn): 45, 65, 90, 115, 135 mg
Caps (pellet filled): 50, 100 mg
Sustained-release microspheres (Arestin): 1 mg (12s)
Oral suspension: 50 mg/5 mL (60 mL); contains 5% alcohol

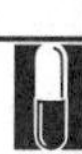

General infections:
Child (8–12 yr): 4 mg/kg/dose × 1 PO, then 2 mg/kg/dose Q12 hr PO; **max. dose:** 200 mg/24 hr
Adolescent and adult: 200 mg/dose × 1 PO, then 100 mg Q12 hr PO
Chlamydia trachomatis/Ureaplasma urealyticum:
Adolescent and adult: 100 mg PO Q12 hr × 7 days
Acne (≥12 yr to adult):
Immediate-release dosage forms: 50–100 mg PO once to twice daily

Continued

For explanation of icons, see p. 364.

MINOCYCLINE *continued*

Acne (≥12 yr to adult):

Extended-release tabs:

45–54 kg: 45 mg PO once daily

55–77 kg: 65 mg PO once daily

78–102 kg: 90 mg PO once daily

103–125 kg: 115 mg PO once daily

126–136 kg: 135 mg PO once daily

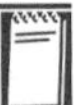

Contraindications: Hypersensitivity to minocycline, tetracyclines, or any other components in the formulation

Warnings/Precautions: **Not** recommended for children younger than 8 years and during the last half of pregnancy because of risk for permanent tooth discoloration. **Use with caution** in renal failure; lower dosage may be necessary. Discontinue use if drug rash with eosinophilia and systemic symptoms (DRESS) occur.

Adverse effects: High incidence rate of vestibular dysfunction (30%–90%). Nausea, vomiting, allergy, increased intracranial pressure (leading to headaches, papilledema, and blurred vision), photophobia, and injury to developing teeth may occur. Hepatitis, including autoimmune hepatitis, liver failure, hypersensitivity reactions (e.g., anaphylaxis, Stevens–Johnson syndrome, erythema multiforme), and lupus-like syndrome have been reported.

Drug interactions: Use with isotretinoin or vitamin A is **not** recommended because of added risk for increased intracranial pressure. May decrease the efficacy of live attenuated oral typhoid vaccine. May increase the effects/toxicity of warfarin. The absorption of the following elements and the absorption of minocycline may be reduced with concomitant administration: aluminum, iron, calcium, magnesium, and zinc.

Drug administration: Administer tablets and pellet-filled capsules 1 hour before or 2 hours after meals. Capsule and extended-release tablets may be administered with or without food. **Do not** give with dairy products.

MOXIFLOXACIN

Avelox, Avelox IV, Moxeza, Vigamox

Antibiotic, quinolone

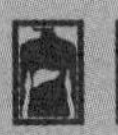
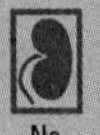
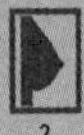
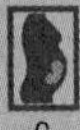
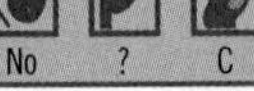

Tabs: 400 mg

Injection, premixed ready-to-use bags: 400 mg in 0.8% saline (250 mL)

Ophthalmic solution:

Moxeza, Vigamox: 0.5% (3 mL)

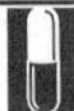

Child: Currently being studied with complicated intraabdominal infections at the following dosages (see www.clinicaltrials.gov for latest update):

2–5 yr: 5 mg/kg/dose PO/IV Q12 hr; **max. dose:** 400 mg/24 hr

6–11 yr: 4 mg/kg/dose PO/IV Q12 hr; **max. dose:** 400 mg/24 hr

12–17 yr:

<45 kg: 4 mg/kg/dose PO/IV Q12 hr; **max. dose:** 400 mg/24 hr

≥45 kg: 400 mg PO/IV once daily

Adult: 400 mg PO/IV once daily

Bacterial conjunctivitis:

Moxeza:

≥4 mo to adult: Instill one drop to affected eye(s) BID × 7 days.

Vigamox:

≥1 yr to adult: Instill one drop to affected eye(s) TID × 7 days.

Continued

MOXIFLOXACIN *continued*

Contraindications: Hypersensitivity to moxifloxacin, quinolones, or any of the components in the formulation

Warnings/Precautions:

IV/PO: **Avoid** use in patients with QT interval prolongation (including taking other medications with the same effect), bradycardia, myocardial ischemia, or uncorrected hypokalemia. Use with corticosteroids may increase risk for tendon rupture. **Use with caution** in seizures. Avoid use in myasthenia gravis; may exacerbate muscle weakness. No dosing adjustment is necessary in renal impairment and mild-to-moderate hepatic insufficiency (Child–Pugh classes A and B). Has **not** been studied in patients with severe hepatic impairment (Child–Pugh class C).

Ophthalmic: **Avoid** wearing contact lens during active infection. Topical use only; **do not** inject this product.

Adverse effects:

IV/PO: GI disturbances, dizziness, and headaches are common. Torsades de pointes, Stevens–Johnson syndrome, severe immune hypersensitivity reaction, tendon rupture, and peripheral neuropathy have been reported.

Ophthalmic: Conjunctivitis, decreased visual acuity, dry eyes, keratitis, ocular discomfort, subconjunctival hemorrhage, and tearing are common.

Drug interactions: Use of class IA (e.g., quinidine, procainamide) and class III (e.g., amiodarone, sotalol) antiarrhythmics should be **avoided.** Antacids and iron, when administered close together, reduce the absorption of moxifloxacin.

Drug administration:

PO: May be taken with or without food. If patient is to receive antacids containing aluminum or magnesium, sucralfate, iron, multivitamins with zinc, or buffered didanosine, administer dose at least 4 hours before or 8 hours after.

IV: For intermittent IV infusion, infuse over 60 minutes with the premixed concentration of 1.6 mg/mL.

Ophthalmic drops: Apply finger pressure to lacrimal sac during and for 1 to 2 minutes after dose application.

MUPIROCIN

Bactroban, Bactroban Nasal, and others

Topical antibiotic

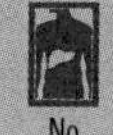
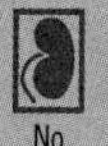
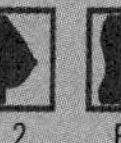

No No 2 B

Ointment: 2% (22, 30 g); contains polyethylene glycol
Cream: 2% (15, 30 g); contains benzyl alcohol
Nasal ointment: 2% (1 g), as calcium salt

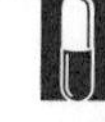

Topical (see remarks):

≥3 mo to adult: Apply small amount TID to affected area × 5–14 days. Ointment may be used in infants ≥2 mo old.

Intranasal (see remarks): Apply small amount intranasally BID × 5–10 days.

Contraindications: Hypersensitivity to mupirocin products

Warnings/Precautions: **Avoid** contact with eyes. Cream is **not** intended for use in lesions more than 10 cm in length or 100 cm^2 in surface area. **Do not** use topical ointment preparation on open wounds because of concerns for systemic absorption of polyethylene glycol.

If clinical response is **not** apparent in 3 to 5 days with topical use, reevaluate infection. Intranasal administration may be used to eliminate carriage of *Staphylococcus aureus,* including MRSA.

Continued

For explanation of icons, see p. 364.

MUPIROCIN *continued*

Adverse effects:

Topical: May cause minor local irritation and dry skin.

Intranasal: Nasal stinging, taste disorder, headache, rhinitis, and pharyngitis may occur.

Drug Interactions: None identified.

Drug administration: **Avoid** contact with eyes.

Topical: May cover treated areas with gauze dressings.

Intranasal: Press nostrils together and release repeatedly for 1 minute to improve drug distribution in the nares. Discard tube after use **(do not reuse)**.

NAFCILLIN

Unipen, Nallpen, and others

Antibiotic, penicillin (penicillinase resistant)

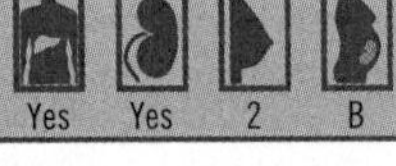

Injection: 1, 2, 10 g; contains 2.9 mEq Na/g drug

Injection, premixed in iso-osmotic dextrose: 1 g in 50 mL, 2 g in 100 mL

Neonate (IM/IV):

≤7 days:

<2 kg: 50 mg/kg/24 hr ÷ Q12 hr

≥2 kg: 75 mg/kg/24 hr ÷ Q8 hr

>7 days:

<1.2 kg: 50 mg/kg/24 hr ÷ Q12 hr

1.2–2 kg: 75 mg/kg/24 hr ÷ Q8 hr

≥2 kg: 100 mg/kg/24 hr ÷ Q6 hr

Infant and child (IM/IV):

Mild-to-moderate infections: 50–100 mg/kg/24 hr ÷ Q6 hr

Severe infections: 100–200 mg/kg/24 hr ÷ Q4–6 hr; give 200 mg/kg/24 hr ÷ Q4–6 hr for staphylococcal endocarditis

Max. dose: 12 g/24 hr

Adult:

IV: 500–2000 mg Q4–6 hr

IM: 500 mg Q4–6 hr

Max. dose: 12 g/24 hr

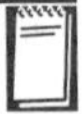

Contraindications: Hypersensitivity to nafcillin, penicillins, or any other components in the formulation. Solutions containing dextrose may be **contraindicated** in patients with known allergy to corn or corn products.

Warnings/Precautions: Allergic cross-sensitivity with penicillin. **Oral route not recommended** because of unpredictable absorption. CSF penetration is poor unless meninges are inflamed. **Use with caution** in patients with combined renal and hepatic impairment (reduce dose by 33%–50%) and cephalosporin hypersensitivity.

Adverse effects: High incidence of phlebitis with IV dosing. May cause rash and bone marrow suppression. Acute interstitial nephritis is rare. Hypokalemia has been reported.

Drug interactions: Nafcillin may increase elimination of cyclosporine and warfarin. Probenecid increases serum nafcillin levels. May cause false-positive urinary and serum proteins.

Drug administration:

IV: IV push, infuse over 5–10 min at a concentration ≤66.7 mg/mL. For intermittent infusion, infuse over 15–60 min at a concentration ≤40 mg/mL (100 mg/mL for fluid-restricted patients).

IM: Dilute with sterile water or NS to 250 mg/mL and immediately administer by deep intragluteal injection.

N

FORMULARY

NAFTIFINE
Naftin Cream, Naftin Gel
Antifungal, allylamine derivative

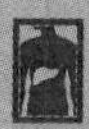 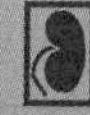 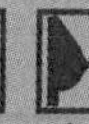 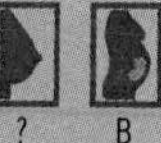

No No ? B

Cream: 1% (30, 60, 90 g), 2% (45 g); contains benzyl alcohol
Gel: 1% (40, 60, 90 g); contains alcohol 52% (v/v)

Adult:

Tinea (reevaluate if no clinical effect after 4 weeks with 1% preparations or after 2 weeks with 2% preparations):

Cream: Gently massage into affected and surrounding skin areas once daily for up to 2 or 4 wk with the 2% or 1% preparations, respectively.

Gel: Gently massage into affected and surrounding skin areas BID (morning and evening).

Contraindications: Hypersensitivity to naftifine products and to any of its components
Warnings/Precautions: Discontinue use if excessive irritation or hypersensitivity develops. Safety and efficacy in children have not been established.
Adverse effects: Burning/stinging, itching, local irritation, dryness, and erythema are common.

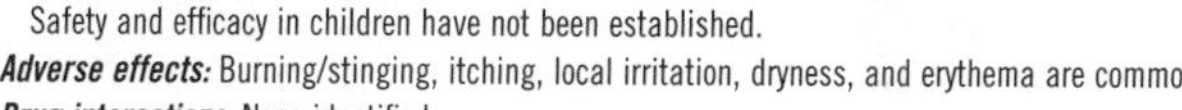

Drug interactions: None identified.
Drug administration: **Avoid** occlusive dressings unless otherwise directed. **Avoid** contact with eyes, nose, mouth, and other mucous membranes. Wash hands after application.

NATAMYCIN
Natacyn
Antifungal (Ophthalmic)

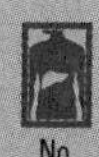 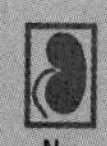 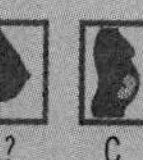

No No ? C

Ophthalmic suspension: 5% (15 mL); contains benzalkonium chloride

Adult:

Fungal keratitis: Instill 1 drop to affected eye(s) Q1–2 hr × 3–4 days, then 1 drop 6–8 times/24 hr. Usual therapy course is 2–3 wk or until resolution of keratitis.

Fungal blepharitis or conjunctivitis: Instill 1 drop to affected eye(s) Q4–6 hr.

Contraindications: Hypersensitivity to natamycin or any component of the formulation
Warnings/Precautions: Reevaluate cause of infection if no improvement is seen after 7–10 days of use. Use of contact lens is not recommended.
Adverse effects: Ocular irritation is common. Chest pain, hypersensitivity reactions, paresthesia, ocular discomfort, abnormal vision, and dyspnea have been reported.
Drug interactions: None identified.
Drug administration: Shake bottle well before each use. Instill drop in lower conjunctival sac by **avoiding** contact with the dropper tip to eye or skin.

NELFINAVIR
Viracept, NFV
Antiviral, protease inhibitor

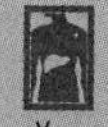 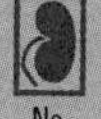 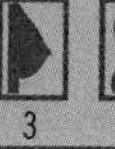

Yes No 3 B

Powder, oral: 50 mg/level scoop (50 mg drug per 1 g powder) (144 g powder per bottle); contains 11.2 mg phenylalanine/g powder

One level teaspoon provides 200 mg nelfinavir.

Four level scoops equivalent to 1 level teaspoon.

Tabs: 250, 625 mg

Continued

For explanation of icons, see p. 364.

NELFINAVIR *continued*

Child 2–13 yr (see remarks): 45–55 mg/kg/dose PO BID (**max. dose:** 1250 mg/dose); or 25–35 mg/kg/dose PO TID (**max. dose:** 750 mg/dose). Alternative dosing tables for tablets and oral powder by weight are as follows:

TABLET DOSING FOR CHILDREN ≥2 YEARS OLD

Weight (kg)	No. of 250-mg Tablets to Provide 45–55 mg/kg/dose PO for BID Administration	No. of 250-mg Tablets to Provide 25–35 mg/kg/dose PO for TID Administration
10–12	2	1
13–18	3	2
19–20	4	2
≥21	4–5*	3†

***Max. dose** for BID dosing is 5 tablets BID.
†**Max. dose** for TID dosing is 3 tablets TID.

ORAL POWDER DOSING FOR CHILDREN ≥2 YEARS OLD

	Amount of Powder to Provide 45–55 mg/kg/dose PO for BID Administration		Amount of Powder to Provide 25–35 mg/kg/dose PO for TID Administration	
Weight (kg)	No. of Level Scoops (50 mg/1 g powder)	No. of Level Teaspoons*	No. of Level Scoops (50 mg/1 g powder)	No. of Level Teaspoons*
9 to <10.5	10	2.5	6	1.5
10.5 to <12	11	2.75	7	1.75
12 to <14	13	3.25	8	2
14 to <16	15	3.75	9	2.25
16 to <18	NR†	NR†	10	2.5
18 to <23	NR†	NR†	12	3
≥23	NR†	NR†	15	3.75

*One level teaspoon contains 200 mg nelfinavir (4 level scoops = 1 level teaspoon).
†Not recommended (NR), use 250-mg oral tablet.

Adolescent and adult: 1250 mg PO BID or 750 mg PO TID. Some adolescents may require higher doses than adults; use of therapeutic drug monitoring to guide appropriate dosing has been suggested.

Contraindications: Hypersensitivity to nelfinavir or any other components in the formulation. Do **NOT** coadminister with alfuzosin, amiodarone, cisapride, lovastatin, simvastatin, midazolam (PO), triazolam, sildenafil, ergot derivatives, quinidine, rifampin, or pimozide.

Warnings/Precautions: Avoid use of oral powder dosage form in patients with phenylketonuria because it contains phenylalanine. **Noncompliance can quickly promote resistant HIV strains.** Use with **caution** in mild hepatic impairment (Child–Pugh class A); **avoid** use in moderate or severe hepatic impairment (Child–Pugh class B or C). Use in children younger than 2 years is not recommended because of high interpatient variability. **Do not use** in combination with astemizole, cisapride, terfenadine, rifampin, St. John's wort, or proton pump inhibitors. Many other drug–drug interactions exist; see earlier Contraindications and also the following sections.

Adverse effects: Diarrhea, leukopenia/neutropenia, rash, anorexia, and abdominal pain are common. Asthenia, lipodystrophy, hyperglycemia, and exacerbation of chronic liver disease may occur.

Continued

NELFINAVIR *continued*

Spontaneous bleeding episodes in hemophiliacs and immune reconstitution syndrome have been reported.

Drug interactions: Nelfinavir is a substrate and inhibitor of CYP 450 3A3/4 and substrate for CYP 450 2C19. Rifampin, rifabutin, nevirapine, azithromycin, phenobarbital, phenytoin, and carbamazepine can decrease nelfinavir levels. Nelfinavir can increase the effects/toxicity of rifabutin, tacrolimus, sirolimus, sildenafil, and hepatically metabolized benzodiazepines (e.g., midazolam); decrease effects/levels of efavirenz, delavirdine, phenytoin, zidovudine, methadone, and oral contraceptive effectiveness (use alternative methods). When used in combination with other protease inhibitors (PIs), nelfinavir and other PI levels may increase. See earlier Contraindications. **Always check the potential for other drug interactions when either initiating therapy or adding new drugs onto an existing regimen.**

Drug administration: Administer all doses with food; **avoid** mixing with acidic foods or juice (may result in poor taste). If didanosine is part of the antiviral regimen, nelfinavir should be administered at least 2 hours before or 1 hour after didanosine. Oral powder dosage form may be mixed with water, milk (including soy), pudding, formula (including soy), or dietary supplements (refrigerated up to 6 hours). Oral tablets may be dissolved and mixed in small amounts of water and consumed immediately (rinse glass with water and drink rinse to ensure complete dose administration).

NEOMYCIN SULFATE

Mycifradin, Neo-Fradin, Neo-Tabs, and others

Antibiotic, aminoglycoside; ammonium detoxicant

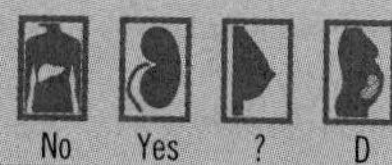

Tabs (Mycifradin, Neo-Tabs): 500 mg (300 mg base)
Oral solution (Neo-Fradin): 125 mg/5 mL; contains parabens

Diarrhea:
Preterm and newborn: 50 mg/kg/24 hr ÷ Q6 hr PO

Hepatic encephalopathy:
Infant and child: 50–100 mg/kg/24 hr ÷ Q6–8 hr PO × 5–6 days; **max. dose:** 12 g/24 hr
Adult: 4–12 g/24 hr ÷ Q4–6 hr PO × 5–6 days

Bowel prep (in combination with erythromycin base):
Child: 90 mg/kg/24 hr PO ÷ Q4 hr × 2–3 days
Adult: 1 g Q1 hr PO × 4 doses, then 1 g Q4 hr PO × 5 doses (Many other regimens exist.)

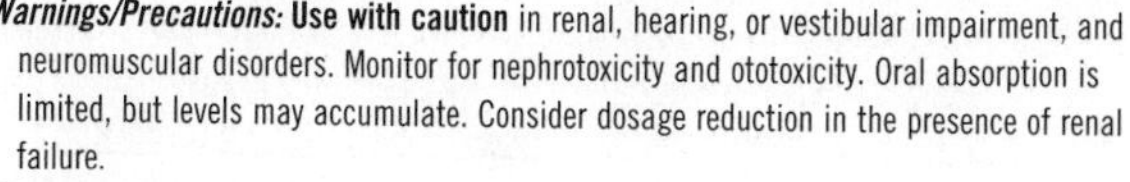

Contraindications: Ulcerative bowel disease or intestinal obstruction; hypersensitivity to neomycin or aminoglycosides

Warnings/Precautions: **Use with caution** in renal, hearing, or vestibular impairment, and neuromuscular disorders. Monitor for nephrotoxicity and ototoxicity. Oral absorption is limited, but levels may accumulate. Consider dosage reduction in the presence of renal failure.

Adverse effects: GI disturbances are common. May cause itching, redness, edema, colitis, candidiasis, or poor wound healing if applied topically. Prevalence of neomycin hypersensitivity has increased.

Drug interactions: May potentiate oral anticoagulants and decrease the absorption of penicillin V, vitamin B_{12}, digoxin, and methotrexate. Increase in adverse effects of other neurotoxic, ototoxic, or nephrotoxic drugs.

Drug administration: Doses may be administered with or without food.

For explanation of icons, see p. 364.

NEOMYCIN/HYDROCORTISONE OTIC PREPARATIONS
NEOMYCIN/POLYMYXIN B/HYDROCORTISONE:
Cortisporin Otic, Cortomycin, and others
NEOMYCIN/COLISTIN/HYDROCORTISONE:
Cortisporin TC Otic, Coly-Mycin S Otic with neomycin and hydrocortisone
Steroid and antibiotic, otic suspension

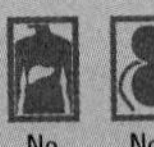
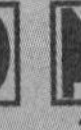
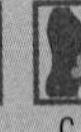
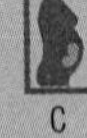

No No 2 C

Otic suspension:
NEOMYCIN/POLYMYXIN B/HYDROCORTISONE: Each 1 mL contains 3.5 mg neomycin base, 10,000 units polymyxin base, and 10 mg (1%) hydrocortisone; may contain metasulfites and propylene glycol (10 mL).
NEOMYCIN/COLISTIN/HYDROCORTISONE: Each 1 mL contains 3 mg colistin sulfate, 3.3 mg neomycin sulfate, 10 mg (1%) hydrocortisone acetate, and 0.5 mg thonzonium bromide; contains 0.002% thimerosal (7.5 mL). See Colistimethate Sodium for IV colistin.

Otitis externa (see Drug Administration section for alternative dosing method):
NEOMYCIN/POLYMYXIN B/HYDROCORTISONE:
Child: Instill 3 drops in affected ear(s) TID–QID up to a **maximum** of 10 days.
Adult: Instill 4 drops in affected ear(s) TID–QID up to a **maximum** of 10 days.

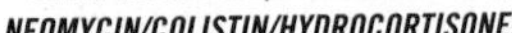

NEOMYCIN/COLISTIN/HYDROCORTISONE:
Child: Instill 4 drops in affected ear(s) TID–QID up to a **maximum** of 10 days.
Adult: Instill 5 drops in affected ear(s) TID–QID up to a **maximum** of 10 days.

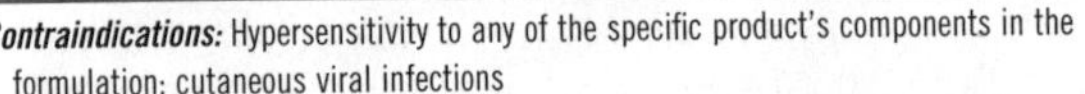

Contraindications: Hypersensitivity to any of the specific product's components in the formulation; cutaneous viral infections
Warnings/Precautions: **Use with caution** with sulfite allergy, perforated tympanic membrane, and chronic otitis media.
Adverse effects: Allergic skin reactions, stinging and burning in the ear, and ototoxicity have been reported. Prevalence of neomycin hypersensitivity has increased.
Drug interactions: None identified.
Drug administration: Clean and dry the external auditory canal with a sterile cotton applicator before dose. Patient should lie with the affected ear upward when instilling drops. Remain in this position for 5 minutes after dosing. Alternatively, a cotton wick saturated with suspension may be inserted into the ear canal. Wick should be remoistened every 4 hours, and the wick should be replaced once every 24 hours.

NEOMYCIN/POLYMYXIN B/± BACITRACIN
NEOMYCIN/POLYMYXIN B:
Neosporin GU irrigant, and others
NEOMYCIN/POLYMYXIN B + BACITRACIN:
Neosporin, Neo To Go, Neo-Polycin, Neosporin Ophthalmic, and others
Topical antibiotic

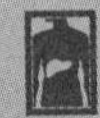
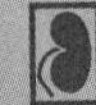
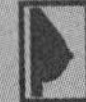
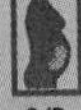
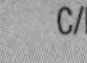

No No ? C/D

NEOMYCIN/POLYMYXIN B:
Solution, GU irrigant: 40 mg neomycin sulfate, 200,000 units polymyxin B/mL (1, 20 mL); multidose vial contains methylparabens
NEOMYCIN/POLYMYXIN B + BACITRACIN:
Ointment, topical (Neosporin, Neo To Go) (OTC): 3.5 mg neomycin sulfate, 400 units bacitracin, 5000 units polymyxin B/g (0.9, 15, 30, 454 g)

Continued

NEOMYCIN/POLYMYXIN B/± BACITRACIN *continued*

Ointment, ophthalmic (Neosporin Ophthalmic): 3.5 mg neomycin sulfate, 400 units bacitracin, 10,000 units polymyxin B/g (3.5 g)

NEOMYCIN/POLYMYXIN B + BACITRACIN:

Child and adult:

Topical: Apply to minor wounds and burns once to twice daily.

Ophthalmic: Apply small amount to conjunctiva Q3–4 hr × 7–10 days, depending on the severity of infection.

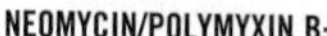

NEOMYCIN/POLYMYXIN B:

Bladder irrigation:

Child and adult: Mix 1 ml in 1000 ml NS and administer via a three-way catheter at a rate adjusted to the patient's urine output. Do not exceed 10 days of continuous use.

Contraindications: Hypersensitivity to neomycin and polymyxin B or any of its components **Avoid** use of bladder irrigant in patients with defects in the bladder mucosa or wall.

Warnings/Precautions: **Do not use** for extended periods. May cause superinfection, delayed healing. Ophthalmic ointments may retard corneal healing. Pregnancy category is a "C" for NEOMYCIN/POLYMYXIN B + BACITRACIN products and "D" for NEOMYCIN/POLYMYXIN B GU irrigation.

Adverse effects: Ophthalmic preparation may cause stinging and sensitivity to bright light. Prevalence of neomycin hypersensitivity has increased.

Drug interactions: None identified.

Drug administration:

Topical: Apply a thin layer to the cleaned affected area. May be covered with a sterile bandage.

Ophthalmic: Instill ointment in lower conjunctival sac by avoiding contact of ointment tip with eye or skin. **Avoid** contamination with the tube.

Bladder irrigation: **Do not** inject irrigant solution. Connect the container to the inflow lumen of the three-way catheter. Connect the outflow lumen via a sterile disposable plastic tube to a disposable plastic collection bag. Continuously rinse the bladder; **do not** interrupt the inflow or rinse solution for more than a few minutes.

NEVIRAPINE

Viramune, Viramune XR, NVP, and others

Antiviral, nonnucleoside reverse transcriptase inhibitor

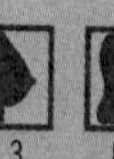

Tabs: 200 mg

Extended-release tabs (Viramune XR): 400 mg

Oral suspension: 10 mg/mL (240 mL); contains parabens

Treatment of HIV (see remarks regarding dosing and presence of rash):

Neonate, infant, and child:

≥15 days to 8 yr old: Start with 200 mg/m²/dose once daily PO × 14 days; if no rash or other side effects, increase to 200 mg/ m²/dose Q12 hr PO (**max. dose:** 200 mg/dose) has been recommended by the Pediatric HIV guidelines (www.hivatis.gov). Alternative FDA-labeled dosage: 150 mg/m²/dose PO (**max. dose:** 200 mg/dose) using the same dosing interval from earlier.

≥8 yr old: Start with 120–150 mg/m²/dose once daily PO × 14 days; if no rash or other side effects, increase to 120–150 mg/ m²/dose Q12 hr PO (**max. dose:** 200 mg/dose).

Adolescent and adult: Start with 200 mg/dose once daily PO × 14 days; if no rash or other side effects, increase to 200 mg/dose Q12 hr.

Continued

For explanation of icons, see p. 364.

NEVIRAPINE *continued*

Nevirapine Extended-Release (Viramune XR):

Adult: 400 mg PO once daily; patients must be initiated with the immediate-release product first. For nevirapine-naïve patients, initiate therapy with 200 mg immediate-release tabs once daily for 14 days (if patient develops a rash during initial 14-day period, do not start extended-release product until rash resolves and do not continue immediate-release lead-in period beyond 28 days). Patients already receiving 200-mg immediate-release tabs Q12 hr may be converted to the extended-release product.

Prevention of vertical transmission during high-risk situations (women who received no antepartum antiretroviral prophylaxis, women with suboptimal viral suppression at delivery, or women with known antiretroviral drug-resistant virus) and in combination with zidovudine:

Newborn: 3 doses (based on birth weight) in the first week of life; Dose 1: within 0–48 hr of birth; Dose 2: 48 hr after Dose 1; Dose 3: 96 hr after Dose 2

Birth weight 1.5–2 kg: 8 mg/dose PO

Birth weight >2 kg: 12 mg /dose PO

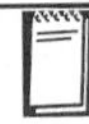

Contraindications: Hypersensitivity to nevirapine or any of its components; moderate-to-severe hepatic impairment (Child–Pugh Class B or C); occupational and nonoccupational postexposure prophylaxis regimens

Warnings/Precautions: **Use with caution** in patients with hepatic or renal dysfunction. **Discontinue therapy** if a severe rash or a rash with fever, blistering, oral lesions, conjunctivitis, or muscle aches occur.

Life-threatening hepatotoxicity has been reported primarily during the first 12 weeks of therapy. Patients with increased serum transaminase or a history of hepatitis B or C infection before nevirapine are at greater risk for hepatotoxicity. Women, including pregnant women, with CD4 counts greater than 250 cells/mm^3 or men with CD_4 counts greater than 400 cells/mm^3 are at risk for hepatotoxicity. Monitor LFTs and CBCs. Noncompliance can quickly promote resistant HIV strains.

If a nonsevere rash without the presence of a transaminase elevation occurs during the first 14 days of therapy, do not increase dose until the rash resolves. If the rash continues beyond 28 days, use an alternative drug. If nevirapine is discontinued for more than 7 days and is restarted, initiate with the once-daily dose for the first 14 days before increasing to BID dosing.

Adverse effects: Skin rash (may be life-threatening, including Stevens–Johnson syndrome; permanently discontinue and never restart), fever, abnormal liver function tests, headache, and nausea are common. Hypersensitivity reactions and hypophosphatemia have been reported. Permanently discontinue and not restart nevirapine if symptomatic hepatitis, severe transaminase elevations, or hypersensitivity reactions occur. See earlier Warnings/Precautions.

Drug interactions: Induces the CYP450 3A4 and 2B6 drug-metabolizing isoenzymes, and causes an autoinduction of its own metabolism within the first 2 to 4 weeks of therapy and has the potential to interact with many drugs. Drug can decrease levels of itraconazole, ketoconazole, maraviroc, methadone, indinavir, ritonavir, saquinavir, and oral/other hormonal contraceptives. Rifampin, rifabutin, and St. John's wort can reduce serum levels of nevirapine and should not be given. Atazanavir + ritonavir, cimetidine, clarithromycin, erythromycin, fosamprenavir, and ketoconazole can increase serum levels of nevirapine and are not recommended for use. **Carefully review the patient's drug profile for other drug interactions each time nevirapine is initiated or when a new drug is added to a regimen containing nevirapine.**

Drug administration: Doses can be administered with food and concurrently with didanosine. If therapy is interrupted longer than 7 days, restart therapy with initial once-daily dosing for 14 days followed by BID dosing.

Extended-release tablets must be swallowed whole and cannot be crushed, chewed, or divided.

NIFURTIMOX
Lampit, Bayer 2502
Antiprotozoal agent

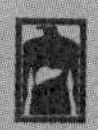
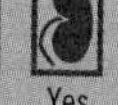
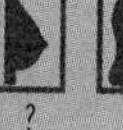
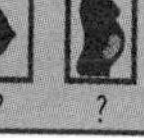

Yes Yes ? ?

AVAILABLE FROM THE U.S. CENTERS FOR DISEASE CONTROL AND PREVENTION (404-639-3670 Monday–Friday 8:00 AM–4:30 PM EST or 404-639-2888 evenings, weekends, or holidays)
Tabs: 30, 120 mg

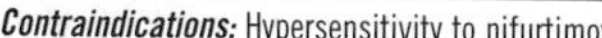

Trypanosomiasis:
Child (duration of treatment: 90 days acute infection and 120 days for chronic infection):
1–10 yr: 15–20 mg/kg/24 hr PO ÷ QID after meals
11–16 yr: 12.5–15 mg/kg/24 hr PO ÷ QID after meals
Adolescent and adult (acute and chronic infections): 8–10 mg/kg/24 hr PO ÷ TID–QID after meals × 90–120 days

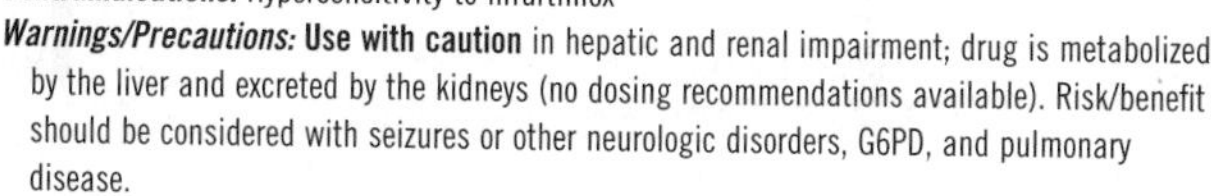

Contraindications: Hypersensitivity to nifurtimox

Warnings/Precautions: **Use with caution** in hepatic and renal impairment; drug is metabolized by the liver and excreted by the kidneys (no dosing recommendations available). Risk/benefit should be considered with seizures or other neurologic disorders, G6PD, and pulmonary disease.

Adverse effects: Anorexia, GI discomfort, rash, cutaneous reactions, and arthralgias are common. Leukopenia, pancytopenia, hemolytic anemia, abnormal LFTs, pulmonary infiltrates, CNS toxicity, and impotence have been reported.

Drug interactions: None identified.

Drug administration: May be taken with meals to minimize GI irritation. Tablets may be crushed and mixed with food.

NITAZOXANIDE
Alinia
Antiprotozoal agent

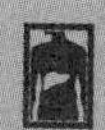
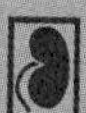
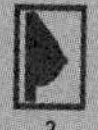
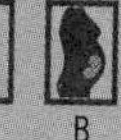

Yes Yes ? B

Oral suspension: 100 mg/5 mL (60 mL); contains sodium benzoate
Tabs: 500 mg; contains soy lecithin

***Diarrhea caused by* Giardia lamblia *or* Cryptosporidium parvum:**
1–3 yr: 100 mg (5 mL) oral suspension Q12 hr PO × 3 days
4–11 yr: 200 mg (10 mL) oral suspension Q12 hr PO × 3 days
≥12 yr and adult: 500 mg tablet Q12 hr PO × 3 days

Hymenolepis nana (dwarf tapeworm):
1–11 yr: Use same dose and duration for diarrhea caused by *Giardia lamblia* or *Cryptosporidium parvum* (see earlier).
≥12 yr and adult: 500-mg tablet once daily or Q12 hr PO × 3 days

Clostridium difficile*–associated diarrhea:*
Adult: 500 mg PO Q12 hr × 7–10 days

Contraindications: Hypersensitivity to nitazoxanide or any other components in the formulation

Warnings/Precautions: **Use with caution** in hepatic or renal dysfunction; studies have not been completed. Has **not** been shown to be superior to placebo for the treatment of diarrhea caused by *Cryptosporidium parvum* in immunocompromised patients, including HIV. Has **not** been studied for *Giardia lamblia* in HIV or immunocompromised patients. Tablets and oral suspension are not bioequivalent; suspension is 70% bioavailable to the tablet.

Continued

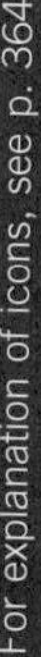
For explanation of icons, see p. 364.

NITAZOXANIDE *continued*

Adverse effects: Abdominal pain, diarrhea, headache, nausea and vomiting are common.

Drug interactions: Drug's metabolite, tizoxanide, is highly protein bound (>99.9%); use caution when used with other highly protein-bound drugs.

Drug administration: Administer all doses with food; drug was administered with food in clinical trials.

NITROFURANTOIN
Furadantin, Macrodantin, Macrobid, and others
Antibiotic

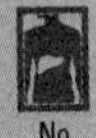 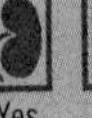 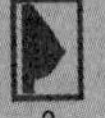 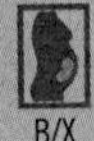
No Yes 2 B/X

Caps (macrocrystals; Macrodantin): 25, 50, 100 mg
Caps (dual-release; Macrobid): 100 mg (25 mg macrocrystal/75 mg monohydrate)
Oral suspension (Furadantin): 25 mg/5 mL (230 mL); contains parabens and saccharin

Child (>1 mo):
Treatment: 5–7 mg/kg/24 hr ÷ Q6 hr PO; **max. dose:** 400 mg/24 hr
UTI prophylaxis: 1–2 mg/kg/dose QHS PO; **max. dose:** 100 mg/24 hr

≥12 yr and adult:
(Macrocrystals): 50–100 mg/dose Q6 hr PO
(Dual-release): 100 mg/dose Q12 hr PO
UTI prophylaxis (macrocrystals): 50–100 mg/dose PO QHS

Contraindications: Hypersensitivity to nitrofurantoin, severe renal disease, infants younger than 1 month, GFR less than 60 mL/min (reduced drug distribution in the urine), active/previous cholestatic jaundice/hepatic dysfunction; and pregnant women at term (38–42 weeks' gestation; pregnancy category changes to "X" at term)

Warnings/Precautions: **Use with caution** in G6PD deficiency, anemia, lung disease, and peripheral neuropathy. Breast-feeding in mothers receiving nitrofurantoin is not recommended in infants younger than 1 month and those with G6PD deficiency.

Adverse effects: GI disturbances and loss of appetite are common. Hypersensitivity reactions, cholestatic jaundice, headache, hepatotoxicity, polyneuropathy, and hemolytic anemia may occur.

Drug interactions: Anticholinergic drugs and high-dose probenecid may increase nitrofurantoin's effects/toxicity. Magnesium salts may decrease the absorption of nitrofurantoin. Causes false-positive urine glucose with Clinitest.

Drug administration: Give with food or milk.

NORFLOXACIN
Noroxin
Antibiotic, quinolone

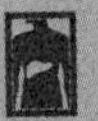 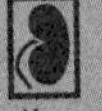 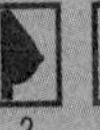 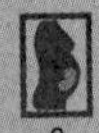
No Yes 2 C

Tabs: 400 mg
Oral suspension: 20 mg/mL 

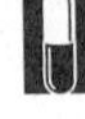

Child:
UTI (limited data in children 5 mo to 19 yr; see remarks): 9–14 mg/kg/24 hr PO ÷ Q12 hr; **max. dose:** 800 mg/24 hr. For UTI prophylaxis, give 2–6 mg/kg/24 hr.

Adult:
UTI: 400 mg PO Q12 hr (× 7–10 days for uncomplicated cases and × 10–21 days for complicated cases)
Prostatitis: 400 mg PO Q12 hr × 28 days

Continued

NORFLOXACIN *continued*

Contraindications: Hypersensitivity to norfloxacin or other quinolones; history of tendinitis or tendon rupture associated with quinolone use

Warnings/Precautions: **Use with caution** in children younger than 18 years, seizures, proarrhythmic conditions, diabetes, patients receiving class Ia or class III antiarrhythmics, and impaired renal function **(adjust dose in renal failure, see Chapter 3).** Like other quinolones, there is concern regarding development of arthropathy. Use with corticosteroids may increase risk for tendon rupture. **Avoid use** in myasthenia gravis; may exacerbate muscle weakness.

Does **not** adequately treat chlamydia co-infections. No longer recommended for gonorrhea by the CDC because of resistance. UTI dosing can be used for BK virus nephropathy in immunocompromised patients.

Adverse effects: GI disturbances, headache, and dizziness are common. QTc prolongation, peripheral neuropathy, myasthenia gravis exacerbation, drug rash with eosinophilia and systemic symptoms (DRESS), seizures, increased intracranial pressure, toxic psychoses, and tendon rupture have been reported.

Drug interactions: Inhibits CYP 450 1A2. May increase serum cyclosporine and theophylline levels, and prolong PT in patients on warfarin. May decrease mycophenolate levels. Probenecid may increase norfloxacin's effects/toxicity. Nitrofurantoin may decrease norfloxacin's antibacterial effects.

Drug administration: Administer oral doses on an empty stomach. If administering with iron-, zinc-, aluminum-, or magnesium-containing products, sucralfate, or buffered didanosine, administer dose 2 hours before or after.

NYSTATIN

Mycostatin, Nilstat, and others

Antifungal agent

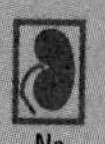
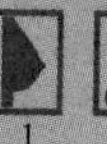
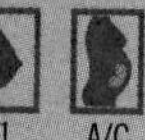

No No I A/C

Tabs: 500,000 units
Oral suspension: 100,000 units/mL (5, 60, 480 mL)
Cream/ointment: 100,000 units/g (15, 30 g)
Topical powder: 100,000 units/g (15, 30 g)
Vaginal tabs: 100,000 units (15s)

Oral:

Preterm infant: 0.5 mL (50,000 units) to each side of mouth QID

Term infant: 1 mL (100,000 units) to each side of mouth QID

Child/adult:

Suspension: 4–6 mL (400,000–600,000 units) swish and swallow QID

Vaginal:

Adolescent and adult: 1 tab QHS × 14 days

Topical: Apply to affected areas BID–QID.

Contraindications: Hypersensitivity to nystatin products

Warnings/Precautions: Treat until 48 to 72 hours after resolution of symptoms. Drug is poorly absorbed through the GI tract. Pregnancy category is an "A" for the vaginal product and "C" for oral and topical products.

Adverse effects: May produce diarrhea and GI side effects, especially with large systemic doses. Local irritation, contact dermatitis, and Stevens–Johnson syndrome have been reported.

Continued

For explanation of icons, see p. 364.

NYSTATIN *continued*

Drug interactions: None identified.

Drug administration:

Oral suspension: Should be swished about the mouth and retained in the mouth as long as possible before swallowing.

Topical: Apply liberally to affected areas.

Vaginal: Insert tablet into applicator with the pointed side up. Tablet may be wetted with warm water or water-soluble lubricating gel. Insert applicator into vagina as far as possible and push the plunger all the way in. Remove applicator and wash with warm, soapy water.

OFLOXACIN

Floxin, Floxin Otic, Ocuflox, and others

Antibiotic, quinolone

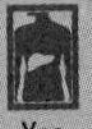
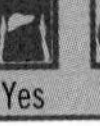
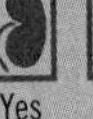
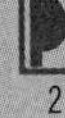
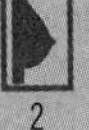
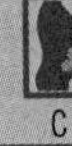
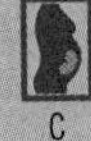

Yes Yes 2 C

Otic solution (Floxin Otic): 0.3% (5, 10 mL)

Ophthalmic solution (Ocuflox): 0.3% (5, 10 mL)

Tabs: 200, 300, 400 mg

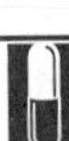

Otic use:

Otitis externa:

6 mo to 12 yr: 5 drops to affected ear(s) once daily × 7days

≥13 yr: 10 drops to affected ear(s) once daily × 7 days

Chronic suppurative otitis media with perforated tympanic membrane:

≥12 yr: 10 drops to affected ear(s) BID × 14 days

Acute otitis media with tympanostomy tubes:

1–12 yr: 5 drops to affected ear(s) BID × 10 days

Ophthalmic use (>1 yr to adult):

Conjunctivitis: 1–2 drops to affected eye(s) Q2–4 hr × 2 days, then QID for an additional 5 days

Corneal ulcer: 1–2 drops to affected eye(s) Q30 min while awake and Q4–6 hr while asleep (awaken) × 2 days, followed by Q1 hr while awake × 5 days, and then QID × 3 days

Systemic use (Adults; see remarks):

Lower respiratory tract and skin infections: 400 mg PO Q12 hr × 10 days

UTI: 200 mg PO Q12 hr × 3–7 days (uncomplicated) or 10 days (complicated)

Prostatitis: 300 mg PO Q12 hr × 6 wk

Contraindications: Hypersensitivity to ofloxacin or other fluoroquinolones

Warnings/Precautions: **Use with caution** in children younger than 18 years, seizures, diabetes, proarrythmic conditions, and in patients receiving class Ia or III antiarrhythmics. Like other quinolones, there is concern regarding development of arthropathy. Use with corticosteroids may increase risk for tendon rupture. **Avoid use** in myasthenia gravis; may exacerbate muscle weakness. **Not recommended** for gonorrhea because of potential resistance.

Adjust dose in severe renal (see Chapter 3) or severe hepatic impairment (**max. dose:** 400 mg/24 hr) with systemic use.

Levofloxacin, the S-isomer of ofloxacin, has replaced systemic ofloxacin because of a more favorable side effect profile.

Adverse effects: Pruritus, rash, GI disturbances, dizziness, headache, and insomnia are common with systemic use. Pruritus, local irritation, taste perversion, dizziness, and earache have been reported with otic use. Ocular burning/discomfort is frequent with ophthalmic use.

Drug interactions: Inhibits CYP450 1A2. May increase effects/toxicity of cyclosporine, theophylline, methylxanthines, warfarin, and glyburide. Antacids containing aluminum, magnesium, and/or

Continued

OFLOXACIN *continued*

calcium, sucralfate, metal cations (e.g., zinc, iron), and didanosine decrease ofloxacin's absorption. Probenecid may increase ofloxacin levels. See earlier Warnings/Precautions.

Drug administration:

PO: Administer oral doses on an empty stomach. If administering with iron, zinc, alluminum- or magnesium-containing products, sulcralfate, or buffered didanosine, administer dose 2 hours before or after.

IV: For intermittent infusion, infuse over 60 minutes at a concentration of 4 mg/mL.

Otic solution: Warm solution by holding the bottle in the hand for 1 to 2 minutes. Cold solutions may result in dizziness. For otitis externa, patient should lie with affected ear upward before instillation and remain in the same position after dose administration for 5 minutes to enhance drug delivery. For acute otitis media with tympanostomy tubes, patient should lie in the same position before instillation and the tragus should be pumped four times after the dose to assist in drug delivery to the middle ear.

Ophthalmic drops: Apply finger pressure to lacrimal sac during and for 1 to 2 minutes after dose application. Remove contact lenses before administration. Lenses may be reinserted 15 minutes after administration.

OSELTAMIVIR PHOSPHATE

Tamiflu

Antiviral

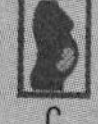

Caps: 30, 45, 75 mg

Oral suspension: 6 mg/mL (60 mL); contains saccharin and sodium benzoate

Treatment of influenza (initiate therapy within 2 days of onset of symptoms):

Neonate:

Pre-term neonate (24–37 weeks' gestation; based on pharmacokinetic data from 20 neonates): 1 mg/kg/dose PO BID

Full-term neonate:

<14 days old: 3 mg/kg/dose PO once daily × 5 days

≥14–28 days old: 3 mg/kg/dose PO BID × 5 days

Child <1 yr: See following table.

Age (mo)	Dosage for 5 days	Volume of Oral Suspension (6 mg/mL)
<3	12 mg PO BID	2 mL
3–5	20 mg PO BID	3.33 mL
6–11	25 mg PO BID	4.2 mL

Child ≥1–12 yr: See following table.

Weight (kg)	Dosage for 5 days	Volume of Oral Suspension (6 mg/mL)
≤15	30 mg PO BID	5 mL
>15–23	45 mg PO BID	7.5 mL
>23–40	60 mg PO BID	10 mL
>40	75 mg PO BID	12.5 mL

≥13 yr and adult: 75 mg PO BID × 5 days

Continued

For explanation of icons, see p. 364.

OSELTAMIVIR PHOSPHATE *continued*

Prophylaxis of influenza (initiate therapy within 2 days of exposure; see remarks):

Child 3 mo to <1 yr: 3 mg/kg/dose PO once daily; alternative dosage based on age:

3–5 mo: 20 mg PO once daily

6–11 mo: 25 mg PO once daily

Child 1–12 yr:

≤15 kg: 30 mg PO once daily

16–23 kg: 45 mg PO once daily

24–40 kg: 60 mg PO once daily

>40 kg: 75 mg PO once daily

≥13 yr and adult: 75 mg PO once daily for a minimum of 7 days and up to 6 wk; initiate therapy within 2 days of exposure.

Contraindications: Hypersensitivity to oseltamivir or any other component of the product

Warnings/Precautions: Currently indicated for the treatment of influenza A and B strains. **Do not use** in children younger than 1 year because of concerns of fatalities related to excessive CNS penetration in 7-day-old rats. Self-injury and delirium in children have been reported. **Adjust dose in renal impairment (see Chapter 3).** Dosage adjustments in severe renal impairment (GFR <10 mL/min) have not been established for either treatment or prophylaxis use. No dosage adjustment is needed for mild-to-moderate hepatic impairment (Child–Pugh score ≤9). The safety and efficacy of repeated treatment or prophylaxis courses have **not** been evaluated.

Prophylaxis use: Oseltamivir is not a substitute for annual flu vaccination. Safety and efficacy have been demonstrated for ≤6 weeks; duration of protection lasts for as long as dosing is continued. Adjust prophylaxis dose if GFR is 10 to 30 mL/min to 75 mg PO every other day for adults.

Adverse effects: Nausea and vomiting generally occur within the first 2 days and are the most common adverse effects. Insomnia, vertigo, seizures, hypothermia, neuropsychiatric events (may result in fatal outcomes), arrhythmias, rash, and toxic epidermal necrolysis have also been reported.

Drug interactions: Probenecid increases oseltamivir levels. Oseltamivir decreases the efficacy of the nasal influenzae vaccine (FluMist; discontinue oseltamivir 48 hours before and do not restart for at least 1 to 2 weeks after FluMist administration.)

Drug administration: Doses may be administered with or without food.

OXACILLIN

Various generic brands

Antibiotic, penicillin (penicillinase resistant)

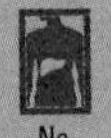
No
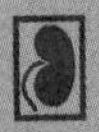
Yes

2
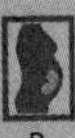
B

Injection: 1, 2, 10 g

Injection, premixed in iso-osmotic dextrose: 1 g/50 mL, 2 g/50 mL

Contains 2.8–3.1 mEq Na per 1 g drug

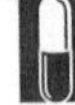

Neonate: IM/IV

≤7 days:

<1.2 kg: 50 mg/kg/24 hr ÷ Q12 hr

1.2–2 kg: 50–100 mg/kg/24 hr ÷ Q12 hr

≥2 kg: 75–150 mg/kg/24 hr ÷ Q8 hr

>7 days:

<1.2 kg: 50 mg/kg/24 hr ÷ Q12 hr

1.2–2 kg: 75–150 mg/kg/24 hr ÷ Q8 hr

≥2 kg: 100–200 mg/kg/24 hr ÷ Q6 hr

Continued

OXACILLIN *continued*

Infant and child (IM/IV): 100–200 mg/kg/24 hr ÷ Q4–6 hr (**max. dose:** 12 g/24 hr); use 200 mg/kg/24 hr for endocarditis or severe infections

Adult (IM/IV): 250–2000 mg/dose Q4–6 hr; use higher end of dosage range for endocarditis or severe infections

Max. dose: 12 g/24 hr

Contraindications: Hypersensitivity to oxacillin and penicillin products

Warnings/Precautions: **Use with caution** with cephalosporin allergy and renal impairment **(adjust dose in renal failure; see Chapter 3).** Use the lower end of the usual dosage range for patients with creatinine clearances <10 mL/min. CSF penetration is poor unless meninges are inflamed.

Adverse effects: Rash and GI disturbances are common. Leukopenia, reversible hepatotoxicity, and acute interstitial nephritis have been reported. Hematuria and azotemia have occurred in neonates and infants with high doses. May cause false-positive urinary and serum proteins.

Drug interactions: Probenecid increases serum oxacillin levels. Tetracycline may antagonize the bactericidal effects of oxacillin.

Drug administration:

IV: For IV push, infuse over 10 min at a concentration ≤100 mg/mL. For intermittent infusion, infuse over 15–30 min at a concentration ≤40 mg/mL.

IM: Dilute with sterile water to 167 mg/mL and inject dose into a large muscle mass.

OXICONAZOLE

Oxistat

Antifungal agent, imidazole

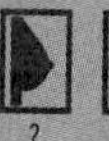

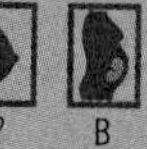

Cream: 1% (30, 60, 90 g)

Lotion: 1% (30, 60 mL)

Both preparations contain propylene glycol, cetyl alcohol, stearyl alcohol, and 0.2% benzoic acid.

≥12 yr to adult:

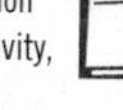

Pityriasis versicolor: Apply cream to affected and surrounding areas once daily × 2 wk.

Tinea corporis, tinea cruris, and tinea pedis: Apply cream or lotion to affected and surrounding areas once daily to twice a day; treat tinea corporis and tinea cruris for 2 weeks and tinea pedis for 1 month.

Contraindications: Hypersensitivity to oxiconazole or any other components in the formulation

Warnings/Precautions: Discontinue use when experiencing a reaction suggestive of sensitivity, or chemical or epidermal irritation.

Hyperpigmented or hypopigmented patches on the trunk extending to the neck, arms, and upper thighs may occur with pityriasis versicolor. Pigment restoration may take months after successful therapy.

Adverse effects: Erythema, pruritus, and burning/stinging sensation are common. Folliculitis, papules, fissure, maceration, rash, and nodules have been reported.

Drug interactions: None identified.

Drug administration: Avoid contact to eyes, vagina, and other mucous membranes. Wash hands after applying dose.

For explanation of icons, see p. 364.

PALIVIZUMAB
Synagis
Monoclonal antibody

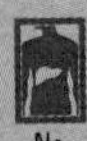
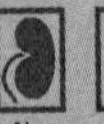
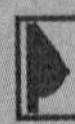
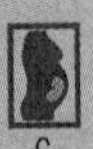

No No ? C

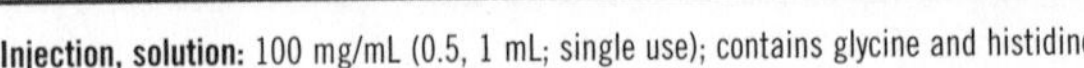

Injection, solution: 100 mg/mL (0.5, 1 mL; single use); contains glycine and histidine

RSV prophylaxis (see latest edition of* AAP Red Book *for most recent indications):
Chronic lung disease ≤2 yr requiring medical therapy within 6 mo of age before RSV season; premature infant [≤28 wk gestation] <12 mo of age; premature infant [29–32 wk gestation] <6 mo of age; hemodynamically significant cyanotic and acyanotic congenital heart disease ≤2 yr; or congenital airway abnormality or neuromuscular disorder <12 mo of age: 15 mg/kg/dose IM monthly just before and during the RSV season

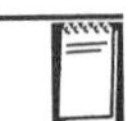

Contraindications: History of a severe reaction to palivizumab or other components to the product

Warnings/Precautions: **Use with caution** in patients with thrombocytopenia or any coagulation disorder because of IM route of administration. IM is currently the only route of administration. RSV season is typically November through April in the Northern Hemisphere but may begin earlier or persist later in certain communities. Palivizumab is currently indicated for RSV prophylaxis in high-risk infants only. Efficacy and safety have **not** been demonstrated for treatment of RSV.

Adverse effects: Rhinitis, rash, pain, increased liver enzymes, pharyngitis, cough, wheeze, diarrhea, vomiting, conjunctivitis, and anemia have been reported at slightly higher incidences when compared with placebo. Anaphylaxis and acute hypersensitivity reactions have been reported (first or subsequent doses).

Drug interactions: Does **not** interfere with the response to routine childhood vaccines (e.g., measles, mumps, rubella, and varicella). May interfere with immunologic-based RSV diagnostic tests such as some antigen detection-based assays. Does not interfere with reverse transcriptase-polymerase chain reaction–based assays.

Drug administration: Each dose should be administered IM in the anterolateral aspect of the thigh. Divide doses with total injection volumes greater than 1 mL. **Avoid** injection in the gluteal muscle because of risk for damage to the sciatic nerve.

PARA-AMINOSALICYLIC ACID
Paser Granules, aminosalicylic acid, PAS
Antituberculosis agent

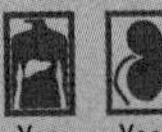
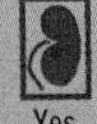
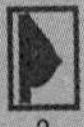
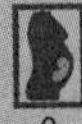
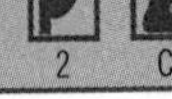

Yes Yes 2 C

Oral granules, delayed release: 4 g/packet; does not contain any sodium or sugar

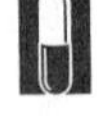

Tuberculosis:
Child (<15 yr or ≤40 kg): 200–300 mg/kg/24 hr PO ÷ BID–QID; **max. dose:** 10 g/24 hr
Adolescent (≥15 yr): 8–12 g/24 hr PO ÷ BID–TID
Adult: 4 g PO TID. Alternatively, 8–12 g/24 hr PO ÷ BID–TID has been recommended.

Contraindications: Hypersensitivity to aminosalicylic acid products and end-stage (severe) renal disease

Warnings/Precautions: **Not recommended** in patients with severe renal failure. **Use with caution** in hepatic insufficiency (drug not well tolerated), peptic ulcer disease, and impaired renal function. Consider maintenance vitamin B_{12} for therapies ≥1 month. Crystalluria may be prevented by maintaining a neutral or an alkaline pH of the urine. **Do not use** product if the package is swollen or the granules are dark brown or purple.

Adverse effects: GI disturbances are common. Immune hypersensitivity reaction, rash with fever, thrombocytopenia, and hepatotoxicity have been reported.

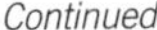

Continued

PARA-AMINOSALICYLIC ACID *continued*

Drug interactions: May reduce the metabolism of isoniazid and decrease the levels of digoxin, rifampin, and vitamin B_{12}.

Drug administration: Sprinkle oral granules on applesauce or yogurt, or mix granules in a glass with an acidic drink such as tomato or orange juice. **Do not use** if packet is swollen or the granules have lost their tan color, turning dark brown or purple. Store granules in the refrigerator or freezer.

PAROMOMYCIN SULFATE
Humatin
Amebicide, antibiotic (aminoglycoside)

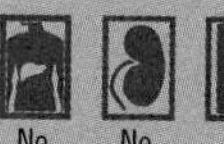
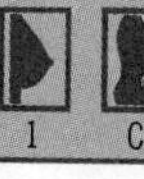

No No 1 C

Caps: 250 mg

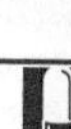

Intestinal amebiasis* (Entamoeba histolytica), Dientamoeba fragilis, *and* Giardia lamblia *infection:
Child and adult: 25–35 mg/kg/24 hr PO ÷ Q8 hr × 7 days

Tapeworm (*Taenia saginata, Taenia solium, Diphyllobothrium latum, *and* Dipylidium caninum*):
Child: 11 mg/kg/dose PO Q15 min × 4 doses
Adult: 1 g PO Q15 min × 4 doses

***Tapeworm* (Hymenolepis nana):**
Child and adult: 45 mg/kg/dose PO once daily × 5–7 days

Cryptosporidial diarrhea:
Adult: 1.5–2.25 g/24 hr PO ÷ 3–6 × daily. Duration varies from 10–14 days to 4–8 wk. Maintenance therapy has also been used. Alternatively, 1 g PO BID × 12 wk in conjunction with 600 mg azithromycin PO once daily × 4 wk has been used in patients with AIDS.

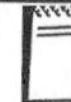

Contraindications: History of hypersensitivity reactions to paromomycin products and intestinal obstruction

Warnings/Precautions: **Use with caution** in ulcerative bowel lesions to avoid renal toxicity via systemic absorption. Drug is generally poorly absorbed and, therefore, **not indicated** for sole treatment of extraintestinal amebiasis.

Adverse effects: GI disturbances are common. Hematuria, rash, ototoxicity, and hypocholesterolemia have been reported. Bacterial overgrowth of nonsusceptible organisms, including fungi, may occur.

Drug interactions: May decrease the effects of digoxin.

Drug administration: Administer doses with or after meals.

PENCICLOVIR
Denavir
Antiviral, topical

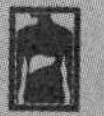
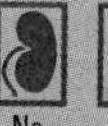
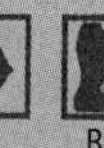
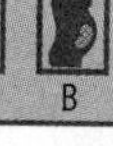

No No ? B

Cream: 1% (1.5, 5 g); contains propylene glycol

Herpes labialis:
≥12 yr and adult: Apply to affected areas Q2 hr while awake × 4 days. Initiate therapy early as possible (during the prodrome or when lesions appear).

Contraindications: Hypersensitivity to penciclovir, famciclovir, or any of its components

Warnings/Precautions: **Not recommended** for use on mucous membranes because of the lack of data. **Avoid** contact with eyes because it can cause irritation. Efficacy has **not** been evaluated in immunocompromised patients and children younger than 12 years.

Continued

For explanation of icons, see p. 364.

PENCICLOVIR *continued*

Adverse effects: Headache and erythema are common. Application-site reaction, rash, taste perversion, and hypesthesia have been reported.

Drug interaction: None identified.

Drug administration: Apply topically to affected lesions of the lips and surrounding skin, and rub gently until the cream disappears.

PENICILLIN G PREPARATIONS—AQUEOUS POTASSIUM AND SODIUM

Pfizerpen and others

Antibiotic, aqueous penicillin

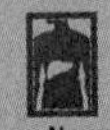
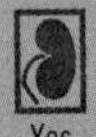
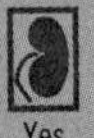
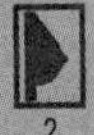
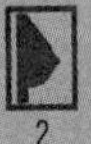
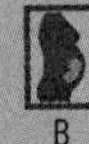
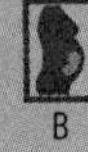
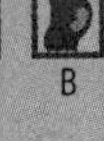

No Yes 2 B

Injection (K⁺): 5, 20 million units (contains 1.7 mEq K and 0.3 mEq Na/1 million units penicillin G)

Premixed frozen injection (K⁺): 1 million units in 50 mL dextrose 4%; 2 million units in 50 mL dextrose 2.3%; 3 million units in 50 mL dextrose 0.7% (contains 1.7 mEq K and 0.3 mEq Na/1 million units penicillin G)

Injection (Na⁺): 5 million units (contains 2 mEq Na/1 million units penicillin G)

Conversion: 250 mg = 400,000 units

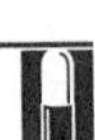

Neonate (IM/IV; use higher end of dosage range for meningitis and severe infections):

≤7 days:

≤2 kg: 50,000–100,000 units/kg/24 hr ÷ Q12 hr

>2 kg: 75,000–150,000 units/kg/24 hr ÷ Q8 hr

>7 days:

<1.2 kg: 50,000–100,000 units/kg/24 hr ÷ Q12 hr

1.2–2 kg: 75,000–150,000 units/kg/24 hr ÷ Q8 hr

≥2 kg: 100,000–200,000 units/kg/24 hr ÷ Q6 hr

Group B streptococcal meningitis:

≤7 days: 250,000–450,000 units/kg/24 hr ÷ Q8 hr

>7 days: 450,000–500,000 units/kg/24 hr ÷ Q4–6 hr

Congenital syphilis (total of 10 days of therapy; if >1 day of therapy is missed, restart the entire course):

≤7 days: 100,000 units/kg/24 hr ÷ Q12 hr IV; increase to following dosage at day 8 of life

>7 days: 150,000 units/kg/24 hr ÷ Q8 hr IV

Infant and child:

IM/IV (use higher end of dosage range for meningitis and severe infections): 100,000–400,000 units/kg/24 hr ÷ Q4–6 hr; **max. dose:** 24 million units/24 hr

Neurosyphilis: 200,000–300,000 units/kg/24 hr ÷ Q4–6 hr IV × 10–14 days; **max. dose:** 24 million units/24 hr

Adult:

IM/IV: 4–24 million units/24 hr ÷ Q4–6 hr

Neurosyphilis: 18–24 million units/24 hr ÷ Q4–6 hr IV × 10–14 days

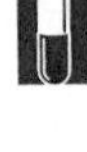

Contraindications: Hypersensitivity to penicillin or any of its components

Warnings/Precautions: **Use with caution** in cephalosporin hypersensitivity. For meningitis, use higher daily dose at shorter dosing intervals. For the treatment of anthrax *(Bacillus anthracis)*, see www.bt.cdc.gov for additional information.

Use penicillin V potassium for oral use. **Adjust dose in renal impairment (see Chapter 3).** Consider the amount of potassium and/or sodium to be provided with the corresponding dosage. Preparations contain potassium and/or sodium salts, which may alter serum electrolytes.

Continued

PENICILLIN G PREPARATIONS—AQUEOUS POTASSIUM AND SODIUM *continued*

Adverse effects: Eosinophilia is common. Anaphylaxis, urticaria, hemolytic anemia, seizures (renal failure, infants, meningitis, and seizure history), interstitial nephritis, and Jarisch–Herxheimer reaction (syphilis) have been reported.

Drug interactions: Tetracyclines, chloramphenicol, and erythromycin may antagonize penicillin's activity.

Probenecid increases penicillin levels. May cause false-positive or negative urinary glucose (Clinitest method), false-positive direct Coombs' test, and false-positive urinary and/or serum proteins.

Drug administration:

IV: For intermittent infusion, infuse over 15–30 min at a concentration 50,000 units/mL for neonates and infants, and 100,000–500,000 units/mL for older patients.

IM: Dilute with sterile water or NS to 50,000–1,000,000 units/mL.

PENICILLIN G PREPARATIONS—BENZATHINE

Bicillin L-A

Antibiotic, penicillin (very-long-acting IM)

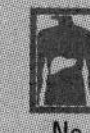 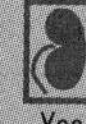 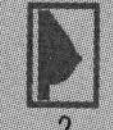 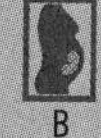

No Yes 2 B

Injection (suspension): 600,000 units/mL (1, 2, 4 mL); contains parabens and povidone

Injection should be IM only.

Group A streptococci:

Infant and child: 25,000–50,000 units/kg/dose IM × 1. **Max. dose:** 1.2 million units/dose ***or***

>1 mo and <27 kg: 600,000 units/dose IM × 1

≥27 kg and adult: 1.2 million units/dose IM × 1

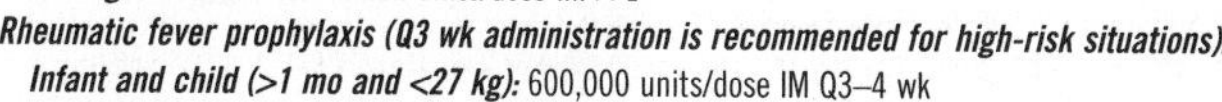

Rheumatic fever prophylaxis (Q3 wk administration is recommended for high-risk situations):

Infant and child (>1 mo and <27 kg): 600,000 units/dose IM Q3–4 wk

Adult: 1.2 million units/dose IM Q3–4 wk

Syphilis (divided total dose into two different injection sites):

Infant and child:

Primary, secondary, and early latent syphilis (<1-yr duration): 50,000 units/kg/dose IM × 1

Late latent, latent with unknown duration syphilis: 50,000 units/kg/dose Q7 days × 3 doses

Max. dose: 2.4 million units/dose

Adult:

Primary, secondary, and early latent syphilis: 2.4 million units/dose IM × 1

Late latent syphilis or latent syphilis of unknown duration: 2.4 million units/dose IM Q7 days × 3 doses

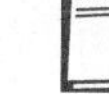

Contraindications: Hypersensitivity to any of the penicillins or any other components in the formulation

Warnings/Precautions: **Use with caution** in renal failure.

FOR INTRAMUSCULAR USE ONLY. Use with caution in asthma, significant allergies, and cephalosporin hypersensitivity. Provides sustained levels for 2 to 4 weeks.

Adverse effects: Rash, urticaria, injection-site reaction, fever, and Jarisch–Herxheimer reaction (syphilis) are common.

Drug interactions: Tetracyclines, chloramphenicol, and erythromycin may antagonize penicillin's activity.

Probenecid increases penicillin levels. May cause false-positive or negative urinary glucose (Clinitest method), false-positive direct Coombs' test, and false-positive urinary and/or serum proteins.

Drug administration: **Deep IM administration only. Do not administer intravenously (cardiac arrest and death may occur) and do not inject into or near an artery or nerve (may result in permanent neurologic damage).** Administer in the midlateral aspect of the thigh for neonates, infants, and small children. Administer in the upper quadrant of the buttock for adults.

For explanation of icons, see p. 364.

PENICILLIN G PREPARATIONS—PENICILLIN G BENZATHINE AND PENICILLIN G PROCAINE

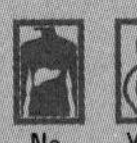 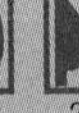 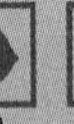 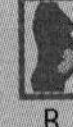

No Yes 2 B

Bicillin C-R, Bicillin C-R 900/300

Antibiotic, penicillin (very-long-acting IM)

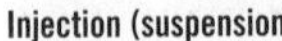

Injection (suspension):

Bicillin CR: 300,000 units PenG procaine + 300,000 units PenG benzathine/mL to provide 600,000 units penicillin per 1 mL (2 mL prefilled syringe)

Bicillin CR (900/300): 150,000 units PenG procaine + 450,000 units PenG benzathine per 1 mL (2 mL prefilled syringe)

All preparations contain parabens and povidone.

Injection should be for IM use only.

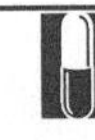

Dosage based on total amount of penicillin.

Group A streptococci:

Child <14 kg: 600,000 units/dose IM × 1

Child 14–27 kg: 900,000–1,200,000 units/dose IM × 1

Child >27 kg and adult: 2,400,000 units/dose IM × 1

Contraindications: Hypersensitivity to procaine or to any penicillin

Warnings/Precautions: **Use with caution** in renal failure, asthma, significant allergies, and cephalosporin hypersensitivity. **Do not use** this product to treat syphilis because of potential treatment failure. The addition of procaine penicillin has not been shown to be more efficacious than benzathine alone. However, it may reduce injection discomfort.

FOR INTRAMUSCULAR USE ONLY; do not administer IV. This preparation provides early peak levels in addition to prolonged levels of penicillin in the blood.

Adverse effects: Injection-site reaction is common. Immune hypersensitivity reaction has been reported.

Drug interactions: Tetracyclines, chloramphenicol, and erythromycin may antagonize penicillin's activity.

Probenecid increases penicillin levels. May cause false-positive or negative urinary glucose (Clinitest method), false-positive direct Coombs' test, and false-positive urinary and/or serum proteins.

Drug administration: **Deep IM administration only. Do not administer IV (cardiac arrest and death may occur), and do not inject into or near an artery or nerve (may result in permanent neurologic damage).** Administer in the midlateral aspect of the thigh for neonates, infants, and small children. Administer in the upper quadrant of the buttock for adults.

PENICILLIN G PREPARATIONS—PROCAINE

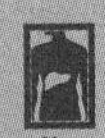 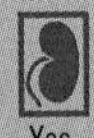 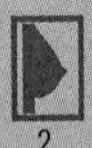 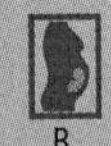

No Yes 2 B

Wycillin and others

Antibiotic, penicillin (long-acting IM)

Injection (suspension): 600,000 units/ml (1, 2 mL); may contain parabens, phenol, povidone, and formaldehyde

Contains 120 mg procaine per 300,000 units penicillin.

Injection should be for IM use only.

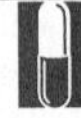

Newborn (see remarks): 50,000 units/kg/dose IM once daily

Infant and child: 25,000–50,000 units/kg/24 hr ÷ Q12–24 hr IM. **Max. dose:** 4.8 million units/24 hr

Adult: 0.6–4.8 million units/24 hr ÷ Q12–24 hr IM

Continued

PENICILLIN G PREPARATIONS—PROCAINE *continued*

Congenital syphilis, syphilis (if >1 day of therapy is missed, restart the entire course):
Neonate, infant, and child: 50,000 units/kg/dose IM once daily × 10 days
Neurosyphilis:
Adult: 2.4 million units IM once daily and 500 mg probenecid Q6 hr PO × 10–14 days (both medications)
Inhalational anthrax: Postexposure prophylaxis (total duration of therapy with all forms of therapy is 60 days; switch to an alternative form of therapy after 2 weeks of procaine penicillin because of the risk for adverse effects):
Child: 25,000 units/kg/dose (**max. dose:** 1.2 million units/dose) IM Q12 hr
Adult: 1.2 million units IM Q12 hr

Contraindications: Hypersensitivity to penicillin/sulfites or procaine
Warnings/Precautions: **Use with caution** in renal failure, neonates (higher incidence of sterile abscess at injection site and risk for procaine toxicity), cephalosporin hypersensitivity, asthma, and significant allergies. No longer recommended for empiric treatment of gonorrhea because of resistant strains. Provides sustained levels for 2 to 4 days. **FOR INTRAMUSCULAR USE ONLY; do not administer IV.**
Adverse effects: Injection-site reaction, rash, and urticaria are common. Immune hypersensitivity reaction has been reported.
Drug interactions: Tetracyclines, chloramphenicol, and erythromycin may antagonize penicillin's activity.
Probenecid increases penicillin levels. May cause false-positive or negative urinary glucose (Clinitest method), false-positive direct Coombs' test, and false-positive urinary and/or serum proteins.
Drug administration: **Deep IM administration only. Do not administer IV (cardiac arrest and death may occur), and do not inject into or near an artery or nerve (may result in permanent neurologic damage).** Administer in the midlateral aspect of the thigh for neonates, infants, and small children. Administer in the upper quadrant of the buttock for adults.

PENICILLIN V POTASSIUM
Veetids and others
Antibiotic, penicillin

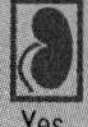
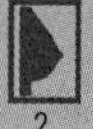
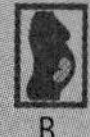

No Yes 2 B

Tabs: 250, 500 mg
Oral solution: 125 mg/5 mL, 250 mg/5 mL (100, 200 mL); may contain saccharin
Contains 0.7 mEq potassium/250 mg drug.
250 mg = 400,000 units

Child: 25–50 mg/kg/24 hr ÷ Q6–8 hr PO. **Max. dose:** 3 g/24 hr
Adolescent and adult: 250–500 mg/dose PO Q6–8 hr
Acute group A streptococcal pharyngitis (use BID dosing regimen ONLY if good compliance is expected):
Child <27 kg: 250 mg PO BID–TID × 10 days
≥27 kg, adolescent and adult: 500 mg PO BID–TID × 10 days
Rheumatic fever prophylaxis and pneumococcal prophylaxis for sickle cell disease and functional or anatomic asplenia (regardless of immunization status):
2 mo to <3 yr: 125 mg PO BID
3–5 yr: 250 mg PO BID; for sickle cell and asplenia, use may be discontinued after 5 years of age if child received recommended pneumococcal immunizations and did not experience invasive pneumococcal infection.

Continued

For explanation of icons, see p. 364.

PENICILLIN V POTASSIUM *continued*

Recurrent rheumatic fever prophylaxis:
Child and adult: 250 mg PO BID

Contraindications: Hypersensitivity to penicillins
Warnings/Precautions: **Use with caution** with cephalosporin hypersensitivity. Penicillin will prevent rheumatic fever if started within 9 days of the acute illness. **Adjust dose in renal failure (see Chapter 3).** GI absorption is better than penicillin G.
Adverse effects: Rash and GI disturbances are common. Hemolytic anemia and immune hypersensitivity reaction have been reported.
Drug interactions: Tetracyclines, chloramphenicol, and erythromycin may antagonize penicillin's activity. Probenecid increases penicillin levels. May cause false-positive or -negative urinary glucose (Clinitest method), false-positive direct Coombs' test, and false-positive urinary and/or serum proteins.
Drug administration: Should be taken 1 hour before or 2 hours after meals. May be administered with food to decrease GI upset.

PENTAMIDINE ISETHIONATE
Pentam 300, NebuPent
Antibiotic, antiprotozoal

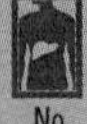
No
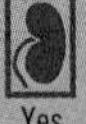
Yes
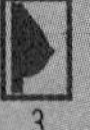
3
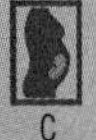
C

Injection (Pentam 300): 300 mg
Inhalation (NebuPent): 300 mg

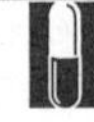

Treatment:
Pneumocystis jiroveci (carinii): 4 mg/kg/24 hr IM/IV once daily × 14–21 days (IV is the preferred route)
Trypanosomiasis (**Trypanosoma** ***gambiense, T. rhodesiense):*** 4 mg/kg/24 hr IM once daily × 7 days
Visceral leishmaniasis (Leishmania donovani, L. infantum, L. chagasi): 4 mg/kg/dose IM once daily or every other day × 15–30 doses
Cutaneous leishmaniasis (**Leishmania** ***[Viannia] panamensis):*** 2–3 mg/kg/dose IM once daily or every other day × 4–7 doses
Prophylaxis:
Pneumocystis jiroveci (formerly carinii):
IM/IV: 4 mg/kg/dose Q2–4 wk
Inhalation
≥5 yr: 300 mg in 6 mL H_2O via inhalation every month. Use with a Respirgard II nebulizer.
Max. single dose: 300 mg

Contraindications: Hypersensitivity to pentamidine or diamidine compounds
Warnings/Precautions: **Use with caution** in ventricular tachycardia, Stevens–Johnson syndrome, and daily doses for more than 21 days. May cause hypoglycemia, hyperglycemia, hypotension (both IV and IM administration), nausea, vomiting, fever, mild hepatotoxicity, pancreatitis, megaloblastic anemia, nephrotoxicity, hypocalcemia, and granulocytopenia. **Adjust dose in renal impairment (see Chapter 3)** with systemic use.
Adverse effects: Rash, nausea, loss of appetite, increased LFTs, and nephrotoxicity (see following Drug Interactions) are common with systemic use. Sterile abscess may occur at IM injection site. Aerosol administration may cause bronchospasm, cough, oxygen desaturation, and dyspnea. See earlier Warnings/Precautions.
Drug interactions: A substrate to CYP P450 2C19. Additive nephrotoxicity with aminoglycosides, amphotericin B, cisplatin, and vancomycin may occur. Avoid use with medications that are high risk for prolonging QTc interval (e.g., thioridazine, pimozide, ziprasidone).

Continued

PENTAMIDINE ISETHIONATE *continued*

Drug administration:

IV: Infuse over 1–2 hr to reduce risk for hypotension at a concentration ≤6 mg/mL.

IM: Reconstitute 300-mg vial with 3 mL sterile water and administer calculated dose by deep IM injection.

Inhalation: Administer with an appropriate-sized (pediatric vs. adult) nebulizer face mask and the Respirgard II nebulizer.

PENTOSTAM

See *Stibogluconate*

PERMETHRIN

Elimite, Acticin, Nix, and many others
Scabicidal agent

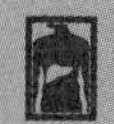
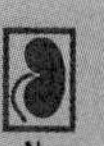
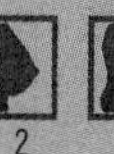
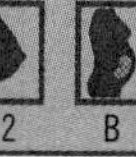

No No 2 B

Cream (Elimite, Acticin): 5% (60 g); contains 0.1% formaldehyde
Liquid cream rinse (Nix-OTC): 1% (60 mL with comb); contains 20% isopropyl alcohol
Lotion (OTC): 1% (60 mL with comb)
Additional permethrin products for use on bedding, furniture, and garments include the following:
Liquid spray (Nix Lice Control Spray): 0.25% (150 mL)
Solution (A200 Lice, Rid): 0.5% (170.1 g or 150 mL)

Pediculus capitis, Phthirus pubis (>2 mo):

Head lice: Saturate hair and scalp with 1% cream rinse after shampooing, rinsing, and towel-drying hair. Leave on for 10 min, then rinse. May repeat in 7 days. May be used for lice in other areas of the body (e.g., pubic lice) in same fashion. If the 1% cream rinse is resistant, the 5% cream may be used after shampooing, rinsing, and towel-drying hair. Leave on for 8–14 hr overnight under a shower cap; then rinse off. May repeat in 7 days.

Scabies: Apply 5% cream from neck to toe (head to toe for infants and toddlers); wash off with water in 8–14 hr. May repeat in 7 days. Use in infants <1 mo is safe and effective when applied for a 6-hr period.

Contraindications: Hypersensitivity to permethrin or chrysanthemums

Warnings/Precautions: May exacerbate pruritus, edema, and erythema. Ovicidal activity generally makes single-dose regimen adequate. However, resistance to permethrin has been reported. For either lice or scabies, instruct patient to launder bedding and clothing. For lice, treat symptomatic contacts only. For scabies, treat all contacts even if asymptomatic. Topical cream dosage form contains formaldehyde, a contact allergen.

Adverse effects: May cause pruritus, hypersensitivity, burning, stinging, erythema, and rash.

Drug administration: Shake well before using. **Avoid** contact with eyes or mucous membranes during application. Dispense one 60-gm cream for one adult or two small children.

PHENAZOPYRIDINE HCL

Pyridium, Azo-Urinary Pain Relief [OTC], and many others
Urinary analgesic

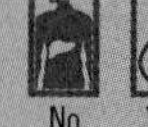
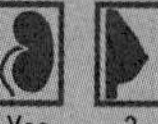
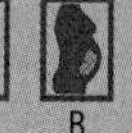

No Yes 3 B

Tabs: 95 mg [OTC], 97.2 mg, 100 mg [OTC and Rx], 200 mg
Oral suspension: 10 mg/mL

Continued

For explanation of icons, see p. 364.

PHENAZOPYRIDINE HCL *continued*

UTI (use with an appropriate antibacterial agent):
Child 6–12 yr: 12 mg/kg/24 hr ÷ TID PO until symptoms of lower urinary tract irritation are controlled or 2 days
Adult: 95–200 mg TID PO until symptoms are controlled or 2 days

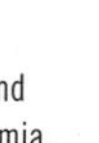

Contraindications: Hypersensitivity to phenazopyridine products and renal insufficiency (GFR <50 mL/min)
Warnings/Precautions: Medication is a urinary analgesic and does **not** treat infections. **Adjust dose in mild renal impairment (see Chapter 3)** and **avoid use** in moderate-to-severe impairment (GFR <50 mL/min).
Adverse effects: Pruritus, rash, GI distress, and headache are common. Colors urine orange and stains clothing. May also stain contact lenses. Anaphylactoid-like reaction, methemoglobinemia, hemolytic anemia, renal toxicity, and hepatic toxicity have been reported, usually at overdosage levels.
Drug interactions: May interfere with urinalysis tests (false-negative) based on spectrometry or color reactions.
Drug administration: Give doses after meals.

PIPERACILLIN
Pipracil and others
Antibiotic, penicillin (extended spectrum)

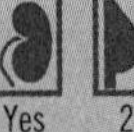 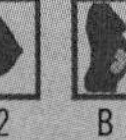 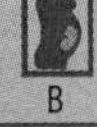
No Yes 2 B

Injection: 2, 3, 4, 40 g
Contains 1.85 mEq Na/g drug.

Neonate, IV:
≤7 days:
≤36 wk of gestation: 150 mg/kg/24 hr ÷ Q12 hr
>36 wk of gestation: 225 mg/kg/24 hr ÷ Q8 hr
>7 days:
≤36 wk of gestation: 225 mg/kg/24 hr ÷ Q8 hr
>36 wk of gestation: 300 mg/kg/24 hr ÷ Q6 hr
Infant and child: 200–300 mg/kg/24 hr IM/IV ÷ Q4–6 hr; **max. dose:** 24 g/24 hr
Cystic fibrosis: 350–600 mg/kg/24 hr IM/IV ÷ Q4–6 hr; **max. dose:** 24 g/24 hr
Adult: 2–4 g/dose IV Q4–6 hr or 1–2 g/dose IM Q6 hr; **max. dose:** 24 g/24 hr

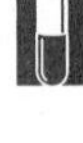

Contraindications: Hypersensitivity to piperacillin, penicillins, or any other components in the formulation
Warnings/Precautions: **Use with caution** in cephalosporin hypersensitivity. Discontinue use if bleeding manifestations should occur. **Adjust dose in renal impairment (see Chapter 3).** Patients with cystic fibrosis have an increased risk for fever and rash. Like other penicillins, CSF penetration occurs only with inflamed meninges.
Adverse effects: Thrombophlebitis, injection-site pain, rash, diarrhea, headache, and fever are common. Seizures (higher doses), prolonged bleeding time, bone marrow suppression, LFT elevations, and acute interstitial nephritis have been reported. See earlier Warnings/Precautions.
Drug interactions: Probenecid increases serum piperacillin levels. May prolong the neuromuscular blockade effects of vecuronium. May falsely lower aminoglycoside serum levels if the drugs are infused close to one another; allow a minimum of 2 hours between infusions to prevent this interaction. Coagulation parameters should be tested more frequently and monitored regularly with high doses of heparin, warfarin, or other drugs that affect blood coagulation or thrombocyte function.

Continued

PIPERACILLIN *continued*

Drug administration:

IV: For IV push, infuse over 3–5 min at a concentration ≤200 mg/mL. For intermittent infusion, infuse over 30–60 min at a concentration ≤20 mg/mL.

IM: Dilute to 400 mg/mL with sterile water, NS, or 0.5% or 1% lidocaine without epinephrine. Assess the potential risk/benefit for using lidocaine as a diluent.

PIPERACILLIN/TAZOBACTAM

Zosyn and others

Antibiotic, penicillin (extended spectrum with β-lactamase inhibitor)

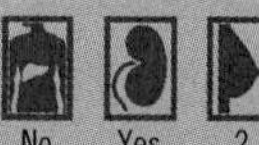
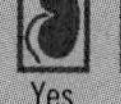
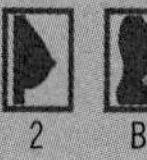

No Yes 2 B

8 : 1 ratio of piperacillin to tazobactam:

Injection, powder: 2 g piperacillin and 0.25 g tazobactam; 3 g piperacillin and 0.375 g tazobactam; 4 g piperacillin and 0.5 g tazobactam; 36 g piperacillin and 4.5 g tazobactam

Injection, premixed in iso-osmotic dextrose: 2 g piperacillin and 0.25 g tazobactam in 50 mL; 3 g piperacillin and 0.375 g tazobactam in 50 mL; 4 g piperacillin and 0.5 g tazobactam in 100 mL

Contains 2.35 mEq Na/g piperacillin.

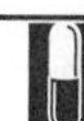

All doses based on piperacillin component.

Neonate: 100 mg/kg/dose at the following intervals:

≤7 days old: Q12 hr

8–28 days old: Q8 hr

Infant <6 mo: 150–300 mg/kg/24 hr IV ÷ Q6–8 hr

Infant >6 mo and child: 300–400 mg/kg/24 hr IV ÷ Q6–8 hr

Adult:

Intraabdominal or soft-tissue infections: 3 g IV Q6 hr

Nosocomial pneumonia: 4 g IV Q6 hr

Cystic fibrosis: See Piperacillin.

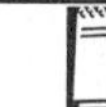

Contraindications: Hypersensitivity to piperacillin, tazobactam, penicillins, or any other components in the formulation.

Warnings/Precautions: **Use with caution** in cephalosporin hypersensitivity or other β-lactamase inhibitors. **Adjust dose in renal impairment (see Chapter 3).** Abnormal platelet aggregation and prolonged bleeding have been reported in patients with renal failure. Patients with cystic fibrosis have an increased risk for fever and rash.

Tazobactam is a β-lactamase inhibitor, thus extending the spectrum of piperacillin. Like other penicillins, CSF penetration occurs only with inflamed meninges.

Adverse effects: GI disturbances, pruritus, rash, and headache are common. See Piperacillin and above Warnings/Precautions section.

Drug interactions: Probenecid increases serum piperacillin levels. May prolong the neuromuscular blockade effects of vecuronium. May falsely decrease aminoglycoside serum levels if the drugs are infused close to one another; allow a minimum of 2 hours between infusions to prevent this interaction. Coagulation parameters should be tested more frequently and monitored regularly with high doses of heparin, warfarin, or other drugs that affect blood coagulation or thrombocyte function.

Drug administration:

IV: Infuse over 30 minutes at a concentration ≤200 mg/mL (piperacillin component); however, concentrations ≤20 mg/mL (piperacillin component) are preferred. Prolonging the dose administration time to 4 hours will maximize the pharmacokinetics/pharmacodynamics properties by prolonging the time of drug concentration above the MIC.

For explanation of icons, see p. 364.

PODOFILOX
Condylox and others
Keratolytic agent

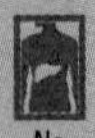 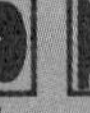 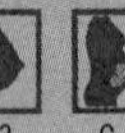 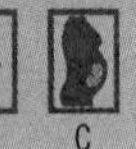

No No 3 C

Topical gel: 0.5% (3.5 mL); contains alcohol
Topical solution: 0.5% (3.5 mL); contains 95% alcohol

Condyloma acuminatum *(external and perianal; see remarks for dosage form specific administration requirements):*
Adult: Apply to affected areas Q12 hr (morning and evening) × 3 consecutive days, then withhold use for 4 consecutive days. This 1-week cycle of treatment may be repeated until there is no visible wart tissue for a **maximum** of 4 cycles. **Limit treatment area to no more than 10 cm² and no more than 0.5 g/24 hr.**

Contraindications: Hypersensitivity or intolerance to podofilox or to any component of the formulation
Warnings/Precautions: **Do not** exceed the recommended method of application, frequency of application, and duration of usage. Safety and efficacy not established for the treatment of mucous membrane warts and in pediatric patients. **Avoid** contact with the eyes.

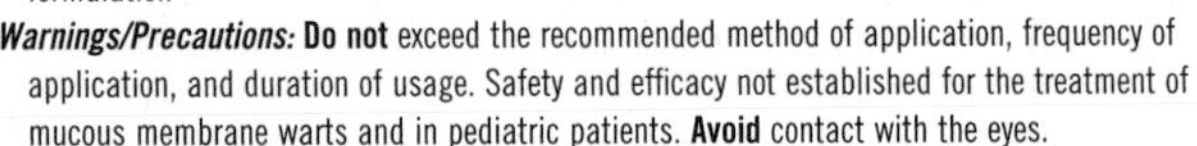

Adverse effects: Pruritus, superficial ulcer of skin, pain, burning sensation, headache, and inflammation are common.
Drug interactions: None identified.
Drug administration: Use the minimum amount necessary to cover lesion by minimizing application to surrounding tissue; allow to dry thoroughly. Do not use occlusive dressings/wrappings.
Topical gel: Apply with applicator tip or finger to genital or anogenital areas. Wash hands thoroughly before and after each application.
Topical solution: Apply with supplied cotton-tip applicator to genital area only. Wash hands thoroughly after each application. Use protective occlusive dressing around wart to prevent contact with unaffected skin.

PODOPHYLLIN/PODOPHYLLUM RESIN
Podocon-25
Keratolytic agent

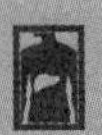 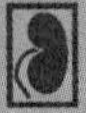 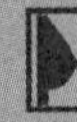 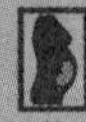 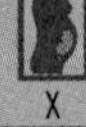

No No X X

Topical liquid: 25% podophyllum resin in tincture of benzoin (15 mL)

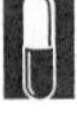

Podophyllin 25% solution should be applied by a physician and not dispensed to a patient. Dilute straight 25% solution with alcohol by one-third to half when applying near mucous membranes. Use concentrations of 5%–10% for very large lesions (>10–20 cm) to minimize toxicity risk.
Adult:
Genital warts: Apply 10%–25% solution sparingly to warts, avoiding contact with healthy tissue. For the first application, leave in contact with skin for no more than 30–40 min; subsequent applications, leave on skin for minimum time to achieve desired results (1–4 hr). After treatment, remove dried medication thoroughly with soap and water or alcohol.

Contraindications: Diabetics, patients using steroids, or patients with poor blood circulation. **Do not** use on bleeding warts, moles, birthmarks, or unusual warts with hair growing from them. Use is contraindicated during pregnancy.
Warnings/Precautions: **For external use only.** Podophyllum is caustic and a severe irritant; **avoid contact with the eyes. Do not** use for perianal or mucous membrane warts. Differentiate wart from squamous cell carcinoma and Bowenoid papulosis; podophyllum is not indicated.

Continued

PODOPHYLLIN/PODOPHYLLUM RESIN *continued*

Adverse effects: Pruritus, superficial skin ulceration, burning sensation, inflammatory disorder, and localized pain are common.

Drug interactions: None identified.

Drug administration: Thoroughly cleanse affected area. Use applicator to apply sparingly to lesion. **Avoid** contact with healthy tissue, eyes, or mucous membranes. After treatment, remove dried medication thoroughly with soap and water or alcohol. Use protective occlusive dressing around wart to prevent contact with unaffected skin.

POLYMYXIN B SULFATE AND BACITRACIN

See *Bacitracin ± Polymyxin B*

POLYMYXIN B SULFATE AND TRIMETHOPRIM SULFATE

Polytrim Ophthalmic Solution and others

Topical antibiotic (ophthalmic preparations listed)

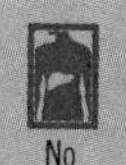
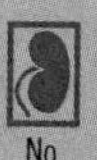
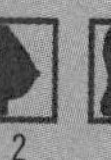

No No 2 C

Ophthalmic solution: Polymyxin B sulfate 10,000 units, trimethoprim sulfate 1 mg/mL (10 mL); some preparations may contain 0.04 mg/mL benzalkonium chloride

≥2 mo and adult: Instill 1 drop in the affected eye(s) Q3 hr (**maximum** of 6 doses/24 hr) × 7–10 days.

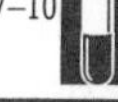

Contraindications: Hypersensitivity to polymyxin, trimethoprim, or any of its components

Warnings/Precautions: **Not indicated** for the prophylaxis or treatment of ophthalmia neonatorum. Prolonged use may result in overgrowth of resistant organisms.

Adverse effects: Local irritation consisting of redness, burning, stinging, and/or itching is common. Hypersensitivity reactions consisting of lid edema, itching, increased redness, tearing, and/or circumocular rash has been reported.

Drug interactions: None identified.

Drug administration: For ophthalmic use only. **Avoid** contaminating the applicator tip. Apply finger pressure to lacrimal sac during and for 1 to 2 minutes after dose application.

POLYMYXIN B SULFATE, NEOMYCIN SULFATE, AND HYDROCORTISONE

Cortisporin Otic, Cortomycin, AK-Spore H.C. Otic, PediOtic, and many other generics

Topical antibiotic (otic and ophthalmic preparations listed)

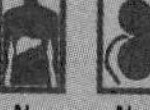
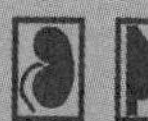
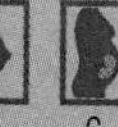
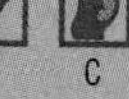

No No 2 C

Otic solution or suspension: Polymyxin B sulfate 10,000 units, neomycin sulfate 5 mg (3.5 mg neomycin base), hydrocortisone 10 mg/mL (10 mL); some preparations may contain thimerosal and metabisulfite.

Ophthalmic suspension: Polymyxin B sulfate 10,000 units, neomycin sulfate 5 mg (3.5 mg neomycin base), hydrocortisone 10 mg/mL (7.5 mL); may contain thimerosal and propylene glycol

Otitis externa:

≥2 yr to adult: 3–4 drops TID-QID × 7–10 days; see remarks for drug administration

Ophthalmic:

Child, adolescent, and adult: Instill 1–2 drops into the affected eye(s) Q3–4 hr.

Continued

For explanation of icons, see p. 364.

POLYMYXIN B SULFATE, NEOMYCIN SULFATE, AND HYDROCORTISONE
continued

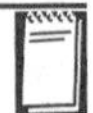

Contraindications: Hypersensitivity to polymyxin B, neomycin, hydrocortisone, or any other components in the formulation. For otic use, **do not use** in cases with perforated eardrum because of possible ototoxicity, and if the external auditory canal disorder is suspected or known to be due to cutaneous viral infection (e.g., HSV or varicella).

Warnings/Precautions: Neomycin may cause sensitization. Prolonged treatment may result in overgrowth of nonsusceptible organisms and fungi.

Otic: **Use with caution** in chronic otitis media and when the integrity of the tympanic membrane is in question. Metabisulfite-containing products may cause allergic reactions to susceptible individuals.

Ophthalmic: **Use with caution** in glaucoma.

Adverse effects: May cause cutaneous sensitization.

Otic: Hypersensitivity (itching, skin rash, redness, swelling, or other sign of irritation in or around the ear) may occur.

Ophthalmic: Blurred vision, burning, and stinging may occur. Increased intraocular pressure and mycosis may occur with prolonged use.

Drug interaction: None identified.

Drug administration: Shake suspension well before use.

Otic: Warm the medication to body temperature before use. Instill drops directly into the affected ear(s). Alternatively, if preferred, a cotton wick may be saturated and inserted into ear canal. Moisten wick with antibiotic every 4 hr. Change wick Q24 hr.

Ophthalmic: **Avoid** contact/contamination with eye dropper tip. Apply finger pressure to lacrimal sac during and for 1–2 min after dose application.

POLYTRIM OPHTHALMIC SOLUTION

See *Polymyxin B Sulfate and Trimethoprim Sulfate*

POSACONAZOLE

Noxafil

Antifungal, triazole

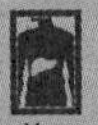
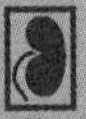
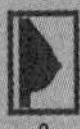
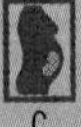

Yes No ? C

Oral suspension: 40 mg/mL (105 mL); with calibrated dosing spoon marked for doses of 2.5 and 5 mL

Child (≥13 yr) and adult:

Treatment of oropharyngeal candidiasis: 100 mg (2.5 mL) PO BID × 1 day, followed by 100 mg PO once daily × 13 days

Treatment of oropharyngeal candidiasis refractory to fluconazole and/or itraconazole: 400 mg (10 mL) PO BID; duration of therapy should be based on severity of the patient's underlying disease and clinical response

Prophylaxis of disseminated candidiasis or aspergillus infection in severely immunocompromised patients: 200 mg (5 mL) PO TID; duration of therapy should be based on recovery from neutropenia or immunosuppression

Chronic granulomatous disease: an open-label, phase II dose finding trial in 12 children 2–16 yr old resulted in adequate drug exposure and safety using the following allometrically derived doses by body weight administered PO Q12 hr (additional studies are needed):

Continued

POSACONAZOLE *continued*

10–14 kg: 120 mg
15–19 kg: 160 mg
20–24 kg: 200 mg
25–29 kg: 220 mg
30–34 kg: 260 mg
35–39 kg: 280 mg
≥40 kg: 300 mg

Contraindications: Hypersensitivity to posaconazole or to any of the excipients. **Avoid** coadministration with ergot alkaloids; and **avoid** CYP3A4 substrates (e.g., terfenadine, astemizole, cisapride, pimozide, halofantrine, or quinidine) because this may increase the plasma concentrations of the drugs, leading to QTc prolongation and rare occurrence of torsades de pointes. Use with HMG-CoA reductase inhibitors (e.g., atorvastatin, lovastatin, and simvastatin) is contraindicated because of risk for rhabdomyolysis.

Warnings/Precautions: **Use with caution** with hepatic impairment (studies have not been completed), hematologic malignancies (may precipitate severe hepatic reactions), hypersensitivity to other azoles, and patients with potentially proarrhythmic conditions. Monitor hepatic function at the start and during the course of therapy. Active against Zygomycetes.

Adverse effects: Abdominal pain, diarrhea, nausea, and vomiting are common. Prolonged QT interval, adrenal insufficiency, cholestasis, hyperbilirubinemia, increased LFTs, liver failure, and seizures have been reported.

Drug interactions: Drug is an inhibitor of the CYP 450 3A4 isoenzyme; may increase the effects/toxicity of atazanavir, cyclosporine, halofantrine, ritonavir, sirolimus **(contraindicated),** tacrolimus, phenytoin, midazolam, rifabutin, vincristine, and vinblastine. See earlier Contraindications section for additional interactions. Drug is primarily metabolized via UDP glucuronidation and a substrate for P-glycoprotein (P-gp) efflux. Rifabutin, phenytoin, efavirenz, fosamprenavir, and cimetidine may decrease posaconazole levels, and use should be **avoided** unless benefit outweighs the risks.

Drug administration: Shake oral suspension well before each use. Administer each dose with a full meal or liquid nutritional supplement for optimal absorption. Consider an alternative antifungal agent if patient is unable to eat a full meal or tolerate an oral nutritional supplement. Use the provided measuring spoon and rinse with water after each use.

POTASSIUM IODIDE
Iosat, Pima, SSKI, ThyroShield, ThyroSafe, and others
Antithyroid agent

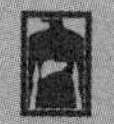
No
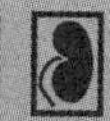
Yes
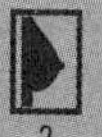
2
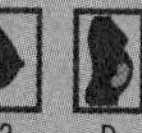
D

Tabs:
ThyroSafe (OTC): 65 mg (50 mg iodine)
Iosat: 130 mg
Syrup (Pima): 325 mg/5 mL (249 mg iodine per 5 mL) (473 mL, 4000 mL)
Oral solution:
ThyroShield (OTC): 65 mg/mL (30 mL); contains parabens and saccharin
Saturated solution (SSKI): 1000 mg/mL (30, 240 mL); 10 drops = 500 mg potassium iodide
Lugol's (strong iodine) solution: potassium iodide 100 mg/mL in combination with iodine 50 mg/mL (120, 473 mL)
Potassium content: 6 mEq (234 mg) K^+/gram potassium iodide

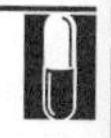

Cutaneous or lymphocutaneous sporotrichosis (treat for 4–6 wk after lesions have completely healed; increase dose until either maximum dose is achieved or signs of intolerance appear):

Continued

For explanation of icons, see p. 364.

POTASSIUM IODIDE *continued*

Child and adult: Start with 250 mg PO TID. Dosages may be gradually increased as tolerated to the following **maximum** dosages:

Child max.: 1250–2000 mg PO TID

Adult max.: 2000–2500 mg PO TID

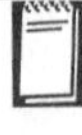

Contraindications: Pregnancy, iodide hypersensitivity, hyperkalemia, hypothyroidism, and iodine-induced goiter

Warnings/Precautions: **Use with caution** in thyroid disease, cardiac disease, and renal failure. May cause acne flare-up. Monitor thyroid function tests. Use in breastfeeding may cause transient hypothyroidism to infant.

Adverse effects: GI disturbance, metallic taste, rash, salivary gland inflammation, headache, lacrimation, and rhinitis are symptoms of iodism. Paresthesia and immune hypersensitivity reaction have been reported.

Drug interactions: Lithium carbonate, antithyroid medications, and iodide-containing medications may have synergistic hypothyroid activity. Potassium-containing medications, potassium-sparing diuretics, and ACE inhibitors may increase serum potassium levels.

Drug administration: Dilute strong iodine solution with large amounts of water, milk, broth, or fruit juice to improve taste. Give with milk or water after meals.

PRAZIQUANTEL

Biltricide

Anthelmintic

 Yes 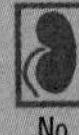 No 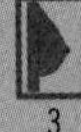 3 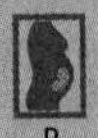 B

Tabs: 600 mg (tri-scored)

Child and adult:

Schistosomiasis:

Schistosoma haematobium, Schistosoma intercalatum, *and* Schistosoma mansoni: 20 mg/kg/dose PO BID × 1 day

Schistosoma japonicum *and* Schistosoma mekongi: 20 mg/kg/dose PO TID × 1 day

Flukes:

Fasciolopsis buski, Heterophyes heterophyes, Metagonimus yokogawai, *and* Metorchis conjunctus: 25 mg/kg/dose PO Q8 hr × 1 day

Nanophyetus salmincola: 20 mg/kg/dose PO Q8 hr × 1 day

Clonorchis sinensis, Opisthorchis viverrini, *and paragonimiasis (e.g.,* Paragonimus westermani*):* 25 mg/kg/dose PO Q8 hr × 2 days

Tapeworms:

Cysticercosis (taenia solium): 100 mg/kg/24 hr PO ÷ Q8 hr × 1 day, then 50 mg/kg/24 hr PO ÷ Q8 hr × 29 days (dexamethasone may be added to regimen for 2–3 days to minimize inflammatory response)

Diphyllobothrium latum, Taenia saginata, Taenia solium, *and* Dipylidium canium: 5–10 mg/kg/dose PO × 1 dose

Hymenolepis nana: 25 mg/kg/dose PO × 1 dose

Contraindications: Hypersensitivity to praziquantel or ocular cysticercosis.

Strong CYP 450 inducers (e.g., rifampin) are contraindicated; consider alternative therapy to praziquantel. If praziquantel is necessary, discontinue rifampin 4 weeks before initiating praziquantel and restart rifampin 1 day after completing praziquantel.

Warnings/Precautions: **Use with caution** in patients with severe hepatic disease, history of seizures, or cardiac irregularities. Hospitalize patients being treated for schistosomiasis or fluke infection associated with cerebral cysticercosis.

Continued

PRAZIQUANTEL *continued*

Adverse effects: Abdominal pain, dizziness, drowsiness, headache, and malaise are common. Seizures, pruritus, cardiac dysrhythmia, eosinophilia, heart block, intracranial hypertension, and increased CSF protein have been reported. Hyperthermia has occurred in patients treated for neurocysticercosis.

Drug interactions: Carbamazepine, phenytoin, rifampin (see Contraindications) and chloroquine may decrease praziquantel's effects. Cimetidine may increase praziquantel's effects. Alcohol may increase CNS depression.

Drug administration: Take with food. **Do not** chew tablets because of bitter taste.

PRIMAQUINE PHOSPHATE
Various generic brands
Antimalarial

No No ? C

Tabs: 26.3 mg (15 mg base)
Oral suspension: 10.52 mg (6 mg base)/5 mL

All doses expressed in milligrams of primaquine base:

Malaria:

Prevention of relapses for Plasmodium vivax or Plasmodium ovale only (initiate therapy during the last 2 weeks of, or following a course of, suppression with chloroquine or comparable drug):

Child: 0.5 mg/kg/dose (**max. dose:** 30 mg/dose) PO once daily × 14 days
Adult: 30 mg PO once daily × 14 days

Prevention of chloroquine-resistant strains (initiate 1 day before departure and continue until 3–7 days after leaving endemic area):

Child: 0.5 mg/kg/dose (**max. dose:** 30 mg/dose) PO once daily
Adult: 30 mg PO once daily

Pneumocystis *jiroveci (carinii) pneumonia (in combination with clindamycin):*

Child: 0.3 mg/kg/dose (**max. dose:** 30 mg/dose) PO once daily × 21 days
Adult: 30 mg PO once daily × 21 days

Contraindications: Granulocytopenia (e.g., rheumatoid arthritis, lupus erythematosus) and bone marrow suppression. **Avoid use** with quinacrine and with other drugs that have a potential for causing hemolysis or bone marrow suppression.

Warnings/Precautions: **Use with caution** in G6PD and NADH methemoglobin-reductase–deficient patients because of increased risk for hemolytic anemia and leukopenia, respectively. Use in pregnancy is **not recommended** by the *AAP Red Book.* Cross-sensitivity with iodoquinol.

Adverse effects: May cause headache, visual disturbances, nausea, vomiting, and abdominal cramps. Hemolytic anemia, leukopenia, and methemoglobinemia have been reported.

Drug interactions: Quinacrine may increase primaquine toxicity; **avoid use.**

Drug administration: Administer all doses with food to mask bitter taste.

PYRANTEL PAMOATE
Antiminth, Reese's Pinworm, Pamix, Pin-Rid, and Pin-X
Anthelmintic

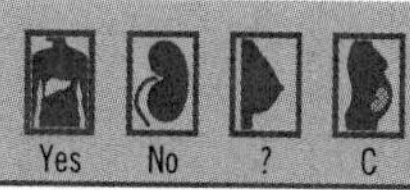

Oral suspension (OTC): 50 mg/mL pyrantel base (144 mg/mL pyrantel pamoate) (30, 60 mL); may contain sodium benzoate, parabens, and saccharin

Continued

For explanation of icons, see p. 364.

PYRANTEL PAMOATE *continued*

Liquid (OTC): 50 mg/mL pyrantel base (144 mg/mL pyrantel pamoate) (30 mL); may contain parabens
Tabs (OTC): 62.5 mg pyrantel base (180 mg pyrantel pamoate)
Chewable tabs (OTC): 250 mg pyrantel base (720.5 mg pyrantel pamoate); contains aspartame

All doses expressed in terms of pyrantel base.
Child (≥2 yr) and adult:
Ascaris (roundworm) and Trichostrongylus: 11 mg/kg/dose PO × 1
Enterobius (pinworm): 11 mg/kg/dose PO × 1. Repeat same dose 2 wk later.
Hookworm or eosinophilic enterocolitis: 11 mg/kg/dose PO once daily × 3 days
Moniliformis: 11 mg/kg/dose PO × 1. Repeat twice 2 weeks apart.
Max. dose (all indications): 1 g/dose

Contraindications: Hypersensitivity to pyrantel or any of its components. **Do not** use in combination with piperazine because of antagonism.
Warnings/Precautions: **Use with caution** in liver dysfunction, anemia, severe malnutrition, and pregnancy. Chewable tablet dosage form contains aspartame. Limited experience in children younger than 2 years.
Adverse effects: May cause nausea, vomiting, anorexia, transient AST elevations, headaches, rash, and muscle weakness.
Drug interactions: May increase theophylline levels. See earlier Contraindications.
Drug administration: Drug may be mixed with milk or fruit juices and may be taken with food.

PYRAZINAMIDE

Pyrazinoic acid amide
Antituberculous agent

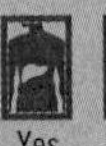 Yes 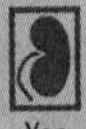 Yes 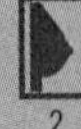 2 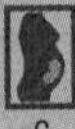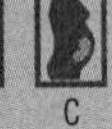 C

Tab: 500 mg
Oral suspension: 10, 100 mg/mL
In combination with isoniazid and rifampin (Rifater):
Tab: 300 mg with 50 mg isoniazid and 120 mg rifampin; contains povidone and propylene glycol

Tuberculosis: Use as part of a multidrug regimen. See latest edition of the* AAP Red Book *for recommended treatment for tuberculosis.
Child:
Daily dose: 30–40 mg/kg/24 hr PO ÷ once to twice daily; **max. dose:** 2 g/24 hr
Twice-weekly dose: 50 mg/kg/dose PO 2 × per week; **max. dose:** 2 g/dose
Adult:
Daily dose: 15–30 mg/kg/24 hr PO ÷ once to twice daily; **max. dose:** 2 g/24 hr
Twice-weekly dose: 50–70 mg/kg/dose PO 2 × per week; **max. dose:** 4 g/dose
Mycobacterium tuberculosis ***in HIV, prophylaxis to prevent first episode:***
Infant and child: Not recommended because of increased risk for severe/fatal hepatotoxicity.
Adolescent and adult: 15–20 mg/kg/24 hr PO once daily × 2 mo in combination with either 600 mg rifampin PO once daily × 2 mo or 300 mg rifabutin PO once daily × 2 mo

Contraindications: Hypersensitivity to pyrazinamide products, acute gout, and severe hepatic damage
Warnings/Precautions: **Use with caution** in patients with renal failure (dosage reduction has been recommended), liver disease, gout, or diabetes mellitus. Monitor LFTs (baseline and periodic) and serum uric acid. The CDC and ATS **do not** recommend the combination of pyrazinamide and

Continued

PYRAZINAMIDE *continued*

rifampin for latent TB infections. For HIV *M. tuberculosis* prophylaxis and treatment, see www.aidsinfo.nih.gov for latest recommendations.

Adverse effects: Hepatotoxicity (dose related, dosages ≤30 mg/kg/24 hr minimize effect), hyperuricemia, GI disturbances, and arthralgia are common. Maculopapular rash, fever, acne, porphyria, dysuria, and photosensitivity may occur.

Drug interactions: May decrease isoniazid levels. **Severe and fatal hepatic toxicity may occur when used with rifampin.** May interfere with Acetest and Ketostix urine test to produce a pink–brown color.

Drug administration: May be taken with or without food or milk. If using the fixed-combination product (Rifater), give 1 hour before or 2 hours after a meal with a full glass of water.

PYRETHRINS WITH PIPERONYL BUTOXIDE
Tisit, A-200, Pronto, RID, Klout and others
Pediculicide

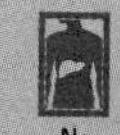
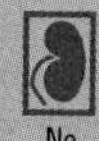
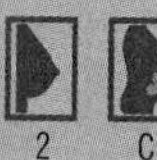

No No 2 C

All products are available without a prescription.
Lotion (Tisit): 0.3% pyrethrins and 2% piperonyl butoxide (59, 118 mL); contains petroleum distillate and equivalent to 1.6% ether
Gel (Tisit): 0.3% pyrethrins and 3% piperonyl butoxide (30 mL)
Shampoo (Tisit, RID, Pronto, A-200, Klout): 0.33% pyrethrins and 4% piperonyl butoxide (60, 120, 240 mL); may contain alcohol and benzyl alcohol
Mousse (RID): 0.33% pyrethrins and 4% piperonyl butoxide (165 mL); contains alcohol

Pediculosis: Apply to hair or affected body area for 10 min, then wash thoroughly and comb with fine-tooth comb or nit-removing comb; repeat in 7–10 days.

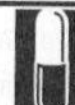

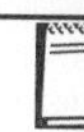

Contraindications: Ragweed hypersensitivity; drug is derived from chrysanthemum flowers

Warnings/Precautions: **Do not use** near eyes, mouth, nose, or vagina. Low ovicidal activity requires repeat treatment. Dead nits require mechanical removal. Wash bedding and clothing to eradicate infestation.

Adverse effects: Local irritation including erythema, pruritus, urticaria, edema, and eczema may occur. Rare immune hypersensitivity reaction has been reported.

Drug interactions: None identified.

Drug administration: For topical use only. **Avoid** vaginal, eye, or facial contact and PO intake. **Avoid** repeat applications in less than 24 hours.

PYRIMETHAMINE
Daraprim
Antiparasitic agent ± sulfonamide antibiotic

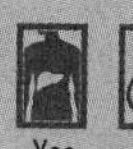
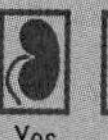
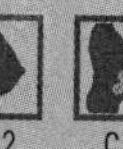
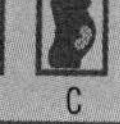

Yes Yes 2 C

Tabs: 25 mg
Oral suspension: 2 mg/mL
Combination product with sulfadoxine (Fansidar) is no longer available in the United States.

Congenital toxoplasmosis (administer with sulfadiazine and leucovorin; see remarks):
Load: 2 mg/kg/24 hr PO ÷ Q12 hr × 2 days
Maintenance: 1 mg/kg/24 hr PO once daily × 2–6 mo, then 1 mg/kg/24 hr 3 ×/wk to complete total 12 mo of therapy

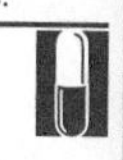

Continued

For explanation of icons, see p. 364.

PYRIMETHAMINE *continued*

Toxoplasmosis (administer with sulfadiazine or trisulfapyrimidines and leucovorin)

Child:

Load: 2 mg/kg/24 hr PO ÷ BID × 3 days; **max. dose:** 100 mg/24 hr

Maintenance: 1 mg/kg/24 hr PO ÷ once to twice daily × 4 wk; **max. dose:** 25 mg/24 hr

Adult: 50–75 mg/24 hr × 3–4 wk depending on response. After response, decrease dose by 50% and continue for an additional 4–5 wk.

Toxoplasma gondii ***(see remarks):***

First episode prophylaxis:

Child ≥1 mo: 1 mg/kg/dose (**max. dose:** 25 mg) PO once daily with dapsone 2 mg/kg PO once daily plus leucovorin 5 mg PO Q3 days

Adolescent and adult: 75 mg PO Q7 days with dapsone 200 mg PO Q7 days plus leucovorin 25 mg PO Q7 days

Recurrence prophylaxis:

Child ≥1 mo: 1 mg/kg/dose (**max. dose:** 25 mg) PO once daily with sulfadiazine 85–120 mg/kg/24 hr PO ÷ BID–QID plus leucovorin 5 mg PO Q3 days

Adolescent and adult: 25–50 mg PO once daily with sulfadiazine 500–1000 mg PO QID, OR clindamycin 300–450 mg PO Q6–8 hr, plus leucovorin 10–25 mg PO once daily

Pneumocystis ***jiroveci (carinii):***

First episode or recurrence prophylaxis:

Adolescent and adult: 50–75 mg PO Q7 days with dapsone (50 mg PO once daily or 200 mg PO Q7days) plus leucovorin 25 mg PO Q7 days.

Contraindications: Hypersensitivity to pyrimethamine products and megaloblastic anemia secondary to folate deficiency

Warnings/Precautions: **Use with caution** in G6PD deficiency, malabsorption syndromes, alcoholism, pregnancy, and renal or hepatic impairment. Pyrimethamine is a folate antagonist. Supplementation with folinic acid leucovorin at 5–15 mg/24 hr is recommended. For congenital toxoplasmosis, see Clin Infect Dis 1994; 18:38–72. Most cases of acquired toxoplasmosis **do not** require specific antimicrobial therapy.

Adverse effects: Rash is common. Glossitis, bone marrow suppression, seizures, and photosensitivity may occur.

Drug interactions: Aurothioglucose, trimethoprim, and sulfamethoxazole may increase risk for blood dyscrasias. Zidovudine and methotrexate may increase risk for bone marrow suppression.

Drug administration: Administer doses with meals.

QUINIDINE GLUCONATE

Quinidine gluconate and various generic brands

Antiarrhythmic, class Ia

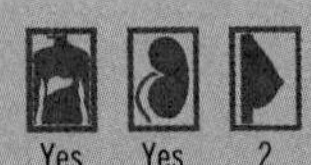

Injection: 80 mg/mL (50 mg/mL quinidine) (10 mL); contains phenol

Slow-release tabs: 324 mg

Quinidine gluconate salt contains 62% quinidine base

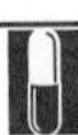

All doses expressed as quinidine gluconate salt.

Malaria (see remarks):

Child and adult (give IV as gluconate; see remarks):

Loading dose: 10 mg/kg/dose (**max. dose:** 600 mg) IV in NS over 1–2 hr followed by maintenance dose. Omit or decrease load if patient has received quinine or mefloquine.

Maintenance dose: 0.02 mg/kg/min IV as continuous infusion until oral therapy can be initiated. If >48 hr of IV therapy is required, reduce dose by 30%–50%.

Continued

QUINIDINE GLUCONATE *continued*

Contraindications: Quinidine, quinine, or cinchona alkaloid hypersensitivity, myasthenia gravis, digitalis intoxication, complete AV block with AV junctional or idioventricular pacemaker, intraventricular conduction defects, and absense of atrial activity

Warnings/Precautions: **Use with caution** in renal insufficiency (15%–25% of drug is eliminated unchanged in the urine), myocardial depression, sick sinus syndrome, G6PD deficiency, and hepatic dysfunction. Continuous monitoring of ECG, blood pressure, and serum glucose are recommended, especially in pregnant women and young children.

To assess for possible idiosyncratic reaction to quinidine, the following test dose of **quinidine sulfate salt** administered several hours before full doses has been recommended.

Child: 2 mg/kg PO × 1

Adult: 200 mg PO × 1

Toxicity indicated by increase of QRS interval by ≥0.02 sec (skip dose or stop drug).

Adverse effects: May cause GI symptoms, hypotension, tinnitus, TTP, rash, heart block, and blood dyscrasias. When used alone, may cause 1 : 1 conduction in atrial flutter leading to ventricular fibrillation. Idiosyncratic ventricular tachycardia may occur with low levels, especially when initiating therapy. Myelosuppression, hepatotoxicity, cardiac dysrhythmia, SLE, and kidney disease have been reported.

Drug interactions: Quinidine is a substrate of cytochrome P 450 3A3/4 and 3A5–7 enzymes, and inhibitor of cytochrome P 450 2D6 and 3A3/4 enzymes. Can cause increase in digoxin levels. Quinidine potentiates the effect of neuromuscular blocking agents, β-blockers, anticholinergics, and warfarin. Amiodarone, antacids, delavirdine, diltiazem, grapefruit juice, saquinavir, ritonavir, verapamil, or cimetidine may enhance the drug's effect. Barbiturates, phenytoin, cholinergic drugs, nifedipine, sucralfate, or rifampin may reduce quinidine's effect.

Drug administration:

IV: Dilute to a concentration ≤16 mg/mL and administer at a rate ≤0.25 mg/kg/min. IV tubing length should be minimized to minimize drug adsorption to PVC tubing.

QUININE SULFATE

Qualaquin and various generic products

Antimalarial agent

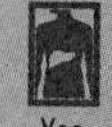
Yes

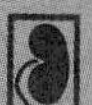
Yes

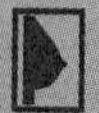
2

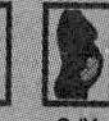
C/X

Caps: 324 mg

Malaria, treatment (chloroquine resistant; in combination with doxycycline, tetracycline, or clindamycin):

Child: 30 mg/kg/24 hr PO ÷ Q8 hr × 3–7 days; **max. dose:** 1944 mg/24 hr

Adult: 648 mg PO Q8 hr × 3–7 days

Babesiosis (in combination with clindamycin):

Child: 30 mg/kg/24 hr PO ÷ Q8 hr × 7–10 days; **max. dose:** 648 mg/dose

Adult: 684 mg PO Q8 hr × 7–10 days

Contraindications: Hypersensitivity to quinine, mefloquine, or quinidine; prolonged QT interval; G6PD deficiency; myasthenia gravis; and optic neuritis

Warnings/Precautions: **Use with caution** in asthma, heart disease, blackwater fever, tinnitus, and hepatic disease. Monitor CBC, platelets, LFTs, blood glucose, and administer ophthalmologic examination. **Reduce dosage** in severe chronic renal failure by administering a single load of 648 mg followed by 12 hr of maintenance doses of 324 mg Q12 hr in adults for malaria (10 mg/kg/dose load followed by 5 mg/kg/dose Q12 hr in children).

Continued

For explanation of icons, see p. 364.

QUININE SULFATE *continued*

Use in the prevention or treatment of nocturnal leg cramps is not recommended by the FDA because serious/life-threatening thrombocytopenia and hemolytic uremic syndrome/thrombotic thrombocytopenic purpura have been reported.

Pregnancy code is an "X" when used at very high doses (optic nerve hypoplasia and deafness to infant); therapeutic doses for malaria is considered safe.

Adverse effects: Rash, hypoglycemia, headache, and GI disturbances are common. DIC, thrombocytopenia, hepatotoxicity, ototoxicity, HUS, and interstitial nephritis have been reported. Chronic renal impairment associated with the development of thrombotic thrombocytopenic purpura have also been reported.

Drug interactions: Quinine is a substrate and inhibitor of cytochrome P 450 3A3/4. May increase levels/effects of digoxin, neuromuscular blocking agents, and oral anticoagulants. Cimetidine, ritonavir, verapamil, and amiodarone may increase serum quinine levels/effects/toxicity. Aminophylline/theophylline, urinary alkalinizers, and mefloquine may increase the effects/toxicity of quinine. Aluminum-containing antacids decrease quinine absorption; cigarette smoking may reduce quinine levels.

Drug administration: **Do not** crush tablets or capsule because of bitter taste. Take with food or milk to minimize GI irritation.

QUINUPRISTIN WITH DALFOPRISTIN
Synercid
Antibiotic, streptogramin

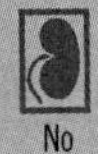
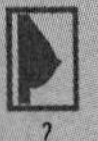
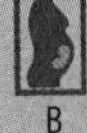

Yes No ? B

Injection: 500 mg (150 mg quinupristin and 350 mg dalfopristin)

Doses expressed in milligrams of combined quinupristin and dalfopristin.

Vancomycin-resistant **Enterococcus faecium** ***(VREF):***

Child <16 yr (limited data), ≥16 yr and adult: 7.5 mg/kg/dose IV Q8 hr

Complicated skin infections:

Child <16 yr (limited data), ≥16 yr and adult: 7.5 mg/kg/dose IV Q12 hr for at least 7 days

VREF endocarditis:

Child and adult: 7.5 mg/kg/dose IV Q8 hr for at least 8 wk

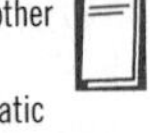

Contraindications: Hypersensitivity to quinupristin/dalfopristin or prior hypersensitivity to other streptogramins

Warnings/Precautions: **Not active** against *Enterococcus faecalis.* **Use with caution** in hepatic impairment; dosage reduction may be necessary with hepatic cirrhosis (Child–Pugh class A or B). **Pediatric studies are incomplete.** Drug is an inhibitor to the cytochrome P 450 3A4 isoenzyme (see Drug Interactions section).

Adverse effects: Pain, burning, inflammation, and edema at the IV infusion site, thrombophlebitis, thrombosis, GI disturbances, rash, arthralgia, myalgia, increased liver enzymes, hyperbilirubinemia, and headache are common. Dose frequency reductions (Q8–12 hr) or discontinuation can improve severe cases of arthralgia and myalgia. Use total body weight for obese patients when calculating dosages.

Drug interactions: **Avoid use** with cytochrome P 450 3A4 substrates, which can prolong QTc interval (e.g., cisapride). May increase the effects/toxicity of cyclosporine, tacrolimus, sirolimus, delavirdine, nevirapine, indinavir, ritonavir, diazepam, midazolam, carbamazepine, methylprednisolone, vinca alkaloids, docetaxel, paclitaxel, quinidine, and some calcium channel blockers.

Drug administration: Drug is compatible with D_5W and incompatible with saline and heparin (avoid using NS or heparin flushes). Infuse each dose over 1 hr using the following **maximum** IV concentrations: peripheral line: 2 mg/mL; central line: 5 mg/mL. If injection site reaction occurs, dilute infusion to <1 mg/mL.

RABIES IMMUNE GLOBULIN (HUMAN)
HyperRAB S/D, Imogam Rabies-HT
Immne globulin, rabies (high titer)

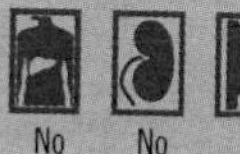
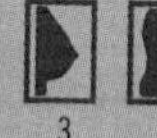
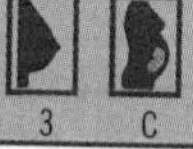

No No 3 C

Injection: 150 IU/mL (2, 10 mL)

Rabies postexposure passive immunization (with rabies vaccine and thorough wound treatment):

Child and adult: 20 IU/kg/dose × 1. See Drug Administration section for method of administration. Dose **must** be administered with or within 7 days of the first dose of rabies vaccine. Individuals previously immunized with rabies vaccine (with good titers) should **NOT** receive rabies immune globulin. **Do not** repeat dose of rabies immune globulin.

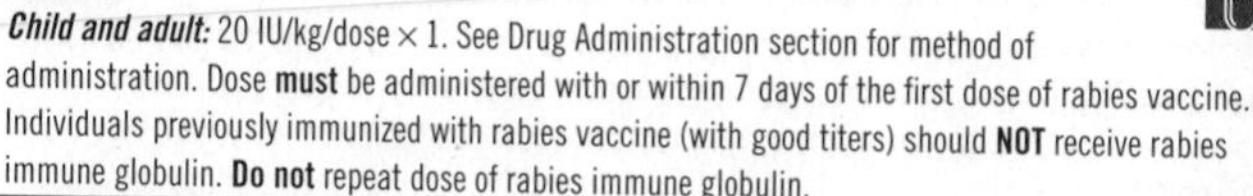

Contraindications: **Should not** be administered in repeated doses once vaccine treatment has been initiated. Repeating the dose may interfere with maximum active immunity expected from the vaccine.

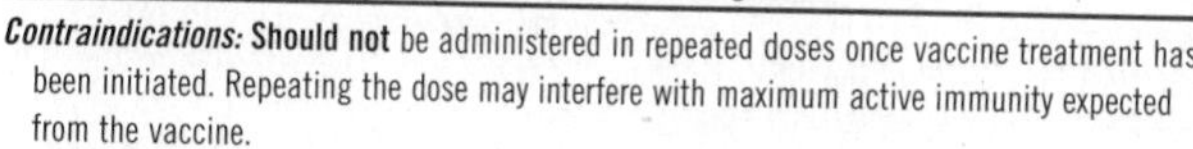

Warnings/Precautions: **Use with caution** in patients with prior systemic reaction (including anaphylaxis) to other human immunoglobulin preparations, thrombocytopenia, or coagulation disorders and isolated immunoglobulin A deficiency.

Adverse effects: Injection site pain, immune hypersensitivity reaction, headache, and fever are common.

Drug interactions: Rabies immune globulin and rabies vaccine should **not** be mixed in the same syringe or injected at the same site. Response of live virus vaccines (e.g., MMR, varicella) may be reduced with rabies immune globulin; **do not** administer live vaccines within 6 months after rabies immune globulin, and revaccination is necessary in patients receiving live vaccine within 14 days before rabies immune globulin.

Drug administration: **Do not** administer IV. **Do not** mix or inject at the same site with rabies vaccine. If possible, infiltrate the entire dose in the area around and into the wound; give the remainder of dose IM distant from vaccine administration.

RALTEGRAVIR
Isentress
HIV-1 integrase strand transfer inhibitor (HIV-1 INSTI)

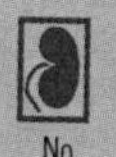
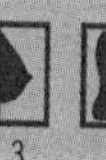
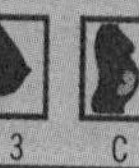

No No 3 C

Chewable tabs: 25, 200 mg; contains phenylalanine
Tabs: 400 mg

Child (2 to <12 yr): Use chewable tablet dosage form by the following weight groups:
- ***10 to <14 kg:*** 75 mg PO BID
- ***14 to <20 kg:*** 100 mg PO BID
- ***20 to <28 kg:*** 150 mg PO BID
- ***28 to <40 kg:*** 200 mg PO BID
- ***≥40 kg:*** 300 mg PO BID

Alternative dosing method:

2 to <6 yr:
- ***≥10 kg:*** 6 mg/kg/dose (**max. dose:** 300 mg/dose) PO BID as chewable tablets

6 to <12 yr:
- ***<25 kg:*** 6 mg/kg/dose (**max. dose:** 300 mg/dose) PO BID as chewable tablets
- ***≥25 kg:*** 6 mg/kg/dose (**max. dose:** 300 mg/dose) PO BID as chewable tablets *or* 400 mg PO BID as tablets

Child ≥12 yr and adult (tablets): 400 mg PO BID; if drug is coadministered with rifampin, give 800 mg PO BID

Continued

For explanation of icons, see p. 364.

RALTEGRAVIR *continued*

Contraindications: Have **not** been determined
Warnings/Precautions: **Use with caution** when using concurrent medications causing myopathy or rhabdomyolysis, or in patients at risk for these effects. See Drug Interactions section for additional information. Immune reconstitution syndrome during the initial treatment period may cause an inflammatory response to indolent or residual opportunistic infections (e.g., MAC, CMV, PCP, VZV). Severe, potentially life-threatening and fatal skin reactions have been reported.
The chewable tablet dosage form has higher bioavailability than regular tablet in healthy adult subjects.
Adverse effects: Nausea, headache, diarrhea, and pyrexia are common. Myocardial infarction, paranoia, anxiety, cerebellar ataxia, anemia, neutropenia, and renal or hepatic failure have been reported.
Drug interactions: Strong inducers of uridine diphosphate glucuronosyltransferase (UGT) 1A1 (e.g., rifampin), efavirenz, etravirine, and tipranavir/ritonavir may decrease raltegravir levels. Omeprazole and atazanavir ± ritonavir may increase raltegravir levels.
Drug administration: May be taken with or without food for either oral dosage form (chewable tablet and tablet).

RETAPAMULIN
Altabax
Antibacterial, pleuromutilin

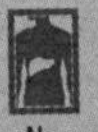 No
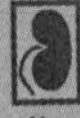 No
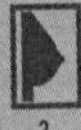 ?
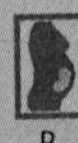 B

Ointment: 1% (15 g)

***Impetigo caused by* S. aureus *(methicillin susceptible) or* S. pyogenes:**
≥9 mo and adult: Apply a thin layer to affected area BID × 5 days.
Maximum dose:
Child: 2% of total body surface area
Adult: 100 cm^2 of total area

Contraindications: Have **not** been determined
Warnings/Precautions: **Discontinue** use if sensitization or severe local irritation occurs. **For external use only; not for** intranasal, ophthalmic, or intravaginal use.
Adverse effects: Application site irritation is common. Pruritus, headache, and diarrhea have been reported. Epistaxis has been reported with use on nasal mucosa.
Drug interactions: Retapamulin is a CYP 3A4 substrate.
Drug administration: Apply a thin layer to affected area. Treated area may be covered with a sterile bandage or gauze dressing.

RIBAVIRIN
Oral: Rebetol, Copegus, Ribasphere, Ribasphere RibaPak, and others
Inhalation: Virazole
Antiviral agent

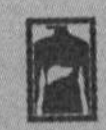 Yes
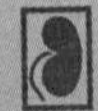 Yes
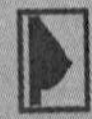 ?
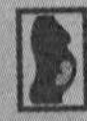 X

Oral solution (Rebetol): 200 mg/5 mL (100 mL); contains sodium benzoate, propylene glycol
Oral caps (Rebetol, Ribasphere): 200 mg
Tabs (Copegus, Ribasphere): 200, 400, 600 mg
Dose-pack (Ribasphere RibaPak):
Ribasphere RibaPak 600: 200 mg AM dose, 400 mg PM dose (14s, 56s)
Ribasphere RibaPak 800: 400 mg AM dose, 400 mg PM dose (14s, 56s)

Continued

RIBAVIRIN *continued*

Ribasphere RibaPak 1000: 600 mg AM dose, 400 mg PM dose (14s, 56s)
Ribasphere RibaPak 1200: 600 mg AM dose, 600 mg PM dose (14s, 56s)
Aerosol (Virazole): 6 g

Chronic hepatitis C (PO, see remarks):
Child (≥3 yr, in combination with interferon alfa-2b at 3 million units 3× per week SC using oral solution or capsule):
25–36 kg: 200 mg BID
37–49 kg: 200 mg QAM and 400 mg QPM
50–61 kg: 400 mg BID
>61–75 kg: 400 mg QAM and 600 mg QPM
>75 kg: Use adult dose
Dosage modification for toxicity: See remarks.
Adult:
Oral capsules in combination with interferon alfa-2b at 3 million units 3× per week SC:
≤75 kg: 400 mg QAM and 600 mg QPM
>75 kg: 600 mg BID
Oral capsules in combination with peginterferon alfa-2b: 400 mg BID
Oral tablets in combination with peginterferon alfa-2a for hepatitis C genotype 1, 4:
≤75 kg: 500 mg BID × 48 wk
>75 kg: 600 mg BID × 48 wk
Oral tablets in combination with peginterferon alfa-2a for hepatitis C genotype 2, 3: 400 mg BID × 24 wk
Oral tablets in combination with peginterferon alfa-2a for hepatitis C any genotype and HIV co-infection: 400 mg BID × 24 wk
Dosage modification for toxicity: See remarks.
Inhalation:
Continuous: Administer 6 g by aerosol over 12 to 18 hours once daily for 3 to 7 days. The 6-g ribavirin vial is diluted in 300 mL preservative-free sterile water to a final concentration of 20 mg/mL. Must be administered with Viratek Small Particle Aerosol Generator (SPAG-2).
Intermittent (for nonventilated patients): Administer 2 g by aerosol over 2 hours TID for 3 to 7 days. The 6-g ribavirin vial is diluted in 100 mL preservative-free sterile water to a final concentration of 60 mg/mL. The intermittent use is **not** recommended in patients with endotracheal tubes.

Contraindications:
ORAL RIBAVIRIN: Pregnancy, significant or unstable cardiac disease, autoimmune hepatitis, hepatic decompensation (Child–Pugh score >6; class B or C), hemoglobinopathies, and creatinine clearance less than 50 mL/min
INHALED RIBAVIRIN: Pregnancy and hypersensitivity to ribavirin or its components
Warnings/Precautions:
ORAL RIBAVIRIN: Used in combination with a specific interferon alfa injection product for hepatitis C. **Use with caution** in preexisiting cardiac disease, pulmonary disease, and sarcoidosis. Suicidal ideation has been reported to be higher in adolescent and pediatric patients. Reduce or discontinue dosage for toxicity as follows:
Patient with no cardiac disease:
Hgb <10 g/dL and ≥8.5 g/dL:
Child: 12 mg/kg/dose PO once daily; may further reduce to 8 mg/kg/dose PO once daily
Adult: 600 mg PO once daily (capsules or solution) or 200 mg PO QAM and 400 mg PO QPM (tablets)

Continued

For explanation of icons, see p. 364.

RIBAVIRIN *continued*

Hgb <8.5 g/dL: Discontinue therapy permanently.

Patient with cardiac disease:

≥2 mg/dL decrease in Hgb during any 4-wk period during therapy:

Child: 12 mg/kg/dose PO once daily; may further reduce to 8 mg/kg/dose PO once daily (monitor weekly)

Adult: 600 mg PO once daily (capsules or solution) or 200 mg PO QAM and 400 mg PO QPM (tablets)

Hgb <12 g/dL after 4 wk of reduced dose: Discontinue therapy permanently.

INHALED RIBAVIRIN: Use for RSV is controversial and not routinely indicated. Aerosol therapy may be considered for selected infants and young children at high risk for serious RSV disease (see recent edition of the *AAP Red Book*). Most effective if therapy is initiated early in course of RSV infection, generally in the first 3 days. **Avoid** unnecessary occupational exposure to ribavirin because of its teratogenic effects. Drug can precipitate in the respiratory equipment especially with mechanical ventilators. Sudden deterioration of respiratory function has been reported.

Adverse effects:

ORAL RIBAVIRIN: Anemia (see dose modification for toxicity), insomnia, depression, anxiety, irritability, fatigue, and GI disturbances are common. Suicidal behavior has been reported. Tinnitus, hearing loss, vertigo, and severe hypertriglyceridemia have been reported in combination with interferon. Pancytopenia has been reported in combination with interferon and azathioprine (azathioprine should be discontinued and not reintroduced). Increased risk for hepatic decompensation with cirrotic chronic hepatitis C patients treated with α inteferons or with HIV co-infection receiving HAART and interferon alfa-2a. Dry mouth and dental/peridontal disorders have been reported with long-term use.

INHALED RIBAVIRIN: Worsening respiratory distress, rash, conjunctivitis, mild bronchospasm, hypotension, anemia, and cardiac arrest may occur.

Drug interactions:

ORAL RIBAVIRIN: May decrease the effects of zidovudine and stavudine; increased risk for lactic acidosis with nucleoside analogues (adefovir, didanosine, lamivudine, stavudine, zalcitabine, or zidovudine).

Drug administration:

ORAL RIBAVIRIN: Administer tablets with food. Capsules and oral solution may be administered with or without food.

INHALED RIBAVIRIN: Administer with SPAG-2 small-particle aerosol generator in a well-ventilated room (≥6 changes/hr). **Do not** mix with other aerosolized medications. Use of one-way valves in inspiratory lines, breathing circuit filter in the expiratory line, and frequent monitoring and filter replacement have been recommended for mechanically ventilated patients.

RIFABUTIN
Mycobutin
Antituberculous agent, rifamycin

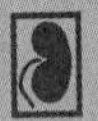 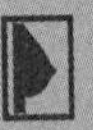 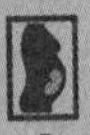

Yes Yes 3 B

Caps: 150 mg
Oral suspension: 20 mg/mL

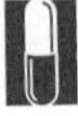

MAC prophylaxis to prevent first episode of opportunistic disease in HIV (see remarks for interactions and www.aidsinfo.nih.gov/guidelines):

≥6 yr and adult: 300 mg PO once daily; doses may be administered as 150 mg PO BID if GI upset occurs

Continued

RIFABUTIN *continued*

MAC prophylaxis for recurrence of opportunistic disease in HIV (in combination with ethambutol and a macrolide antibiotic [clarithromycin or azithromycin]):

Infant and child: 5 mg/kg/24 hr PO once daily; **max. dose:** 300 mg/24 hr

Adolescent and adult: 300 mg PO once daily; doses may be administered as 150 mg PO BID if GI upset occurs

MAC treatment:

Child: 10–20 mg/kg/24 hr PO once daily; **max. dose:** 300 mg/24 hr as part of a multidrug regimen for severe disease

Adolescent and adult: 300 mg PO once daily; may be used in combination with azithromycin and ethambutol

In combination with nonnucleoside reverse transcriptase inhibitors:

With efavirenz and no concomitant protease inhibitor: 450 mg PO once daily or 600 mg PO 3× per wk

With nevirapine: 300 mg PO 3× per wk

In combination with protease inhibitors:

With amprenavir, indinavir, or nelfinavir: 150 mg PO once daily or 300 mg PO 3× per wk

With ritonavir boosted regimens (e.g., saquinavir/ritonavir or lopinavir/ritonavir): 150 mg PO every other day or 150 mg PO 3× per wk

Mycobacterium tuberculosis ***opportunistic disease in HIV (alternative to rifampin):***

Child:

Treatment: 10–20 mg/kg/24 hr (**max. dose:** 300 mg/kg/24 hr) PO once daily or 2–3 times weekly

Adolescent and adult:

Prophylaxis: 300 mg PO once daily × 4 mo

Treatment: 300 mg PO once daily or two to three times weekly as part of a multidrug regimen. For concomitant nonnucleoside reverse transcriptase inhibitor and protease inhibitor use, use the earlier adolescent/adult dosing recommendations for MAC treatment.

Contraindications: Clinically significant hypersensitivity to rifabutin or to any other rifamycins

Warnings/Precautions: Should **not** be used for MAC prophylaxis with active TB. **Use with caution** in renal and hepatic impairment. **Adjust dose in renal impairment (see Chapter 3).**

Adverse effects: GI distress, discoloration of skin and body fluids (brown–orange color), and rash are common. May permanently stain contact lenses. Uveitis can occur when using high doses (>300 mg/24 hr in adults) in combination with macrolide antibiotics. Bone marrow suppression and SLE have been reported.

Drug interactions: Induces cytochrome P 450 3A isoenzyme and is structurally similar to rifampin (similar drug interactions; see Rifampin). Clarithromycin, fluconazole, itraconazole, nevirapine, and protease inhibitors increase rifabutin levels. Efavirenz may decrease rifabutin levels. May decrease effectiveness of dapsone, delavirdine, nevirapine, amprenavir, indinavir, nelfinavir, saquinavir, itraconazole, warfarin, oral contraceptives, digoxin, cyclosporine, ketoconazole, and narcotics.

Drug administration: Doses may be administered with food if patient experiences GI intolerance.

RIFAMPIN

Rimactane, Rifadin, and others

Antibiotic, antituberculous agent, rifamycin

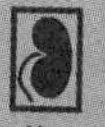

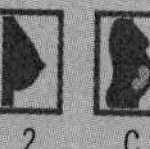

Yes Yes 2 C

Caps: 150, 300 mg

Oral suspension: 10, 15, 25 mg/mL

Injection: 600 mg

Continued

For explanation of icons, see p. 364.

RIFAMPIN *continued*

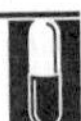

Staphylococcus aureus *infections (as part of synergistic therapy with other antistaphylococcal agents):*

0–1 mo:

IV: 10–20 mg/kg/24 hr ÷ Q12 hr

PO: 10–20 mg/kg/dose Q24 hr

>1 mo: 10–20 mg/kg/24 hr ÷ Q12 hr IV/PO; **max. dose:** 600 mg/24 hr

Prosthetic valve endocarditis: 15–20 mg/kg/24 hr IV/PO ÷ Q8 hr

Adult: 300–600 mg Q12 hr IV/PO

Prosthetic valve endocarditis: 300 mg Q8 hr IV/PO for a minimum of 6 wk in combination with antistaphylococcal penicillin with or without gentamicin

Tuberculosis: (see latest edition of the *AAP Red Book* for duration of therapy and combination therapy). Twice-weekly therapy may be used after 1 to 2 months of daily therapy.

Infant, child, and adolescent:

Daily therapy: 10–20 mg/kg/24 hr ÷ Q12–24 hr IV/PO

Twice weekly therapy: 10–20 mg/kg/24 hr PO twice weekly

Max. daily dose: 600 mg/24 hr

Adult:

Daily therapy: 10 mg/kg/24 hr once daily PO

Twice-weekly therapy: 10 mg/kg/24 hr twice weekly

Max. daily dose: 600 mg/24 hr

Opportunistic disease in HIV:

Infant and child:

Mycobacterium tuberculosis *prophylaxis for first episode (drug choice for INH-resistant strains and alternative drug choice for INH-sensitive strains):* 10–20 mg/kg/24 hr PO once daily (**max. dose:** 600 mg/24 hr) × 4–6 mo

Mycobacterium tubercolosis *treatment:* 10–20 mg/kg/24 hr PO once daily (**max. dose:** 600 mg/24 hr) in combination with INH, pyrazinamide, and ethambutol × 8 wk as the intensive phase; followed by the continuation phase with just INH

Baronellosis treatment (CNS disease, bacillary peliosis, osteomyelitis, severe infections): 20 mg/kg/24 hr ÷ once daily to BID IV/PO (**max. dose:** 600 mg/24 hr) with erythromycin or doxycycline

Prophylaxis for* Neisseria meningitidis *(see latest edition of the* AAP Red Book *for additional information):

0–1 mo: 10 mg/kg/24 hr ÷ Q12 hr PO × 2 days

>1 mo: 20 mg/kg/24 hr ÷ Q12 hr PO × 2 days

Adult: 600 mg PO Q12 hr × 2 days

Max. dose (all ages): 1200 mg/24 hr

Prophylaxis for* Haemophilus influenzae *(see latest edition of the* AAP Red Book *for additional information):

0–1 mo: 10 mg/kg/dose Q24 hr PO × 4 days

>1 mo: 20 mg/kg/dose (**max. dose:** 600 mg) Q24 hr PO × 4 days

Adult: 600 mg PO Q24 hr × 4 days

Contraindications: Hypersensitivity to rifampin or other rifamycins; in combination with atazanavir, darunavir, fosamprenavir, saqunavir (± ritonavir), or tipranavir

Warnings/Precautions: **Never use** as monotherapy except when used for prophylaxis. Patients with latent tuberculosis infection should **not** be treated with rifampin and pyrazinamide because of the risk for severe liver injury. Use is **not** recommended in porphyria. **Use with caution** in diabetes. Penetrates well into body fluids (see adverse effects), including CSF. **Adjust dose in renal failure (see Chapter 3).** Reduce dose in hepatic impairment.

Continued

RIFAMPIN *continued*

Adverse effects: May cause GI irritation, allergy, headache, fatigue, ataxia, muscle weakness, confusion, fever, hepatitis, transient LFT abnormalities, blood dyscrasias, interstitial nephritis, and elevated BUN and uric acid. Causes red discoloration of body secretions such as urine, saliva, and tears (which can permanently stain contact lenses).

Drug interactions: Induces hepatic enzymes (CYP 450 2C9, 2C19, and 3A4), which may decrease plasma concentration of digoxin, corticosteroids, buspirone, benzodiazepines, fentanyl, calcium channel blockers, β-blockers, cyclosporine, tacrolimus, itraconazole, ketoconazole, voriconazole, oral anticoagulants, barbiturates, and theophylline. May reduce the effectiveness of oral contraceptives and antiretroviral agents (protease inhibitors and nonnucleoside reverse transcriptase inhibitors). Hepatotoxicity is a concern when used in combination with pyrazinamide or ritonavir-boosted saquinavir. See Contraindications section for other interactions.

Drug administration:

IV: For intermittent infusion, infuse over 0.5–3 hr at a concentration ≤6 mg/mL. **Do not** administer IM or SQ.

PO: Give 1 hour before or 2 hours after meals. Contents of the oral capsule may be mixed with applesauce or jelly.

RIFAPENTINE
Priftin
Antibiotic, antituberculosis agent, rifamycin

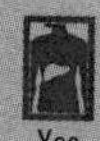
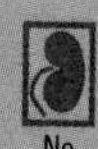
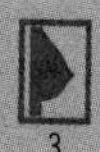
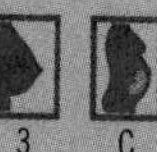

Yes No 3 C

Tabs: 150 mg

Pulmonary tuberculosis:

≥12 yr and adult:

Intensive phase: 600 mg PO twice weekly (with an interval of no less than 72 hr between doses) × 2 mo in combination with other susceptible antitubercular drugs

Continuation phase: 600 mg PO Q7 days × 4 mo in combination with other susceptible antitubercular drug.

Latent tuberculosis:

Child ≥12 yr: PO once weekly dose × 3 mo by weight:

10–14 kg: 300 mg

14.1–25 kg: 450 mg

25.1–32 kg: 600 mg

32.1–49.9 kg: 750 mg

≥50 kg: 900 mg

Adult: 900 mg PO once weekly × 3 mo in combination with isoniazid. Alternative PO once weekly dose × 3 mo adjusted for body weight; use the earlier weight-based dosing for child ≥ 12 yr.

Contraindications: History of hypersensitivity to any rifamycins (e.g., rifampin and rifabutin)

Warnings/Precautions: Hepatotoxicity of other antituberculosis drugs (e.g., isoniazid, pyrazinamide) used in combination should be taken into account. **Use with caution** in liver disease, abnormal LFTs, and hyperbilirubinemia. The CDC does **not** recommend use with HIV-infected patients because of increased risk for TB relapse. Use is **not** recommended in porphyria. Discolors body fluids/tissues red–orange; stains contact lenses and dentures. Drug is extensively protein bound, primarily to albumin.

A pharmacokinetic evaluation revealed lower drug exposure in children when compared with adults at comparable weight-normalized (mg/kg) doses. This suggests larger weight-normalized doses for children; additional studies are needed.

Continued

For explanation of icons, see p. 364.

RIFAPENTINE *continued*

Adverse effects: Hyperuricemia, arthralgia, pyogenic proteinuria, elevated ALT/AST, and red–orange body fluid discoloration are common.

Drug interactions: Induces CYP450 3A4 and 2C8/9 isoenzymes. May decrease the effects of antiretroviral protease inhibitors, oral and other systemic hormonal contraceptives (use alternative nonhormonal contraception), carbamazepine, chloramphenicol, corticosteroids, cyclosporine, delavirdine, fluconazole, voriconazole, warfarin, and other CYP450 3A4 substrates.

Drug administration: Take with or without food.

RIFAXIMIN
Xifaxan
Rifamycin antibiotic

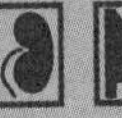
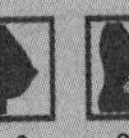
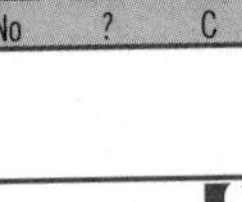

Yes No ? C

Tabs: 200, 550 mg
Oral suspension: 20 mg/mL

Traveler's diarrhea caused by noninvasive strains of* Escherichia coli*:
Child ≥12 and adult: 200 mg PO TID × 3 days
Clostridium difficile*–associated diarrhea:*
Adult: 200–400 mg PO BID–TID × 14 days
See package insert for dosing information for noninfectious conditions such as hepatic encephalopathy and irritable bowel syndrome.

Contraindications: Hypersensitivity to rifaximin, any component of the product, or other rifamycin antimicrobial agents (e.g., rifampin, rifabutin, rifaximin)

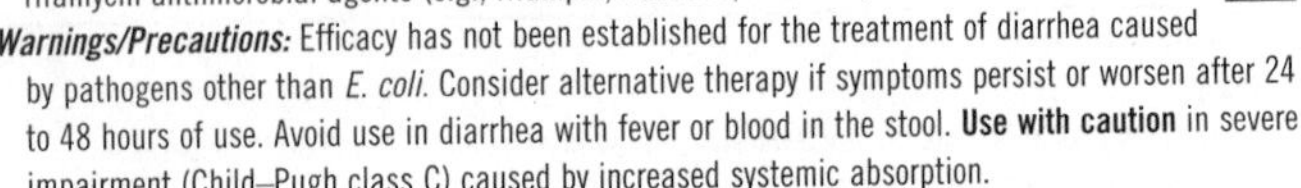

Warnings/Precautions: Efficacy has not been established for the treatment of diarrhea caused by pathogens other than *E. coli.* Consider alternative therapy if symptoms persist or worsen after 24 to 48 hours of use. Avoid use in diarrhea with fever or blood in the stool. **Use with caution** in severe impairment (Child–Pugh class C) caused by increased systemic absorption.

Adverse effects: Peripheral edema, abdominal pain, constipation, flatulence, nausea, vomiting, rectal tenesmus, defecation urgency, ascites, dizziness, headache and fatigue are common. Immune hypersensitivity reaction has been reported. Prolonged use may result in fungal or bacterial superinfection, including *C. difficile*–associated diarrhea.

Drug interaction: May decrease the effects of warfarin. Rifaximin may decrease the effects of BCG and sodium picosulfate; consider alternative therapy.

Drug administration: Doses may be administered with or without food.

RILPIVIRINE
Edurant
In combination with emtricitabine and tenofovir as Complera
Antiviral, nonnucleoside reverse transcriptase inhibitor

No No 3 B

Tab: 25 mg
In combination with emtricitabine and tenofovir as Complera:
Tabs: 25 mg rilpivirine + 200 mg emtricitabine + 300 mg tenofovir

HIV:
Adult: 25 mg PO once daily

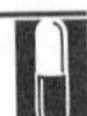
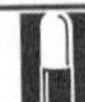

Complera (combination product):
Adult: one tablet PO once daily

Continued

RILPIVIRINE *continued*

Contraindications: Concurrent use with carbamazepine, dexamethasone (>1 dose), oxcarbazepine, phenobarbital, fosphenytoin, phenytoin, primidone, proton pump inhibitors (e.g., omeprazole, lansoprazole, pantoprazole), rifabutin, rifampin, rifapentine, or St. John's wort. These medications will decrease levels/effect of rilpivirine.

Warnings/Precautions: Immune reconstitution syndrome may exacerbate autoimmune disorders such as Graves disease, polymyositis, and Guillain–Barre syndrome. Concomitant use with delavirdine, efavirenz, etravirine, and nevirapine are not recommended because of increased levels/toxicity of rilpivirine. Avoid use with drugs with high risk for QTc prolongation.

Has not been evaluated in severe hepatic impairment (Child–Pugh class C); dosage adjustment is not needed in renal impairment (unlikely for dialysis) and mild-to-moderate hepatic impairment (Child–Pugh class A or B).

Adverse effects: Rash, depression, headache, insomnia, and elevations in ALT/SGPT and AST/SGOT liver enzymes, low-density lipoprotein cholesterol, and serum cholesterol are common. Suicidal ideation, abnormal dreams, GI discomfort, fat redistribution, and glomerulonephritis have been reported.

Drug interaction: Drug is a substrate for CYP 450 3A4.

Dastinib, ivacaftor, ketoconazole, and lopinavir may increase rilpivirine levels/effects. Deferasirox and tocilizumab may decrease rilpivirine levels. Always check the potential for other drug interactions when either initiating therapy or adding new drugs onto an existing regimen. See Contraindications, Warnings/Precautions, and Drug Administration sections for additional interactions.

Drug administration: Administer doses with meals. If didanosine is included in the antiviral regimen, administer rilpivirine 4 hours before or 2 hours after didanosine. If coadministered with antacids containing aluminum, magnesium, or calcium, administer rilpivirine at least 4 hours before or 2 hours after taking the antacid. If coadministered with histamine-2 receptor antagonist (e.g., cimetidine, famotidine, ranitidine), administer rilpivirine at least 4 hours before or 12 hours after taking the histamine-2 receptor antagonist.

RIMANTADINE
Flumadine and others
Antiviral agent

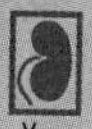
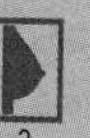
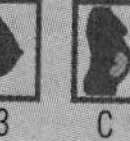

Yes Yes 3 C

Tabs: 100 mg

Influenza A prophylaxis (for at least 10 days after known exposure; usually for 6 to 8 weeks during influenza A season or local outbreak; see remarks):

Child:

- ***1–9 yr:*** 5 mg/kg/24 hr PO once daily; **max. dose:** 150 mg/24 hr
- ***≥10 yr:***
  - ***<40 kg:*** 5 mg/kg/24 hr PO ÷ BID; **max. dose:** 150 mg/24 hr
  - ***≥40 kg:*** 100 mg/dose PO BID

Adult: 100 mg PO BID

Influenza A treatment (within 48 hours of illness onset; see remarks):

Use the earlier prophylaxis dosage × 5–7 days.

Contraindications: Amantadine or rimantadine hypersensitivity

Warnings/Precautions: Resistance to influenza A and recommendations against the use for treatment and prophylaxis have been reported by the CDC. Check with local microbiology laboratories and the CDC for seasonal susceptibility/resistance.

Continued

FORMULARY

For explanation of icons, see p. 364.

RIMANTADINE *continued*

Individuals immunized with live attenuated influenza vaccine (e.g., FluMist) should not receive rimantadine prophylaxis for 14 days after the vaccine. Chemoprophylaxis does not interfere with immune response to inactivated influenza vaccine. **Use with caution** in seizures and in renal or hepatic insufficiency; dosage reduction may be necessary.

Preferred over amantadine for influenza because of lower incidence of adverse effects. **A dosage reduction of 50% has been recommended in severe hepatic or renal impairment (see Chapter 3).** Patients with severe renal impairment have been reported to have an 81% increase in systemic exposure. Have not been fully evaluated in children younger than 1 year. Use is recommended in stem cell transplant patients and treatment indication in chidren younger than 13 years despite insufficient data and lack of FDA approval, respectively.

Adverse effects: GI disturbance, xerostomia, dizziness, headace, insomnia, and nervousness are common. CNS disturbances are less than with amantadine. Urinary retention may occur.

Drug interactions: Anticholinergic agents and CNS stimulants may increase adverse effects.

Drug administration: May give with or without food.

RITONAVIR
Norvir
Antiviral, protease inhibitor

Yes No 3 B

Tabs: 100 mg
Caps, soft gel: 100 mg; contains alcohol
Oral solution: 80 mg/mL (240 mL); contains alcohol (43.2% vol/vol), popylene glycol (26.6% wt/vol), and saccharin

Child ≥1 mo (see remarks): Start at 250 mg/m²/dose Q12 hr PO, then increase dose by 50 mg/m²/dose Q12 hr increments at 2- to 3-day intervals up to 400 mg/m²/dose Q12 hr as tolerated. Usual dosage range is 350–400 mg/m²/dose Q12 hr.

Max dose: 600 mg/dose BID

Adolescent and adult: Start at 300 mg/dose Q12 hr PO. To minimize nausea and vomiting, increase by 100 mg per increments up to 600 mg/dose Q12 hr over 5 days as tolerated.

If used in combination with other protease inhibitors as a pharmacokinetic enhancer, 100–400 mg/dose Q12 hr PO.

Contraindications: Hypersensitivity to ritonavir or any other components in the formulation. Contraindications also include coadministration of the following drugs that could result in potential serious and/or life-threatening reactions such as cardiac arrhythmias, prolonged or increased sedation, and respiratory depression: alfuzosin, amiodarone, cisapride, ergot derivatives, flecainide, lovastatin, pimozide, propafenone, quinidine, St. John's wort, sildenafil (pulmonary hypertension), midazolam (PO), and triazolam. Significantly reduces voriconazole levels.

Warnings/Precautions: **Use with caution** in liver impairment. Dose titration schedule is recommended to minimize risk for adverse effects. Immune reconstitution syndrome may exacerbate autoimmune disorders such as Graves disease, polymyositis, and Guillain–Barre syndrome. Noncompliance can quickly promote resistant HIV strains. **Avoid** using oral liquid dosage form with amprenavir solution because of large amounts of ethanol and propylene glycol. Use **not** recommended with fluticasone propionate, sildenafil, vardenafil, tadalafil, disopyramide, mexiletine, fluoxetine (serotonin syndrome), nefazodone, β-blockers, lovastatin, simvastatin, and other HMG-CoA reductase inhibitors because of increase risk for toxicity and adverse effects. Significant drug–drug interactions exist; see Contraindications and Drug Interactions sections.

Continued

RITONAVIR *continued*

Dose reduction is necessary when used with atazanavir, darunavir, fosamprenavir, saquinavir, and tipranavir. Should not be used in neonates with a postmenstrual age of less than 44 weeks because of the alcohol and propylene glycol excipients in the oral solution dosage form.

Adverse effects: Nausea, vomiting, diarrhea, headache, abdominal pain, anorexia, asthenia, and paresthesias are common. Increases in liver enzymes, triglycerides, cholesterol, and serum glucose may also occur. GI side effects may be greater with tablets compared with the soft-gel capsules dosage form. Spontaneous bleeding in patients with hemophilia, pancreatitis, Stevens–Johnson syndrome, and other severe allergic reactions, hepatic dysfunction (especially with multiple concomitant medication and/or advanced AIDS), and hepatitis have been reported.

Drug interactions: Inhibits and is metabolized by the CYP450 2D6 and 3A4 microsomal enzyme to cause many drug interactions. Drug may increase the levels and adverse effects of carbamazepine, clarithromycin, calcium channel blockers, colchicine, digoxin, cyclosporine, tacrolimus, sirolimus, desipramine, ketoconazole, rifabutin, trazodone, warfarin, and other protease inhibitors. St. John's wort and rifampin may reduce the effects of ritonavir. Theopylline, bosentan, methadone, ethinyl estradiol (PO or transdermal contraception), phenytoin, and valproic acid, lamotrigine, and atovaquine levels/effects may be reduced. **Always check the potential for other drug interactions when either initiating therapy or adding new drugs onto an existing regimen.** See Contraindications and Warnings/Precautions sections for additional interactions.

Drug administration: Administer doses with food to assure absorption. If didanosine is included in the antiretroviral regimen, space the administration of two drugs by 2 hours. Store both capsules and oral solution in the refrigerator. Oral solution can be kept at room temperature if used within 30 days and must be kept in its original container. Administering doses with milk, chocolate milk, pudding, or ice cream may enhance compliance in children. Oral solution may be mixed with chocolate milk, Ensure, or Advera within 1 hour of dosing.

SAQUINAVIR MESYLATE
Invirase
Antiviral agent, protease inhibitor

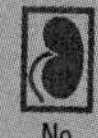
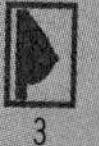
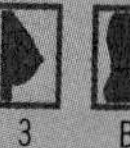

Yes No 3 B

Caps, hard gel: (Invirase): 200 mg
Tabs: 500 mg

Child >2 and <16 yr:

In combination with ritonavir for treatment experienced (limited data): 50 mg/kg/dose (**max. dose:** 1000 mg/dose) PO BID with the following ritonavir dose:

5 to <15 kg: ritonavir 3 mg/kg/dose PO BID
15 to <40 kg: ritonavir 2.5 mg/kg/dose PO BID
≥40 kg: 100 mg PO BID

In combination with lopinavir and ritonavir for salvage therapy (limited data):

≥7 and <16 yr: 750 mg/m^2/dose or 50 mg/kg/dose PO BID; **max. dose:** 1600 mg/dose

Adolescent (≥16 yr) and adult (see Drug Administration in remarks):

In combination with ritonavir 100 mg PO BID: 1000 mg PO BID
In combination with lopinavir 400 mg and ritonavir 100 mg PO BID: 1000 mg PO BID

Contraindications: Saquinavir products and their components, complete AV block without implanted pacemakers (present or risk for), congenital long QT syndrome, refractory hypokalemia or hypomagnesemia, and severe hepatic impairment. Coadministration of the following drugs could result in potential serious and/or life-threatening reactions such as

Continued

For explanation of icons, see p. 364.

SAQUINAVIR MESYLATE *continued*

cardiac arrhythmias, prolonged or increased sedation, and respiratory depression: alfuzosin, amiodarone, bepridil, dofetilide, flecainide, propafenone, quinidine, astemizole, terfenadine, ergot derivatives, cisapride, pimozide, trazodone, sildenafil, midazolam, and triazolam. Rifampin may result in treatment failure and hepatotoxicity. Lovastatin and simvastatin may result in rhabdomyolysis.

Warnings/Precautions: **Use with caution** in hepatic failure. Use **only** in combination with ritonavir or ritonavir/lopinavir. Use **not** recommended with St. John's wort, salmeterol, bosentin, tadalafil, colchicine, or garlic capsules. Significant drug–drug interactions exist; see Contraindications and Drug Interactions sections. Noncompliance can quickly promote resistant HIV strains. Use sunscreen or protective clothing to prevent photosensitivity reactions. When using in combination with ritonavir, doses more than 400 mg PO BID for either ritonavir or saquinavir may be associated with risk for increased adverse effects.

A baseline ECG should be performed before initiation of therapy, and consider ongoing monitoring when necessary.

Adverse effects: Diarrhea, GI discomfort, nausea, paresthesias, skin rash, lipid abnormalities, and headache are common. Spontaneous bleeding in hemophiliacs, hyperglycemia, exacerbation of chronic liver disease, and body fat redistribution without serum lipid abnormalities have been reported.

Drug interactions: Drug inhibits and is metabolized by the CYP450 3A4 drug metabolizing enzyme and is P-glycoprotein substrate. Increased levels and/or toxicity may occur with the following concurrent medications: calcium channel blockers, clindamycin, cyclosporine, lidocaine, tacrolimus, dapsone, and quinidine. Rifabutin, niverapine, carbamazepine, dexamethasone, phenobarbital, and phenytoin can decrease saquinavir levels. Delavirdine, ketoconazole, grapefruit juice, and other protease inhibitors may increase saquinavir levels. **Always carefully review patient's medication profile for other potential drug–drug interactions.**

Drug administration: Administer doses with food or within 2 hours after a meal. Should not be administered at the same time with ritonavir.

Patients who are unable to swallow capsules may empty the capsules contents and mix with 15 mL sugar syrup or sorbitol syrup, *or* 3 teaspoons of jam. Stir with spoon for 30 to 60 seconds and administer the full amount.

SELENIUM SULFIDE
Selsun and others
Topical antiseborrheic agent

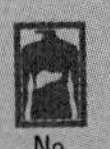
No
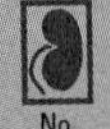
No
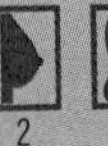
2
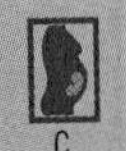
C

Lotion/shampoo: 1% [OTC] (120, 210, 325, 420 mL); some shampoo products are available with conditioner
Topical lotion: 2.5% (120 mL)
Topical aerosol foam: 2.25% (70 g)

≥2 yr and adult:
Seborrhea/dandruff: Massage 5–10 mL 1% or 2.5% into wet scalp and leave on scalp for 2–3 min. Rinse thoroughly and repeat. Shampoo twice weekly × 2 wk. Maintenance applications once every 1–4 wk.
Tinea versicolor: Apply 2.5% lotion to affected areas of skin. Allow to remain on skin × 30 min for children and 10 min for adults. Rinse thoroughly. Repeat once daily × 7 days. Follow with monthly applications for 3 mo to prevent recurrences.

Continued

SELENIUM SULFIDE *continued*

Contraindications: Hypersensitivity to selenium sulfide or any other components in the formulation

Warnings/Precautions: **Do not** use for tinea versicolor during pregnancy. Safety of the 2.5% lotion has **not** been established in infants. **Avoid** contact with eyes, genital areas, and skin folds. Shampoo may be used for tinea capitis to reduce risk for transmission to others (does **not** eradicate tinea infection).

For tinea versicolor, 15%–25% sodium hyposulfite or thiosulfate (Tinver lotion) applied to affected areas BID × 2–4 wk is an alternative. Topical antifungals (e.g., clotrimazole, miconazole) may be used for small, focal infections.

Adverse effects: Local irritation, hair loss, mild contact dermatitis, and hair discoloration are common.

Drug interactions: None identified.

Drug administration: For topical use; **do not** use on broken or inflamed areas. Rinse hair and skin thoroughly after use and discontinue use if sensitivity reactions occur. **Avoid contact** with eyes, genital areas, and skin folds. Rinse hands and body well after treatment.

SERTACONAZOLE NITRATE
Ertaczo
Topical antifungal

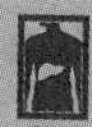
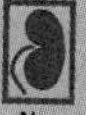
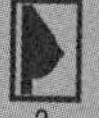
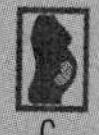

No No 2 C

Topical cream: 2% (30, 60 g)

Tinea:

Child 2–16 yr: Apply to affected area once daily × 2 wk.
Adult: Apply to affected area BID × 28 days.

Tinea pedis:

Child ≥12 yr and adult: Apply between toes and surrounding area BID × 4 wk.

Contraindications: Hypersensitivity to sertaconazole, other imidazoles, or any other components in the formulation

Warnings/Precautions: Discontinue use of drug when skin irritation/sensitivity occurs. **Avoid contact** with eyes, mouth, or vagina.

Adverse effects: Contact dermatitis, dry skin, burning skin, application site reaction, and skin tenderness may occur. Increase in serum aminotransferase has been reported.

Drug interactions: None identified.

Drug administration: Apply to affected area and to surrounding healthy skin. Skin should be dry before applying dose and wash your hands after each application. **Avoid** using an occlusive dressing and contact to the eyes, mouth, vagina, or other mucous membranes.

SILVER SULFADIAZINE
Silvadene, Thermazene, SSD Cream, SSD AF Cream, and others
Topical antibiotic

Yes Yes 3 B

Cream: 1% (20, 25, 50, 85, 400, 1000 g); contains methylparabens

≥2 mo: Cover affected areas completely once daily to BID. Apply cream to a thickness of 1/16 inch using sterile technique.

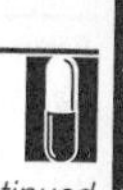

Continued

For explanation of icons, see p. 364.

SILVER SULFADIAZINE *continued*

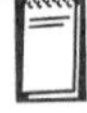

Contraindications: Hypersensitivity to silver, sulfonamide products, or any other components in the formulation; premature infants and infants ≤2 months of age because of concerns of kernicterus; and pregnancy (approaching term)

Warnings/Precautions: **Use with caution** in G6PD and renal and hepatic impairment. Significant systemic absorption may occur in severe burns.

Adverse effects: Pruritus, rash, and local skin irritation are common. Bone marrow suppression, hemolytic anemia, and interstitial nephritis have been reported.

Drug administration: Applied under sterile conditions for topical use to affected areas. Whenever necessary, reapply cream to any areas from which it has been removed by patient activity. Dressing may be used but is **not** necessary. **Not** for ophthalmic use. Discard product if cream has darkened.

SPECTINOMYCIN

Trobicin

Antibiotic, aminoglycoside

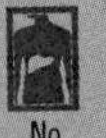 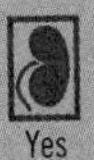 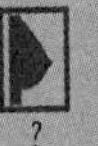 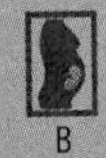

No Yes ? B

Injection: 2 g with 3.2 mL diluent may contain 0.9% benzyl alcohol

Drug may not be available in the United States.

Uncomplicated gonorrhea (consider adding a macrolide):

Child < 45 kg: 40 mg/kg IM × 1; **max. dose:** 2 g/dose

Child ≥ 45 kg and ≥8 yr old, and adult: 2 g IM × 1

Disseminated gonorrhea (for patients allergic to β-lactams and fluoroquinolones):

≥45 kg and ≥8 yrs old: 2 g IM Q12 hr × 7 days; alternatively may treat × 24–48 hr and switch to an oral alternative

Contraindications: Hypersensitivity to spectinomycin or any other components in the formulation

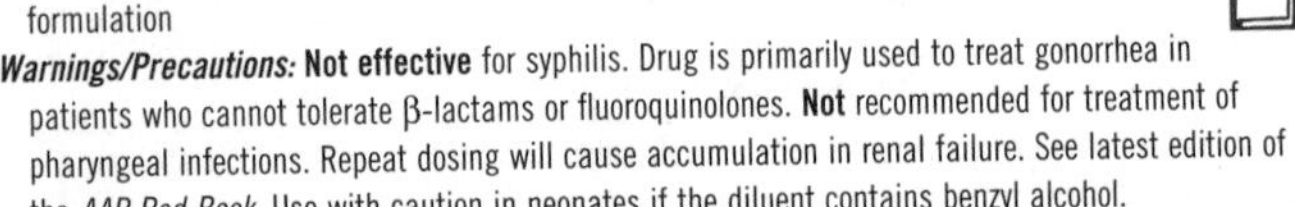

Warnings/Precautions: **Not effective** for syphilis. Drug is primarily used to treat gonorrhea in patients who cannot tolerate β-lactams or fluoroquinolones. **Not** recommended for treatment of pharyngeal infections. Repeat dosing will cause accumulation in renal failure. See latest edition of the *AAP Red Book*. Use with caution in neonates if the diluent contains benzyl alcohol.

Adverse effects: Vertigo, malaise, nausea, anorexia, chills, fever, urticaria, and injection site pain may occur.

Drug interactions: None identified.

Drug administration: **IM use only.** Inject deep into the upper outer quadrant of the gluteal muscle with a 20-gauge needle is recommended.

SPINOSAD

Natroba

Topical antiparasitic, pediculocide

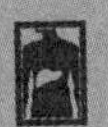 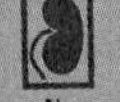 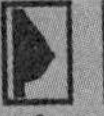 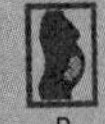

No No 2 B

Topical suspension: 0.9% (120 mL); contains benzyl alcohol, isopropyl alcohol

Head lice:

Child ≥ 6 mo and adult: Apply sufficient amount to cover dry scalp and completely cover dry hair (**max. dose:** 120 mL). Leave on for 10 min and then rinse thoroughly with warm water. If live lice is present after 7 days, dose may be repeated.

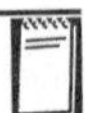

Contraindications: Hypersensitivity to spinosad or any other components in the formulation

Warnings/Precautions: Use is not recommended for infants younger than 6 months because the preparation contains benzyl alcohol. **Not** for oral, ophthalmic, or intravaginal use.

Adverse effects: Application site erythema is common.

Continued

SPINOSAD *continued*

Alopecia, dry skin, and skin exfoliation have been reported. Ocular erythema may occur.

Drug interactions: None identified.

Drug administration: Shake bottle immediately before each use. Apply sufficient amounts to cover dry scalp and rub gently until the scalp is thoroughly moistened (follow specific instructions in the dosing section).

Avoid contact with eyes, mouth, vagina, or other mucous membranes.

STAVUDINE

Zerit, d4T, and generics

Antiviral agent, nucleoside analogue reverse transcriptase inhibitor

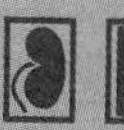
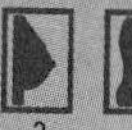
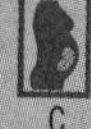

Yes Yes 3 C

Caps: 15, 20, 30, 40 mg

Oral solution: 1 mg/mL (200 mL); may contain methylparabens and propylparabens

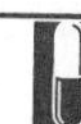

Neonate ≤13 days: 0.5 mg/kg/dose PO Q12 hr

Neonate ≥14 days, infant, and child <30 kg: 1 mg/kg/dose PO Q12 hr; ***max. dose:*** 30 mg PO Q12 hr

Adolescent ≥30 kg and adult:

30–60 kg: 30 mg PO Q12 hr

>60 kg: 40 mg PO Q12 hr

Contraindications: Hypersensitivity to stavudine or any other components contained in the formulation

Warnings/Precautions: Fatal lactic acidosis with hepatic steatosis with or without pancreatitis has been reported with use of nucleoside analogue alone or in combination therapy. The combination of stavudine and didanosine in pregnant women may result in fatal lactic acidosis or pancreatitis. Patients should be monitored for fat redistribution, lipoatrophy, or lipodystrophy.

Use with **caution** in liver disease. **Adjust dosage in renal impairment (see Chapter 3).**

Adverse effects: Headache, GI discomfort, lipoatrophy, and rash are common. Peripheral neuropathy, pancreatitis, lipodystrophy, lactic acidosis, severe hepatomegaly, and elevated liver enzymes have been reported.

Drug interactions: Should **not** be given in combination with zidovudine (AZT) because of poor antiviral effect. Drugs associated with peripheral neuropathy (e.g., chloramphenicol, dapsone, metronidazole) may increase risk for this side effect; see Warnings/Precautions.

Drug administration: Doses may be administered with or without food. *Oral solution:* Shake well before measuring each dose and keep refrigerated (30-day stability after initial reconstitution).

STIBOGLUCONATE

Pentostam, pentavalent antimony

Antiparasitic agent (leishmaniasis)

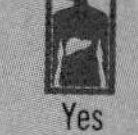
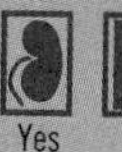
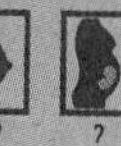
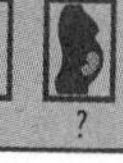

Yes Yes ? ?

AVAILABLE FROM THE U.S. CENTERS FOR DISEASE CONTROL AND PREVENTION (404-639-3670 Monday–Friday 8:00 AM–4:30 PM EST or 404-639-2888 evenings, weekends, or holidays)

Injection: 100 mg pentavalent antimony/mL; contains sodium

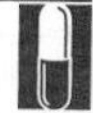

Leishmaniasis:

Child and adult: 20 mg/kg/24 hr IM/IV once daily with the following durations of therapy:

Cutaneous: for 20 days

Visceral and mucosal: for 28 days

Continued

For explanation of icons, see p. 364.

STIBOGLUCONATE *continued*

Contraindications: Hypersensitivity to stibogluconate

Warnings/Precautions: **Use with caution** in mild-to-moderate renal or hepatic insufficiency, pneumonia, cardiac disease, tuberculosis, and ECG abnormalities. **Avoid** concomitant use of alcohol and medications that are hepatotoxic or cause QT interval prolongation. Majority of dose excreted in urine; no specific renal impairment guidelines exist. Monitor baseline and weekly ECG, creatinine, transaminase, lipase, amylase, and CBCs. Hold therapy if QTc >0.5 sec, transaminase ≥4–5 times upper normal limit, and moderately severe clinical pancreatitis.

Adverse effects: Myalgia/arthralgia (use nonsteroidal anti-inflammatory agent), nausea, vomiting, abdominal pain, fatigue, elevated LFTs, T-wave changes on ECG, and depressed levels of hemoglobin, WBCs, and platelets are common. Rare severe cardiotoxicity has been reported.

Drug administration:

IM: Give undiluted drug (100 mg/mL) IM.

IV: Dilute patient-specific dose with 50 mL D_5W or NS; smaller volumes of diluent may be used for smaller drug doses. Administer over at least 10 minutes.

STREPTOMYCIN SULFATE

Various generics

Antibiotic, aminoglycoside; antituberculous agent

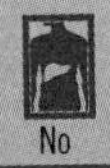
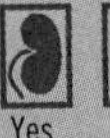
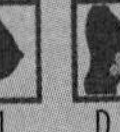
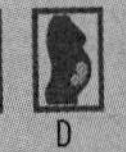
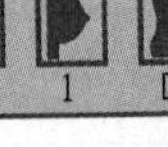

Powder for injection: 1 g

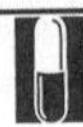

General dosing with other agents to which organism is sensitive:

Newborn: 10–20 mg/kg/24 hr IM ÷ Q12–24 hr

Infant: 20–30 mg/kg/24 hr IM ÷ Q12 hr

Child: 20–40 mg/kg/24 hr IM ÷ 6–12 hr

Adult: 1–2 g/24 hr IM ÷ 6–12 hr; **max. dose:** 2 g/24 hr

Tuberculosis: (use as part of multidrug regimen; see latest edition of* AAP Red Book*)

Infant, child, and adolescent:

Daily therapy: 20–40 mg/kg/24 hr IM once daily

Max. daily dose: 1 g/24 hr

Twice-weekly therapy: 20–40 mg/kg/dose IM twice weekly under direct observation

Max. daily dose: 1.5 g/24 hr

Adult:

Daily therapy: 15 mg/kg/24 hr IM once daily

Max. daily dose: 1 g/24 hr

Twice-weekly therapy: 25–30 mg/kg/dose IM twice weekly under direct observation

Max. daily dose: 1.5 g/24 hr

Brucellosis (see latest edition of the* AAP Red Book*):

Child ≥ 7 yr: 1 g/dose IM once daily (15 mg/kg/dose if ≤50 kg) × 14 days with doxycycline 100 mg PO BID (5 mg/kg/dose if ≤40 kg) × 45 days

Adult: 15 mg/kg/dose (**max. dose:** 1 g/dose) IM once daily × 2–3 wk in combination with doxycycline 100 mg PO BID × 4–6 wk

Tularemia:

Child: 30 mg/kg/24 hr IM ÷ Q8–12 hr; **max. dose:** 2 g/24 hr × 10–14 days

Adult: 1–2 g/24 hr IM ÷ Q8–12 hr × 7–14 days and until afebrile for 5–7 days

Plague:

Child and adult: 30 mg/kg/24 hr IM ÷ Q8–12 hr; **max. dose:** 2 g/24 hr × 10–14 days

Continued

STREPTOMYCIN SULFATE *continued*

Contraindications: Hypersensitivity to streptomycin, aminoglycosides, and sulfites

Warnings/Precautions: **Use with caution** in preexisting vertigo, tinnitus, hearing loss, and neuromuscular disorders. Monitor auditory status. Concomitant neurotoxic, ototoxic, or nephrotoxic drugs and dehydration may increase risk factors for toxicity. Concomitant use of anesthesia or muscle relaxants increases risk for neuromuscular blockade and respiratory paralysis. **Adjust dose in renal insufficiency (see Chapter 3).**

Therapeutic levels: Peak 15–40 mg/L, trough: <5 mg/L. Recommended serum sampling time at steady state: trough within 30 min before the third consecutive dose and peak 30–60 min after the administration of the third consecutive dose. Therapeutic levels are not achieved in CSF.

Adverse effects: Drug-induced eosinophilia, facial paresthesia, and fever are common. May cause bone marrow suppression, other neurologic problems, CNS depression (in infants with dosages exceeding recommended limits), nephrotoxicity, ototoxicity, myocarditis, and serum sickness.

Drug interactions: Ototoxicity is potentiated with ethacrynic acid and furosemide. See Warnings/Precautions for additional interactions.

Drug administration: **Drug is administered via deep IM injection only.** The preferred site is the upper outer quadrant of the buttock (e.g., gluteus maximus) or midlateral thigh.

SULCONAZOLE
Exelderm
Antifungal agent, imidazole

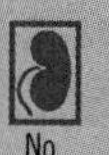
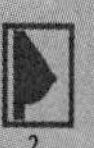
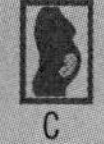

No No ? C

Topical cream: 1% (15, 30, 60 g)
Topical solution: 1% (30 mL)

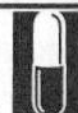

Adult: Apply sparingly to affected and surrounding areas once to twice daily. Tinea cruris, tinea corporis, and tinea versicolor should be treated for 3 wk and tinea pedis for 4 wk to reduce the risk for recurrence.

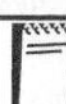

Contraindications: Hypersensitivity to sulconazole, azole antifungals, or any other components in the formulation

Warnings/Precautions: **Discontinue** use if irritation develops. **External use only; avoid** contact with eyes. Safety and effectiveness in children has not been established.

Adverse effects: Itching, burning/stinging, and redness are common. Immune hypersensitivity reaction has been reported.

Drug interactions: None identified.

Drug administration: Gently massage to affected and surrounding areas; **avoid** contact with the eyes.

SULFACETAMIDE SODIUM, OPHTHALMIC
Bleph 10, Sulfamide, and various generic products
Ophthalmic antibiotic, sulfonamide derivative

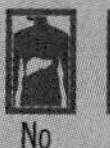
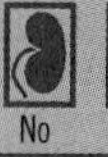
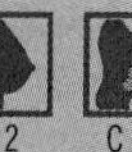

No No 2 C

Ophthalmic solution: 10% (5, 15 mL); may contain methylparaben and propylparaben
Ophthalmic ointment: 10% (3.5 g); may contain phenylmecuric acetate

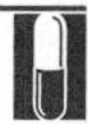

Ophthalmic (usual duration of therapy for ophthalmic use is 7–10 days):

>2 mo and adult:

Ointment: Apply 0.5-inch ribbon into conjunctival sac Q3–4 hr and QHS initially, and reduce the dosing frequency with adequate response.

Drops: 1–2 drops Q2–3 hr to affected eye(s) initially and reduce the dosing frequency with adequate response

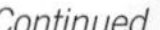

Continued

For explanation of icons, see p. 364.

SULFACETAMIDE SODIUM, OPHTHALMIC *continued*

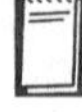

Contraindications: Hypersensitivity to sulfonamides or to any ingredient of the preparation

Warnings/Precautions: Hypersensitivity reactions between different sulfonamides can occur regardless of route of administration.

Adverse effects: Local irritation, stinging, burning, conjunctival hyperemia, excessive tear production, and eye pain are common. Rare toxic epidermal necrolysis and Stevens–Johnson syndrome have been reported.

Drug interactions: Sulfacetamide preparations are incompatible with silver preparations.

Drug administration:

Drops: Apply finger pressure to lacrimal sac during and for 1 to 2 minutes after dose application to reduce risk for systemic absorption. **Avoid** contact with the tip of the container.

Ointment: Apply 0.5-inch ribbon of ointment into conjunctival sac by avoiding contact of ointment tip with eye or skin.

SULFADIAZINE

Various generic products

Antibiotic, sulfonamide derivative

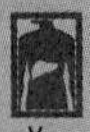 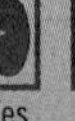 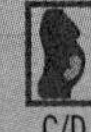

Yes Yes 3 C/D

Tabs: 500 mg

Oral suspension: 100, 200 mg/mL

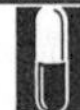

Infant ≥2 mo and child: 75 mg/kg/dose or 2000 mg/m²/dose PO × 1, followed by 150 mg/kg/24 hr or 4000 mg/m²/24 hr PO ÷ Q4–6 hr (**max. dose:** 6000 mg/24 hr)

Adult: 2–4 g/24 hr PO ÷ Q4–8 hr

Congenital toxoplasmosis (administer with pyrimethamine and folinic acid; see pyrimethamine for dosage information) (from Clin Infect Dis 18:38, 1994):

Infant: 100 mg/kg/24 hr PO ÷ BID × 12 mo

Toxoplasmosis (administer with pyrimethamine and folinic acid; see pyrimethamine for dosage information):

Infant ≥2 mo and child: 100–200 mg/kg/24 hr PO ÷ Q6 hr × 3–4 wk; **max. dose:** 6000 mg/24 hr

Adult: 4–6 g/24 hr PO ÷ Q6 hr × 3–4 wk

Prophylaxis for recurrence of* Toxoplasa gondii *with HIV (prior to Toxoplasma encephalitis, with pyrimethamine):

Infant and child: 85–120 mg/kg/24 hr ÷ Q6–12 hr; **max. dose:** 4 g/24 hr

Rheumatic fever prophylaxis:

≤27 kg: 500 mg PO once daily

>27 kg: 1000 mg PO once daily

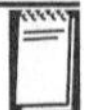

Contraindications: Hypersensitivity to sulfadiazine and other sulfonamides, or porphyria

Warnings/Precautions: **Use with caution** in premature infants and infants younger than 2 months because of risk for hyperbilirubinemia, G6PD deficiency, and in hepatic or renal dysfunction (30%–44% eliminated in urine). Maintain hydration to prevent crystalluria and stone formation. Pregnancy category changes from C to D if administered near term.

Adverse effects: Fever, rash, photosensitivity, GI disturbances, hepatitis, SLE-like syndrome, vasculitis, bone marrow suppression and hemolysis (patients with G6PD deficiency), and Stevens–Johnson syndrome may occur.

Drug interactions: May cause increased effects of warfarin, methotrexate, thiazide diuretics, uricosuric agents, and sulfonylureas. Large quantities of vitamin C or acidifying agents (e.g., cranberry juice) may cause crystalluria.

Drug administration: Take on an empty stomach with water (at least 8 ounces for adults).

S

FORMULARY

SULFAMETHOXAZOLE AND TRIMETHOPRIM

Trimethoprim-sulfamethoxazole (TMP-SMX); Bactrim, Septra, Sulfatrim, and others

Antibiotic, sulfonamide derivative

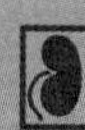
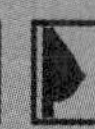
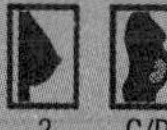
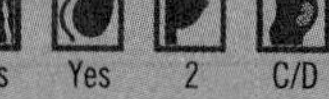

Yes Yes 2 C/D

Tabs (regular strength): 80 mg TMP/400 mg SMX
Tabs (double strength): 160 mg TMP/800 mg SMX
Oral suspension: 40 mg TMP/200 mg SMX per 5 mL (100, 480 mL)
Injection: 16 mg TMP/mL and 80 mg SMX/mL (5, 10, 30 mL); some preparations may contain propylene glycol and benzyl alcohol

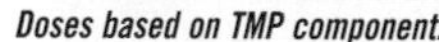
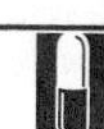

Doses based on TMP component.

Minor-to-moderate infections (PO or IV):
- ***Child:*** 8–12 mg/kg/24 hr ÷ BID
- ***Adult (>40 kg):*** 160 mg/dose BID

Severe infections (PO or IV):
- ***Child and adult:*** 20 mg/kg/24 hr ÷ Q6–8 hr

UTI prophylaxis:
- ***Child:*** 2–4 mg/kg/24 hr PO once daily

Pneumocystis jiroveci *(formerly* carinii*) pneumonia:*
- ***Treatment (PO/IV):*** 20 mg/kg/24 hr ÷ Q6–8 hr × 21 days
- ***Prophylaxis (PO or IV):***
  - ***≥1 mo and child:*** 150 mg/m^2/24 hr ÷ BID for 3 consecutive days/wk; **max. dose:** 320 mg/24 hr
  - ***Adult:*** 160 mg once daily or 160 mg 3 days/wk

Traveler's diarrhea:
- ***Adult:*** 160–320 mg PO Q12 hr × 5 days

Contraindications: Sulfonamide or trimethoprim hypersensitivity, and megaloblastic anemia caused by folate deficiency

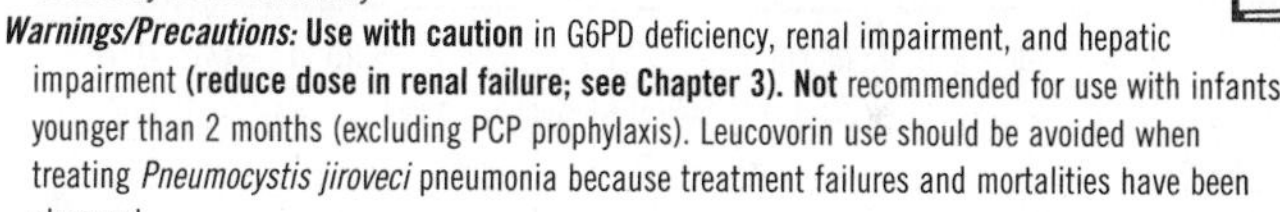

Warnings/Precautions: **Use with caution** in G6PD deficiency, renal impairment, and hepatic impairment **(reduce dose in renal failure; see Chapter 3). Not** recommended for use with infants younger than 2 months (excluding PCP prophylaxis). Leucovorin use should be avoided when treating *Pneumocystis jiroveci* pneumonia because treatment failures and mortalities have been observed.

Do not use drug at term during pregnancy. Pregnancy risk factor changes to "D" if administered near term. Assure adequate hydration.

Adverse effects: May cause kernicterus in newborns. Blood dyscrasias, crystalluria, glossitis, renal or hepatic injury, GI irritation, rash, Stevens–Johnson syndrome, hemolysis in patients with G6PD deficiency. Hyperkalemia may appear in HIV/AIDS patients treated for *Pneumocystis jiroveci.*

Drug interactions: Increases effects/toxicity of warfarin, methotrexate and sulfonylureas, phenytoin, digoxin, and thiopental. Decreases cyclosporine levels. See Warnings/Precautions section for additional drug interactions.

Drug administration:

IV: For intermittent infusion, infuse over 60 to 90 minutes at a concentration 0.64 to 1.6 mg/mL. Stability of diluted IV solution is inversely related to concentration, ranging from 1 to 6 hours.

PO: Administer doses on an empty stomach with adequate hydration.

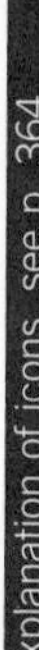
For explanation of icons, see p. 364.

SULFANILAMIDE
AVC Vaginal
Antifungal, sulfonamide

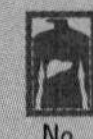 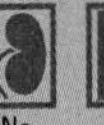 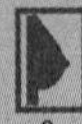 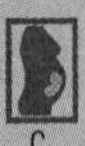
No No 3 C

Vaginal cream: 15% (120 g); contains propylparaben, methylparaben

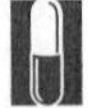

Candida albicans *vulvovaginitis:*
Adult: Insert one applicatorful (~6 g) intravaginally once to twice daily × 30 days.

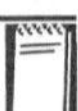

Contraindications: Hypersensitivity to sulfanilamide or any other components in the formulation
Warnings/Precautions: Sulfanilamide is not considered a preferred or alternative therapy for uncomplicated vulvovaginitis as other agents are preferred. Refrain from intercourse during treatment because sexual partner may experience irritation.
Adverse effects: Local vaginal burning and discomfort may occur. Sulfonamide-related reactions such as severe dermatologic reactions (e.g., Stevens–Johnson syndrome, TEN), hepatic necrosis, sulfonamide allergy, and blood dyscrasias (e.g., agranulocytosis, anemia) have been reported regardless of administration route.
Drug interactions: None identified.
Drug administration: Douching with a suitable solution before dose administration may be recommended for hygienic purposes. Wash hands before use. Gently insert applicator full of cream high into the vagina. Remain lying down for 30 minutes after administration. Wash applicator with soap and water after each use.

SURAMIN
Antrypol, Arsobal, Bayer 205, Belganyl, Fourneau 309, Germanin, Mel B, Moranyl, Naphuride
Antiprotozoal, anthelmintic agent

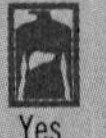 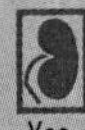 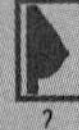 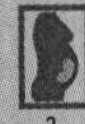 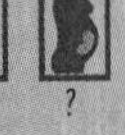
Yes Yes ? ?

AVAILABLE FROM THE U.S. CENTERS FOR DISEASE CONTROL AND PREVENTION (404-639-3670 Monday–Friday 8:00 AM–4:30 PM EST or 404-639-2888 evenings, weekends, or holidays)
Injection: 1 g

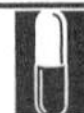

Test dose (for all indications):
Child: 10–20 mg/kg/dose IV × 1; **max. dose:** 200 mg/dose
Adult: 100–200 mg IV × 1

Typanosomiasis (IV, initiate 24 hours after the administration and tolerance of the aforementioned test dose):
Child: 10–20 mg/kg/dose on days 1, 3, 7, 14, and 21
Adult:
Early stage: 20 mg/kg/dose (**max. dose:** 1 g/dose) on days 1, 3, 7, 14, and 21. Alternatively, 20 mg/kg/dose weekly until a total dose of 5 g is achieved may be given. Patients in poor general condition should receive approximately one quarter of the normal dose.
Late stage: 10 mg/kg/dose Q5 days for a total of 12 doses. This is given in combination with tryparsamide at a dose of 30 mg/kg/dose (**max. dose:** 2 g/dose) IV Q5 days for 12 doses. If needed, a second treatment course may be repeated 1 mo later.

Onchocerciasis (IV, usually following a 23- to 32-day course of diethylcarbamazine as an alternative to ivermectin):
Child: Following the administration and tolerance of the aforementioned test dose, initiate 20 mg/kg/dose Q weekly × 5 weeks 1 week after the test dose.

Continued

SURAMIN *continued*

Adult: Following the administration and tolerance of the aforementioned test dose, treatment with the full dose may be started 1 week after. A total dose of 66.7 mg/kg should be administered in six incremental weekly doses apportioned as follows: 3.3 mg/kg/dose week one, 6.7 mg/kg/dose week two, 10 mg/kg/dose week three, 13.3 mg/kg/dose week four, and 16.7 mg/kg/dose weeks 5 and 6.

Max. daily dose for all indications:

Child: 20 mg/kg/24 hr

Adult: 1–1.5 g/24 hr

Contraindications: Hypersensitivity to suramin or any other components in the formulation

Warnings/Precautions: **Administer a test dose before initiating therapy;** significant immediate reactions consist of nausea, vomiting, shock, and loss of consciousness (0.1–0.3% incidence rate). **Use with caution** in renal and hepatic impairment (**avoid** use in severe impairment), peripheral neuritis, and malnourished/debilitated patients. Prolonged use in ocular onchocerciasis may result in degenerative changes to the optic disk and retina.

Eliminated primarily in the urine very slowly; no specific renal impairment dosing guidelines are available. Drug may be absorbed by the liver to cause hepatic damage and is highly protein bound (99.7%). Monitor CBC, creatinine, and urinalysis.

Adverse effects: Arthritis, nephrotoxicity with transient albuminuria, maculopapular eruptions, headache, palmarplantar hyperesthesias, praesthesias, peripheral neuropathy, pruritus, relative adrenal insufficiency, and urticaria are common. Blood dyscrasias, exfoliative dermatitis, hepatitis, jaundice, and occular effects (e.g., lacrimation, optic atrophy, palpebral edema, photophobia, stomatitis, and prostration) have been reported.

Drug interactions: None identified.

Drug administration: Reconstitute vial with sterile water to a 10% (100 mg/mL) concentration and administer by slow IV injection within 30 minutes of reconstitution.

TELAPREVIR
Incivek
Antiviral, protease inhibitor

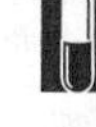

Tabs: 375 mg (28-day pack)

Chronic hepatitis C (genotype 1; in combination with peginterferon alfa and ribavirin):

Adult: 750 mg PO TID (spaced every 7–9 hr) × 12 wk; continue treatment through week 48 with peginterferon alfa and ribavirin if HCV-RNA is ≤1000 units/mL at weeks 4 and/or 12. Discontinue 3-drug regimen at treatment week 4 or 12 if viral RNA levels >1000 units/mL. Discontinue peginterferon alfa and ribavirin therapy if RNA levels are confirmed detectable (>10–15 unit/mL) at treatment week 24.

Contraindications: Hypersensitivity to telaprevir or any component of the formulation. Coadministration with strong CYP 450 3A inducers or drugs that are highly dependent on CYP 450 3A for clearance with a narrow therapeutic index (e.g., alfuzosin, atorvastatin, cisapride, ergot derivatives, lovastatin, midazolam, pimozide, rifampin, sildenafil/tadalafil [for treatment of pulmonary hypertension], simvastatin, St. John's wort, and triazolam). Women who are or may become pregnant; male partners of pregnant women; and combination treatment with ribavirin.

Warnings/Precautions: Severe skin reactions (some fatal) have been reported when taken in combination with peginterferon alfa and ribavirin for chronic hepatitis C; patient should be instructed of this reaction and when to seek medical care. Hemoglobin should be monitored at baseline, and at least at weeks 2, 4, 8, and 12 during combination therapy and as clinically

Continued

For explanation of icons, see p. 364.

TELAPREVIR *continued*

appropriate. Use of a sensitive real-time PCR assay for HCV-RNA with a lower limit of quantification of ≤25 IU/mL and a lower limit of HCV-RNA detection of ~10–15 IU/mL is recommended.

Do not use in moderate-to-severe hepatic impairment (Child–Pugh class B/C). No dosage adjustment needed for mild renal (CrCl >50 mL/min) and hepatic (Child–Pugh class A) impairments. Use with **caution** with moderate-to-severe renal impairment as the pharmacokinetics have not been evaluated in CrCl ≤50 mL/min and hemodialysis.

Pregnancy category changes to "X" when used with ribavirin.

Adverse effects: Rash, pruritus, fatigue, anemia, anorectal discomfort/pain, diarrhea, nausea, vomiting, hemorrhoids, and altered taste perception are common. Stevens–Johnson syndrome, TEN, and drug hypersensitivity syndrome have been reported.

Drug interactions: Drug is a major substrate and strong inhibitor for CYP 450 3A4 and P-glycoprotein.

See Contraindications and Warnings/Precautions sections for additional interactions. May increase effects/toxicity of alprazolam, amiodarone, atazanavir, bosentan, budesonide (all routes of administration), carbamazepine, clarithromycin, colchicine, systemic corticosteroids, digoxin, fluticasone, rifabutin, propafenone, flecainide, quinidine, and triazolam. May decrease the effects of darunavir/ritonavir, efavirenz, and fosamprenavir/ritonavir. Atazanavir, bosentan, carbamazepine, systemic corticosteroids, darunavir/ritonavir, efavirenz, fosamprenavir/ritonavir, lopinavir, phenobarbital, phenytoin, and rifabutin may decrease telaprevir's effects. Macrolide antibiotics (e.g., clarithromycin) may increase telaprevir's effects.

Drug administration: Take doses with a meal and space doses every 7 to 9 hours.

TELAVANCIN
Vibativ
Glycopeptide

No Yes ? C

Injection: 250, 750 mg; contains cyclodextrin

Complicated skin and skin structure infection:
Adult: 10 mg/kg/dose IV Q24 hr × 1–2 wk

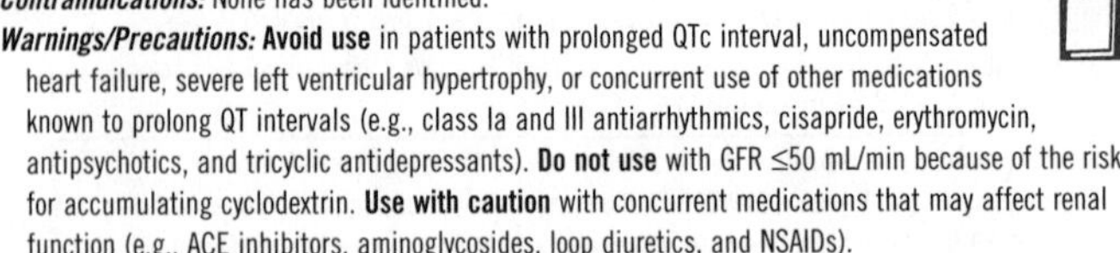

Contraindications: None has been identified.

Warnings/Precautions: **Avoid use** in patients with prolonged QTc interval, uncompensated heart failure, severe left ventricular hypertrophy, or concurrent use of other medications known to prolong QT intervals (e.g., class Ia and III antiarrhythmics, cisapride, erythromycin, antipsychotics, and tricyclic antidepressants). **Do not use** with GFR ≤50 mL/min because of the risk for accumulating cyclodextrin. **Use with caution** with concurrent medications that may affect renal function (e.g., ACE inhibitors, aminoglycosides, loop diuretics, and NSAIDs).

Adverse developmental outcomes have been observed in animals. All women of childbearing potential should have a serum pregnancy test before use with effective contraception.

Adverse effects: Nausea, altered taste perception, vomiting, and foaming of the urine are common. Prolonged cardiac QT interval, rash, infusion-related reactions, and renal impairment have been reported.

Drug interactions: Medications that may affect renal function and prolong QT intervals; see Warnings/Precautions section. May falsely increase clotting factor times (e.g., PT, INR, aPTT, ACT, Xa).

Drug administration: IV over 1 hour. Infusion-related reactions have been reported and may be abated by slowing or stopping the drug infusion.

TELBIVUDINE
Tyzeka
Antiviral, nucleoside reverse transcriptase inhibitor

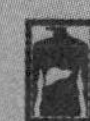 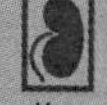 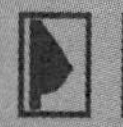 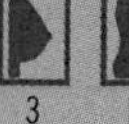 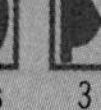 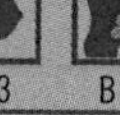

Yes Yes 3 B

Tabs: 600 mg
Oral solution: 100 mg/5 mL; each 600 mg dose contains approximately 47 mg sodium

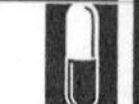

Chronic hepatitis B:
≥16 yr and adult: 600 mg PO once daily

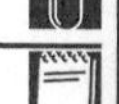

Contraindications: Concomitant use with pegylated interferon alfa-2a; hypersensitivity to telbivudine or any other components in the formulation

Warnings/Precautions: Lactic acidosis and severe hepatomegaly with steatosis (some fatal) have been reported; risk is higher in women, obesity, or with prolonged use of nucleoside reverse transcriptase inhibitor use. Myopathy, rhabdomyolysis, and peripheral neuropathy may occur. Suspend therapy if any of the above adverse events are present.

Severe acute exacerbations of hepatitis B after discontinuation can occur; monitor hepatic function closely for several months after discontinuation. **Adjust dose in renal impairment (see Chapter 3).**

Adverse effects: Fatigue, increased creatine kinase, ALT, headache, cough, diarrhea, GI discomfort, nausea, pharyngolaryngeal pain, arthralgia, pyrexia, rash, back pain, dizziness, myalgia, and insomnia are common.

Drug interactions: Increased risk for peripheral neuropathy when used with interferon alfa-2a.

Drug administration: Doses may be taken with or without food.

TELITHROMYCIN
Ketek
Ketolide

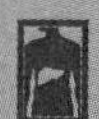 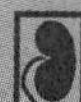 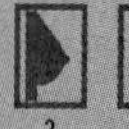 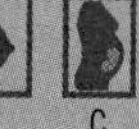

Yes Yes ? C

Tabs: 300, 400 mg

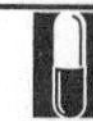

Community-acquired pneumonia:
Adult: 800 mg PO once daily × 7–10 days

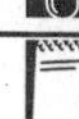

Contraindications: Hypersensitivity to telithromycin, other macrolide antibiotics, or any other components in the formulation. History of hepatitis or jaundice caused by telithromycin or other macrolide antibiotics. Concurrent use with cisapride, pimozide, or vasopressin; or colchicine with renal or hepatic impairment. Presence of myasthenia gravis; may result in exacerbations and fatal respiratory failure.

Warnings/Precautions: **Do not use** with QT interval prolongation and other proarrhythmic conditions (e.g., hypokalemia, hypomagnesemia, bradycardia). **Avoid** use with the following medications: cisapride, ergot derivatives, rifampin, atorvastatin, lovastatin, simvastatin, and other medications that may prolong QT interval (class Ia and III antiarrhythmics). Monitor for hepatic injury because hepatic injury/failure has been observed. Visual disturbances such as blurred vision, difficulty in focusing, diplopia, and accommodation slowness have been reported.

Reduce doses in renal impairment (see Chapter 3). Medication is no longer indicated for use in acute bacterial sinusitis and acute bacterial exacerbations of chronic bronchitis because of unfavorable benefits to risks.

Adverse effects: Diarrhea, nausea, vomiting, headache, dizziness, and abnormal vision are common. Loss of consciousness by a vagal syndrome has been reported. See Warnings/Precautions for additional adverse effects.

Continued

For explanation of icons, see p. 364.

TELITHROMYCIN *continued*

Drug interactions: Telithromycin is a major substrate and inhibitor to CYP 450 3A4, minor substrate to CYP 1A2, and weak inhibitor of CYP 2D6. Azole antifungals (e.g., ketoconazole, itraconazole), diltiazem, and diazepam may increase telithromycin levels/effects. CYP 450 3A4 inducer may decrease telithromycin's effects.

Telithromycin may increase the effects/toxicity of benzodiazepines (e.g., diazepam, midazolam), digoxin, diltiazem, buspirone, carbamazepine, cyclosporine, metoprolol, phenytoin, sirolimus, tacrolimus, narcotic analgesics, theophylline, verapamil, and warfarin, whereas it may decrease the effects of sotalol. See Contraindications and Warnings/Precautions sections for additional interactions.

Drug administration: Doses may be taken with or without food.

TENOFOVIR DISOPROXIL FUMARATE
Viread, PMPA, TDF
Antiviral agent, nucleoside analogue reverse transcriptase inhibitor

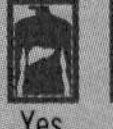
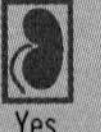
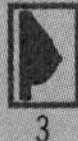
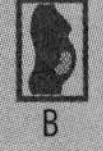
Yes Yes 3 B

Tabs (as tenofovir disoproxil fumarate): 150, 200, 250, 300 mg
Oral powder (as tenofovir disoproxil fumarate): 40 mg/g (60 g); one level scoop = 40 mg tenofovir disoproxil fumarate
In combination with emtricitabine as Truvada:
Tabs: 300 mg tenofovir disoproxil fumarate and 200 mg emtricitabine
In combination with emtricitabine and efavirenz as Atripla:
Tabs: 300 mg tenofovir disoproxil fumarate, 200 mg emtricitabine, and 600 mg efavirenz

Dosage based on tenofovir disoproxil fumarate:
HIV treatment:
Child ≥2–12 yr: 8 mg/kg/dose PO once daily; **max. dose:** 300 mg/dose. Alternative weight-based dosing tables by dosage forms:
Oral powder for child ≥2 yr old:

Weight (kg)	No. of Level Scoops of Powder (mg drug) Administered Once Daily*
10 to <12	2 (80 mg)
12 to <14	2.5 (100 mg)
14 to <17	3 (120 mg)
17 to <19	3.5 (140 mg)
19 to <22	4 (160 mg)
22 to <24	4.5 (180 mg)
24 to <27	5 (200 mg)
27 to <29	5.5 (220 mg)
29 to <32	6 (240 mg)
32 to <34	6.5 (260 mg)
34 to <35	7 (280 mg)
≥35	7.5 (300 mg)

*One level scoop provides 40 mg tenofovir disoproxil fumarate.

Oral tablets for child ≥2 yr and weighing ≥17 kg:

Weight (kg)	Tablet Dosage Administered Once Daily
17 to <22	150 mg
22 to <28	200 mg
28 to <35	250 mg
≥35	300 mg

Continued

TENOFOVIR DISOPROXIL FUMARATE *continued*

Child ≥12 yr and adult (≥35 kg): 300 mg PO once daily
Adult in combination with didanosine: 300 mg PO once daily with the following didanosine dosage:
<60 kg: Didanosine delayed-release capsule 200 mg PO once daily is recommended.
≥60 kg: Didanosine delayed-release capsule 250 mg PO once daily is recommended.
Adult in combination with atazanavir: 300 mg atazanavir boosted with 100 mg ritonavir should be in combination with 300 mg tenofovir, all as PO once daily.

Truvada (HIV treatment and preexposure prophylaxis):
Child ≥12 yr and adult (≥35 kg):
GFR ≥50 mL/min and not receiving hemodialysis: 1 tab PO once daily
GFR 30–49 mL/min and not receiving hemodialysis: 1 tab PO Q48 hr
GFR <30 mL/min or receiving hemodialysis: Use not recommended

Atripla (HIV treatment):
Child ≥12 yr and adult (≥40 kg):
GFR ≥50 mL/min: 1 tab PO once daily on an empty stomach. Patients weighing ≥50 kg and receiving rifampin should have an additional 200 mg/24 hr efavirenz.
GFR <50 mL/min: Use not recommended.

Chronic hepatitis B:
Child <12 yr: Safety and efficacy have not been established.
Child ≥12 yr and adult (≥35 kg): 300 mg PO once daily

Contraindications: Hypersensitivity to tenofovir or any other components in the formulation.
Do not use Truvada for preexposure prophylaxis with unknown or positive HIV-1 status.

Warnings/Precautions: Lactic acidosis and severe hepatomegaly with steatosis have been reported especially in women with obesity, prior liver disease, or prolonged nucleoside exposure. Severe acute exacerbation of hepatitis may occur in patients with HBV when tenofovir is discontinued. Bone mineral density assessment should be considered for patients with history of bone fractures or other risk for osteoporosis or bone loss; use of calcium and vitamin D supplementation may be beneficial. Autoimmune disorders (e.g., Graves disease, polymyositis, and Guillain-Barré syndrome) and angioedema may occur with immune reconstitution syndrome.

Use with caution in renal impairment; reduce dose (see Chapter 3). If using combination product, review other medications.

Truvada: Use in preexposure prophylaxis is only for HIV-negative status before initiating with periodic monitoring (minimum Q3mo), and with GFR ≥60 mL/min.

Atripla: Use not recommended with moderate-to-severe hepatic impairment.

Adverse effects: Nausea, diarrhea, vomiting, and flatulence are common. May cause decreased bone mineral density, lactic acidosis, severe hepatomegaly with steatosis (see Warnings/Precautions) and renal tubular dysfunction (monitor renal status).

Adults treated for chronic hepatitis B and decompensated liver disease frequently experienced abdominal pain, pruritus, insomnia, pyrexia, and the aforementioned common adverse effects.

Drug interactions: Coadministration with drugs that reduce renal function or compete for active tubular secretion (e.g., Cidofovir, acyclovir, valacyclovir, ganciclovir, valganciclovir) may increase tenofovir levels. Tenofovir may increase didanosine levels and decrease atazanavir levels.

Drug administration:

Tabs: Doses may be administered with or without food; high-fat meals may increase absorption. The combination product, Atripla, should be administered on an empty stomach. When coadministered with didanosine, administer delayed-release didanosine capsules under fasted conditions or with a light meal, and administer buffered didanosine tablets under fasted conditions.

Oral powder: Use supplied measuring scoop when measuring doses. Mix powder with 2 to 4 oz of soft food such as applesauce, baby food, or yogurt, and swallow immediately to avoid the bitter taste. **Do not** mix with any liquid because the powder will not mix.

For explanation of icons, see p. 364.

TERBINAFINE
Lamisil, Terbinex, Lamisil AT
Antifungal, allylamine

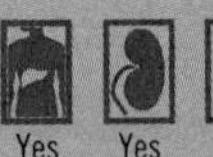
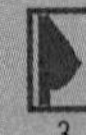
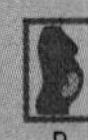
Yes Yes 3 B

Oral suspension: 25 mg/mL
Oral granules: 125-mg packets (42s), 187.5-mg packets (14s, 42s)
Tabs: 250 mg
Terbinex Kit: 250 mg (30s, 42s) with Eco-Formula nail enhancer
Topical solution or spray (Lamisil AT [OTC]): 1% (30 mL); contains propylene glycol and ethanol
Topical cream (Lamisil AT [OTC] and other generics): 1% (15, 30 g); contains benzyl alcohol
Topical gel (Lamisil AT) [OTC]: 1% (6, 12 g); contains benzyl alcohol

Child (dosage is not well established, but the following have been recommended):
"Standard" dose:
10–20 kg: 62.5 mg PO once daily
21–40 kg: 125 mg PO once daily
>40 kg: 250 mg PO once daily
"High" dose:
10–15 kg: 125 mg PO once daily
16–25 kg: 187.5 mg PO once daily
>25 kg: 250 mg PO once daily
Tinea capitis (≥4 yr and adolescent) using the oral granule dosage form sprinkled on pudding or other soft nonacidic foods (e.g., mashed potatoes; do not use applesauce):
<25 kg: 125 mg PO once daily
25–35 kg: 187.5 mg PO once daily
>35 kg: 250 mg PO once daily
Recommended duration of therapy for tinea capitis is 6 wk or 2–8 wk (*Trichophyton* species for 2–4 wk, *Microsporum* species for 2–8 wk).
Onychomycosis (child and adolescent; limited data):
10–20 kg: 62.5 mg PO once daily
21–40 kg: 125 mg PO once daily
>40 kg: 250 mg PO once daily
Recommended duration of therapy for onychomycosis is 6–12 wk (fingernail for 6 wk, toenail for 12 wk).
Adult: 250 mg PO once daily; for fingernail onychomycosis, use for 6 wk and for toenail onychomycosis use for 12 wk.
Topical:
≥12 yr and adult:
Tinea pedis: Apply topical cream, gel, or solution to affected areas once daily for at least 1 wk, but not to exceed 4 wk.
Tinea versicolor: Apply the topical cream or solution to affected areas once daily × 7 days.
Tinea corporis or tinea cruris:
Cream: Apply to affected areas once to twice daily for at least 1 wk, but not to exceed 4 wk.
Gel or solution: Apply to affected areas once daily × 7 days.

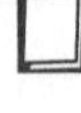

Contraindications: Hypersensitivity to terbinafine or to any other components of the formulation
Warnings/Precautions:
PO: Rare hepatotoxicity, including hepatic failure, has been reported in patients with or without preexisting liver disease. Should **not** be used in chronic or active liver disease because the drug is extensively metabolized by the liver and specific hepatic impairment dosing recommendations are **not** currently available. Baseline ALT and AST are recommended.

Continued

TERBINAFINE *continued*

Not recommended in patients with GFR less than 50 mL/min because the drug has extensive renal excretion (no dose modification information available). **Use with caution** in immunodeficiency because of reports of neutropenia (consider monitoring CBC for therapies longer than 6 wk).

Topical: **Do not** use on nails, scalp, in or near the mouth or eyes, or for vaginal yeast infections.

Adverse effects:

PO: GI disturbances, headache, abnormal LFTs, rash, urticaria, pruritus, and taste disturbances are common and are generally mild and transient. Psoriasiform eruptions or exacerbation of psoriasis, acute exanthematous pustulosis, and precipitation and exacerbation of lupus erythematous have been reported. See Warning/Precautions.

Topical: Localized burning/irritation, itching, skin exfoliation, and rash may occur.

Drug interactions:

PO: Cimetidine increases terbinafine levels, but rifampin significantly decreases terbinafine levels. Terbinafine may increase the effects/toxicity of dextromethorphan and caffeine but decreases cyclosporine levels. Inhibits CYP 450 2D6 and may increase the effects/toxicity of drug metabolized by this enzyme (e.g., β-blockers, class 1C antiarrhythmics, selective serotonin reuptake inhibitors, and MAO inhibitors type B).

Drug administration:

PO: Take with or without food.

Topical: Clean and dry affected areas before dose application. Apply to affected area and surrounding skin. Wash hands after each use.

TERCONAZOLE
Terazol 3, Terazol 7, and other generics
Antifungal agent, triazole

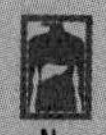

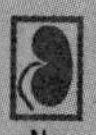

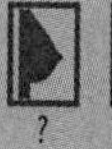

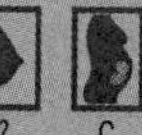

Vaginal cream:
- **Terazol 7 and generics:** 0.4% (45 g with or without applicator)
- **Terazol 3 and generics:** 0.8% (20 g with or without applicator)

Vaginal suppository:
- **Terazol 3 and generics:** 80 mg (3s)

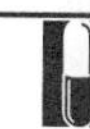

Candidal vulvovaginitis:

Cream:
- ***0.4%:*** 1 applicator full intravaginally QHS × 7 days
- ***0.8%:*** 1 applicator full intravaginally QHS × 3 days

Vaginal suppository: 1 suppository intravaginally QHS × 3 days

Contraindications: Hypersensitivity to terconazole or to any of the components of the cream or suppository

Warnings/Precautions: **Avoid** use in first trimester of pregnancy. The 0.8% vaginal cream should not be used during pregnancy unless the benefits outweigh the risks to the fetus. **Do not** use or retreat if sensitization, irritation, fever, chills, or flu-like symptoms occur. Components in the suppository dosage form may weaken certain rubber or latex products used in vaginal contraceptive diaphragms and condoms.

Adverse effects: Abdominal, musculoskeletal, and vaginal pain, and headache are common. Fever, chills, and vaginal discomfort may occur. Photosensitivity reactions have been reported after repeated dermal application under conditions of artificial UV light.

Drug interactions: None identified.

Continued

For explanation of icons, see p. 364.

TERCONAZOLE *continued*

Drug administration: Wash hands before use. Gently insert suppository or applicator full of cream high into the vagina at bedtime. Remain lying down for 30 minutes after administration. Wash applicator with soap and water after each use. Use sanitary napkin or minipad to prevent staining of clothing. **Do not** use tampons.

TETANUS IMMUNE GLOBULIN
HyperTET S/D
Immune globulin, tetanus (high titer)

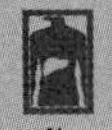 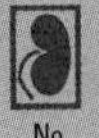 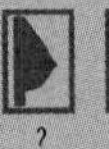 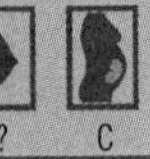
No No ? C

Injection, prefilled syringe for IM use only: 250 units/mL (~1 mL); contains 15%–18% protein; preservative and latex free

Tetanus prophylaxis for patients with incomplete (<3 doses of absorbed tetanus toxoid) or unknown immunization status:
<7 yr: 4 units/kg or 250 units IM × 1
≥7 yr and adult: 250 units IM × 1
Treatment of active tetanus (early symptoms), see latest* AAP Red Book *for additional information and alternatives when product is unavailable:
Child (optimum therapeutic dose has not been established): Some experts recommend 500 units IM × 1, although others have recommended 3000–6000 units IM × 1.
Adult: 500–6000 units IM × 1

Warnings/Precautions: **Use with caution** in hypersensitivity to immune globulin products, IgA deficiency (contains trace amounts of Ig A), thrombocytopenia, or other contraindications to IM injections. Like other plasma products, the risk for transmission of blood-borne viral agents may occur. **For IM injections only;** intradermal skin tests should **NOT** be used.
Immune globulin intravenous (IgIV) contains antibodies to tetanus and may be considered an alternative to tetanus Ig if tetanus Ig is not available; 200–400 mg/kg/dose IV of IgIV has been recommended.

Adverse effects: Injection-site pain is common. Angioedema, nephrotic syndrome, and anaphylaxis have been reported.

Drug interactions: May interfere with the response to live viral vaccines such as measles, mumps, polio, varicella, and rubella; defer these vaccines until approximately 3 months after dose of Ig.

Drug administration: Administer by deep IM injection. Should be administered with Td toxoid but at different extremities and with a separate syringe.

TETRACYCLINE HCL
Various generics
Antibiotic

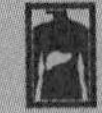 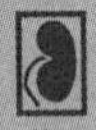 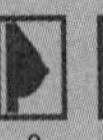 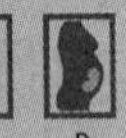
Yes Yes 2 D

Caps: 250, 500 mg
Oral suspension: 25 mg/mL

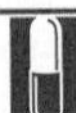

Do not use in children <8 yr old.
Child ≥8 yr: 25–50 mg/kg/24 hr PO ÷ Q6 hr; **max. dose:** 3 g/24 hr
Adult: 1–2 g/24 hr PO ÷ Q6–12 hr
Acne vulgaris: 250 mg PO every other day to 500 mg PO once daily

Continued

TETRACYCLINE HCL *continued*

Contraindications: Hypersensitivity to any tetracycline derivatives

Warnings/Precautions: **Not** recommended in patients younger than 8 years because of tooth staining and decreased bone growth, and in pregnancy because these adverse effects may occur in the fetus. The risk for these adverse effects are highest with long-term use. **Avoid** prolonged exposure to sunlight.

Generally used for treating Rocky Mountain Spotted fever and other Rickettsial diseases, Lyme disease, mycoplasmal disease, Legionella, and moderate-to-severe acne vulgaris in children older than 8 years, adolescents, and adults.

Never use outdated tetracyclines because they may cause Fanconi-like syndrome. **Adjust dose in renal failure (see Chapter 3).**

Adverse effects: GI disturbances, rash, and photophobia are common. Hepatotoxicity, stomatitis, fever, paresthesia, pseudotumor cerebri, and superinfection have been reported.

Drug interactions: May decrease the effectiveness of oral contraceptives, increase serum digoxin levels, and increase effects of warfarin. Use with methoxyflurane increases risk for nephrotoxicity, and use with isotretinoin is associated with pseudotumor cerebri.

Drug administration: Give 1 hour before or 2 hours after meals.

Do not give with dairy products or with any divalent cations (i.e., Fe^{2+}, Ca^{2+}, Mg^{2+}).

THALIDOMIDE
Thalomid
Immunomodulator

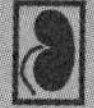 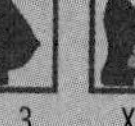 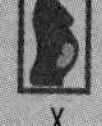

No No 3 X

Caps: 50, 100, 150, 200 mg
Oral suspension: 20 mg/mL

Drug can only be prescribed by health care providers registered with the STEPS program and dispensed by pharmacists registered with the STEPS program (1-888-423-5436).

Erythema nodosum leprosum:

Child ≥12 yr and adult: 100–300 mg PO QHS and at least 1 hr after the evening meal. Use lower end of dosing range for patients weighing <50 kg. May use 400 mg PO QHS for severe cases. Continue until signs and symptoms have subsided, usually around 2 wk, and dosage may be tapered off in 50-mg decrements at 2- to 4-wk intervals. Patients requiring prolonged maintenance therapy to prevent recurrence or who have failed the tapering process should be maintained on a minimum dose to control symptoms. Tapering should be attempted every 3–6 mo in decrements of 50 mg at 2- to 4-wk intervals.

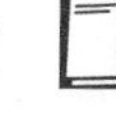

Contraindications: Hypersensitivity to thalidomide products, pregnancy (highly teratogenic), sexually active males not using latex condom (risk to fetus from semen of males taking thalidomide unknown), and women of childbearing potential **NOT** using two forms of contraception.

Warnings/Precautions: Women of childbearing potential should have a pregnancy test (sensitivity of at least 50 mIU/mL) performed within 24 hours before starting therapy and periodically during therapy. Reported teratogenic effects have included amelia, phocomelia, hypoplasticity of the bones, absence of bones, mortality (~40%), external ear abnormalities, congenital heart defects, and alimentary tract, urinary tract, and genital malformations. **Use with caution** in peripheral neuropathy (especially with other medications with the same side effect), seizures, neutropenia, HIV, and multiple myeloma. **Avoid** hazardous activities, operating machinery, or driving, because it may cause drowsiness. Patients with neoplastic or inflammatory disorders have increased risk for thrombotic events.

Continued

For explanation of icons, see p. 364.

THALIDOMIDE *continued*

Dosing in hepatic dysfunction have **not** been established. Therapy should not be initiated or continued with ANCs ≤750/mm³.

Adverse effects: Edema, rash, hypocalcemia, constipation, nausea, leukopenia, confusion, somnolence, and tremor are common. Steven–Johnson syndrome, TEN, teratogenesis, neutropenia, thrombotic disorder, and peripheral neuropathy may occur. Seizures and pulmonary embolism have been reported.

Drug interactions: Alcohol, barbiturates, chlorpromazine, and reserpine may enhance sedative effects. Dexamethasone may increase risk for TEN. Docetaxel may increase risk for venous thromboembolism. Zoledronic acid and pamidronate may increase risk for renal dysfunction. Darbepoetin alpha increases thrombogenic state in patients with myelodysplastic syndrome.

Drug administration: Take with water in the evening, at least 1 hour after a meal. Avoid excessive handling of capsules.

TICARCILLIN WITH CLAVULANATE

Timentin

Antibiotic, penicillin (extended spectrum with β-lactamase inhibitor)

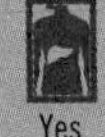
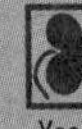
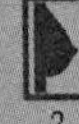
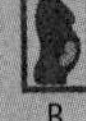

Yes Yes 2 B

Injection: 3.1 g (3 g ticarcillin and 0.1 g clavulanate) (3.1, 31 g); contains 4.51 mEq Na^+ and 0.15 mEq K^+ per 1 g drug

Premixed injection: 3.1 g (3 g ticarcillin and 0.1 g clavulanate) in 100 mL; contains 18.7 mEq Na^+ and 0.5 mEq K^+ per 100 mL

All doses are based on ticarcillin component.

Neonate (IV):

≤7 days:

<2 kg: 150 mg/kg/24 hr ÷ Q12 hr

≥2 kg: 225 mg/kg/24 hr ÷ Q8 hr

>7 days:

<1.2 kg: 150 mg/kg/24 hr ÷ Q12 hr

≥1.2–2 kg: 225 mg/kg/24 hr ÷ Q8 hr

>2 kg: 300 mg/kg/24 hr ÷ Q8 hr

Term neonate and infant <3 mo: 200–300 mg/kg/24 hr IV ÷ Q4–6 hr

Infant ≥3 mo and child <60 kg:

Mild-to-moderate infections: 200 mg/kg/24 hr IV ÷ Q6 hr

Severe infections: 300 mg/kg/24 hr IV ÷ Q4–6 hr

Max. dose: 18–24 mg/24 hr

Cystic fibrosis: 300–600 mg/kg/24 hr IV ÷ Q4–6 hr; **max. dose:** 24 g/24 hr

Adult: 3 g/dose IV Q4–6 hr IV

UTI: 3 g/dose IV Q6–8 hr

Max. dose: 18–24 g/24 hr

Contraindications: Hypersensitivity to penicillins

Warnings/Precautions: **Use with caution** with cephalosporin hypersensitivity and CHF (high sodium content). Activity similar to ticarcillin except that β-lactamase inhibitor broadens spectrum to include *Staphylococcus aureus* and *Haemophilus influenzae.* Like other penicillins, CSF penetration occurs only with inflamed meninges. Ticarcillin elimination is prolonged with impaired hepatic and/or renal function **(adjust dosage in renal impairment; see Chapter 3).**

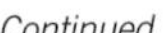

Continued

TICARCILLIN WITH CLAVULANATE *continued*

Adverse effects: Thrombophlebitis, headache, and immune hypersensitivity reaction are common. May also cause decreased platelet aggregation, bleeding diathesis, hypernatremia, hematuria, hypokalemia, hypocalcemia, allergy, and increased AST. Hemorrhagic cystitis has been reported.

Drug interactions: Probenecid increases ticarcillin levels. May cause false-positive results for urine protein and serum Coombs' tests. **Do not mix** with aminoglycosides in the same solution.

Drug administration: For intermittent IV infusion, infuse over 30 minutes at a concentration ≤100 mg/mL; concentrations ≤50 mg/mL are preferred. If patient is receiving concomitant aminoglycoside therapy, separate ticarcillin/clavulanate from aminoglycoside by at least 1 hour; separate by at least 2 hours if aminoglycoside serum levels are being sampled before and after an aminoglycoside dosage.

TIGECYCLINE

Tygacil

Antibiotic, glycylcycline

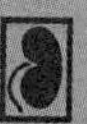
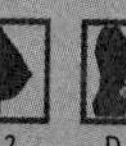

Yes No ? D

Injection: 50 mg; contains 100 mg lactose

Child:

8–11 yr (limited data): A phase II ascending-dose study recommends 1.2 mg/kg/dose IV Q12 hr to attain PK/PD target (AUC/MIC ratio) similar to that attained in adults who received 50 mg Q12 hr.

≥12 yr (limited data): 1.5 mg/kg/dose (**max. dose:** 100 mg/kg/dose) IV × 1, followed by 1 mg/kg/dose (**max. dose:** 50 mg/dose) IV Q12 hr

Adult: 100 mg IV × 1, followed by 50 mg IV Q12 hr with the following durations of therapy:

Skin, skin structure, or intraabdominal infection: 5–14 days

Community-acquired pneumonia: 7–14 days

Contraindications: Hypersensitivity to tigecycline

Warnings/Precautions: Glycylcycline antibiotics are structurally similar to tetracyclines and may have similar adverse effects. **Not** recommended in patients younger than 8 years because of tooth staining and decreased bone growth, and in pregnancy because these side effects may occur in the fetus. Currently not approved for use in hospital-acquired pneumonia (including ventilator-associated) or diabetic foot infection.

Use with caution with known hypersensitivity to tetracyclines, pancreatitis, and hepatic impairment (Child–Pugh class C: reduce maintenance dose to 25 mg IV Q12 hr).

Adverse effects: Diarrhea, nausea, and vomiting are common. Injection-site reactions, acute pancreatitis, anaphylactoid reactions, hepatic dysfunction/failure, vaginitis, somnolence, and taste perversion have been reported.

Drug interactions: PT and other suitable anticoagulation tests should be monitored if used with warfarin. May reduce the effectiveness of oral contraceptives.

Drug administration: For intermittent infusion, infuse over 30 to 60 minutes at a concentration ≤1 mg/mL.

For explanation of icons, see p. 364.

TINIDAZOLE
Tindamax and others
Antiprotozoal agent, nitroimidazole

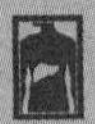 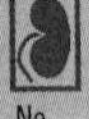 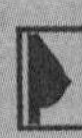 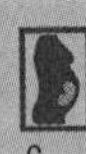 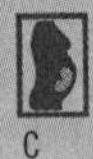
Yes No 3 C

Tabs: 250, 500 mg
Oral suspension: 67 mg/mL

Child (≥3 yr):
Amebiasis **(Entamoeba histolytica),** ***intestinal:*** 50 mg/kg/dose PO once daily × 3 days
Amebic liver abscess: 50 mg/kg/dose PO once daily × 3–5 days
Giardia lamblia: 50 mg/kg/dose PO × 1
Max. dose ***(all indications):*** 2 g/dose

Adult:
Amebiasis **(Entamoeba histolytica),** ***intestinal:*** 2 g PO once daily × 3 days
Amebic liver abscess: 2 g PO once daily × 3–5 days
Giardia lamblia, ***or*** **Trichomonas vaginalis** ***(treat patient and sexual partner at the same time):*** 2 g PO × 1

Contraindications: Hypersensitivity to tinidazole or other nitroimidazole derivatives (e.g., metronidazole). Do not use during first trimester of pregnancy. For use during lactation, interruption is recommended during therapy and for 3 days after the last dose.

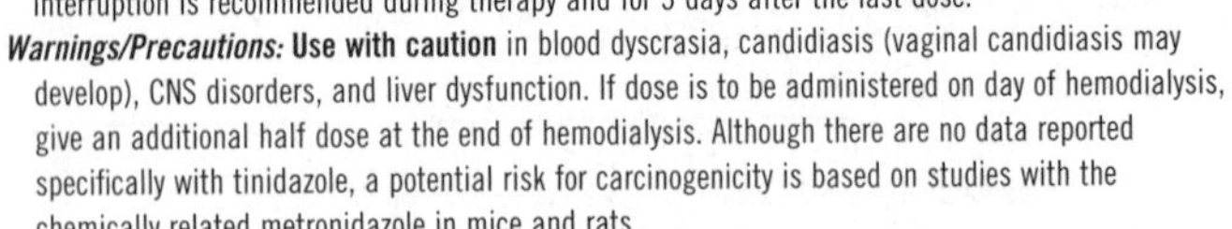

Warnings/Precautions: **Use with caution** in blood dyscrasia, candidiasis (vaginal candidiasis may develop), CNS disorders, and liver dysfunction. If dose is to be administered on day of hemodialysis, give an additional half dose at the end of hemodialysis. Although there are no data reported specifically with tinidazole, a potential risk for carcinogenicity is based on studies with the chemically related metronidazole in mice and rats.

Adverse effects: Constipation, epigastric discomfort, indigestion, loss of appetite, nausea, taste sense alterations, vomiting, cramps, asthenia, dizziness, headache, malaise, and fatigue are common. Seizures, peripheral neuropathy, urticaria, Stevens–Johnson syndrome, tongue discoloration, darkened urine, and palpitations have been reported.

Drug interactions: Although studies are incomplete and tinidazole is chemically related to metronidazole, it may enhance the effects of warfarin and other oral coumarin anticoagulants, alcohols, disulfiram, lithium, phenytoin, cyclosporin, tacrolimus, and fluorouracil, and drugs that induce CYP3A4 liver enzymes; cholestyramine, and oxytetracycline may reduce tinidazole's effects. CYP3A4 inhibitors may increase tinidazole's effects/toxicity.

Drug administration: Give doses with food to minimize GI side effects. **Avoid** consumption of alcoholic beverages and preparations containing ethanol or propylene glycol during therapy and 3 days afterward.

TIOCONAZOLE
1-Day, Vagistat-1
Antifungal agent, imidazole

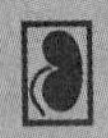 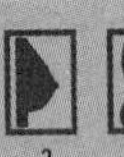 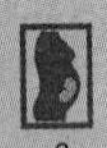
No No ? C

Vaginal ointment (OTC): 6.5% (4.6 g in a prefilled applicator)

≥12 yr and adult: one applicator full (4.6 g of 6.5% ointment) intravaginally once, preferably at bedtime

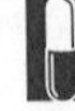

Contraindications: Hypersensitivity to tioconazole or imidazole antifungal agents
Warnings/Precautions: **Do not use** in patients who are pregnant, have diabetes, or have HIV. Most patients experience relief of symptoms within 7 days after the administration of the single dose.

Continued

TIOCONAZOLE *continued*

Components in the suppository dosage form may weaken certain rubber or latex products used in vaginal contraceptive diaphragms and condoms. Wait 3 days after treatment to resume use of condoms and diaphragms.

Adverse effects: Burning, discomfort, rash, and itching are common. Abdominal pain, headache, dysuria, and nocturia have been reported.

Drug interactions: Bleeding or bruising may occur when used with warfarin.

Drug administration: Wash hands before use. Gently insert applicator full of cream high into the vagina at bedtime. Remain lying down for 30 minutes after administration. Use sanitary napkin or minipad to prevent staining of clothing. **Do not** use tampons.

TIPRANAVIR

Aptivus, TPV

Antiviral agent, protease inhibitor

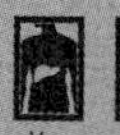

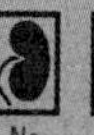

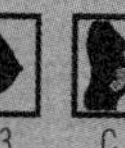

Yes No 3 C

Oral solution: 100 mg/1 mL (95 mL; with 5 mL dispensing syringe); contains propylene glycol and vitamin E 116 IU/mL

Caps (liquid filled): 250 mg; contains 7% dehydrated alcohol

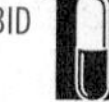

Child (2–18 yr): 14 mg/kg/dose or 375 mg/m^2/dose PO BID with ritonavir 6 mg/kg/dose PO BID

Max. dose: tipranavir: 500 mg/dose and ritonavir 200 mg/dose

Children who become intolerant or develop toxicity with the above dosage may have their dosage reduced to 12 mg/kg/dose or 290 mg/m^2/dose tipranavir PO BID with 5 mg/kg/dose or 115 mg/m^2/dose ritonavir PO BID

Adult: 500 mg PO BID with 200 mg ritonavir PO BID

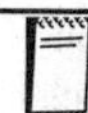

Contraindications: Hypersensitivity to tipranavir or other components of the formulation; moderate-to-severe hepatic impairment (Child–Pugh class B or C). Concomitant administration with drugs that are highly dependent on CYP 3A clearance such as alfuzosin, amiodarone, astemizole, bepridil, cisapride, ergot derivatives, flecainide, lovastatin, midazolam, pimozide, propafenone, quinidine, sildenafil, simvastatin, terfenadine, and triazolam.

Warnings/Precautions: Potential cross-sensitivity with sulfa-allergic patients. Coadministration with St. John's wort and HMG-CoA reductase inhibitors (e.g., lovastatin, simvastatin) are **not** recommended because of causing reductions in tipranavir levels and increasing risk for myopathy and rhabdomyolysis, respectively. Reports of intracranial hemorrhage, hepatitis, and hepatic decompensation have resulted in some fatalities. Autoimmune disorders (e.g., Graves disease, polymyositis, and Guillain-Barré syndrome) have also been reported with immune reconstitution. **Use with caution** in hepatic impairment (primary route of metabolism; no dose reduction recommendations available), hemophilia type A or B, diabetes or hyperglycemia, and in patients at risk for increased bleeding from trauma, surgery, or other medical conditions, or who are receiving medications known to increase the risk for bleeding, such as antiplatelet agents or anticoagulants.

Tipranavir should always be administered in combination with ritonavir and is currently indicated in adults who are highly treatment experienced or have HIV-1 strains resistant to multiple PIs, and who have evidence of viral replication. LFTs should be obtained at baseline and monitored frequently.

Do not take additional vitamin E supplements if taking the oral liquid dosage form (contains vitamin E).

Continued

TIPRANAVIR *continued*

Adverse effects: GI disturbances, fatigue, headache, rash, vomiting, and elevated LFTs, cholesterol, and triglycerides are common in children and adults. Rash occurs more frequent in children than adults. Fat redistribution, immune reconstitution syndrome, hepatitis, hepatic decompensation, and elevated transaminases in patients with hepatitis B or C, or already elevated transaminates have been reported. See earlier Warnings/Precautions.

Drug interactions: Substrate and inhibitor of cytochrome P450 3A. May reduce levels of amprenavir, lopinavir, saquinavir, raltegravir, and valproic acid. Carbamazepine, phenobarbital, phenytoin, and rifampin may decrease effects of tipranavir. Ritonavir boosts tipranavir levels and is also a substrate and inhibitor of CYP P450 3A. See earlier Contraindications and Warnings/Precautions sections. Always check the potential for other drug interactions when either initiating therapy or adding new drugs onto an existing regimen.

Drug administration: **Drug is always given in combination with ritonavir.** Administer all doses with a meal or light snack. If given together, separate dose from didanosine by at least 2 hours.

TOBRAMYCIN

Nebcin, Tobrex, AKTob, TOBI, TOBI Podhaler, and others

Antibiotic, aminoglycoside

No Yes 2 B/D

Injection: 10, 40 mg/mL; may contain phenol and bisulfites
Premixed injection: 80 mg in 100 mL NS
Powder for injection: 1.2 g; preservative free
Ophthalmic ointment (Tobrex, AKTob): 0.3% (3.5 g)
In combination with dexamethasone (TobraDex): 0.3% tobramycin with 0.1% dexamethasone (3.5 g); contains 0.5% chlorbutanol
Ophthalmic solution (Tobrex): 0.3% (5 mL)
In combination with dexamethasone: 0.3% tobramycin with 0.1% dexamethasone (2.5, 5, 10 mL); contains 0.01% benzalkonium chloride and EDTA
Nebulizer solution: 300 mg/5 mL (TOBI, preservative free) (56s), 170 mg/3.4 mL (mixed in 0.45% NS, preservative free, use with eFlow/Trio nebulizer
Powder for inhalation (TOBI Podhaler): 28 mg capsules (224 capsules in 4 weekly packs)

Initial empiric dosage; patient-specific dosage defined by therapeutic drug monitoring (see remarks):

Neonate, IM/IV (see following table):

Postconceptional Age (wk)	Postnatal Age (days)	Dose (mg/kg/dose)	Interval (hr)
≤29*	0–7	5	48
	8–28	4	36
	>28	4	24
30–33	0–7	4.5	36
	>7	4	24
34–37	0–7	4	24
	>7	4	18–24
≥38	0–7	4	24[†]
	>7	4	12–18

*Or significant asphyxia, PDA, indomethacin use, poor cardiac output, reduced renal function.
[†]Use Q36 hr interval for HIE patients receiving whole-body therapeutic cooling.

Continued

TOBRAMYCIN *continued*

Child: 7.5 mg/kg/24 hr ÷ Q8 hr IV/IM

Cystic fibrosis (if available, use patient's previous therapeutic mg/kg dosage):

Conventional Q8 hr dosing: 7.5–10.5 mg/kg/24 hr ÷ Q8 hr IV

High-dose extended-interval (once-daily) dosing: 10–12 mg/kg/dose Q24 hr IV

Adult: 3–6 mg/kg/24 hr ÷ Q8 hr IV/IM

Ophthalmic:

Tobramycin:

Child and adult:

Ophthalmic ointment: Apply 0.5-inch ribbon of ointment into conjunctival sac(s) BID–TID; for severe infections, apply Q3–4 hr.

Ophthalmic drop: Instill 1–2 drops of solution to affected eye(s) Q4 hr; for severe infections, instill 2 drops Q30–60 min initially, then reduce dosing frequency.

Tobramycin with dexamethasone:

≥2 yr and adult:

Ophthalmic ointment: Apply 0.5-inch ribbon of ointment into conjunctival sac(s) TID–QID.

Ophthalmic drop: Instill 1–2 drops of solution to affected eye(s) Q2 hr × 24–48 hr, then 1–2 drops Q4–6 hr.

Inhalation:

Cystic fibrosis prophylaxis therapy:

≥6 yr and adults:

TOBI: 300 mg Q12 hr administered in repeated cycles of 28 days on drug followed by 28 days off drug

Use with eFlow/Trio nebulizer: 170 mg Q12 hr administered in repeated cycles of 28 days on drug followed by 28 days off drug

TOBI Podhaler: Four 28-mg capsules Q12 hr administered in repeated cycles of 28 days on drug followed by 28 days off drug.

Contraindications: Hypersensitivity to aminoglycosides or any other components in the formulation

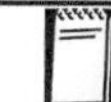

Warnings/Precautions: **Use with caution** in combination with neurotoxic, ototoxic, or nephrotoxic drugs; anesthetics or neuromuscular blocking agents; preexisting renal, vestibular, or auditory impairment; and in patients with neuromuscular disorders.

Higher doses are recommended in patients with cystic fibrosis, neutropenia, or burns. **Adjust dose in renal failure (see Chapter 3).** Monitor peak and trough levels.

Therapeutic peak levels with conventional Q8 hr dosing:

6–10 mg/L in general

8–10 mg/L in pulmonary infections, neutropenia, osteomyelitis, and severe sepsis

Therapeutic trough levels with conventional Q8 hr dosing: <2 mg/L. Recommended serum sampling time at steady state for conventional Q8 hr dosing: trough within 30 min before the third consecutive dose and peak 30–60 min after the administration of the third consecutive dose.

Therapeutic peak and trough goals for high-dose extended-interval dosing for cystic fibrosis:

Peak: 20–40 mg/L; recommended serum sampling time at 30–60 min after the administration of the first dose.

Trough: <1 mg/L; recommended serum sampling time within 30 min before the second dose.

Serum levels should be rechecked with changing renal function, poor clinical response, and at a minimum of once weekly for prolonged therapies.

An individualized peak concentration to target a peak/MIC ratio of 8–10 : 1 may be applied to maximize bacteriocidal effects. For initial dosing in obese patients, use an adjusted body weight (ABW). ABW = Ideal body weight + 0.4 (total body weight – ideal body weight).

Continued

TOBRAMYCIN *continued*

Pregnancy category is a "D" for injection and inhalation routes of administration, and a "B" for the ophthalmic route.

Adverse effects: May cause ototoxicity, nephrotoxicity, and neuromuscular blockade. Vertigo, myelotoxicity, and hypomagnesemia have been reported. Serious allergic reactions including anaphylaxis and dermatologic reactions including exfoliative dermatitis, toxic epidermal necrolysis, erythema multiforme, and Stevens–Johnson syndrome have been reported rarely.

Inhalation use: Transient voice alteration, bronchospasm, dyspnea, pharyngitis, and increase cough may occur. Transient tinnitus has been reported.

Drug interactions: **Ototoxic effects synergistic with furosemide.** See Warnings/Precautions section.

Drug administration:

IV: Infuse over 30–60 min at a concentration ≤10 mg/mL. Administer β-lactam antibiotics at least 1 hr before or after gentamicin.

IM: Use either undiluted commercial products of 10 or 40 mg/mL.

Ophthalmic:

Drops: Apply finger pressure to lacrimal sac during and for 1–2 min after dose application.

Ointment: Instill ointment in lower conjunctival sac by avoiding contact of ointment tip with eye or skin.

Inhalation: For use with other medications in cystic fibrosis, use the following order of administration: bronchodilator first, chest physiotherapy, other inhaled medications (if indicated), and tobramycin last.

TOBI: Use PARI LC Plus nebulizer and a DeVilbiss Pulmo-Aide compressor. Treatment period is usually over 15 min. Disinfecting your nebulizer parts (except tubing) by boiling in water every other treatment day has been recommended.

eFlow nebulizer: Dose may be diluted with NS up to a total volume of 4 mL. Treatment period is usually over 10–12 min.

TOLNAFTATE

Tinactin, Aftate, and many others

Antifungal agent

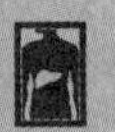
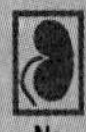
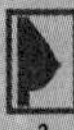
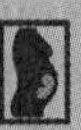
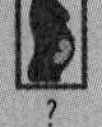

No No ? ?

Topical aerosol spray [OTC]: 1% (128, 150 g); may contain 29% vol/vol or 41% wt/wt alcohol
Topical aerosol powder [OTC]: 1% (133 g); contains 11% vol/vol alcohol and talc
Cream [OTC]: 1% (15, 30, 114 g)
Topical powder [OTC]: 1% (45, 60, 108 g)
Topical solution [OTC]: 1% (10, 30 mL)

Child (≥2 yr) and adult:

Topical: Apply 1–3 drops of solution or small amount of gel, liquid, cream, or powder to affected areas BID–TID for 2–4 wk.

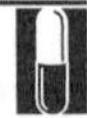

Contraindications: Hypersensitivity to tolnaftate

Warnings/Precautions: **Avoid** eye contact. **Do not use** for nail or scalp infections. **Not** recommended in children younger than 2 years. **Discontinue use if sensitization develops.**

Adverse effects: May cause mild irritation and sensitivity. Contact dermatitis has been reported.

Drug interactions: None identified.

Drug administration: Wash and dry affected area before drug application and **avoid** contact with eyes. Apply enough medicine to cover affected area. When treating foot infections, use liberal quantities of powder to affected areas and apply to socks and shoes. When using the aerosolized liquid or powder dosage form, use a 6- to 10-inch distance when applying dose.

TRIFLURIDINE
Viroptic, trifluorothymidine
Antiviral agent, ophthalmic

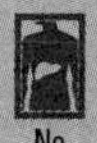 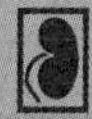 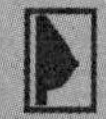 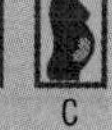
No No ? C

Ophthalmic solution: 1% (7.5 mL); contains 0.001% thimerosal

Herpes simplex keratitis:
≥6 yr and adult: Instill 1 drop onto the cornea of the affected eye(s) Q2 hr while awake (**max. dose:** 9 drops/24 hr) until corneal ulcer has completely reepithelialized followed by 1 drop Q4 hr while awake (**max. dose:** 5 drops/24 hr) for an additional 7 days. **Do not exceed** 21 days of continuous therapy.

Contraindications: Hypersensitivity reactions or chemical intolerance to trifluridine or any of its components

Warnings/Precautions: Has **not** shown to be effective in the prophylaxis of herpes simplex keratoconjunctivitis and epithelial keratitis. Although safety and efficacy in ophthalmic infections caused by vaccinia virus have not been established, the drug also is recommended for the treatment and prevention of ocular vaccinia infections that occur as a complication of smallpox vaccination.

Adverse effects: May cause mild transient local irritation of the conjunctiva and cornea and palpebral edema. Superficial punctate keratopathy, epithelial keratopathy, hypersensitivity reaction, stromal edema, and increased intraocular pressure have been reported.

Drug interactions: None identified.

Drug administration: Apply directly onto the cornea and avoid touching the tip of the dropper. Apply finger pressure to lacrimal sac during and for 1 to 2 minutes after dose application. Store drops in the refrigerator.

TRIMETHOPRIM
Proloprim, Primsol, TMP, and various generics
Anti-infective, folate antagonist

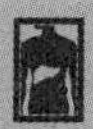 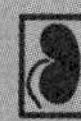 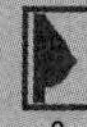 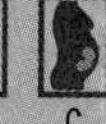
Yes Yes 2 C

Tab: 100 mg
Oral solution: 10 mg/mL 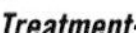
Primsol: 50 mg/5 mL (473 mL); contains propylene glycol, sodium benzoate

Acute otitis media:
≥6 mo: 10 mg/kg/24 hr ÷ Q12 hr PO × 10 days

UTI:
Treatment:
Infant and child <12 yr: 4–6 mg/kg/24 hr ÷ Q12 hr PO × 10 days
≥12 yr and adult: 100 mg Q12 hr PO or 200 mg Q24 hr PO × 10 days
Prophylaxis:
≥12 yr and adult: 100 mg PO once daily

Pneumocystis ***jiroveci (carinii) pneumonia, mild-to-moderate, treatment:***
≥12 yr and adult: 15 mg/kg/24 hr ÷ TID PO × 21 days with dapsone (<13 yr: 2 mg/kg/dose PO once daily and ≥13 yr: 100 mg PO once daily)

Contraindications: Hypersensitivity to trimethoprim and in those with documented megaloblastic anemia because of folate deficiency

Warnings/Precautions: **Use with caution** in patients with possible folate deficiency and impaired hepatic or renal function **(see Chapter 3). Discontinue use** if the count of any formed blood element is significantly reduced. Folates may be administered concomitantly without interfering with antibacterial action.

Continued

For explanation of icons, see p. 364.

TRIMETHOPRIM *continued*

Adverse effects: Pruritus and rash are common. Fever, headache, bone marrow suppression, and elevated liver enzymes, BUN, and serum creatinine may occur. Rare immune hypersensitivity reaction (e.g., TEN, Stevens–Johnson, and exfoliative dermatitis) and aseptic meningitis have been reported.

Drug interactions: Inhibits CYP 450 2C8 and 2C9 isoenzymes. May increase the effects/toxicity of phenytoin, cyclosporin, dapsone, procainamide, rifampin, and warfarin. Use with other folate antagonists (e.g., methotrexate, pyrimethamine) may increase risk for megaloblastic anemia. May falsely increase creatinine determination measured by Jaffe alkaline picrate method, and may falsely interfere with serum methotrexate assay (bacterial dihydrofolate reductase methods).

Drug administration: Give on an empty stomach. If GI upset occurs, give with milk or food.

TRIMETHOPRIM AND SULFAMETHOXAZOLE

See *Sulfamethoxazole and Trimethoprim*

TRIMETREXATE GLUCURONATE

NeuTrexin

Anti-infective agent, folate antagonist

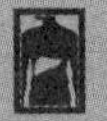
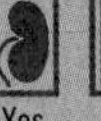
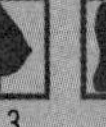
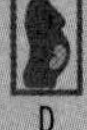

Yes Yes 3 D

Powder for injection: 25, 200 mg

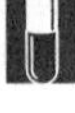

Pneumocystis jiroveci ***pneumonia, moderate/severe (limited data in children):*** 45 mg/m²/dose IV over 60–90 min once daily × 21 days with leucovorin 20 mg/m²/dose IV over 5–10 min or PO Q6 hr × 24 days. If using oral leucovorin, round dose up to the next highest 25-mg increment.

Alternative trimetrexate and leucovorin dosing by body weight:

Body Weight (kg)	Trimetrexate Glucuronate Dose (mg/kg/dose IV once daily)	Leucovorin Dose (mg/kg/dose IV/PO Q6 hr)*
<50	1.5	0.6
50–80	1.2	0.5
>80	1	0.5

*With oral use, round up to the next highest 25-mg increment.

Dose modifications for hematologic toxicity:

Hematologic Toxicity Dosage Modification for Trimetrexate Glucuronate and Leucovorin

Toxicity Grade	Neutrophils (polys and bands) (mm³)	Platelets (mm³)	Trimetrexate Dose (mg/m²/dose IV once daily)	Leucovorin Dose (mg/m²/dose IV/PO Q6 hr)*
1	>1000	>75,000	45	20
2	750–1000	50,000–75,000	45	40
3	500–749	25,000–49,999	22	40
4	<500	<25,000	If days 1–9: discontinue†; if day 10–21: interrupt up to 96 hr‡	40

*With oral use, round up to the next highest 25-mg increment.

†Maintain leucovorin therapy for an additional 72 hr after discontinuing trimetrexate.

‡If counts recover within 96 hr, resume at trimetrexate dosage at respective toxicity grade level and maintain leucovorin therapy at 40 mg/m²/dose IV/PO Q6 hr. Discontinue trimetrexate if counts do not improve to grade 3 or less within 96 hr of interruption and continue leucovorin therapy for an additional 72 hr after discontinuing trimetrexate.

Continued

TRIMETREXATE GLUCURONATE *continued*

Contraindications: Clinically significant hypersensitivity to trimetrexate, leucovorin, or methotrexate

Warnings/Precautions: **Must be used** with concurrent leucovorin to avoid potentially serious or life-threatening toxicities. **Use with caution** in alcoholic patients, ulcerative disorders of the GI tract, impaired hematologic reserve, patients receiving myelosuppressive drugs, and impaired hepatic and renal **(see Chapter 3)** function. Permanently discontinue use if severe hypersensitivity reactions occur.

Adverse effects: Rash, nausea, vomiting, and stomatitis are common. Myelosuppression, hepatotoxicity, and nephrotoxicity may occur. Consider alternative safer drugs with pregnancy.

Drug interactions: Enzyme-inhibiting medications such as erythromycin, cimetidine, rifampin, rifabutin, ketoconazole, clotrimazole, miconazole, and fluconazole may increase risk for trimetrexate toxicity. Zidovudine should be discontinued during trimetrexate therapy to allow use of full therapeutic doses. Vaccination with live virus vaccines (e.g., MMR, varicella, rotavirus) may result in severe and fatal infections.

Drug administration: For intermittent infusion, infuse over 60 to 90 minutes at a concentration 0.25 to 2 mg/mL diluted in D_5W. Concomitant leucovorin therapy must extend for 72 hours past the last dose of trimetrexate to prevent toxicities.

UNDECYLENIC ACID

Elon Dual Defense Anti-Fungal Formula, Fungoid AF, Goordochom, Caldesene, Cruex, and many others

Antifungal agent

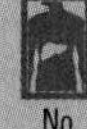
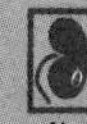
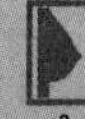
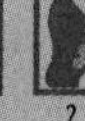
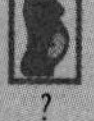

No No ? ?

Topical solution [OTC]: 25% (30 mL); may contain alcohol
Topical powder [OTC]: 10% (45, 60, 120 g), 12% (60 g), 25% (45 g)
Topcial spray [OTC]: 10% (51, 100, 155.9 g), 19% (54, 105, 165 g)
Topical cream [OTC]: 8% (60 g; contains 0.05% pramoxine), 10% (42 g; contains aloe and PEG-100), 20% (15 g; contains parabens)
Soap [OTC]: 97.5 g

Child ≥2 yr and adult:

Tinea corporis and tinea pedis: Apply topically BID to clean dry area × 4 wk.

Contraindications: Hypersensitivity to undecylenic acid

Warnings/Precautions: **For external use only.** Product has **not** been proved effective on the scalp or nail. Cream and solution dosage forms are primarily used. Powders are generally used as adjunctive therapy or as primary therapy for very mild conditions.

Adverse effects: Skin irritation and rash are common. Hypersensitivity has been reported.

Drug interactions: None identified.

Drug administration: **Avoid** contact with eyes or other mucous membranes. **Do not** inhale powder. Clean affected area with soap and warm water and dry thoroughly. Apply thin layer over affected area. For tinea pedis, pay attention to spaces between the toes. **Do not** apply to blistered, raw, or oozing areas of skin or over deep wounds or puncture wounds.

For explanation of icons, see p. 364.

VALACYCLOVIR
Valtrex and others
Antiviral agent

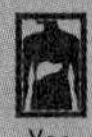 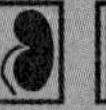 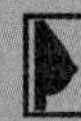 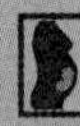
Yes Yes 1 B

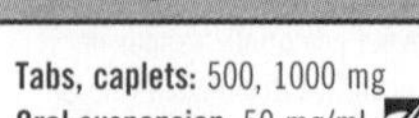

Tabs, caplets: 500, 1000 mg
Oral suspension: 50 mg/mL

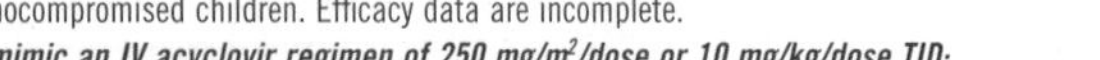

Child: Recommended dosages based on steady-state pharmacokinetic data in immunocompromised children. Efficacy data are incomplete.

To mimic an IV acyclovir regimen of 250 mg/m²/dose or 10 mg/kg/dose TID:
30 mg/kg/dose PO TID or alternatively by weight:
4–12 kg: 250 mg PO TID
13–21 kg: 500 mg PO TID
22–29 kg: 750 mg PO TID
≥30 kg: 1000 mg PO TID

To mimic a PO acyclovir regimen of 20 mg/kg/dose 4 or 5 times a day:
20 mg/kg/dose PO TID or alternatively by weight:
6–19 kg: 250 mg PO TID
20–31 kg: 500 mg PO TID
≥32 kg: 750 mg PO TID

Chickenpox (immunocompetent patient):
2 to <18 yr: 20 mg/kg/dose PO TID × 5 days; **max. dose:** 1 g/dose TID

Herpes zoster (see remarks):
Adult (immunocompetent): 1 g/dose PO TID × 7 days within 48–72 hr of onset of rash

Genital herpes:
Adolescent and adult:
Initial episodes: 1 g/dose PO BID × 10 days
Recurrent episodes: 500 mg/dose PO BID × 3 days
Suppressive therapy: 500–1000 mg/dose PO once daily × 1 yr, then reassess for recurrences. Patients with <9 recurrences/yr may be dosed at 500 mg/dose PO once daily × 1 yr

Herpes labialis (cold sores; initiated at earliest symptoms):
≥12 yr and adult: 2 g/dose PO Q12 hr × 1 day

Contraindications: Hypersensitivity or intolerance to valacyclovir, acyclovir, or any component of the formulation

Warnings/Precautions: This prodrug is metabolized to acyclovir and L-valine with better oral absorption than acyclovir. Valacyclovir **CANNOT** be substituted for acyclovir on a one-to-one basis. **Use with caution** in hepatic or renal insufficiency **(adjust dose; see Chapter 3).** Thrombotic thrombocytopenic purpura/hemolytic uremic syndrome has been reported in patients with advanced HIV infection and in bone marrow and renal transplant recipients.

For initial episodes of genital herpes, therapy is most effective when initiated within 48 hours of symptom onset; no efficacy data are available if therapy initiated more than 72 hours after rash onset. Therapy should be initiated immediately after the onset of symptoms in recurrent episodes (no efficacy data when initiating therapy more than 24 hours after onset of symptoms). Data are not available for use as suppressive therapy for periods longer than 1 year.

Adverse effects: Nausea, abdominal pain, and headache are common in adults. Headache is common in children. See Warnings/Precautions section and Acyclovir for additional information. Aggressive behavior, agitation, mania, sedation, and tremors have been reported.

Drug interactions: Probenecid or cimetidine can reduce the rate of conversion to acyclovir. Use with mycophenolate may increase risk for neutropenia. See Acyclovir for additional drug interactions.

Drug administration: Doses may be given with or without food. Maintain adequate hydration while on therapy.

VALGANCICLOVIR
Valcyte
Antiviral agent

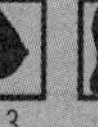

Tabs: 450 mg
Oral solution: 50 mg/mL (100 mL)
Oral suspension: 60 mg/mL

Neonate and infant:

Symptomatic congenital CMV (from pharmacokinetic [PK] data in 8 infants 4–90 days old [mean, 20 days] and 24 neonates 8–34 days old): 15–16 mg/kg/dose PO BID produced simlar serum levels to IV ganciclovir 6 mg/kg/dose BID. Additional PK, safety, and efficacy studies are required.

Child:

CMV prophylaxis in kidney or heart transplantation: Once-daily PO dosage is calculated with the following equation: ***daily mg dose (max. dose: 900 mg) = 7 × BSA × CrCl, where BSA is determined by the Mosteller equation and CrCl is determined by a modified Schwartz equation (max. value:*** 150 mL/min/1.73 m^2).

Mosteller BSA (m^2) equation: square root of [(height [cm] × weight [kg]) ÷ 3600]

Modified Schwartz (mL/min/1.73 m^2) equation (max. value = 150 mL/min/1.73 m^2): k × height (cm) ÷ serum creatinine (mg/dL); where k = 0.45 if patient is 4 mo to <2 yr old, or k = 0.55 for boys 2 to <13 yr old and girls 2–16 yr old, or k = 0.7 for boys 13–16 yr old.

CMV prophylaxis in liver transplantation (limited data based on a retrospective review in 10 patients; mean age, 4.9 + 5.6 yr): 15–18 mg/kg/dose PO once daily × 100 days after transplantation resulted in one case of asymptomatic CMV infection detected by CMV antigenemia at day 7 of therapy. This patient then received a higher dose of 15 mg/kg/dose BID until three consecutive negative CMV antigenemia were achieved. The dose was switched back to a prophylatic regimen at day 46 posttransplant.

Adolescent and adult:

CMV retinitis:

Induction therapy: 900 mg PO BID × 21 days with food

Maintenance therapy: 900 mg PO once daily with food

CMV prophylaxis in heart, kidney, and kidney–pancreas transplantation: 900 mg PO once daily starting within 10 days of transplantation until 100 days after heart or kidney–pancreas transplantation, or until 200 days after kidney transplantation

Contraindications: Hypersensitivity to valganciclovir or ganciclovir; ANC <500 mm^3; platelets <25,000 mm^3; hemoglobin <8 g/dL; and patients on hemodialysis

Warnings/Precautions: This prodrug is metabolized to ganciclovir with better oral absorption than ganciclovor. Valganciclovir **CANNOT** be substituted for ganciclovir on a one-to-one basis. **Use with caution** in renal insufficiency **(adjust dose; see Chapter 3),** preexisting bone marrow supression, or receiving myelosuppressive drugs or irradiation. Has not been evaluated in hepatic impairment.

May impair fertility in men and women; use effective contraception during and for at least 90 days after therapy. **Not** indicated in preventing CMV disease in liver transplant patients.

Adverse effects: Headache, fever, insomnia, peripheral neuropathy, diarrhea, vomiting, abdominal pain, neutropenia, anemia, and thrombocytopenia are common. See Ganciclovir for additional information.

Drug interactions: Immunosuppressive agents may increase hematologic toxicities. May increase the risk for seizures with imipenem/cilastatin. May increase didanosine and zidovudine levels, whereas

Continued

For explanation of icons, see p. 364.

VALGANCICLOVIR *continued*

didanosine and zidovudine may decrease ganciclovir levels. See Ganciclovir for additional information.

Drug administration: All doses are administered with food. **Do not** break or crush tablet. **Avoid** direct contact with broken or crushed tablets with the skin or mucous membranes.

VANCOMYCIN
Vancocin and others
Antibiotic, glycopeptide

No Yes 2 C/B

Injection: 0.5, 0.75, 1, 5, 10 g
Premixed injection: 500 mg/100 mL in dextrose; 750 mg/150 mL in dextrose, 1000 mg/200 mL in dextrose (iso-osmotic solutions)
Caps: 125, 250 mg
Oral solution: 25 mg/mL

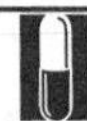

Initial empiric dosage; patient-specific dosage defined by therapeutic drug monitoring (see remarks):

Neonates, IV (see following table for dosage interval):

Bacteremia: 10 mg/kg/dose
Meningitis, pneumonia: 15 mg/kg/dose

Postmenstrual Age (wk)*	Postnatal Age (days)	Dosage Interval (hr)
≤29	0–14	18
	>14	12
30–36	0–14	12
	>14	8
37–44	0–7	12
	>7	8
≥45	All	6

*Postmenstrual age = gestational age + postnatal age.

Infant, child, adolescent, and adult, IV:

Age	General Dosage	CNS Infections, Endocarditis, Osteomyelitis, Pneumonia, and MRSA Bacteremia
1 mo to 12 yr old	15 mg/kg Q6 hr	20 mg/kg Q6 hr
Adolescent	15 mg/kg Q6–8 hr	20 mg/kg Q6–8 hr
Adult	15 mg/kg Q8–12 hr	20 mg/kg Q8–12 hr

Clostridium difficile ***colitis:***

Child: 40–50 mg/kg/24 hr ÷ Q6 hr PO × 7–10 days

Max. dose: 500 mg/24 hr; higher **maximum** of 2 g/24 hr has also been used

Adult: 125 mg/dose PO Q6 hr × 7–10 days; dosages as high as 2 g/24 hr ÷ Q6–8 hr have also been used

Endocarditis prophylaxis for GU or GI (excluding esophageal) procedures (complete all antibiotic dose infusion(s) within 30 minutes of starting procedure):

Moderate-risk patients allergic to ampicillin or amoxicillin:

Child: 20 mg/kg/dose IV over 1–2 hr × 1

Continued

VANCOMYCIN *continued*

Adult: 1 g/dose IV over 1–2 hr × 1

High-risk patients allergic to ampicillin or amoxicillin:

Child and adult: Same dose as moderate-risk patients plus gentamicin 1.5 mg/kg/dose (**max. dose:** 120 mg/dose) IV/IM × 1

Intrathecal/ intraventricular (use preservative-free preparation):

Neonate: 5–10 mg once daily

Child: 5–20 mg once daily

Adult: 10–20 mg once daily

Contraindications: Hypersensitivity to vancomycin products

Warnings/Precautions: **Avoid** IM injection and rapid IV infusions (see following Drug Administration section). **Use with caution** in renal impairment **(adjust dose; see Chapter 3)**, preexisting hearing loss, and concomitant nephrotoxic/ototoxic drugs or anesthetics. Low concentrations of the drug may appear in CSF with inflamed meninges. Use total body weight for obese patients when calculating dosages.

Toxicity relationship with serum levels has not been clearly established, but nephrotoxicity has been reported in approximately 14% of pediatric patients using the recommended higher serum trough concentrations found in adult guidelines for efficacy and modern versions of the drug's formulation. Earlier impure version of the drug ("Mississippi Mud") may have been more toxic.

Although current extrapolated adult guidelines suggest measuring only trough levels, an additional postdistributional level may be useful in characterizing enhanced/altered drug clearance for quicker dosage modification to attain target levels; this may be useful for infants with known faster clearance and patients in renal compromise. Consult a pharmacist. The following therapeutic trough level recommendations are based on the assumption that the pathogen's vancomycin MIC is ≤1 mg/L.

Indication	Goal Trough Level
Uncomplicated skin and soft-tissue infection, non-MRSA bacteremia, febrile neutropenia	10–15 mg/L
CNS infections, endocarditis, pneumonia, osteomyelitis, MRSA bacteremia	15–20 mg/L

Peak level measurement (20–50 mg/L) has also been recommended for patients with burns, clinically nonresponsive in 72 hr of therapy, persistent positive cultures, and CNS infections (≥30 mg/L). See Chapter 6 for additional information.

Recommended serum sampling time at steady state: trough within 30 minutes before the fourth consecutive dose and peak 60 minutes after the administration of the fourth consecutive dose. Infants with faster elimination (shorter $T_{1/2}$) may be sampled around the third consecutive dose.

Metronidazole (PO) is the drug of choice for *C. difficile* colitis; vancomycin should be avoided because of the emergence of vancomycin-resistant enterococcus. Vancomycin is NOT absorbed via the oral route of administration. Pregnancy category B is assigned with the oral route of administration.

Adverse effects:

IV: Nausea, vomiting, and drug-induced erythroderma are common. "Red man syndrome" associated with rapid IV infusion may occur. Allergic reactions (including drug rash with eosinophilia and systemic symptoms [DRESS]), neutropenia, and immune-mediated thrombocytopenia have been reported. Greater risk for nephrotoxicity risk has been associated with higher doses and serum concentrations (≥15 mg/L), and receiving furosemide in the intensive care unit.

PO: Nausea, abdominal pain, and hypokalemia (greater in adults older than 65 years) are common. Nephrotoxicity and ototoxicity have been reported.

Continued

VANCOMYCIN *continued*

Drug interactions:

IV: Ototoxicity and nephrotoxicity may occur and may be exacerbated with concurrent use of aminoglycosides, loop diuretics, or cisplatin. Use with anesthetics has been associated with erythema and histamine-like flushing in children. May enhance neuromuscular blockade with nondepolarizing muscular relaxants.

PO: None identified.

Drug administration:

IV: For intermittent infusion, infuse over 60 min or a **maximum rate** of 10 mg/min (whichever is longer) at a concentration ≤5 mg/mL. Infusion may be extended to 120 min if 60-min infusion is not tolerated. Diphenhydramine is used to reverse infusion-related red man syndrome.

PO: Oral solution may be further diluted with water or with flavoring syrup to improve taste.

Intraventricular/intraventricular: Dilute 1-g vial with preservative-free NS to a concentration of 20 mg/mL.

VARICELLA ZOSTER IMMUNE GLOBULIN (HUMAN)

VariZig, VZIG

Hyperimmune globulin, varicella zoster

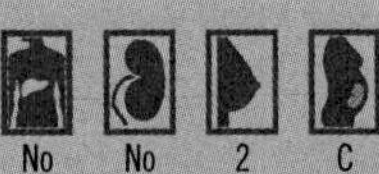

Injection: 125 units vial; each vial contains 60–200 mg human immunoglobulin G, 0.1 M glycine, 0.04 M sodium chloride, and 0.01% polysorbate 80. A vial of 8.5 mL of sterile diluent is provided.

Dose should be given within 48 hr of varicella exposure and no later than 96 hr after exposure.

IM (preferred route) or IV (see remarks):

≤2.1 kg: 62.5 units
2.1–10 kg: 125 units
10.1–20 kg: 250 units
20.1–30 kg: 375 units
30.1–40 kg: 500 units
>40 kg: 625 units
Max. dose: 625 units/dose

If patient is at high risk and reexposed to varicella more than 3 weeks after a prior dose, another full dose may be given.

Contraindications: Hypersensitivity to immune globulin products or any components to the formulation, severe thrombocytopenia (IM injection), IgA-deficient individuals, and known immunity to varicella zoster virus.

Warnings/Precautions: Dose should be given within 48 hours of exposure and no later than 96 hours after exposure. See latest *AAP Red Book* for additional information. As with other products pooled from human plasma, product may contain unknown infectious agents that are not screened for. Hyperviscosity of the blood may increase risk for thrombotic events. IM route is preferred over IV in patients with preexisting respiratory conditions. This product does not contain a sucrose stabilizer.

Adverse effects: Local discomfort, redness, and swelling at the injection site, headache, and rash are common. Myalgia, rigors, fatigue, nausea, and flushing have been reported.

Drug interactions: Interferes with immune response to live virus vaccines such as measles, mumps, and rubella; defer administration of live vaccines ≥6 months after VZIG dose.

Drug administration: Reconstituted product may be stored up to 12 hours at 2–8°C.

IM: Dilute each vial with 1.25 mL sterile diluent for a final concentration of 100 units/mL. Administer IM into the anterolateral aspect of the thigh for infants and small children, and into the deltoid muscle or anterolateral aspect of the thigh for older children and adults. **Avoid**

Continued

VARICELLA ZOSTER IMMUNE GLOBULIN (HUMAN) *continued*

injection into gluteal region because of risk for sciatic nerve injury. **Do not exceed age-specific single-maximum IM injection volume;** separate injections may be necessary.

IV: Dilute each vial with 2.5 mL sterile diluent for a final concentration of 50 units/mL. Administer IV dose over 3 to 5 minutes.

VORICONAZOLE
Vfend and others
Antifungal, triazole

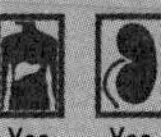
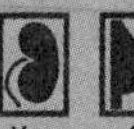
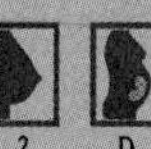

Yes Yes ? D

Tabs: 50, 200 mg; contains povidone
Oral suspension: 40 mg/mL (75 mL); contains sodium benzoate
Injection: 200 mg; contains 3200 mg sulfobutyl ether β-cyclodextrin (SBECD)

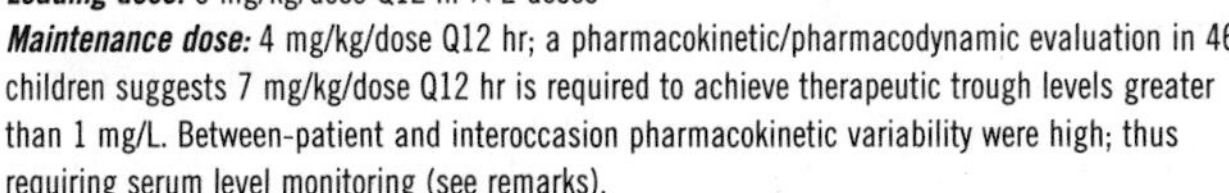

IV:

2–11 yr (pediatric dosing not well established; see remarks):

Loading dose: 6 mg/kg/dose Q12 hr × 2 doses

Maintenance dose: 4 mg/kg/dose Q12 hr; a pharmacokinetic/pharmacodynamic evaluation in 46 children suggests 7 mg/kg/dose Q12 hr is required to achieve therapeutic trough levels greater than 1 mg/L. Between-patient and interoccasion pharmacokinetic variability were high; thus requiring serum level monitoring (see remarks).

Invasive aspergillosis: 5–7 mg/kg/dose Q12 hr

≥12 yr and adult:

Loading dose: 6 mg/kg/dose Q12 hr × 2 doses

Maintenance dose:

Candidemia: 3–4 mg/kg/dose Q12 hr

Invasive aspergilosis or other serious fungal infection: 4 mg/kg/dose Q12 hr; if patient unable to tolerate, reduce dose to 3 mg/kg/dose Q12 hr

PO:

2–11 yr: The following oral dosages are currently being investigated in phase III clinical trials (see www.clinicaltrials.gov):

Invasive aspergillosis, serious* Candida *infections, esophageal candidiasis, and other rare molds (including 12–14 yr weighing <50 kg): 9 mg/kg/dose Q12 hr PO; **max. initial dose:** 350 mg Q12 hr

Prophylaxis in pediatric acute leukemia (up to 15 yr old): 6 mg/kg/dose Q12 hr PO × 2 doses, followed by 4 mg/kg/dose Q12 hr PO

≥12 yr and adult (see remarks):

Invasive aspergillosis/Fusarium/Scedosporium/and other serious infections:

<40 kg: 100 mg PO Q12 hr; if response is inadequate, increase to 150 mg PO Q12 hr (if unable to tolerate, reduce dose by 50-mg increments to a minimum of 100 mg Q12 hr)

≥40 kg: 200 mg PO Q12 hr; if response is inadequate, increase to 300 mg PO Q12 hr (if unable to tolerate, reduce dose by 50-mg increments to a minimum of 200 mg Q12 hr)

Esophageal candidiasis (treat for a minimum 14 days and until 7 days after resolution of symptoms):

<40 kg: 100 mg PO Q12 hr; if response is inadequate, dose may be increased to 150 mg PO Q12 hr (if unable to tolerate, reduce dose by 50-mg increments to a minimum of 100 mg Q12 hr)

≥40 kg: 200 mg PO Q12 hr; if response is inadequate, dose may be increased to 300 mg PO Q12 hr (if unable to tolerate, reduce dose by 50-mg increments to a minimum of 200 mg Q12 hr)

Continued

For explanation of icons, see p. 364.

VORICONAZOLE *continued*

Contraindications: Hypersensitivity to voriconazole or its excipients and other azoles. **Do not use** with other CYP 450 3A4 substrates that can lead to prolonged QTc interval (e.g., cisapride, pimozide, and quinidine). Concomitant administration with rifampin, carbamazepine, long-acting barbiturates, ritonavir, efavirenz, rifabutin, and St. Johns's wort can decrease voriconazole levels/effects. Concomitant administration with sirolimus, efavirenz, rifabutin, and ergot alkaloids may result in increased levels/toxicity of these drugs.

Warnings/Precautions: **Use with caution** in severe hepatic disease and galactose intolerance. **Avoid** strong direct sunlight during therapy and warn patients of potential visual disturbances (blurred vision, photophobia, visual acuity, and color changes). Women of childbearing potential should use effective contraception during treatment. Currently approved for use in invasive aspergillosis, Candidal esophagitis, and *Fusarium* and *Scedosporium apiospermum* infections.

Adjust dose in hepatic impairment by decreasing only the maintenance dose by 50% for patients with a Child–Pugh class A or B. **Do not** use IV dosage form for patients with GFR <50 mL/min because of accumulation of the cyclodextrin excipient; switch to oral therapy if possible.

Therapeutic levels: trough: 1–5.5 mg/L. Levels less than 1 mg/L have resulted in treatment failures and levels greater than 5.5 mg/L have resulted in neurotoxicity such as encephalopathy. Recommended serum sampling time: obtain trough within 30 min before a dose. Steady state is typically achieved after 5 to 7 days of initiating therapy.

Adverse effects: Common negative side effects include GI disturbances, fever, headache, hepatic abnormalities, photosensitivity, rash (6%), and visual disturbances (30%). Serious but rare side effects include anaphylaxis, liver or renal failure, and Stevens–Johnsons syndrome. Pancreatitis has been reported in children.

Drug interactions: Drug is a substrate and inhibitor for CYP 450 2C9, 2C19 (major substrate), and 3A4 isoenzymes. In addition to the interactions mentioned in the Contraindications section, voriconazole may increase the effects/toxicity of cyclosporine, methadone, tacrolimus, warfarin, coumarin products, statins, benzodiazepines, calcium channel blockers, sulfonylureas, vincristine, and vinblastine. Patients receiving concurrent phenytoin should increase their voriconazole maintenance doses (IV: 5 mg/kg/dose Q12 hr; PO: double the usual dose).

Drug administration: Administer IV over 1–2 hr with a **maximum rate** of 3 mg/kg/hr at a concentration ≤5 mg/mL. Administer oral doses 1 hr before and after meals.

ZANAMIVIR
Relenza
Antiviral

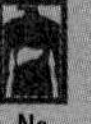
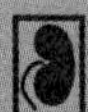
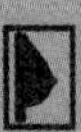
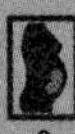

No No ? C

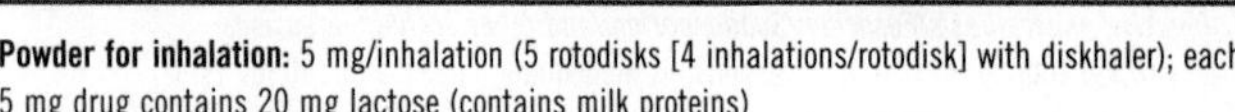

Powder for inhalation: 5 mg/inhalation (5 rotodisks [4 inhalations/rotodisk] with diskhaler); each 5 mg drug contains 20 mg lactose (contains milk proteins)

Treatment of uncomplicated influenza (initiate therapy within 2 days of onset of symptoms):

Child ≥7 yr and adult:

Day 1: 10 mg inhaled (as two 5-mg inhalations) BID (2–12 hr between the first two doses) × 2 doses

Days 2–5: 10 mg inhaled (as two 5-mg inhalations) Q12 hr × 4 days

Prophylaxis of influenza:

Child ≥5 yr and adult: 10 mg inhaled (as two 5-mg inhalations) once daily for the following duration:

After household exposure (initiate therapy within 1.5 days after the onset of index case signs and symptoms): 10 days

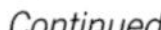

Continued

ZANAMIVIR *continued*

Control of outbreaks in long-term-care facilities or hospitals: Minimum of 14 days continuing up to 1 wk after last known case

Community outbreaks (only for adolescent and adult; initiate therapy within 5 days of outbreak): 10 mg once daily × 28 days

Contraindications: Hypersensitivity to any component of the formulation (contains milk proteins)

Warnings/Precautions: Currently indicated for the treatment of influenza A and B strains. **Not recommended** for patients with underlying respiratory diseases (e.g., asthma or COPD) because bronchospasm may occur and efficacy could not be demonstrated. **Discontinue** use if bronchospasm or decline in respiratory function occurs. Monitor for signs of abnormal behavior as neuropsychiatric symptoms have been reported in postmarketing studies (primarily from Japan).

Adverse effects: May cause nasal discomfort, cough, diarrhea, nausea, headache, facial edema, throat/tonsil discomfort, and pain. Allergic reactions involving oropharyngeal edema and serious skin rashes have been reported; discontinue therapy if this occurs. Vasovagal-like episodes have been reported shortly after dose administration. See Warnings/Precautions.

Drug interactions: None identified.

Drug administration: See package insert for specific instructions for using the rotodisk/diskhaler system. The dry powder inhalation dosage form cannot be used safely by a nebulizer or mechanical ventilation. If patient is concurrently using a bronchodilator, use the bronchodilator before taking zanamivir.

ZIDOVUDINE

Retrovir, AZT

Antiviral agent, nucleoside analogue reverse transcriptase inhibitor

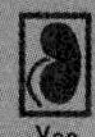
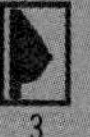
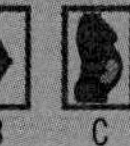

Yes Yes 3 C

Caps: 100 mg
Tabs: 300 mg
Oral syrup: 50 mg/5 mL (240 mL); contains 0.2% sodium benzoate
Injection: 10 mg/mL (20 mL)
In combination with lamivudine (3TC) as Combivir:
Tabs: 300 mg zidovudine + 150 mg lamivudine
In combination with abacavir and lamivudine (3TC) as Trizivir:
Tabs: 300 mg zidovudine + 300 mg abacavir + 150 mg lamivudine

HIV treatment:

Premature neonate:

Gestational Age (wk)	Oral (PO) Dosage	IV Dosage*
<30	2 mg/kg/dose Q12 hr, increase to 3 mg/kg/dose Q12 hr at 4 wk of age	1.5 mg/kg/dose Q12 hr, increase to 2.3 mg/kg/dose Q12 hr at 4 wk of age
30–34	2 mg/kg/dose Q12 hr, increase to 3 mg/kg/dose Q12 hr at postnatal age of 15 days	1.5 mg/kg/dose Q12 hr, increase to 2.3 mg/kg/dose Q12 hr at postnatal age of 15 days
≥35	4 mg/kg/dose Q12 hr	3 mg/kg/dose Q12 hr

*Convert to PO route when possible.

Continued

ZIDOVUDINE *continued*

Full-term neonate:
PO: 4 mg/kg/dose Q12 hr
IV: 3 mg/kg/dose Q12 hr
Child ≥4 wk to <18 yr
PO (for ≥4 kg; use oral syrup dosage form to provide accurate dosing):
4 to <9 kg: 24 mg/kg/24 hr PO ÷ BID–TID
≥9 to <30 kg: 18 mg/kg/24 hr PO ÷ BID–TID
≥30 kg: 600 mg/24 hr PO ÷ BID–TID
Alternative body surface area dosing: 480 mg/m^2/24 hr PO ÷ BID–TID; **max. dose:** 600 mg/24 hr
IV:
Child >6 wk to <12 yr (use until PO route is possible):
Intermittent IV: 120 mg/m^2/dose Q6 hr
Continuous IV infusion: 20 mg/m^2/hr
Child ≥12 yr and adolescent (use until PO route is possible): 1 mg/kg/dose IV Q4 hr
Adult:
PO: 200 mg/dose TID, or 300 mg/dose BID; **max dose:** 600 mg/24 hr
Combivir: 1 tablet PO BID
Trizivir (≥40 kg): 1 tablet PO BID
IV: 1 mg/kg/dose Q4 hr
Prevention of vertical transmission:
14–34 wk of pregnancy (maternal dosing):
Until labor: 600 mg/24 hr PO ÷ BID–TID
During labor: 2 mg/kg/dose IV over 1 hr followed by 1 mg/kg/hr IV infusion until umbilical cord clamped
Term neonate to infant <6 wk: 2 mg/kg/dose Q6 hr PO or 1.5 mg/kg/dose Q6 hr IV over 60 min. Begin within 12 hr after birth and continue until 6 wk of age.
Premature infant: Use earlier premature infant dosing table for HIV treatment.

Contraindications: Hypersensitivity to zidovudine or any other of its components
Warnings/Precautions: **Use with caution** in patients with impaired renal or hepatic function. Neutropenia and severe anemia have occurred in patients with advanced HIV. Lactic acidosis and severe hepatomegaly with steatosis, including fatal cases, have been reported. Macrocytosis is noted after 4 wk of therapy and can be used as an indicator of compliance. Immune reconstitution syndrome has been reported.
Dosage reduction may be necessary in severe renal impairment (GFR <15 mL/min) and in hepatic dysfunction.
Adverse effects: Most common include anemia (may require dose interruption), granulocytopenia, nausea, and headache (dosage reduction, erythropoietin, filgrastim/G-CSF, or discontinuance may be required depending on event). Seizures, confusion, rash, myositis, myopathy (use >1 yr), hepatitis, and elevated liver enzymes have been reported. See Warnings/Precautions.
Drug interactions: **Do not** use in combination with stavudine because of poor antiretroviral effect. Effects of interacting drugs include increased toxicity (acyclovir, trimethoprim-sulfamethoxazole), increased hematologic toxicity (ganciclovir, interferon-α, marrow suppressive drugs), and granulocytopenia (drugs that affect glucuronidation). Methadone, atovaquone, cimetidine, valproic acid, probenecid, and fluconazole may increase levels of zidovudine, whereas nelfinavir, ritonavir, rifampin, rifabutin, and clarithromycin may decrease levels.
Drug administration:
IV: **Do not** administer IM. IV form is incompatible with blood product infusions and should be infused over 1 hour (intermittent IV dosing) at a concentration ≤4 mg/mL diluted in 5% dextrose.
PO: Oral doses may be administered with or without food.

Index

Page numbers that are followed by f indicate figures.
Page numbers that are followed by t indicate tables.
Page numbers in *italics* indicate formulary information.

G